# PUBLIC HEALTH LAW

**Kenneth R. Wing**
*Professor of Law*
*Seattle University School of Law*

**Wendy K. Mariner**
*Professor of Law*
*Boston University School of Public Health,*
*School of Medicine & School of Law*

**George J. Annas**
*Edward R. Utley Professor & Chair*
*Health Law, Bioethics & Human Rights Department*
*Boston University School of Public Health,*
*School of Medicine & School of Law*

**Daniel S. Strouse**
*Professor of Law & Faculty Fellow*
*Center for the Study of Law, Science & Technology*
*Sandra Day O'Connor College of Law*
*Arizona State University*

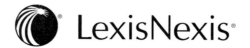

## Library of Congress Cataloging-in-Publication Data

Public health law / by Kenneth R. Wing . . . [et al.].
    p. cm.
Includes index.
ISBN 1-4224-0641-5 (hard cover)
1. Public health laws — United States — Cases. I. Wing, Kenneth R., 1946-
KF3775.A7P83 2007
344.7304 — dc22

2007003071

LexisNexis and the Knowledge Burst logo are trademarks of Reed Elsevier Properties Inc, used under license. Matthew Bender is a registered trademark of Matthew Bender Properties Inc. Copyright © 2007 Matthew Bender & Company, Inc., a member of the LexisNexis Group. All Rights Reserved.

Editorial Offices
744 Broad Street, Newark, NJ 07102 (973) 820-2000
201 Mission St., San Francisco, CA 94105-1831 (415) 908-3200
701 East Water Street, Charlottesville, VA 22902-7587 (434) 972-7600
www.lexis.com

*With thanks to Nancy Ammons, Stephanie Wilson, Brook Assefa, Aaron Bass, Amy Condon, Julie Kamerrer, Hajung Lee, Angela Macey-Cushman, Sophia Palmer, Coreen Schnepf, Britnye Segraves, Jason D. Smith, and Aimee Welch for their assistance, and particular thanks to Leonard Glantz for his original contributions to these materials.*

# PREFACE

Our primary purpose in writing and editing these materials is to prepare a textbook that can be used in a law school-based course called Public Health Law. We envision Public Health Law as an upper level course, one that is offered to second or, preferably, third year law students who have already had some exposure to constitutional law, administrative law, and other basic law school courses that provide useful background. We also envision this course as a supplement to, but nonetheless distinct from, Health Law, Law and Medicine, and other health-related offerings that may be in a law school's curriculum.

Just what should a course on public health law be about? We think that Public Health Law should be offered and taught as an introduction to the various governmental programs and activities that fall under the general rubric of public health, the problems that they are intended to address, and the unique legal and political issues that arise as these efforts are pursued. For some students, Public Health Law may mark the first step towards a career that focuses on public health or health policy. For others, it may be an introduction to matters that they may only occasionally encounter in their professional lives. But for anyone who takes this course, we think Public Health Law will provide useful if not necessary preparation for a range of legal and political controversies that they are certain to confront, one way or another, regardless of their legal career paths. Public health has been, is, and always will be, central to the lives of all Americans, and indeed, all humans, no matter where in the world they live.

Most law students, like most Americans, have only a vague awareness of the various programs and institutions that make up the nation's public health infrastructure; they generally know even less about public health activities, the types of problems that they are intended to address, and the legal and political controversies that may arise when public health efforts are carried out. A good course on Public Health Law will have to educate law students as to what is public health law, but it will have to teach them, first and foremost, what is public health. In this sense public health law is applied law, i.e., all areas of the law applied to the activities we know as public health.

As will be reviewed in Chapter One of these materials, there is an ongoing and lively debate in both academic and professional circles over the definitional limits of public health and the kinds of issues and problems that should appropriately be considered within its purview. Some of this debate reflects important political and ideological concerns; some of it is a by-product of "turf" wars and jurisdictional disputes between agencies and various levels of government. But in large part it is a reflection of the breadth of the factors that can influence the health of the American population, ranging from environmental influences to social and cultural biases to individual lifestyle choices.

This debate, its origins, and its implications are all important to a full understanding of public health issues and problems. In an introductory course, however, we think the proper way to define public health, at least initially, should be much more discrete and focused. In the most basic sense, public health refers to the federal, state, and local governmental efforts to maintain and protect the health of the general population. There is an array of public health agencies, laboratory and research facilities, and other institutional arrangements that are generally referred to as the "public health infrastructure." That infrastructure is staffed by a variety of professionals that could be regarded as the "public health workforce": epidemiologists, statisticians, toxicologists and other scientists; health service providers and educators; inspectors; and various law enforcement officials at all levels of government. What they do ranges from the mundane to the exotic: from organizing programs to try to prevent teenage smoking to enforcing health standards in occupational settings to confronting outbreaks of novel contagious diseases.

Activities under the banner of public health have been responsible for some of the most startling and dramatic advances in the nation's health, yet many have taken place only on the periphery of the public's vision. Public health workers often labor in the shadow of their more visible, and usually more highly paid and appreciated, medical colleagues. The surgeon who develops a new procedure may be front page news, while the county's epidemiologist whose vigilance prevents the next SARS-type virus from entering the community — and, in doing so, saves far more lives than her medical counterpart — may draw little or no public recognition at all.

At the other extreme, some public health matters can dominate the American public's attention, even at the expense of more important problems, as happens when threats of terrorist activities, real or imagined, spark public fears of biological or chemical attacks and overshadow patient safety initiatives.

Public health represents an imperfectly coordinated network of people, institutions, disciplines, and activities, some of which are highly visible and familiar, but many of which are neither fully understood nor appreciated by most Americans.

In some respects, this bi-polar impression is inherent in the nature of public health. Population-based analysis, the hallmark of public health thinking and activities, rarely focuses on the individual. Rather, the public health professional usually focuses on the needs of the population taken as a whole and measures success accordingly. As one consequence, the individuals whose lives are affected by public health efforts are often unaware of their good fortune, since public health aims at prevention rather than treatment. Even in extreme cases, where efforts such as quarantine or isolation are thought necessary to prevent catastrophic results, the individual whose life or well-being is spared is seldom identified other than as a statistic. Indeed, the only individual who may be fully aware of these efforts is the one who must bear the burden necessary to produce the public benefit; and even that individual may have little appreciation of the public health justification for what is being done or why — or even who is responsible.

Public health's limited visibility among Americans also can be traced to its peculiar history. An occasionally blurred but distinctive division between those health-related activities that are carried out by the government, "public health," and medical care and related activities that take place primarily in the private sector, "private medicine," was established early in the nation's social and political history and has been persistent throughout the evolution of the American health care system. In fact, that division between public health activities by the government and medicine delivered through largely private actors and institutions is one of the reasons that the term "system" is only partially descriptive of the way Americans receive their health care. Moreover, it is surely one of the features that make American health care uniquely American. That division also has taken a toll on public health programs and the people who carry them out, not only in terms of the appreciation that they receive from the American public, but also in terms of the funding of activities that are identified as falling on the public health side of that division. In this regard, perhaps the strangest, though not uncommon, view of public health is that it is "medicine for poor people."

## Organization and Structure of PUBLIC HEALTH LAW

To provide the materials that we think are necessary to teach a law school-based Public Health Law course in an effective way, we have organized this book to provide a set of introductory readings, first on the history and scope of public health, then on the basic constitutional principles that define the scope and limits of government power, followed by a series of case studies of specific public health problems. Each case study chapter focuses on one particular set of public health problems and analyzes the legal and political parameters within which these problems can and should be addressed. We have attempted to select problems that are each important in their own right. But the particular problems also have been selected because of the more generalized lessons they illustrate — lessons that can be applied to other public health problems. We have tried to order these chapters in a way that develops basic themes and highlights recurring issues and paradigms, with the final chapter bringing many of these together in an integrated way.

The first chapter begins with some historical examples of public health in the United States in excerpts from Charles Rosenberg, George Rosen, and Jim Murphy, chronicling encounters among 18th, 19th, and early 20th century Americans and some of the major public health problems of their respective eras: epidemics of yellow fever, cholera, and tuberculosis. The foundations for American public health institutions and programs were laid in large part by the efforts of local, state, and federal governments to respond to these epidemics. We have included a short excerpt from Leonard Cole's book, *The Anthrax Letters*, because it describes a contemporary public health menace, and also because it implicitly references a new dimension found in public health problems in the 21st century: the possibility that today's Americans may be encountering infectious diseases or other biological hazards that are intentionally released into their lives. We have also included an excerpt from the 2001 Institute of Medicine Report because it is the best recent assessment of the public health system in the United States, the public health related problems facing Americans, and some of the important issues that will determine whether we can effectively respond to these problems. We have further included a critical commentary on the earlier 1988 IOM report on public health because it was a much less successful treatment of the field and helps students understand some of the basic problems of defining the field of public health itself, as well as what counts as a public health agency. We have closed Chapter One with a portion of Wendy Mariner's article *Public Health: Beyond Emergency Preparedness* discussing some of the reasons why the definition of public health has been broadened in contemporary policy debates and some directions it may take in the future.

Chapter Two is an introduction to the constitutional foundations of public health law. Using classic public health cases, Chapter Two reviews some basic constitutional principles describing the powers of the federal and, in particular, the state and local governments in matters concerning the public's health. It also reviews principles concerning the distribution of power among the branches of government and among levels of government. In its section on abortion, it broadens this discussion to include the relationship of medical practice to public health, and the limits of the state's authority to protect the health of individuals, especially pregnant women, against their wills. Most fundamentally, this chapter outlines the basic issues that must be addressed in judicial, legislative, and administrative decisions that attempt to strike a balance between individual rights and the power of the government when it acts to protect the public's health.

Chapter Three presents a series of case studies involving the use of quarantine and isolation to control the spread of contagious disease, from a local outbreak to an epidemic. It begins with the measures that have been used to respond to tuberculosis and HIV infection, and moves to the potential use of such measures to respond to outbreaks of SARS or pandemic influenza, and anticipating how the states, the federal government, and the rest of us may react if and when the nation is required to respond to some large-scale disease outbreak. Because deciding what prevention or control measures to use depends importantly on the nature of each disease and how it is transmitted, the chapter offers some essential background on each disease examined. And, since medical treatment can prevent the further spread of some diseases, it also briefly reviews basic constitutional principles concerning the right to make treatment decisions. Chapter Three closes with an introduction to emergency preparedness for bioterrorism and epidemics, subjects which are revisited in Chapter Eight.

Chapter Four examines public health surveillance, how government agencies collect and use information to solve public health problems. Sound public health policy depends on good information, and advances in research methods, electronic medical records, information technology, and data linkage make all kinds of health information easily accessible. These advances also raise increasingly difficult questions about when and why government agencies can obtain personally identifiable information. The chapter examines possible conflicts between protecting privacy and protecting public health in key examples of surveillance programs, from contagious diseases to DNA banking. As public health moves into areas historically reserved to physicians and biomedical researchers, it tests the value of the law's protection of individual autonomy and control of one's personal information.

Chapter Five reviews the on-going health problems associated with smoking and other uses of tobacco products and the various ways in which the local, state, and federal governments have attempted to reduce the impact of tobacco on the public's health. Of particular significance here is the fact that the government's interest in reducing the use of tobacco is justified only in part by the impact of smoking on non-smokers; the greater health problems associated with smoking are self-inflicted by the smoker: the growing list of illnesses and disabilities associated with tobacco use. Also of particular interest is the fact that some public health strategies for reducing smoking raise unique constitutional issues. As local, state, and federal anti-smoking programs attempt to reduce smoking through educational campaigns and efforts to limit the advertising or promotion of tobacco — eschewing more draconian forms of tobacco regulation — they must surmount the more difficult constitutional barriers to government regulation of what is considered speech; somewhat ironically, lesser constitutional constraints would apply if the government were to more directly regulate or prohibit altogether the use of tobacco. In addition, Chapter Five considers the role of private litigation in influencing public health policy.

Chapter Six considers public health promotion and education primarily in the context of two related problems: drug abuse and obesity. In doing so, the chapter raises important questions concerning the scope and nature of appropriate public health strategies. Drug testing, for example, can be part of either a criminal or civil approach to reduce drug abuse. The constitutional constraints on each approach, as well as their effectiveness in improving health, are examined in several examples of drug testing programs. Is the proper response to these problems better education or should the government more directly regulate individual behavior? For that matter, in the case of obesity, is the problem, public health or otherwise, obesity *per se*, or is the growing rate of obesity in the American population merely one measure of a more fundamental lack of good health? Chapter Six attempts to document the problem we currently label "obesity," both in the United States and elsewhere in the world, and considers the range of local, state, and federal public health responses that are currently under consideration. Chapter Six also reviews in some depth the so-called "cheeseburger lawsuits"; at the least, these privately initiated lawsuits are one vehicle for evaluating the underlying causes of obesity and the circumstances under which causal links may be found between obesity in consumers and various actions by food producers that encourage consumption.

Chapter Seven considers an important but politically volatile problem: the private ownership of guns and the consequent impact on the public's health. As reviewed in the articles that begin the chapter, the data concerning the increasing number of people injured or killed by guns are sobering. The definitional problem from a public health perspective is not so much assessing the magnitude of the risks, but determining the proper remedial focus: Is the widespread availability of guns *per se* the problem or is it the behavior of gun owners? Should public health policy focus on the fact that some guns may be unsafe or defectively designed or, alternatively, should strategies be developed to prevent the improper distribution of guns or to train or educate potential gun users? As argued in the article by Lott, it is even possible that what is needed is more, not fewer, guns in circulation. Complicating the analysis of each of these issues is the unique constitutional status of gun ownership. As demonstrated in the cases excerpted in Chapter Seven, the private ownership and use of guns are protected, to some as yet not completely defined extent, by both the federal and the state constitutions. As a result, fashioning remedial public health responses to gun violence must be done within potentially restrictive constitutional barriers. Chapter Seven also reviews some of the lawsuits brought by local governments seeking to achieve various gun control measures through the courts, as well as some of the privately initiated lawsuits that have attempted to limit indirectly the use and distribution of guns.

Chapter Eight could be regarded as an introduction to the "new public health" had the term not already been adopted in earlier eras (as discussed in Chapter One). The threat of bioterrorism, the possibility of an intentional release of a biological agent capable of causing thousands of casualties, has had a fundamental impact on public health in the United States and the way Americans think about the government's public health-related responsibilities. As reflected in the articles that begin the chapter, 9/11 was the beginning of a new way to think about public health, now termed "public health preparedness," which includes mock exercises, new research priorities and facilities, and much more interaction between public health workers and law enforcement officials. Simultaneously, lawyers are attempting to increase the level of what could be called our "public health legal preparedness," reviewing the existing legal apparatus that would be required if massive quarantine measures and other interventions were thought to be necessary to effectively respond to a bioterrorism attack. More and more, however, public health professionals are recognizing that public health is inherently a global concern, and the global HIV/AIDS pandemic has led directly to the founding of a new global field of public health law, termed "health and human rights" (although these two terms are sometimes used in reverse order). The chapter and the book conclude with an introduction to the international legal scene of public health, as well as with suggestions of how the law can be used to promote public health globally, with special attention to the meaning of "the right to health" in international law. It is also stressed that insofar as public health is best considered as an activity focused on populations and prevention and that as important as damage control is after a bioterrorist attack, more important is taking effective steps to try to prevent the attack in the first place.

Each chapter includes references to additional and supplemental materials, and provides citations to websites and other sources for updating these materials. The notes accompanying each section of the chapters outline the issues and questions that we think are important and that should be the focus of an introductory, law school-based Public Health Law course. Obviously there are many ways to teach such a course. Much of the organization and emphasis of any particular course will depend upon such matters as the other courses offered in a law school's curriculum, the particular interests of the course instructor, and current events.

One thing that we particularly recommend is that any introductory Public Health Law course be taught using examples from the law school's jurisdiction. Public health law is, in very large part, built on the laws of each state; any particular course should do so as well. This also makes sense pedagogically, as it allows for a more finely tuned discussion of some of the problems concerning statutory interpretation and administrative law. We also have found that this increases the practical relevance of the material for most of our students.

We try to highlight the international dimensions of each of the problem areas covered in these materials. In some cases, the public health problems we face as Americans are nearly dwarfed by their counterparts in other countries; for example, however problematic the new drug-resistant tuberculosis may become in the United States, the implications for resource-poor countries are overwhelming. We are not sure how much class-time should be devoted to the international dimensions of each problem reviewed in these materials. We are sure we would be remiss to overlook them altogether — even if we can offer little more than an introduction and a reminder to our students that we should at least maintain some comparative perspective.

These materials are a work in progress, much like contemporary public health itself. We expect to be constantly amending and updating them in the next several years. We hope we will be doing so in response to the comments and suggestions we receive from others who have the opportunity to read or use them. You can reach us through the publisher or contact us directly at our home schools.

Ken Wing
*Seattle University School of Law*

Wendy Mariner
*Boston University School of Public Health, School of Medicine,
and School of Law*

George Annas
*Boston University School of Public Health, School of Medicine,
and School of Law*

Dan Strouse
*Sandra Day O'Connor College of Law
Arizona State University*

# SUMMARY TABLE OF CONTENTS

# TABLE OF CONTENTS

# ACKNOWLEDGMENTS

Annas, George J., *Bioterror and "Bioart" — A Plague o' Both Your Houses*, 354 NEW ENG. J. MED. 2715 (2006). Copyright © 2006 by George J. Annas. Reprinted with permission.

Annas, George J., *Blinded by Terrorism: Public Health and Liberty in the 21st Century*, 13 HEALTH MATRIX 33, 50–52, 60 (2003). Copyright © 2003 by George J. Annas. Reprinted with permission.

Annas, George J., *Control of Tuberculosis: The Law and the Public's Health*, 328 NEW. ENG. J. MED. 585 (1993). Copyright © 1993 by George J. Annas. Reprinted with permission.

Annas, George J., Op/Ed, BOSTON GLOBE, Oct. 8, 2005, at A15. Copyright © 2005 by George J. Annas. Reprinted with permission.

Annas, George J., *Puppy Love: Bioterrorism, Civil Rights, and Public Health*, 55 FLA. L. REV. 1171, 1182-90 (2003). Copyright © 2003. Reprinted with permission of the author and the *Florida Law Review*.

Annas, George J., *The Statue of Security: Human Rights and Post-9/11 Epidemics*, 28 J. HEALTH L. 319 (2005). Copyright © 2005 by George J. Annas. Reprinted with permission.

Barbera, Joseph, et al., *Large-Scale Quarantine Following Biological Terrorism in the United States*, 286 JAMA 2711 (2001). Copyright © 2001 JAMA, The Journal of the American Medical Association. Reprinted with permission.

BARRY, JOHN M., THE GREAT INFLUENZA: THE EPIC STORY OF THE DEADLIEST PLAGUE IN HISTORY 2–5 (2004). Copyright © 2004 by John M. Barry. Reprinted with permission.

Berkelman, Ruth L., et al., *Public Health Surveillance*, in 2 OXFORD TEXTBOOK OF PUBLIC HEALTH 759, 759-60 (Roger Detels et al., eds., 4th ed. 2002). Copyright © 2002 Oxford University Press. Reprinted with permission.

BROWNELL, KELLY & HORGEN, KATHERINE BATTLE, FOOD FIGHT 3–13 (2004). Copyright © 2004 McGraw-Hill Companies. Reprinted with permission.

CHEMERINSKY, ERWIN, CONSTITUTIONAL LAW: PRINCIPLES AND POLICIES 452 (1997). Copyright © 1997 by Erwin Chemerinsky. Reprinted with permission.

Cohen, Hillel, et al., *The Pitfalls of Bioterrorism Preparedness: the Anthrax and Smallpox Experiences*, 94 AM. J. PUB. HEALTH 1667 (2004). Copyright © 2004. Reprinted with permission of the author and the American Public Health Association.

COLE, LEONARD A., THE ANTHRAX LETTERS vii-ix (2003). Copyright © 2003 by the National Academy of Sciences, courtesy of the National Academies Press, Washington, D.C. Reprinted with permission.

Daynard, Richard A., Howard, P. Tim & Wilking, Cara L., *Private Enforcement: Litigation as a Tool to Prevent Obesity*, 25 J. PUB. HEALTH POL'Y 408–14 (2004). Copyright © 2004. Reprinted with permission of the authors.

KLUGER, RICHARD, ASHES TO ASHES XI-XIX (1996). Copyright © 1996 by Richard Kluger. Used by permission of Alfred A. Knopf, a division of Random House, Inc.

LOTT, JR., JOHN R., MORE GUNS, LESS CRIME: UNDERSTANDING CRIME AND GUN CONTROL LAWS 160-166 (2d ed. 2000). Copyright © 2000 University of Chicago Press. Reprinted with permission of the publisher.

Mariner, Wendy K., *Law and Public Health: Beyond Emergency Preparedness*, 38 J. HEALTH L. 251–68 (2005). Copyright © 2005. Reprinted with permission of the author.

Mariner, Wendy K., *Medicine and Public Health: Crossing Boundaries*, 10 J. HEALTH CARE L. & POL'Y 101 (2007). Copyright © 2007. Reprinted with permission of the author.

Mariner, Wendy K., *Mission Creep: Public Health Surveillance and Medical Privacy*, 86 B.U. L. REV. (forthcoming 2007). Copyright © 2007. Reprinted with permission of the author.

Moulton, Anthony, Gottfried, Richard N., Goodman, Richard A., Murphy, Anne M. & Rawson, Raymond D., *What is Public Health Legal Preparedness?*, 31 J.L. MED. & ETHICS 672, 674 (2003). Copyright © 2003 The American Society of Law, Medicine & Ethics. Reprinted with permission.

MURPHY, JIM, AN AMERICAN PLAGUE: THE TRUE AND TERRIFYING STORY OF THE YELLOW FEVER EPIDEMIC OF *1793* 135–39 (2003). Copyright © 2003 by Jim Murphy. Reprinted by permission of Clarion Books, an imprint of Houghton Mifflin Company. All rights reserved.

Parmet, Wendy, *AIDS and Quarantine: The Revival of an Archaic Doctrine*, 14 HOFSTRA L. REV. 53, 55–71 (1985). Copyright © 1985. Reprinted with permission of the Hofstra Law Review Association.

PBS, A HISTORY OF QUARANTINE. Copyright © 2004 Public Broadcasting Service (PBS). Available at www.pbs.org/wgbh/nova/typhoid/quarantine.html. Reprinted with permission.

Roche, Patricia A., *DNA and DNA Banking, in* 1 ENCYCLOPEDIA OF PRIVACY 174, 174–177 (William G. Staples ed., 2007). Copyright © 2007. Reproduced with permission of Greenwood Publishing Group, Inc., Westport, CT.

Roche, Patricia A., *Genetic Information and Testing, in* 1 ENCYCLOPEDIA OF PRIVACY 252, 252–256 (William G. Staples ed., 2007). Copyright © 2007. Reproduced with permission of Greenwood Publishing Group, Inc., Westport, CT.

ROSEN, GEORGE, PREVENTIVE MEDICINE IN THE UNITED STATES *1900–1975* 25–36 (1975). Copyright © 1975 Watson Publishing Int'l. Reprinted with permission.

ROSENBERG, CHARLES, THE CHOLERA YEARS 1–7, 101–08, 110–11, 114–17, 120 (1962). Copyright © 1962 University of Chicago Press. Reprinted with permission of the publisher.

# Chapter 1

# AN INTRODUCTION TO PUBLIC HEALTH IN THE UNITED STATES

## A.  AMERICAN PUBLIC HEALTH . . . PAST

### 1.  Cholera in the 19th Century

In *The Cholera Years*, Charles Rosenberg chronicled the medical and social impact of the three major cholera epidemics that swept through 19th century America in 1832, 1849, and 1866. As he emphasized, each period had its own set of theories about and responses to the dreaded disease, reflecting contemporary religious, medical, and social understandings of illness as well as prevailing political and economic values. Seen in 1832 as the divine wages of sin (intemperance, sloth, impiety) and squalor (the disease disproportionately affected America's poorest — Irish immigrants living in filthy urban tenements, and African-Americans), cholera was eventually regarded in more scientific and less moralistic tones in the 1860s; and while effective governmental programs for sanitation and other public health measures would ultimately grow out of such crises, for Americans neither the willingness nor the ability to respond in the most (perhaps the only) effective way — collectively — was easily achieved.

Rosenberg's story of cholera, focusing heavily though not exclusively on the disease in New York City, is really a story of 19th century America. Yet it is hard to avoid drawing parallels to American reactions to the public health problems that now are described — with only slight exaggeration — as equivalent to the 19th century epidemics of which cholera was just one.

The immediately-following excerpt is from the Introduction to Rosenberg's book. The next one describes the epidemic of 1849 in some detail, and its impact on pre-industrialized and pre-scientific America.

### CHARLES ROSENBERG, THE CHOLERA YEARS
#### 1–7, 101–08, 110–11, 114–17, 120 (1962)

* * *

There has not been an active case of cholera in the United States for almost 50 years, and to the present-day American physician it is no more than a chapter in a textbook of tropical medicine. To his 19th century counterpart, it was a soul-trying and sometimes fatal reality.

Cholera was the classic epidemic disease of the 19th century, as plague had been of the 14th. When cholera first appeared in the United States in 1832,

1

yellow fever and smallpox, the great epidemic diseases of the previous two centuries, were no longer truly national problems. Yellow fever had disappeared from the North, and vaccination had deprived smallpox of much of its menace. Cholera, on the other hand, appeared in almost every part of the country in the course of the century. It flourished in the great cities, New York, Cincinnati, Chicago; it crossed the continent with the Forty-Niners; its victims included Iowa dirt farmers and New York longshoremen, Wisconsin lead miners and Negro field hands.

Before 1817, there had probably never been a cholera epidemic outside the Far East; during the 19th century, it spread through almost the entire world. Of all epidemic diseases, only influenza in the 20th century has had a more extensive odyssey.

Cholera could not have thrived where filth and want did not already exist; nor could it have traveled so widely without an unprecedented development of trade and transportation. The cholera pandemics were transitory phenomena, destined to occupy the world stage for only a short time — the period during which public health and medical science were catching up with urbanization and the transportation revolution. Indeed, cholera was to play a key role in its own banishment from the Western world; the cholera epidemics of the 19th century provided much of the impetus needed to overcome centuries of governmental inertia and indifference in regard to problems of public health.

It was not easy for survivors to forget a cholera epidemic. The symptoms of cholera are spectacular; they could not be ignored or romanticized as were the physical manifestations of malaria and tuberculosis. The onset of cholera is marked by diarrhea, acute spasmodic vomiting, and painful cramps. Consequent dehydration, often accompanied by cyanosis, gives to the sufferer a characteristic and disquieting appearance: his face blue and pinched, his extremities cold and darkened, the skin of his hands and feet drawn and puckered. "One often," recalled a New York physician, "thought of the Laocoön, but looked in vain for the serpent." [The reference is to a famous statue that depicts the agonized death, by sea serpent, of a mythological priest (Laocoon) and his two sons, in divine punishment for Laocoon's having warned the Trojans about the wooden horse and throwing his spear into its side]. Death may intervene within a day, sometimes within a few hours of the appearance of the first symptoms. And these first symptoms appear with little or no warning.

The abrupt onset and fearful symptoms of cholera made Americans apprehensive and reflective — as they were not by the equally deadly, but more deliberate, ravages of tuberculosis or malaria. "To see individuals well in the morning & buried before night, retiring apparently well & dead in the morning is something which is appalling to the boldest heart." It is not surprising that the growing public health movement found in cholera an effective ally.

It was not until 1883 that Robert Koch, directing a German scientific commission in Egypt, isolated the organism that causes cholera — *Vibrio comma*, a motile, comma-shaped bacterium. Once they find their way into the human intestine, these vibrios are capable of producing an acute disease, which, if untreated, kills roughly a half of those unfortunate enough to contract it. Cholera, like typhoid, can be spread along any pathway leading to the human digestive tract. Unwashed hands or uncooked fruits and vegetables, for example, are frequently responsible for the transmission of the disease, though sewage-contaminated water supplies have been the cause of the most severe, widespread and explosive cholera epidemics.

. . .[C]holera returned to the United States four times after its initial appearance in 1832–34. After this two-year visit, North America was free of the disease until the winter of 1848–49. Between 1849 and 1854, however, no 12-month period passed without cholera appearing in some part of the United States. Then the disease disappeared as abruptly as it had in 1834; it was not to return until 1866.

Thirty-four years are a short time in man's history. Yet few historians would question the significance or magnitude of the changes effected in American society between 1832 and 1866. Comparatively little, however, has been written in a systematic attempt to define the dimensions of this social change or to describe the nature of the processes which brought it about.

. . . .

Perhaps most striking of the changes in America between 1832 and 1866 was the dissipation of the piety still so characteristic of many Americans in the Age of Jackson. The evangelical fervor of this earlier generation had been eroded by a materialism already present in 1832, but seemingly triumphant by 1866. Habits of thought and patterns of rhetoric had changed as well. A more critical and empirical temper had begun to replace the abstract rationalism of an earlier day. In medicine, for example, thoughtful physicians scorned those concepts which could not be expressed in tables and percentages. The most skeptical disavowed traditional therapy and relied upon the body's natural powers to triumph over disease. This "positivistic" temper of thought and expression infiltrated the pulpit and editorial page as well as the laboratory and consultation room. Cholera, a scourge of the sinful to many Americans in 1832, had, by 1866, become the consequence of remediable faults in sanitation. Whereas ministers in 1832 urged morality upon their congregations as a guarantor of health, their forward-looking counterparts in 1866 endorsed sanitary reform as a necessary prerequisite to moral improvement. There could be no public virtue without public health.

The means of improving the public health seemed clear enough. Clean streets, airy apartments, a pure supply of water, were certain safeguards against epidemic disease. And, by 1866, advocates of sanitary reform could in justification of their programs point to the discovery of John Snow, a London physician, that cholera was spread through a contaminated water supply. The matter-of-fact, empirical approach to epidemiology which enabled Snow to confirm his theory of the disease's transmission would have been rare a century before. He had, as well, new theories of disease causation, of the very nature of disease, available to him. Cholera in 1849, for example, was assumed by the great majority of physicians to be a specific disease, whereas in 1832, most practitioners had still regarded cholera as a vague atmospheric malaise and had vigorously disavowed the very existence of specific disease entities.

In 1832, most Americans regarded the United States as a land of health, virtue and rustic simplicity. Cities seemed often unnatural and perhaps ultimately undesirable excrescences in our otherwise green and pleasant realm. By 1866, this was no longer the case. America's cities had grown immensely in size and significance; they could be deplored, but no longer ignored. But though the existence of the city might be inevitable, its evils were not. The willingness to accept the city and its continued growth was an indispensable step in the finding of appropriate solutions to the problems such growth created. Flight to the country was no longer in 1866, as it had been to many in 1849, an acceptable solution to urban problems. A pure water supply, adequate sanitation, and a reliable police force were necessary if the dangerous and unhealthful conditions of city life were to be ameliorated.

When in the spring of 1832 Americans awaited cholera, they reassured themselves that this new pestilence attacked only the filthy, the hungry, the ignorant. There seemed few such in the United States. In the spring of 1866, when Americans again prepared themselves for an impending cholera epidemic, they expected no such exemption. North America had nurtured slums as squalid as any of those festering in the Old World. The inhabitants, moreover, were not the pious, cleanly, and ambitious Americans of an earlier generation. Filthy, illiterate peasants could expect no greater exemption from cholera in Boston than that which they had received in Ireland. America was no longer a city set upon a hill. The piety which sustained such a belief and the confidence which this belief engendered were both disappearing. Americans were adjusting to life on the plain.

. . . .

## VI.   THE EPIDEMIC: 1849

. . . .

Cholera, like revolution, had swept through Europe in 1848. Spreading outward from its Ganges homeland, the disease had, in a half-dozen years, visited almost every part of Asia, Europe and the Middle East . . . In the fall of 1848, as in the Spring of 1832, cholera poised at the Atlantic.

Realistic Americans assumed that this barrier would not long protect the United States. The course of the epidemic was the same as it had been in 1832, except that the Atlantic was now crossed more rapidly, more frequently, and by larger ships. With cholera in London and Edinburgh in October, diarist George Templeton Strong commented resignedly, it would doubtless be in New York before the New Year.

By mid-October, the medically sophisticated had already begun to notice forerunners of cholera in the atmosphere. Insects swarmed, influenza and diarrheas were epidemic, and the usual diseases of winter failed to respond to treatment. In this tainted air, the decades' accumulation of filth that polluted houses, streets and yards was more than ordinarily pernicious. To allow the continued existence of such breeding places of pestilence seemed inexcusable, and moribund health boards and street-cleaning committees were attacked for their chronic inactivity. . . .

. . . New Englanders were especially soothed by a plausible new theory, which held that cholera flourished only in areas underlain by limestone. Perhaps this explained how granite-bound New England escaped so lightly in

1832. Most reassuring of all was the unshaken conviction that the United States was the most prosperous, pious and enlightened of nations. Cholera's ancestral home was India, its natural victims a dirty, ignorant and fatalistic people.

There was little doubt in the minds of medical men, however, that cholera could thrive wherever there was sufficient filth. And no extraordinary sensibilities were required to see and smell the potential death in America's cities and villages. Few communities could provide their citizens with a reliable supply of water; sanitation and waste disposal were everywhere inadequate. Pigs, dogs and goats still provided the only effective sanitation in many American cities. . . .

The hogs roamed everywhere. In New York, pig-napping became a recognized trade (practiced by men who toured the city in wagons, scooping up unwatched pigs and selling them to butchers). In Little Rock, Arkansas, the porkers filled the streets and had, as one editor put it, begun to "dispute the sidewalks with other persons." Such whimsy could not be shared by the parents of children killed or mutilated by foraging pigs.

. . . .

On the morning of December 2, 1848, the "New York" rode at anchor off Staten Island. Aboard were over 300 steerage passengers, all of whom had been exposed to cholera below decks. Prudence and public opinion alike demanded their quarantine.

But where? America's greatest port possessed no facilities adequate to quarantine 50, let along 300, immigrants. After 15 years without cholera or yellow fever, New York's quarantine had become little more than an administrative gesture. Only the customs warehouses were large enough to accommodate so many people, and these were hurriedly converted into barrack-like hospital wards.

Such improvisations were small improvement over the holds of the "New York." Before the New Year, sixty of the immigrants had fallen ill; more than 30 had died. And over half of those originally quarantined had, as the health officer put it, "eloped," scaling the walls and making for New York or New Jersey in small boats. Within a week, cases began to appear in New York City itself, in the most crowded and dirty of the immigrant boardinghouses.

Apprehensive interest turned suddenly to alarm, for it seemed that New York, like Moscow, might be scourged by cholera despite the cold of winter. Newspapers that printed cholera remedies were sold out within hours of publication. Both the New York Academy of Medicine and the Board of Health held special meetings within 24 hours of the discovery of the first cases. While the Academy of Medicine spent most of its time condemning the incompetence of the board, the board authorized the mayor to take whatever steps should be necessary to have the streets cleaned. A committee was also chosen to arrange for the establishment of cholera hospitals.

For the moment, these hospitals were not needed. The bitter cold of January brought the city a momentary reprieve, and there were no more new cases. . . .

Winter temperatures limited the disease to the lower South. Few doubted, however, that spring and the opening of navigation would spread cholera throughout the Mississippi Valley. Quarantines had proved themselves useless; cleanliness alone seemed to offer protection. City councils and local health boards were urged to have streets and houses cleaned and limed. "Another spring will bring the cholera among us," warned a Milwaukee editor, "sweeping like the Angel of Death over our firesides."

. . .

Twenty Orange Street was not one of New York's fashionable addresses. Thirty yards from the front door was the Five Points, a focus of infection during the 1832 cholera epidemic, and still the most filthy and dangerous crossroads of a rough and sprawling port. A tenement two doors up from 20 Orange Street housed one hundred and six hogs.

The poor and the criminal lived in Orange Street, and of these, only the most miserable tenanted its dark and oozing cellars. In the Spring of 1849, James Gilligan, a laborer when he worked, lived with four women in a room ten or 12 feet square in the rear basement of 20 Orange Street. The door had fallen from its hinges; the sashes of its two small windows were empty. There was no bed, no chair or table — with the exception of two empty barrels, no movable furniture at all. Across these barrels, the door was laid. This served as a table, and from it the five tenants ate the spoiled ham purchased at two or three cents a pound which was their usual fare.

Gilligan became ill on Friday, May 11. A habitual drinker, he thought little of his persistent cramps and vomiting. And by Saturday he felt better. On Monday the 14th, a local physician was notified that two of the women living in the cellar with Gilligan had sickened, as well, complaining of severe cramps, vomiting and diarrhea. Early Monday morning, Dr. Herriot made his way through the airless backyard, which provided the only access to the rear basement of 20 Orange Street, lowered his head, and stepped down into the cellar. When his eyes had become accustomed to the dark, a scene macabre even for the Five Points confronted him. Three bodies, one male and two female, lay on the floor, a few rags separating them from the decaying earthen floor. Two of the three died before evening. By this time, another woman in the cellar had been taken ill, and she, too, died before morning.

Dr. Seth Greer, the city's resident physician, was notified early that morning. It was clear to him after he had visited 20 Orange Street — as clear as it had been to Dr. Herriot — that these unfortunates had died of cholera. And so he reported to the Board of Health. This was the 15th of May.

Most New Yorkers were not overly alarmed. It did not seem surprising to those more comfortably situated that such wretches should die "like rotten sheep." Degraded by rum and breathing impure air, they would have succumbed had cholera never existed. Testy old Philip Hone noted on Saturday, the 19th, that the cases thus far reported had all been in Orange Street, "where water never was used internally or externally, and the pigs were contaminated by the contact of the children."

The Board of Health was in a quandary. Despite intermittent efforts beginning in December, the board had not, by May, been able to establish even one cholera hospital. Fear and avarice had made it almost impossible to rent any sort of building. In desperation, Bedloe's Island, even steamboats and barges had been suggested as possible hospitals. But ship-owners had proved as intractable as landlords: barges as well as houses would be permanently tainted in the public mind by their temporary use as cholera hospitals. By May, after five months of search, the only building which the board could confidently rely upon was the colored public school — and this prospective hospital possessed no sanitary facilities, not even facilities to heat water. On May 16, the day after hearing the report from Orange Street, the board established its first cholera hospital. It was the second floor of a tavern and ordinarily used for meetings and militia drills. Even this crude loft was obtained only at an exorbitant rent and after a mob, threatening to burn down the building, had been dispersed.

Before the epidemic had run its course, four of the city's public schools had been converted into makeshift hospitals, their desks ripped out and replaced by cots. But even these quasi-public buildings were not acquired without a struggle. The stigma of having once served as a cholera hospital could never be erased. . . .

The disease soon spread from the Five Points. Alarmed New Yorkers demanded that the Board of Health contain the disease before it invaded every part of the city. And by the end of June, the Board of Health had enacted what seemed to be a comprehensive anti-cholera program. The alderman and assistant alderman of each ward were authorized to hire four inspectors to help enforce the health ordinances — at a salary not to exceed $2.00 a day. The sale of fruits, vegetables and fish from open carts was forbidden; and owners of filthy tenements were ordered to have them cleaned immediately.

    . . . .

It seemed inevitable that the mid-summer heat would force into luxuriant growth the already well-established rootings of the disease. (Even the air seemed to have lost its elasticity, one observer noted — as it had done in the summer of 1832.) And, editorialists commented acidly, there was little chance of cholera subsiding while the streets of New York were still covered with filth and garbage.

Such fears were soon justified. In July, the case rate began steadily and abruptly to rise. A week after the 4th, 85 new cases and 30 deaths were reported. The weather, too, had grown steadily warmer, and business declined as New Yorkers left and provincial merchants feared to enter the plague-ridden city. By the 14th of July, only one theater remained open. At least two dozen churches had, before the month ended, closed their doors, as well.

Though deaths increased, the city's streets were still filthy, still patrolled by pigs and dogs. Garbage still encrusted cellars and yards. It seemed clear that the city fathers were either ignorant or incompetent. As early as May 25, William Cullen Bryant's *Evening Post* had charged the municipal authorities with criminal neglect. The *Herald*, too, was quick to attack the "culpable neglect and imbecility" of the Board of Health.

Nor were such attacks unjustified. Things simply did not get done — despite the statutory power of the Board of Health "to do or cause to be done anything, which, in their opinion, may be proper to preserve the health of the city." The members of the Common Council who constituted the Board of Health were ill-prepared to implement such wide and ill-defined powers. Precedent and traditional penury determined that so vague a grant of power would be construed in the narrowest fashion. New York aldermen were, moreover, notoriously immune to the promptings of civic morality. . . . Even when the harried councilmen did attempt to enforce a regimen of strict cleanliness, they met with continual obstruction. Conflicts arose between city and state authorities, between the Board of Health and the Commissioners of the Alms-House, between the board and the president of the Croton Water Board. Equally discouraging was the recalcitrant attitude of the average householder. In an admission of impotence, the Board of Health finally resorted, as it had 17 years earlier, to requesting the city's clergymen to urge upon their congregations the sanitary regulations, which the board had shown itself unable to enforce. Even the best of efforts, however, could not have overcome the inertia of generations.

. . . .

April had been cruel, breeding cholera in dozens of American cities and villages. River and lake steamers sowed the disease at scores of landings, while the railroads, which already crisscrossed the Northwest, discharged cholera at points even more remote. The pestilence often flared up among immigrant barge and steamboat passengers, debilitated by long sea voyages, hungry, dirty and huddled together on decks so crowded that even the sick could not lie down. Armed men discouraged attempts to land and bury the cholera dead. Bodies were lowered unceremoniously overboard, and drifted ominously past river and lake towns.

. . . .

By May, the disease had appeared as far north as Kenosha, Wisconsin. In hundreds of towns and cities, the outbreak of the first cholera case was expected daily. Newspapers in the smallest and most remote of communities were filled with demands for cleanliness, for the banishment of pigs, and for the establishment of hospitals. Managers of New England cotton mills distributed cholera tracts to their employees. Milwaukee built special bathhouses for arriving immigrants, while other town councils distributed chloride of lime to the poor.

It was in the infant cities of the West, with no adequate water supply, primitive sanitation, and crowded with a transient population, that the disease was most severe. St. Louis lost a tenth of her population. Cincinnati suffered almost as severely, Sandusky even more severely than St. Louis. Sextons, undertakers, even the horses in St. Louis were exhausted in the Sisyphean task of removing and burying the dead. Carts and furniture wagons served as makeshift hearses, and many of the dead came finally to an informal rest in the woods or on Mississippi sand bars. . . .

. . . .

There was little that could be done. Municipal health boards found their rudimentary powers insufficient to prevent or mitigate the epidemic. Indeed, many towns possessed no health board; in a greater number, they existed more in statute than reality — except during epidemics. New York, like most states, had no public health legislation. The law providing for local boards of health, passed as an emergency cholera measure in June, 1832, had expired by limitation the following year. It took more than good intentions to clean a town or city; and cleanliness, physicians agreed, was the only guarantee of immunity from cholera.

Even the largest cities lacked administrative tools. Attempts to effect sanitary reforms were in many cities, as in New York, paralyzed by the politically expedient contract system. In Baltimore, a local physician remarked, the only effectual scavenger was a heavy shower. Not even Boston, well-governed by standards of the time, was able to thoroughly clean its narrow and ill-graded courts, lanes, and alleys. The filth disinterred from cellars and cesspools was piled in streets or dumped in rivers — and, to the horror of a Boston railroad man, on his tracks. Despite the menace of cholera, many communities were unwilling or unable to enact coercive legislation and to force citizens to clean their property. In Vincennes, householders were "earnestly urged," in Galena "earnestly requested," to clean and lime their premises. In even the most authoritarian of communities, the penalty for nonobservance of sanitary regulations was modest, at most a $50.00 fine or 30 days in jail. And even these mild penalties were rarely imposed.

Money too was lacking. Most Americans were unwilling to be taxed or otherwise inconvenienced at the behest of some health board. In a city as large as Chicago, unpaid volunteers enforced sanitary regulations. New York, like many other communities, entrusted city council members with much of the responsibility for enforcing such ordinances. But, as an early chronicler of Milwaukee commented: "human nature predominates in an Alderman — and self-preservation is the first law of nature."

. . . .

Cholera still seemed a disease of poverty and sin; lechery, gluttony, or alcoholism could as appropriately as cholera be entered on the death certificates of its victims. The deaths of the moral, the prudent, the respectable were usually ignored. . . .

\* \* \*

## 2.  Tuberculosis in the 20th Century

As its title suggests, the book from which the next excerpt is taken is primarily intended to document the evolution of what some experts might call preventive medicine and others might call public health: the peculiar mix of public and private sector activities that emerged as Americans attempted to solve the major health problems of the early 20th century. As Rosen asks in his preface, why have some forms of preventive action been effective while others have not? Why have preventive measures been applied only in some instances? Why does accurate knowledge of disease etiology not necessarily lead to effective prevention? The answers to these questions raise a familiar theme, visible also in Rosenberg's work: Both disease and its prevention (or treatment) must be viewed in a social, political, and historical context.

Rosen's book also develops another recurring theme: the contrast between a preventive (and some would say necessarily collective) approach to maintaining health, and an approach that relies primarily on curative, patient-by-patient medical care.

The following excerpt is a description of the evolution of the understanding and eventually the prevention and treatment of tuberculosis, one of the major success stories of American disease-control in the early 20th century.

## GEORGE ROSEN, PREVENTIVE MEDICINE IN THE UNITED STATES 1900–1975
### 25–36 (1975)

\* \* \*

. . . Tuberculosis is for the most part an endemic disease, protean in its manifestations, slow and insidious in its progress, selecting its victims from among those whose resistance is diminished, and thriving in deprived bodies. In this connection, it must be emphasized that living and working conditions are highly important in determining the tuberculosis experience of a population. Throughout the 19th Century and beyond, the disease overwhelmingly affected urban communities. An urban community is a complicated structure within which no single factor operates alone to cause tuberculosis. As a result, it is not easy to separate and weigh the interlocking, interdependent causative elements. One of the best studies of this problem was made by F.C.S. Bradbury, who, in 1930-31, investigated the high incidence of tuberculosis in the towns of Jarrow and Blaydon in England. Bradbury concluded that the most important social factors were poverty, undernourishment and overcrowding in dwellings. Poverty compels people to skimp on food, and to live in overcrowded rooms. It must be emphasized, however, that while poverty and tuberculosis can be closely linked in an ugly alliance, poor people need not become tubercular. Poverty, poor housing, overcrowding, and malnutrition are important but secondary. The primary factor is the presence of an individual with an open [that is, active and infectious] case of the disease. In a community where tuberculosis is widely prevalent, most people from time to time come in contact with the pathogenic organism. On the whole, occasional fortuitous contacts are quite unimportant. Much more significant is close and regular contact over extended periods, as between husband and wife, parent and child, or other household members such as lodgers or servants. Contacts of this kind can also occur in places of employment, schools or institutions such as mental hospitals. In such circumstances, lack of previous exposure to tuberculosis is an important predisposing factor. . . .

On March 4, 1882, Robert Koch announced his discovery of the tubercle bacillus as the etiologic agent of tuberculosis. The concept of tuberculosis as a disease entity, originally set up on purely clinical and pathological-anatomical grounds, was now confirmed by bacteriological evidence. The implications of this discovery for community action were soon recognized in Great Britain, France and several other European countries, nor did the United States remain uninfluenced by these developments. As early as 1899, a report prepared by Hermann M. Biggs, J. Mitchell Prudden and H.P. Loomis, consulting pathologists to the New York City Health Department, emphasized the preventability of tuberculosis, and recommended surveillance of the disease by the department, as well as education of the public concerning its nature. In 1894, the department began to require reporting of cases of tuberculosis by institutions, and, in 1897, reporting by physicians. Similar efforts were undertaken at about the same time by local health officers and physicians in other communities.

Up to this point, however, the war against tuberculosis was a matter for the professional. The mobilization of the forces of the community for the control of a disease was first undertaken in the United States during the same decade. The discovery of the potentialities of broad community organization as a means of controlling disease was to have far-reaching significance for the entire community health program. . . .

. . . Initial attempts to produce active or passive immunization had failed, nor had any specific therapy been developed. Koch's announcement in 1890 of a preparation from tubercle bacilli as a curative and preventive agent for tuberculosis soon led to disappointment when experience showed that it was useless and even dangerous. There was agreement, however, on the value of tuberculin, as Koch's preparation was called, for diagnosis, and it remained in use for this purpose. Nevertheless, this immunological limitation was counterbalanced by increasing knowledge of the characteristics of the causal agent, and of the routes by which it was transmitted. . . . Tubercle bacilli were transmitted through infected sputum either as droplets expelled by coughing or as dust particles after expectorated sputum had dried. Even though these views were only partly correct, they emphasized the danger of careless expectoration of sputum, *e.g.*, on floors or into handkerchiefs, and provided a rationale for preventive measures.

Central to the prevention of tuberculosis was avoidance of exposure to infection, thus interrupting the chain of transmission. This principle, interruption of transmission by separating the affected individuals from others, and, thus, rendering them ineffective as sources of the pathogenic microbe, was not new. Introduced in Europe during the Middle Ages, initially to combat leprosy and then plague, it had given rise to an important tool of primary prevention, the practice of quarantine. Owing to ignorance or inadequate knowledge of the etiology and epidemiology of communicable diseases, however, quarantine measures were of only questionable effectiveness until the beginning of the 20th Century. The microbiological discoveries made it possible for health authorities to act with greater discrimination in carrying out preventive procedures. By establishing the incubation period in a given disease, the number of days required for isolation could be set more exactly. Similarly, by showing how water or food transmitted disease under given conditions, control measures could be undertaken more effectively. The first decade of the 20th Century thus had a solid, expanding scientific basis for the control of a number of communicable diseases, and throughout succeeding decades up to the present advances in these terms have continued.

. . . .

The strategy for an attack on tuberculosis, aimed at its prevention, developed within the context described above. A specific biologic enemy was known, the tubercle bacillus, as were its social allies that fostered the spread of the disease: depressed living standards, poor, overcrowded housing, unsanitary and unhealthful conditions at work, undernourishment, and precarious economic circumstances. . . . The strategy employed to fight tuberculosis may be characterized as socio-medical. In order to know the extent of the problem, compulsory reporting of cases of tuberculosis was necessary. Physicians and hospitals caring for such patients were to register them with the appropriate health agency, a municipal or county health department. To dispel ignorance and fear of the disease, and to achieve support for measures of compulsion, the general public had to be informed about its nature, transmission and means of control. Education was also required for patients and their families, particularly with respect to personal habits and hygiene. Furthermore, sanatoria were needed for the isolation and care of tuberculous patients, and clinics to examine those who had had contact with active cases or who were suspected of having the disease. Finally, to obtain legislation establishing such facilities and to secure the removal of the social evils contributing to the propagation of tuberculosis, public support had to be rallied and effectively organized.

The campaign against tuberculosis was undertaken by physicians, social workers and public spirited citizens in a crusading spirit, and it is certainly not a matter of chance that military terms pervade the publicity employed by the anti-tuberculosis movement. At first, the chief aims were early discovery and isolation of cases so as to prevent the spread of infection, to strike at the germ by finding and treating the early case. These aims were pursued as vigorously as possible, but it gradually became clear that matters were not so simple. Findings that early infection was widespread among urban inhabitants, and that most infected individuals did not develop recognizable disease [i.e., many otherwise healthy people can be infected and have no outward signs of illness] led to an increased emphasis on environmental factors involving public and personal hygiene, including clean streets, fresh air, proper nutrition, pure food and personal cleanliness, what Ida M. Cannon called the "hygienic gospel."

. . . .

Since bovine tuberculosis [a highly contagious form of TB typically found in cows and deer that can be transmitted to other mammals, including humans] caused about one-fifth to a quarter of the cases in infants and children, it was evident that bovine tubercle bacilli played a significant role in the etiology of childhood tuberculosis, and that prevention had to deal with the bovine source by breaking the chain of transmission. This aim could be achieved in two ways, by eliminating bovine tuberculosis in cattle, and by pasteurizing milk. Both approaches were pursued. Although dairy inspection had begun in Newark, New Jersey, as early as 1882, and pasteurization about a decade later, the movement was slow. Chicago enacted a compulsory pasteurization ordinance in 1909, the first such law in the United States. New York followed in 1910. . . .

The elimination of bovine tuberculosis by killing tuberculous animals and recompensing the owners was started in 1917 as a national program under the Department of Agriculture. By employing systematic tuberculin testing, prompt slaughtering of infected animals, thorough disinfection and appropriate procedures for the movement of cattle, the reactor rate of tested cattle fell from 4.9 percent in 1918 to 0.08 percent in 1965.

The campaign to eradicate bovine tuberculosis, particularly through the increasing practice of pasteurization, had a significant impact on the transmission of other communicable diseases. Milk as a vehicle for the transmission of typhoid fever had first been incriminated in 1857. . . . That year, at the International Medical Congress in London, Ernest Hart reported 50 epidemics of typhoid fever, 15 epidemics of scarlet fever and 4 epidemics of diphtheria attributed to this cause. In 1909, the U.S. Public Health Service issued its famous Bulletin 56, which listed 500 outbreaks of milk-borne disease between 1880 and 1907. These epidemics were noted when they were severe, as in Boston between 1907 and 1911 when the city had five milk-borne outbreaks (diphtheria, scarlet fever, typhoid fever, and "tonsillitis," probably streptococcal sore throat). But as Rosenau pointed out in 1912, these outbreaks were not always reported. . . .

Obviously, a preventive measure such as pasteurization intended to provide uncontaminated milk was an attack not on one disease or one health problem, but rather on several. Such measures, of which the effects ramify in several directions, can reinforce the action of other procedures and approaches for combating specific diseases or problems. . . .

In bovine tuberculosis, the pathogenic organism could be attacked directly by destroying the infected host or by treating the product, milk, so as to render it safe for consumption. These methods could be applied because the force of law eventually coincided with the economic interests of the cattle and the dairy industries. Since these methods were inapplicable to human beings, the alternative was to find the early case, segregate the patient in a sanatorium or by teaching the patient and the family to observe strict hygienic practices so as to prevent transmission, and to follow-up the contacts. These aims were implemented through programs of case-finding, and by establishing diagnostic clinics and sanatoria. By the 1920s, it had been recognized in principle that tuberculosis prevention and control was a governmental responsibility exercised at the municipal, county and state levels. . . . However, the implementation of the principle left much to be desired. A survey by the Public Health service in 1923 of activities in 100 municipalities led to the conclusion that the diagnostic clinics were insufficient in number and inefficiently administered. Furthermore, in most states, the number of sanatorium beds was wholly inadequate to meet the needs. In fact, some cities and counties did not have half enough beds. Not only were the facilities for diagnosed cases inadequate, but physicians were limited in their ability to detect early tuberculosis by the available diagnostic methods. This was also a transitional period in medical education, a period in which there were numerous physicians who had not been properly taught to recognize manifestations of early pulmonary tuberculosis. There were still others whose approach was limited by their socio-economic views. In Muncie, Indiana, for example, the local Anti-tuberculosis Association maintained a weekly chest clinic to which physicians from the County Medical Society donated their services with the proviso that the clinic should be available only to those too poor to pay privately. Until the early 1930s x-rays were used unsystematically and sporadically for the detection of early tuberculosis. Mass survey techniques had not yet been developed. With the introduction of cheap paper films around 1931 and miniature photo-roentgen films after 1936, low cost mass chest x-ray surveys became possible. Such surveys became an important function of health departments, another indication that official health agencies were taking over the task of controlling tuberculosis. Assistance was given to many communities by the U.S. Public Health Service. Acceptance of mass x-ray services by labor unions, business executives and the general public led to surveys of occupational groups, selected community groups considered to be at high risk, and after World War II, from about 1946 to 1953, to a number of large city surveys. During this period, chest x-ray programs were started in general hospitals on all admissions and proved productive. During the same period, three chemotherapeutic agents were introduced, streptomycin in 1947, para-aminosalicylic acid in 1949 and isonazid in 1952 with the result that the pattern of tuberculosis prevention and control began to change markedly. Sanatoria and special hospitals closed since no prolonged stays in institutions were required, tuberculosis specialists disappeared or no longer limited their work to the disease, the voluntary associations saw the handwriting on the wall and expanded their scope to include respiratory diseases, and health departments rearranged their priorities so that activities concerned with tuberculosis were downgraded. The amount of tuberculosis in the United States declined, but the disease did not disappear.

. . . .

The outbreak of the First World War interrupted the great Atlantic migration, which, since the 1880s, had brought millions of Europeans to the United States where they settled largely in urban centers. The cessation of immigration during the war years and the restrictive legislation of 1921 and 1924 were undoubtedly important factors in changing the circumstances of the foreign born. As the flow of new immigrants was cut down to a trickle, the foreign born and even more so their children tended to improve their mode of life under the influence of economic and educational factors. As they moved up the economic ladder, even if only moderately, there was an increasing tendency to move out of the areas of initial settlement into sections with better housing. Between 1920 and 1930, a growing trend appeared toward less clustering of the foreign born in ethnic neighborhoods. Many of those involved in this process of change were younger persons of the native born generations, with a greater earning capacity and, thus, able to afford a higher standard of living. Although the depression of the 1930s retarded these tendencies, they revived toward the end of the decade coincident with the outbreak of World War II and continued after the war.

During the same period, housing was being improved. By 1937, central heating, hot and cold running water, and interior installed toilets and baths were commonplace essentials in millions of houses. Nonetheless, such advances were uneven; overcrowding in houses and living conditions conducive to ill health were still present. . . .

As the disease declined, living conditions improved though not equally in all segments of communities, even when the inhabitants were of the same ethnic stock. Unfavorable conditions persisted in the socially remote sectors where living standards were low, for example, among Negroes in urban centers, the majority of whom lived on the lowest economic level, affected not only by poor housing, but also by inadequate nutrition and lack of other basic necessities. The role of nutrition as a probable factor in the evolution of tuberculosis has already been mentioned, but it must also be emphasized that special attention began to be given to the nutritional status of the population between the two World Wars. The necessity to safeguard health while conserving food during the First World War led to the production of increased supplies of protective foods and a growing recognition of their value. Improved methods of producing and distributing perishable foods made protective foods more easily available in urban communities. Furthermore, the development of more effective advertising and merchandising methods for fruits, vegetables, milk and other products led to their increased use. The growth of chain stores, cafeterias and restaurants also facilitated the distribution of perishable food to consumers. At the same time, in the 1920s, interest in improving the nutrition of children and of mothers during the childbearing period was furthered by the [federal] Maternal and Infancy Act. Attention to nutrition was further stimulated by the world economic crisis of 1929–1936, when widespread malnutrition followed on the heels of mass unemployment, as well as by the special needs of the Second World War with its attendant food shortages, rationing and the necessity for protecting workers in industry, as well as women and children. After 1935, the Federal Surplus Commodities Corporation provided food for school lunches, and by the end of 1938, 45 states and the District of Columbia were participating in this activity. In May 1939, the Food Stamp Plan was inaugurated to supply families on relief and those with low incomes with food. In 1939 and 1941, a total of $135,000,000 was available for the distribution of agricultural surpluses through the stamp plan, through relief agencies, and for school lunches. These activities undoubtedly had a beneficial effect on the nutritional status of a large segment of the American population, thus, contributing to the continuing decline of tuberculosis.

. . . .

. . . Discussing the great increase in tuberculosis in Europe after the Second World War, Johannes Holm . . . added another significant factor. According to Holm, the marked rise was due to malnutrition which lowered resistance; overcrowded living conditions in the large cities, and a low standard of personal hygiene because facilities for cleanliness and hygiene were nonexistent, thus enabling tubercle bacilli to appear, *and* the disorganization of the antituberculosis program in many European countries.

The implication of Holm's analysis is that a fundamental element in any practical program of disease prevention is the existence of an organized institutional framework within which it can be implemented. If such a structured context does not exist, or is inadequate, or is disrupted as happened in Europe, it is difficult if not impossible to carry out a coherent and consistent preventive program. In fact, this is one of the difficulties in the United States today with respect to cardiovascular disease, neoplasms, and a number of other health problems. . . . To put the matter in another way, one reason why the socioeconomic conditions of the Depression did not materially affect the continuing decline of tuberculosis was the existence of a well developed preventive program which was being carried out within a coherent institutional arrangement comprising official health agencies, voluntary organizations and medical practitioners. . . .

\* \* \*

### 3.   Yellow Fever After World War II

Like Rosenberg's tale of cholera, Murphy's book (as its title suggests) is the story of another of America's battles with fast-spreading epidemic diseases, in this case the yellow fever epidemics that struck in the late 1700s and early 1800s. It is a story worth reading, both for its place in public health's history and for its confirmation of many of the same lessons about Americans and their characteristic responses to such crises. In an epilogue, Murphy also considers a much later encounter with yellow fever (and malaria, among many other infectious diseases), incident to the construction of the Panama Canal in the early 1900s. The Panama experience has been shared virtually everywhere in the world where the primary source of such diseases could be encountered: *Aedes aegypti*, your friendly (and, if you are unlucky) neighborhood mosquito.

Yellow fever is caused by a virus, often producing only mild symptoms, which, however, progress from high fever and chills, to vomiting, and after what appears to be a stage of remission, kidney failure (and, therefore, the appearance that the victim is turning yellow), and death. During the 18th century epidemics, mortality rates ran as high as 50 percent of those who developed symptoms. Even today there is no known cure. There is, however, an effective vaccine, although it carries the potential for serious side effects.

Murphy's choice to close his story of yellow fever with a brief review excerpted below of the public health measures taken in the post-World War II period to combat mosquito-borne diseases illustrates some important lessons that, unfortunately, have been only partially appreciated.

### JIM MURPHY, AN AMERICAN PLAGUE: THE TRUE AND TERRIFYING STORY OF THE YELLOW FEVER EPIDEMIC OF 1793
#### 135–39 (2003)

\* \* \*

The Havana and Panama campaigns controlled yellow fever and the *Aedes aegypti* mosquito in those regions, but they did not eliminate the disease completely. It continued to terrorize numerous cities, especially in Central and South America. Finally, in 1947, the Pan American Sanitary Bureau (later renamed the Pan American Health Organization) decided to eradicate the mosquito — and, thus, the disease — in the entire Western Hemisphere.

Along with destroying breeding areas, adult mosquito populations were also attacked with the widespread use of the pesticide dichlorodiphenyltrichloroethane, better known as DDT, much of it sprayed from planes. By 1962, 21 countries declared themselves free of *Aedes aegypti*, and the world seemed very close to ending yellow fever forever. That was when problems began to develop in the United States.

First, experts in mosquito control complained that Congress had not budgeted enough money for the campaign to succeed. Virtually every southern state was infested with *Aedes aegypti*, these experts pointed out, but funds would run out before the job of eradicating the mosquitoes was half completed.

Second, concern about the health risks and environmental problems associated with the use of DDT increased during the 1960s. These fears were given a public platform with the publication of Rachel Carson's *Silent Spring* in 1962. In this groundbreaking book, the author tackled many emerging ecological concerns, such as the environmental dangers associated with radiation. But it was the use of DDT, and its potential health risks to both animals and humans, that grabbed the public's attention.

The book became a best seller and convinced many citizens and politicians of the dangers posed by indiscriminate spraying of DDT and other chemicals. The use of DDT would be banned in the United States in 1972, but the anti-mosquito campaign had died long before that.

Actually, Carson had predicted that the campaign would fail even if the spraying continued as mosquito-control experts wanted. "Spraying kills off the weaklings," she explained. "The only survivors are insects that have some inherent quality that allows them to escape harm. These are the parents of the new generation, which, by simple inheritance, possess all the qualities of toughness inherent in its forebears." In other words, super-mosquitoes were being created that were capable of resisting DDT.

Careful testing established that it takes about seven years for this new mosquito to emerge and replace the old one. In addition, the same evolutionary process happens when newer pesticides, such as malathion, Sevin or permethrin, are used.

As this new pesticide-resistant *Aedes Aegypti* gradually reestablished itself in Central and South America, another problem was noted. Because the old mosquito — and with it the disease — had been absent so long, hardly anyone had built up an immunity to yellow fever. As a result, hundreds of millions of people were now susceptible to getting yellow fever and other deadly diseases carried by *Aedes aegypti*.

An even more alarming problem was that several mosquito-borne diseases had begun to change. Malaria was the first in which a change was observed. Prior to the 1960s, a number of drugs, such as atabrine and chloroquine, had been developed that effectively treated this illness. Unfortunately, patients would often use only enough of these medicines to reduce the symptoms, saving the rest for future bouts of the disease. Many of the microscopic parasites that produced malaria would survive the sub-lethal dose and produce offspring capable of withstanding a full dose of the medicine.

This drug-resistant type of malaria began to appear among U.S. troops during the Vietnam War, in which more soldiers were incapacitated by the disease than by battle wounds. Despite the introduction of different, more powerful drugs, the new kind of malaria spread across Asia, then to Africa, and eventually to South America. Today, ten percent of the world's population suffers from malaria every year, resulting in almost three million deaths. In the time it takes to read this sentence, another person has died of malaria.

It's clear now that mosquitoes, animals and human disease go together. We know that the virus that causes West Nile encephalitis is carried by birds that travel up and down the east coast of the United States, and that mosquitoes feed on them and then give the disease to humans. *Aedes albopictus*, better known as the Asian tiger mosquito, sucks the blood of both animals and humans and is capable of carrying a wide variety of viruses, including dengue fever, eastern equine encephalitis, West Nile encephalitis, and La Crosse encephalitis, all serious illnesses and all potentially lethal to humans. In fact, of the 2500 kinds of mosquitoes that infest the world, almost 400 of them are capable of transmitting diseases to humans.

"No animal on earth," assert mosquito experts Andrew Spielman and Michael D'Antonio, "has touched so directly and profoundly the lives of so many human beings. . . . With their glassy wings, delicate legs and seemingly fragile bodies, mosquitoes are, nevertheless, a powerful, even fatal, presence in our lives."

Which brings us back to *Aedes aegypti* and yellow fever. The disease exists anywhere there are monkey populations, as does the pesticide-resistant mosquito that can transport the disease to humans. As new roads are cut into virgin rain forests, more and more people enter areas where they can become infected. A car ride takes that newly infected person to a major city, where more *Aedes aegypti* mosquitoes wait to feed on him, then carry the disease to another and another and another person. A plane ride carries one of these infected persons to a new country, where still more *Aedes aegypti* wait to feed and fly off.

Two factors make the situation especially dire in the United States. First, no company here has produced the vaccine in recent years. If the disease invaded a large city and a call went out for hundreds of thousands of doses of the vaccine, it would take months to produce it. The Institute of Medicine studied the situation in 1992 and estimated that an outbreak of yellow fever in a city like New Orleans would infect 100,000 people and kill at least 10,000 of them before it could be brought under control.

Second, despite years of research, there is still no cure for yellow fever. While modern medicines can lessen the impact the disease has on the human body, once a person has yellow fever, he or she will have to endure most of the horrible symptoms that Philadelphia's people suffered in 1793 [the primary subject of Murphy's book].

"Once urban transmission begins in the American region," Duane Gubler, a director at the Centers for Disease Control, warns, "it's probably going to spread very rapidly throughout the region to other urban centers and then from there to Asia and the Pacific." In other words, yellow fever is a "modern-day time bomb. We're just sitting here waiting for it to happen."

The situation is the kind that produces nightmares in thoughtful people. Yet, the history of yellow fever offers hope. We know, for instance, that [in Philadelphia in 1793] Benjamin Rush was alert enough to recognize the disease before it had spread much beyond Water Street and sounded an alert. Modern doctors should be able to spot yellow fever and issue warnings even sooner.

We know, too, that the anti-mosquito breeding campaigns in Cuba and Panama were very effective in halting the infections and that massive insecticide campaigns can control the populations of *Aedes aegypti*. Prompt warning and fast (if unpleasant) action have kept yellow fever and related diseases in check over recent decades, as well, and the same will be true in the future. Meanwhile, dedicated scientists develop theories and test them, hoping to discover a safe and effective cure.

Yet, if the history of yellow fever tells us anything, it is that this is a struggle with no real end. Yellow fever, as we know it now, might be conquered, but another version of the disease will eventually emerge to challenge us again. And when it does, we will have to overcome our fears and be prepared to confront it.

* * *

## 4.  Anthrax

In *The Anthrax Letters*, excerpted below, Leonard Cole documents the unfolding of what some experts have labeled the first bioterrorist attack on American soil: the deliberate distribution of anthrax spores through the U.S. mail, apparently targeting the publishers of *The National Enquirer*, but also infecting scores of postal employees and others who had contact with them. Cole's basic thesis is that these sorts of incidents cannot be investigated as crimes and by law enforcement, but are public health emergencies, requiring the rapid and effective response of public health officials as well. Whether that response is ready and available, Cole strongly hints, is doubtful. For that matter, the perpetrator of the crime has never been identified (although Cole offers some strong hints as to that identity).

The excerpt here, from the prologue, describes anthrax, its effects, and the possible scenarios that may flow from its release.

### LEONARD A. COLE, THE ANTHRAX LETTERS
vii–ix (2003)

* * *

Anthrax bacteria are as murderous as South American flesh-eating ants. An army of ants, traveling in the millions, can decimate an immobilized individual by devouring his flesh layer by layer. Death is gradual and agonizing. Anthrax bacilli can do to the body from within what the ants do from without. They attack everywhere, shutting down and destroying the body's functions from top to bottom. The organisms continue to multiply and swarm until there is nothing left for them to feed on. In two or three days, a few thousand bacilli may become trillions. At the time of death, as much as 30 percent of a person's blood weight may be live bacilli. A microscopic cross section of a blood vessel looks as though it is teeming with worms.

. . . .

Concern about anthrax is as old as the Bible. Primarily a disease of animals, it is thought to have been the fifth of the 10 biblical plagues visited by God on the ancient Egyptians for refusing freedom to the Jews. As recounted in

Exodus, horses, donkeys, camels, cattle, and sheep were struck "with a very severe pestilence." After their carcasses were burned, the virulence of the anthrax germs persisted, for the soot caused "boils on man and beast throughout the land of Egypt."

In recent years, anthrax spores have been deemed among the most likely of biological weapons because they are hardy, long lived and, if inhaled, utterly destructive. A victim is unlikely to know he is under attack. As with other biological agents, anthrax germs are odorless and tasteless, and lethal quantities can be so tiny as to go unseen.

Every three seconds or so, a human being inhales and exhales about a pint of air. Each cycle draws in oxygen to fuel the body and releases carbon dioxide, the gaseous waste product. The inhaled air commonly carries with it floating incidentals such as dust, bacteria and other microscopic particles. If a particle is larger than five microns, it is likely to be blocked from reaching deep into the lungs by the respiratory tract's mucus and filtration hairs. If smaller than one micron, a particle is too small to be retained and is blown out during exhalation. An anthrax spore may be one micron wide and two or three microns long, just the right size to reach deep into the respiratory pathway.

A spore is so tiny that a cluster of thousands, which would be enough to kill someone, is scarcely visible to the naked eye. A thousand spores side by side would barely reach across the thin edge of a dime. Once inhaled, the spores are drawn into the bronchial tree where they travel through numerous branches deep in the lungs. Near the tip of the branches are microscopic sacs called alveoli. It is in these sacs that inhaled oxygen is exchanged with carbon dioxide.

Stationed among the alveoli are armies of defender cells called macrophages. These cells sense foreign micro-invaders and engulf them. A pulmonary macrophage normally destroys its inhaled captive and taxis it to the lymph nodes in the mediastinum, the area between the lungs. But in the case of anthrax, spores may transform into active, germinating organisms before the macrophage can affect them. The bacteria then can reproduce and release toxin that destroys the macrophage. Thus, in a perverse turnabout, the anthrax bacteria, like soldiers in the Trojan horse, can burst out of their encirclement, into the lymph and blood systems.

An infected person at first is unaware that a gruesome cascade is under way. Although the onslaught is relentless, symptoms do not appear immediately. Fluids that have begun to accumulate in the mediastinum gradually pry the lungs apart. Breathing becomes increasingly difficult, and, after a few days, a person feels as if his head is being held underwater, permitted to bob up for a quick gulp of air and then pushed under again.

The agony works its way through the body. Nausea gives way to violent, bloody vomiting. Joints are so inflamed that flexing an arm or leg becomes an act of torment. Bloody fluids squeeze between the brain and skull, and the victim's face may balloon out beyond recognition. The tightening vice around the brain causes excruciating pain and delirium. Survival depends on being provided appropriate antibiotics before the bacteria have released so much toxin that the body cannot recover. If inhalation anthrax is not treated in time, almost all victims suffer a tortured death. One organ after another is decimated — the lungs, the kidneys, the heart — until life is sucked away.

It is because of such ghastly effects that anthrax and other biological agents have been prohibited as weapons by international agreement. The treaty that bans their development or possession by nations, the 1972 Biological Weapons Convention, uniquely describes their use as "repugnant to the conscience of mankind." Yet, despite this widely accepted moral precept, a germ weapon is seen by some not as a shameful blight but as a preferred instrument of terror.

* * *

# NOTES AND QUESTIONS

**1.** The excerpts from Rosenberg, Rosen, Murphy, and Cole are only selections from what is a rich literature that could be called "public health history." Other works that are both well-written and informative include: JOHN M. BARRY, THE GREAT INFLUENZA: THE EPIC STORY OF THE GREATEST PLAGUE IN HISTORY (2004); HOWARD MARKEL, WHEN GERMS TRAVEL: SIX MAJOR EPIDEMICS THAT HAVE INVADED AMERICA SINCE 1900 AND THE FEARS THEY HAVE UNLEASHED (2004); MARILYN CHASE, THE BARBARY PLAGUE: THE BLACK DEATH IN VICTORIAN SAN FRANCISCO (2003); BARRON H. LERNER, CONTAGION, CONTAINMENT: CONTROLLING TUBERCULOSIS ALONG THE SKID ROAD (1998); HOWARD MARKEL, QUARANTINE! EAST EUROPEAN JEWISH IMMIGRANTS AND THE NEW YORK CITY EPIDEMICS OF 1892 (1997); JUDITH WALZER LEAVITT, TYPHOID MARY: CAPTIVE TO THE PUBLIC'S HEALTH (1996); & JOHN ETTLING, THE GERM OF LAZINESS (1981) (a chronicle of the discovery of the health and social consequences of hook worm disease among low income Southerners).

For an excellent, concise history of the field of public health, see Elizabeth Fee's chapter, *The Origins and Development of Public Health in the United States*, in 1 OXFORD TEXTBOOK OF PUBLIC HEALTH, 35–54 (R. Detels et al., eds., 3d ed. 1997).

**2.** Cholera, of course, is not the only disease to be explained through the lens of time-specific social values; apparent differences in the social impact of a disease are frequently used to defend or advance prevalent beliefs or norms. For example, during yellow fever epidemics in the pre-Civil War South, it sometimes appeared that African-Americans were less susceptible to the disease, or contracted milder or non-fatal cases. It was not difficult for some observers to seize upon this perception as a justification for slavery: after all, didn't it prove that slaves, rather than whites, were best "suited" for demanding outdoor physical labor — precisely the environment in which (we later came to recognize) exposure to disease-carrying mosquitoes was most likely to occur? This kind of thinking became known as the "medical pro-slavery" argument. *See generally* Jo Ann Carrigan, *Notes and Documents: Privilege, Prejudice, and the Stranger's Disease in Nineteenth Century New Orleans*, XXXVI(4) J. SOC. HIST. 568 (1970). Can you think of contemporary examples of this phenomenon?

**3.** Charles Rosenberg states emphatically that "in the history of public health in the United States, there is no date more important than 1866, no event more significant than the organization of the Metropolitan Board of Health. For the first time, an American community had successfully organized itself to conquer an epidemic." ROSENBERG, THE CHOLERA YEARS, *supra*, at 193. The creation of an effective Board of Health is attributable to the enactment of a New York state law (Act of Feb. 26, 1866, Ch. 74, 1866 N.Y. Laws 114) implementing new scientific knowledge, advances in public administration, and a collective commitment to reform. For a fascinating political history of the enactment of the law and the first years of the Board's activities, see JAMES C. MOHR, THE RADICAL REPUBLICANS AND REFORM IN NEW YORK DURING RECONSTRUCTION 61–85, 86–111 (1973).

In a course on public health law, this seminal state legislation provides an opportunity to consider in depth the ways in which legislative and administrative law can be extremely effective tools in the promotion of public health. Many of the law's policy innovations exist, in modern form, in a wide range of public health legislation today. As you read this note, consider those that still seem familiar.

The state law created "The Metropolitan Sanitary District of the State of New York," which was geographically co-extensive with the existing metropolitan police district. Simultaneously, it consolidated the new Sanitary District's four gubernatorially-appointed Commissioners (plus the health officer of the Port of New York) with the four existing police commissioners, to form a "super-agency," the Metropolitan Board of Health — thereby harnessing together, at the outset, public health power with law enforcement capabilities. The linkage was not only structural, but operational as well: the Board of Health and police commission were to cooperate in the promotion of public health and safety, and the latter were required to enforce and execute the "sanitary rules, regulations and . . . orders" of the Board. Violations of the new law or orders of the Board, obstruction or interference with execution of a Board order, and willful failure to obey such an order constituted misdemeanors.

Both the police and the Board's inspectors were authorized to arrest anyone who committed "any act or thing forbidden by this act, or by any law or ordinance," or resisted enforcement of a Board order; such offenses were misdemeanors. The Board itself was given power to order the arrest of a violator; its order had the same effect as a judicially-ordered arrest warrant. Such an arrestee was to be taken before a magistrate and treated as one arrested for a misdemeanor. The law seemed to contemplate that, in the course of trying to decide whether to have someone arrested, the Board could seek the assistance of a trial court in compelling persons to testify, and in production of records.

In the modern era, the linkage of civil force with public health policy is considerably more controversial; but against the mid-19th Century urban backdrop, it was quite understandable.

The new law sought to displace the tradition of political cronyism, noted by Rosenberg, with mechanisms designed to ensure that public health would be professionalized — newly grounded in scientific expertise and administrative capability, supported by adequate funding, and comparatively insulated from politics. For example, of the four Sanitary Commissioners on the Board, three were required to be physicians. Commissioners enjoyed fixed 4-year terms, were prohibited from simultaneously holding "political or municipal office," and were removable by the Governor for "dereliction of duty." The Board was authorized to appoint a chief executive officer — an "experienced and skillful" physician — to execute Board orders and supervise Board employees. Ten of the fifteen health inspectors whom the statute authorized the Board to employ were to be physicians, and the rest to be selected for "the practical knowledge of scientific or sanitary matters . . . which may especially qualify them." Along with a provision authorizing the sanitary inspection of all forms of property, the law conferred on the Board power to engage persons to render "sanitary engineering service, and to make or supervise practical and scientific investigations and examinations . . . requiring engineering skill, and to prepare plans and reports relative thereto." Lawyers were expressly included in the movement toward professionalization of public health services: the Board was authorized to "take such legal advice and employ such attorneys" as necessary. Funded by the state, the Board's annual budget was to be set by the Board in consultation with the Mayors and Comptrollers of New York City and Brooklyn. Finally, the Board enjoyed borrowing authority (subject to gubernatorial approval) to ensure its solvency pending the availability of needed governmental appropriations.

Of particular importance were the substantive powers granted to the Board. First, all powers previously allocated to other health agencies were transferred to and consolidated in the new Board and all other existing offices and governmental entities "relating to public health" (save the Port of New York's Health Officer and its Board of Quarantine Commissioners) were simultaneously abolished. But beyond consolidation, new powers were specified that had particular relevance to the problems of urban sanitation and filth (vividly described by Rosenberg) that characterized American cities at mid-century.

The Board was authorized to declare that any "building, erection, excavation, premises, business, pursuit, matter or thing, or the sewerage, drainage or ventilation thereof" which, in its "opinion," was "in a condition or in effect dangerous to life or health," constituted a "public nuisance" — and thereupon to order it "removed, abated, suspended, altered or otherwise improved or purified. . . ." The Board could also order "any [dangerous or detrimental] substance, matter or thing. . .left in any street, alley, water, excavation, building, erection, place or grounds ( . . . public or private) . . . to be speedily removed to some proper place. . . ." These and other broad powers over property were accompanied by procedural protections — e.g., a requirement that the Board make reasonable efforts to serve the owner with notice of the finding and proposed remedy, and an opportunity for the owner to stay the order for long enough to provide a "reasonable and fair opportunity to be heard" before the Board, after which the Board might rescind, modify, or reaffirm its original order. The Board was authorized to levy costs of execution against those responsible for violations to impose liens, and to seek judgment against any individual violator notwithstanding that others might also be partly accountable. Moreover, the law imposed on a broad category of owners, lessees and others the duty to keep a physical premise "in such manner that it shall not be dangerous or prejudicial to life or health."

The new law also conferred on the Board other broadly-applicable public health powers, and imposed other duties. It authorized the Board to "remove or cause to be removed to a proper place [of its choosing] . . . any person sick with small pox or other contagious disease." (This is what is termed "isolation" in public health parlance. Interestingly, the law contains no express quarantine power authorizing sequestration of those thought to have been exposed to contagious disease and thus perhaps infectious themselves, even though not yet ill). The Board was empowered to "take measures, and supply agents, and afford inducements and facilities" for "general and gratuitous vaccination and disinfection" and to "afford medical relief to and among the poor," all "as in its opinion the protection of the public health may require." The Board was required to make an annual report of vital statistics — births, deaths, and marriages — and to engage in mutual information-sharing with the Port of New York health authorities and with local health authorities throughout the state. The law made a tentative foray into what is now known as public-health surveillance (*see* Chapter Four, *infra*), requiring the Board to use "all reasonable means for ascertaining the existence and cause of disease or peril to life or health, and for averting the same," and requiring the Board — so far as it was able "without serious expense" — to "gather and preserve such information and facts relating to deaths, disease and health [from the district and the state at large] as may be useful in the discharge of its duties. . . ."

Since at least the early 1930s, it has been an established feature of American law that administrative agencies — which derive their powers and duties exclusively from legislative enactments — exercise policymaking discretion in implementing the statutes that create and govern them. This is justified by agencies' specialized expertise, the generality or ambiguity that frequently characterizes their governing statutes, the institutional infeasibility of legislatures' "administering" programs, changes in circumstances over time that require legal adaptation, and other factors. Such discretion is a practical necessity in the lawmaking process, and many deem it a virtue. Well before the mid-20th Century rise of the "modern administrative state," however, the law creating the Metropolitan Board of Health expressly conferred this kind of discretion on the Board, empowering it to "enact such by-laws, rules and regulations as it may deem advisable, in harmony with the provisions and purposes of this act . . . for the regulation of the action of said Board . . . in the discharge of its . . . duties, and for the protection of life and public health"; and, "from time to time," to "alter, annul or amend the same." Further, it empowered courts to enforce such rules. Finally, the legislation employed a procedural safeguard that would become commonplace in 20th Century efforts to control the potentially-arbitrary exercise of administrative discretion: it required the Board to publish such rules in advance of their taking effect.

If administrative discretion is in general a positive (or at least necessary) aspect of American lawmaking, how far should it go? Consider carefully the following power, which the law granted to the new Board of Health in the event of one kind of extreme circumstance:

> [I]n the presence of great and imminent peril to the public health . . . by reason of impending pestilence, it shall be the duty of said Board to

take such measures and to do and order, and cause to be done, such acts and make such expenditures (beyond those duly estimated for or provided) for the preservation of the public health (though not herein elsewhere or otherwise authorized) as it may in good faith declare the public safety and health to demand, and the Governor of the State shall also in writing approve. But the exercise of this extraordinary power shall also, so far as it involved such excessive expenditures, require the written assent of at least six members of the Board. And such peril shall not be deemed to exist except when, and for such period of time, as the Governor of the State, together with said board, shall declare by proclamation the same to exist or continue.

Ch. 74, §16, 1866 NY. Laws 114, 131. What is the scope of the Board's power under this provision? What procedural and substantive limitations on that power do you find in this passage? Are they sufficient? Too constraining? In an "emergency," however defined, who should be making decisions which — as this law forthrightly concedes — are "not herein elsewhere or otherwise authorized"? By what standards? Compare this provision with the authorities created, in a gubernatorially-declared emergency, under the Model State Health Emergency Powers Act, presented and discussed *infra* in Chapter Three, Section F. How different are the two? How similar?

## B.  AMERICAN PUBLIC HEALTH . . . PRESENT AND FUTURE

In 1988, the Institute of Medicine (IOM)[1] issued a report entitled *The Future of Public Health*, strongly criticizing the nation's public health infrastructure, and the capacity of local, state, and federal agencies to respond to the nation's pressing health needs; the report also delineated a long list of public health issues and problems that needed to be addressed.

The 1988 report spawned a number of reform efforts both within and without government (see Note 5, *infra*, for examples and references), and some public and political attention — but a questionable amount of progress or remediation. In 2001, following the events of September 11, the Centers for Disease Control and Prevention (CDC) and a number of other health-related government agencies asked the IOM to update the 1988 report. Unstated but clearly included in that request was a mandate to be more "inclusive"; that is, IOM was asked to extend its evaluation beyond the traditional public health infrastructure and to include medical care providers and other private actors within the broader "public health system."

The net result echoed the original message of the 1988 report. The assessment of the readiness of local, state, and federal agencies to deal with the various public health problems facing the nation was no more flattering. But a new element in the analysis was the report's use of the terms "public health"

---

[1] The Institute of Medicine is a private organization of academics and other professionals created by the National Academy of Sciences in 1970. The National Academy of Sciences is a private, nonprofit corporation created under a congressional charter in 1893 to act as an advisor to the federal government.

and "health" virtually synonymously, at least when defining the health-related problems of Americans and in assessing their underlying causes. Moreover, in assessing what needed to be done, the report attempted to bridge the distinction between medicine and public health and between the private and public sectors, projecting solutions that would require cooperative "partnerships" among not only the various public health agencies of government but also with private medical care providers and institutions, employers, even the media. Indeed, virtually everyone was given some responsibility for the problems and some role in their potential solution. The result is a document of continuing importance, at many levels. The excerpts from the 2003 report that follow are illustrative of the tone as well as the content of that report.

## INSTITUTE OF MEDICINE, THE FUTURE OF THE PUBLIC'S HEALTH IN THE 21ST CENTURY
### 20–32, 46–66 (2002)

\* \* \*

### ACHIEVEMENT AND DISAPPOINTMENT

The health of the American people at the beginning of the 21st Century would astonish those living in 1900. By every measure, we are healthier, live longer, and enjoy lives that are less likely to be marked by injuries, ill health, or premature death. In the past century, infant mortality declined and life expectancy increased. Vaccines and antibiotics made once life-threatening ailments preventable or less serious; and homes, workplaces, roads, and automobiles became safer. In addition to the many health achievements facilitated by public health efforts such as sanitation and immunization, unparalleled medical advances and national investment in health care also have contributed to improvements in health outcomes. . . .

[Nonetheless] despite the nation's wealth, expenditures for health care and research, and scientific and technical accomplishments, the United States is not fully meeting its potential in the area of population health. For years, the life expectancies of both men and women in the United States have lagged behind those of their counterparts in most other industrialized nations. . . . In 1998, the United States also ranked 28th in infant mortality among 39 industrialized nations. In the area of chronic disease, reported incidence rates in 1990 for all cancers in males and females were highest in the United States among a group of 30 industrialized nations. Some birth defects that appear to have links to environmental factors are increasing. The prevalence of obesity and chronic diseases like diabetes are increasing, and infectious disease constitutes a growing concern because of newly recognized or newly imported agents like West Nile virus, the emergence of drug-resistant pathogens, and the all-too-real threat of bioterrorism.

. . . .

### ISSUES THAT MAY SHAPE THE NATION'S HEALTH

Because health is the result of many interacting factors, it stands in the balance between economic, political, and social priorities and is caught in the middle of necessary and important tensions between rights and responsibilities — individual freedoms and community or social needs, regulation, and free enterprise. These tensions pose complicated questions. How can the public's health be maintained in the face of infectious disease threats without compromising individual privacy and confidentiality? Or how can a vibrant, prosperous economy be supported without sacrificing health to pollutants or to occupational hazards? How can society balance the individual desire to pursue the pleasures of life (*e.g.*, food) with scientific evidence about health risk? Alternatively, how are increased employment, better housing, health benefits, and an improved standard of living in a community achievable in the absence of economic development? . . .

. . . [H]ealth is part individual good served by medicine and part public good secured by public health activities. Instead of complementary and collaborating systems, however, the two disciplines, their institutional cultures, their agencies and organizations, and the public's opinion of them have often been deeply divergent; and the individual focus of one and population focus of the other have become further reinforced and polarized. Often it has been harder to motivate and accomplish the long-term changes needed in the broad environments that influence health status because of the potential of immediate "silver bullet" solutions that can address poor personal health once it occurs. . . .

The personal health and health care agenda has dominated the nation's health concerns and policy for quite some time. In fact, the majority of funding in the health care delivery system is public, and there is a major public investment in biomedical research, yet the United States has failed to make the same level of commitment to population-based health promotion and disease prevention as it has to clinical care and research and biomedical technologies. . . . However, with the resurgence of infectious disease and the escalation of chronic diseases, as well as the new-found awareness of the multiple determinants of population health and the potential impact of macro-level and even global threats to health, the necessity of population-oriented approaches has become clearer. It has also been recognized that the infrastructure and capacity for such approaches must be permanent and sustained by resources equitably distributed between the governmental public health agencies in their partners and the biomedical and personal health care system.

. . . .

. . . [T]here are a number of systemic problems that may provide additional explanations for the shortcomings of America's health attainment. . . . [G]overnmental public health agencies, the backbone of any public health system, still suffer from grave under-funding, political neglect, and continued exclusion from the very forums in which their expertise and leadership are most needed to assure an effective public health system. The governmental public health infrastructure [also] is built on a legal foundation replete with obsolete and inconsistent laws and regulations, and a great deal of public health law is not coordinated among states and territories. . . . A similar fragmentation and lack of coordination is evident in the fact that responsibility for health issues is dispersed across several departments in the federal government and across federal, state and local governments. . . . Additionally, the public health workforce is inadequate in terms of preparation for practice, as well as number, partly because of local budgetary restrictions.

Governmental public health agencies are plagued by deficiencies in the very tools and resources that are essential to assuring population heath. . . . [M]any state public health laboratories are unable to keep pace with the needs for the monitoring and tracking of known infectious agents and become overwhelmed in the wake of new health threats such as the anthrax attacks and the appearance of the West Nile virus. . . . The resurgence of tuberculosis (TB) in the late 1980s offers a cautionary tale about what can happen when the public health infrastructure is not sustained. The success of TB prevention and treatment programs led to decreased funding and even dismantling of TB control as a routine public health activity. In the late 1980s, a resurgence of TB was beginning as a result of anti-microbe resistance, untreated immigrants, and the HIV/AIDS epidemic. The weakening of TB surveillance activities led to a massive spike in the prevalence of the disease and a renewed threat to the health of the public. [See discussion of the prevalence of TB in the United States in the Notes to Chapter Three, Section B[1].]

. . . .

For nations to improve the health of their populations, some have cogently argued, they need to move beyond clinical interventions with high-risk groups. [Medicine and health care have a limited role] that does little to prevent people from becoming sick in the first place, and [private medicine] typically has disregarded issues related to disparities in access to and quality of preventive and treatment services. Personal health care is only one, and perhaps the least powerful, of several types of determinants of health, among which are also included genetic, behavioral, social, and environmental factors. . . .

\* \* \*

UNDERSTANDING POPULATION HEALTH AND ITS DETERMINANTS

. . . .

Three realities are central to the development of effective population-based prevention strategies. First, disease risk is . . . a continuum rather than a dichotomy. There is no clear division between risk for disease and no risk for disease with regard to levels of blood pressure, cholesterol, alcohol consumption, tobacco consumption, physical activity, diet and weight, lead exposure, and other risk factors. . . . for many social and environmental conditions. . . . Any population model of prevention should be built on the recognition that there are degrees of risk rather than just two extremes of exposure (i.e., risk and no risk).

The second reality is that most often only a small percentage of any population is at the extremes of high or low risk. The majority of people are in the middle of the distribution of risk. [Yet an] exposure of a large number of people to a small risk can yield a more absolute number of cases of a condition than exposure of a small number of people to a high risk. This relationship argues for the development of strategies that focus on the modification of risk for the entire population rather than for specific high-risk individuals. [The resulting approach is often termed] the "prevention paradox" because it brings large benefits to the community but offers little to each participating individual. . . . [S]uch strategies would move the entire distribution of risk to lower levels to achieve maximal population gains [but are difficult to achieve based on appeals to individual self-interest.]

The third reality . . . is that an individual's risk of illness cannot be considered in isolation from the disease risk for the population to which he or she belongs. Thus, someone in the United States is more likely to die prematurely from a heart attack than someone living in Japan, because the population distribution of high cholesterol in the United States as a whole is higher than the distribution in Japan. Applying the population perspective to a health measure means asking why a population has the existing distribution of a particular risk, in addition to asking why a particular individual got sick. This is critical, because the greatest improvements in a population's health are likely to derive from interventions based on [answers to] the first question . . . American society experienced this approach to disease prevention and health promotion in the early 20th century, when measures were taken to promote sanitation and food and water safety, and in more recent policies on seat belt use, unleaded gasoline, vaccination, and water fluoridation. . . .

. . . .

Understanding and ultimately improving a population's health rests not only on understanding this population perspective, but also on understanding the ecology of health and the interconnectedness of the biological, behavioral, physical, and socio-environmental domains. . . . The last several decades of research have resulted in a deeper understanding, not only of the physical dimensions of the environment that are toxic, but also a broad range of related conditions in the social environment that are factors in creating poor health. . . .

. . . .

## THE PHYSICAL ENVIRONMENT AS A DETERMINANT OF HEALTH

. . . Improved water, food, and milk sanitation, reduced physical crowding, improved nutrition, and central heating with cleaner fuels were the developments most responsible for the great advances in public health achieved during the 20th Century. These advantages of a developed nation are taken for granted, but, in fact, could deteriorate without adequate support of the governmental public health infrastructure.

Environmental health problems, historically local in their effects and short in duration, have changed dramatically within the last 25 years. Today's problems are also persistent and global. Together, global warming, population growth, habitat destruction, loss of green space, and resource depletion have produced a widely acknowledged environmental crisis. These long-term environmental problems are not amenable to quick technical fixes, and their resolution will require community and societal engagement. . . .

The importance of "place" to health status became increasingly clear in the last decades of the 20th century. The places in which people work and live have an enormous impact on their health. The characteristics of place include the social and economic environments, as well as the natural environment (*e.g.*, air, water) and the built environment, which may include transportation, buildings, green spaces, roads, and other infrastructure. Environmental hazards in workplaces and communities may range from tobacco smoke to pesticides to toxic housing. Rural areas may present increased health risks from pesticides and other environmental exposures. . . .

. . . Although rural Americans experience certain health-related disadvantages . . . some of the health effects of the inner city (*i.e.*, decay and crime) are often dramatic and may be related to broader social issues. The "urban health penalty" — the "greater prevalence of a large number of health problems and risk factors in cities than in suburbs and rural areas" — has been frequently discussed and studied. A variety of political, socioeconomic, and environmental factors shape the health status of cities and their residents by influencing health behaviors such as exercise, diet, sexual behavior, alcohol and substance use. The negative environmental aspects of urban living — toxic buildings, proximity to industrial parks, and a lack of parks or green spaces, among others — likely affect those who are already at an economic and social disadvantage because of the concentration of such negative aspects in specific pockets of poverty and deprivation. Urban dwellers may experience higher levels of air pollution, which is associated with higher levels of cardiovascular and respiratory disease. People who live in aging buildings and in crowded and unsanitary conditions may also experience increased levels of lead in their blood, as well as asthma and allergies. . . .

. . . .

## THE SOCIAL DETERMINANTS OF HEALTH

. . . Among the greatest advances in understanding the factors that shape population health over the last two decades . . . has been the identification of social and behavioral conditions that influence morbidity, mortality, and functioning.

. . . .

A strong and consistent finding of epidemiological research is that there are health differences among socioeconomic groups. Lower mortality, morbidity, and disability rates among socio-economically advantaged people have been observed for hundreds of years; and in recent decades, these observations have been replicated using various indicators of socioeconomic status (SES) and multiple disease outcomes. . . . Furthermore, educational differentials in mortality have increased in the United States over the past three decades, leading to a growing inequality, even though mortality rates have dropped for all groups.

. . . .

A striking finding that emerges from analyses of occupation- and area-based income measures is the graded and continuous nature of the association between socioeconomic position and mortality, with differences persisting well into the middle socioeconomic ranges. . . .

Although many of the studies that focused on occupation-, education- or area-level SES showed a gradient that is virtually linear, studies that focus on income often show somewhat different results. For example, the association between (increasing) income and (decreasing) mortality is clearly curvilinear, with the decline in the mortality rate with increasing income greatest among those in groups earning less than $25,000 per year and with the decline with increasing income being much less among those earning between $25,000 and $60,000 per year. This curvilinear relationship suggests diminishing returns of income as one approaches the highest income categories, although some association may persist. This curvilinear association between income and health is what lays the framework for findings that more egalitarian societies (i.e., those with a less steep differential between the richest and the poorest) have better average health, because a dollar at the bottom "buys" more health than a dollar at the top. Whether SES has a linear or curvilinear relationship with health has enormous implications for understanding both the etiologic associations and the policy implications of this research. In either case, however, it is important to note that a "threshold" model focused exclusively on the very poorest segments and ignoring others near the bottom and the working poor will not address the relatively poor population health outcomes for the U.S. population as a whole. The major reason for this is because there are groups in the moderate risk categories of working poor and working class who contribute disproportionately large numbers to death rates and poor health outcomes.

. . . There is ample evidence that SES is strongly related to access to and the quality of preventive care, ambulatory care, and high-technology procedures; but health care appears to account for a small percentage of variation in health status among different SES groups. . . . [S]imilar gradients persist in countries with universal coverage, such as the United Kingdom.

Despite the past century's great advances in sanitation, which have contributed to the sharp increase in life expectancy observed among all socioeconomic groups, the socioeconomic gradient in health status persists. It has been proposed, and to some extent documented, that the gap in health status by SES may still be attributable to the effects of crowded and unsanitary housing, air and water pollution, environmental toxins, an inadequate food supply, poor working conditions, and other such deficits that have historically affected and that still disproportionately affect those in the lower socioeconomic strata. . . .

Considerable evidence links low SES to adverse psychosocial conditions. People in lower socioeconomic positions are not only more materially disadvantaged, but also have higher levels of job and financial insecurity; experience more unemployment, work injuries, lack of control, and other social and environmental stressors; report fewer social supports; and, more frequently, have a cynically hostile or fatalistic outlook.

There is more often, especially in the United States, a striking and consistent association between SES and risk-related health behaviors such as cigarette smoking, physical inactivity, a less nutritious diet, and heavy alcohol consumption. This patterned behavior response has led [some experts] to speak of situations that place people "at risk of risks." Understanding why "poor people behave poorly" requires recognition that specific behaviors formerly attributed exclusively to individual choice have been found to be influenced by the social context. . . . Both physical and social environments place constraints on individual choice. Over time, those with more economic and social resources have tended to adopt health-promoting behaviors and reduce risky behaviors at a faster rate than those with fewer economic resources.

Socioeconomic disparities in health in the United States are large, are persistent, and appear to be increasing over recent decades, despite the general improvements in many health outcomes. The most advantaged American men and women experience levels of longevity that are the highest in the world. However, less advantaged groups experience levels of health comparable to those of average men and women in developing nations of Africa and Asia or to Americans about half a century ago. Furthermore, these wide disparities coupled with the large numbers of people in these least-advantaged groups contribute to the low overall health ranking of the United States among developed, industrialized nations. A major opportunity for us to improve the health of the U.S. population rests on our capacity to either reduce the numbers of the most disadvantaged men, women, and children in the highest risk categories or to reduce their risks for poor health.

A substantial body of research documents the relationship between racial and ethnic disparities and differences in health status. Numerous studies have shown that minority populations may experience burdens of disease and health risk at disproportionate rates because of complex and poorly understood interactions among socioeconomic, psychosocial, behavioral, and health care-related factors. Although Americans in general experienced substantial improvements in life expectancy at all ages throughout the 20th century, substantial gaps in life expectancy, morbidity and functional status remain between white and minority populations. Life expectancy at birth for African Americans in 1990 was the same as that for whites in 1950. Even after controlling for income, African-American men and women have lower life expectancies than white men and women at every income level. When indicators of SES are considered, these differences, which are often substantial across a diversity of health outcomes, are commonly reduced but remain significant. . . . This phenomenon has led researchers to investigate the health effects of discrimination itself. . . . Additionally . . . there is significant health status differentiation or "hidden heterogeneity" within, for instance, Asian-American and Pacific Islander populations. . . .

. . . .

The association between social connectedness and health has received much attention in recent years. Concepts of social connectedness relate to social integration at the broadest level, social networks, social support, and loneliness. Social connectedness may be conceptualized as a social characteristic related to civic trust and social capital. . . .

. . . [P]eople who are isolated or disconnected from others are at increased risk of dying prematurely from various causes, including heart disease, cerebrovascular disease, cancer, and respiratory and gastrointestinal conditions. Studies of large cohorts of people enrolled in health maintenance organizations or occupational cohorts of people also report that social integration is critical to survival, although it may not be as critical an influence on the onset of disease.

Powerful epidemiological evidence supports the notion that social support, especially intimate ties and the emotional support provided by them, is associated with increased survival and a better prognosis among people with serious cardiovascular disease. The lack of social support, expressed in terms of conflict or loss of intimate ties, is also associated with health outcomes and risk factors such as neuroendocrine changes in women, high blood pressure, elevated plasma catecholamine concentrations, and autonomic activation. . . .

. . . .

Two decades of research show that the workplace not only generates adverse health effects due to economic circumstances such as downsizing and unemployment or to work conditions such as job demands, control, latitude, and threatened job loss, but also generates protective health effects such as social ties that may help counteract the physical and mental adverse effects of work stressors. . . .

. . .

Social characteristics of individuals are closely related to health. Among the most important findings to emerge from public health research over recent years is the extent to which characteristics of areas exert independent effects on health. This ecological approach has been rediscovered and is now embedded in a multilevel framework. The major idea is that characteristics of places — neighborhoods, schools, work sites, and even nations — carry with them health risks for the individuals who live in those environments. The health risk conferred by these places is above and beyond the risk that individuals carry with them. Thus, we might view characteristics of physical environments (*e.g.*, parks and buildings), as well as social environments (*e.g.*, levels of inequality and civic trust) as truly properties of places, not individuals. . . .

* * *

## Wendy K. Mariner, *Law and Public Health: Beyond Emergency Preparedness*
### 38 J. HEALTH L. 251–68 (2005)

* * *

Public health has been both broadly and narrowly defined, usually as a function of its political influence. Broad definitions offer a more accurate description, as in the classic definition by C.E.A. Winslow:

> Public Health is the science and art of preventing disease, prolonging life, and promoting physical health and efficiency through organized community effort for the sanitation of the environment, the control of communicable infections, the education of the individual in personal hygiene, the organization of medical and nursing services for the early diagnosis and preventive treatment of disease, and the development of the social machinery to insure everyone a standard of living

adequate for the maintenance of health, so organizing these benefits as to enable every citizen to realize his birthright of health and longevity.

This broad description still accurately depicts the wide range of activities of people who work in the field of public health. It is also consistent with the broad range of laws enacted in the name of public health. Given such a broad scope, public health might be equated with any public policy that serves in any way to prevent physical or mental harm or to maintain or improve health. This may pose some definitional problems for those seeking a unifying vision of public health. But, the fact that different groups working within public health define their own territory more narrowly should not deter lawyers from recognizing the broad scope of issues relevant to health.

Six trends in public health demonstrate how the field of public health is changing today, in some ways going back to its roots, in others expanding well beyond them.

## 1.   Social Determinants of Health

. . . The field of "social hygiene" began with the nineteenth century recognition that environmental hazards, as well as poor personal hygiene, could cause illness. Sanitary engineers, perhaps the first real public health workers, eliminated cholera and other water-borne diseases by creating systems for sewerage and purifying the water supply; other infectious diseases by regulating waste at animal slaughter houses and dockyards and pasteurizing milk; and dramatically reduced tuberculosis by cleaning up slum housing. Many public health pioneers were social reformers, who sought to reduce the hazardous living and working conditions in nineteenth century cities and factories. Their motives varied, from genuine concern for the disadvantaged, to the economic benefits of hiring healthier workers, to forestalling class rebellion by the poorer classes.

. . . Today, empirical research offers growing evidence that socioeconomic factors, such as the distribution of wealth and income, political inequality, education, employment, and housing, can affect health. Known as the "social determinants of health," these factors recall the concerns of early public health reformers and remind us that contagious disease is not the sole threat to health in the United States. Attention to the social determinants of health poses a challenge to defining public health as a unified or recognizable field. On one hand, scholars in public health have made significant contributions to research identifying social and environmental factors affecting the health of populations. As a practical matter, it may be difficult, if not impossible, to improve health significantly in the future without addressing the social factors. . . . On the other hand, including housing, employment, and political inequality may spread the health sphere so thin that it ceases to have any discernible limits. Some critics argue that research on wealth as it affects health is still too crude to produce useful information for making policy and there are dangers in medicalizing so many social issues. Nonetheless, it is increasingly difficult to avoid recognizing how broad social policies, such as those concerning drug abuse and homelessness, affect health. It should be possible to study and identify the effect of factors external to individuals without necessarily making it the responsibility of health professionals to devise or implement solutions. Only if such factors are investigated can their effects be accurately understood.

## 2. Medicine and Public Health

People in public health have traditionally distinguished their field from medicine by emphasizing that physicians treat individual patients while public health practitioners "treat" entire populations. This distinction, however, is rapidly blurring. It is true that the population-based approach had as much or more success than physicians did with their patients until shortly after World War II, when federal support for hospital construction and medical research fueled the development of modern medical science. The growth of medical technology, beginning with new vaccines and drugs, enabled physicians to save patients' lives, and medicine was rewarded with the mantle of scientific and political superiority.

Nonetheless, medicine and public health have often worked in synergistic ways, both to identify opportunities for research and to translate new technologies into practice. Discovery of bacteria and the germ theory by researchers gave public health its first scientific credibility, as laboratories began to identify specific causes of disease. Medical research also produced the vaccines that enabled public health immunization programs to eradicate or control many infectious diseases, and physicians and nurses, in private practice as well as public clinics, administered the vaccines. Public health research on the distribution of HIV infection in the early 1980s helped academic scientists target their research to identify the virus and also helped practicing physicians counsel their patients about how to prevent transmission of the infection. Public health screening programs, like those for cholesterol or diabetes, are intended to encourage people to get medical care to control their condition. These are only a few examples of essential and productive links between medicine and public health.

Artificial separation of public health and medicine may have more to do with economics and political influence than substance. Until very recently, physicians have been the dominant professionals in health policy, and medicine (and medical research) has received the vast majority of public and private funding. Physicians still play most primary leadership roles in public health. Public attention to public health has waxed and waned, usually rising in response to a crisis, such as, recently, the September 11 attacks, the anthrax letters, severe acute respiratory syndrome (SARS), the recall of Vioxx, and possible avian influenza. Historically, public health has received only a tiny fraction of national expenditures for health, and its share has not risen substantially even with additional post-September 11 funding. Public health tends to be defined by its general goal, improving health, not by the methods it employs, which are legion. Physicians also pursue health as a goal, but the medical profession is defined by a universal method of training for physicians. Similarly, the legal profession is defined by a universal method of training for lawyers. Professions typically are identified by a common (if complex) methodology and knowledge base. These skills can be used to achieve many different goals. In contrast, people who work in public health are trained in many different skills that use very different methodologies. They are united only by the goal they use their skills to achieve — health.

A related distinction between public health and medicine lies in the difference between defining health goals in terms of an entire population (whether defined by geography, sex, or race, for example) as opposed to an individual patient. Success in public health depends on improving the health of the entire population, which can only be measured in aggregate statistics, such as life expectancy and rates of mortality, disease, and disability. Physicians deal with one patient at a time and measure success patient by patient. Although physicians want to save lives and prevent or cure disease, they have an obligation to do what the individual believes to be in her own best interest. Thus, physicians are also successful when their patients succeed in making their own decisions. This kind of individual "success" does not necessarily count as success in public health terms. Patients who refuse life-saving therapy because they find it too burdensome may adversely affect population mortality rates. Public health programs that focus on aggregate outcomes for a population cannot account for individual values in the same manner as medicine.

Nevertheless, some occupational groups within medicine and public health have greater affinity with each other than with other specialists in their own field. For example, academic researchers have similar research methods and values, whether they conduct laboratory experiments with cells or epidemiological studies using large databases. They may have more in common with each other than with practitioners who provide clinical services to patients. Physicians who treat patients in private practice and public health workers who offer substance abuse treatment use similar methods to help individuals, just as physicians and public health workers who offer preventive services share similar methods and concerns. Indeed, a substantial proportion of public health expenditures are for individual healthcare services.

It is difficult to disentangle these professions from one another simply by looking at what people do. This suggests that, whether they acknowledge it or not, public health and medicine are already integrated to a remarkable degree, primarily by the methodology they use, and that it would be both disingenuous and counterproductive to insist on separation.

## 3.   Health Promotion: External and Internal Risks to Health

Public health successes in eradicating or controlling contagious diseases in the nineteenth and mid-twentieth centuries, coupled with research on the causes of disease may have combined to produce another trend — health promotion. In the past, public health programs were most successful at preventing or controlling infectious diseases. The goal was to protect the population from external sources of disease. Relatively straightforward measures, like purifying the water supply, creating sewage systems, monitoring the food supply, and encouraging immunization, dramatically reduced the threat of immediately life-threatening diseases. Ironically, perhaps, these important successes left public health programs with less to do and less public support and funding.

The top four leading causes of death today in the United States are heart disease, cancers, stroke, and chronic respiratory diseases, with accidental injuries in fifth place. Unlike infectious diseases, these problems lack a single viral or bacterial cause. Rather, they may result from multiple factors, including genetic predisposition, diet, personal behaviors, exposure to environmental or occupational hazards and dangerous products, as well as social, economic, and political factors. In addition, chronic diseases develop over a long period, often decades. There are few single interventions that completely prevent or cure a chronic disease comparable to those for an infectious disease. Prevention is multifaceted and success uncertain. The public is likely to think first of medicine, not public health, as the profession with the most expertise in chronic diseases and the most to offer, primarily in the form of curative medical therapies. At the same time, however, the many factors contributing to chronic disease, coupled with their increasing prevalence, may have encouraged the field of public health to characterize such diseases as public health problems.

As the types of diseases affecting Americans changed, the public health field shifted its attention to health promotion, encouraging public education about the causes of chronic diseases, as well as regulations that reduce environmental risks. Given the complex causes of many chronic diseases, one might expect public health programs to focus renewed attention on the full range of social determinants of health. There have been some attempts to educate the public about hazardous working conditions or housing. The mapping of the human genome increased awareness of genetic predispositions to certain diseases. So far, however, most public health campaigns, from education to advocacy for new laws, have focused on the risks to health that arise from personal behaviors, such as a high fat diet, lack of physical exercise, smoking cigarettes, and violence. This emphasis on personal risk behaviors lends support to those who wish to characterize the primary problems in public health as the personal responsibility of individuals themselves, rather than as problems that require societal solutions. Rather than making the world safer for people, it seeks to have people protect themselves from risks in the world as it exists.

The trend toward changing personal behavior coincides with renewed concern about the rising cost of healthcare and a political climate that emphasizes personal responsibility and discourages reliance on public benefit programs. If people change their behavior in ways that improve their health, they are less likely to need expensive medical care. Employers have adopted policies forbidding their employees from smoking or drinking at home as well as on the job. While such policies can be justified as encouraging healthy behavior, they are often initiated primarily to reduce health insurance costs.

Public awareness of how to improve one's health is usually a good thing. If health policy targets personal behavior to the exclusion of more influential causes of ill health, however, it may prove ineffective. Public education programs require a long-term commitment to public education. Moreover, programs that depend on individuals to change their behavior are typically less effective than programs that remove risks from the external environment.

Health promotion programs increasingly target conditions that, unlike contagious diseases, affect only the individual. Both diabetes and obesity have been declared "epidemics," giving a new meaning to the term. It also moves the field of public health farther from any concentration on preventing the spread of disease (from one place or person to another person), and places it squarely beside medicine in the effort to improve the health of an individual for his own sake.

## 4.   Federalization of Public Health

Public health practitioners often think of public health as primarily a local and state endeavor. The Institute of Medicine perpetuated this view in its influential 1988 report by defining public health activities as by and for the community and confining the community to the state, city, or town level, barely mentioning national or international activities. It is true that, when the country began, most governmental efforts to prevent disease were carried out by local officials, but the federal government was never entirely absent from the field. After all, it was the federal government that sent federal public health officials to try to control the spread of plague in San Francisco at the turn of the twentieth century. By the late twentieth century, the federal government had moved decisively into public health and medicine, with legislation such as Medicare and Medicaid, the Occupational Safety and Health Act of 1970, and the Clean Air and Clean Water Acts. Indeed, many of the most important public health achievements have come from federal legislation.

Today, countless public health programs are influenced, if not controlled, by a federal government agency. Despite recent Supreme Court decisions limiting the scope of congressional authority under the Commerce Clause, the federal government retains ample power. Even with block grants and decentralization, the federal government controls the shape and direction of many state and local public health programs through the power of its purse. Most states enacted laws requiring drivers to wear seatbelts when having those laws in place became a prerequisite for the state to receive certain federal highway funds. Similarly, most states enacted laws raising the minimum age for drinking alcoholic beverages to twenty-one years in order to qualify for federal highway funding. Title X funding for family planning programs is subject to specific requirements for how funds are spent. Many state disease-reporting systems might not exist without federal funding from the Centers for Disease Control and Prevention (CDC), and such funding is increasingly tied to legislative requirements. As states face declines in tax revenues and pressure for more services, they may have to rely on federal financial assistance to carry out many of their basic programs. Thus, today, it is often difficult to disentangle federal from state control over even, ostensibly, state public health programs.

After September 11, 2001, as part of the war on terror, the federal government has asserted even greater influence in matters that affect public health — as a matter of national security subject to federal jurisdiction. Even if the states remain primarily responsible for carrying out public health activities, they will often take their cue from Washington, DC.

## 5.   Globalization of Health

Increasing interdependence among global economies is pushing the public health field more firmly into the international sphere. As companies expand their operations around the world, they are beginning to recognize the need for consistent international standards in product safety, environmental controls, and occupational hazards. Sales of goods over the internet raise questions about which product safety standards and marketing rules should apply. Climate change and natural disasters require a coordinated global response from many countries. Disasters like the December 2004 Tsunami create financial and logistical challenges, from identifying the dead to housing and feeding the displaced, that no single country can meet alone. Even war is increasingly recognized as an international public health concern, which requires multinational efforts to provide for the health and safety of civilians, who are often targets of military or terrorist violence. Here, especially, the international human rights movement has brought attention to the positive relationship between human health and respect for human rights.

People in public health are rightly paying more attention to these global issues. Research itself is increasingly international, with scientists in different countries sharing insights and techniques to study everything from genetic diseases to management. As in the United States, affinities tend to follow the subject matter rather than the professional category.

Infectious diseases that cross national borders no longer exhaust the subject matter of global health concerns, but they remain firmly on the radar. Global travel and migration make it relatively easy for viruses and parasites to become world travelers, as SARS' leap from Hong Kong to Toronto demonstrated. Although SARS proved to be less hardy than feared, with most deaths in Canada occurring among people infected before the disease was recognized and most infections occurring in the hospital, a new virus might be more lethal, especially if the population has no natural immunity and no vaccine or treatment is available. For example, if the avian influenza virus (H5N1), which has ravaged poultry stocks in Southeast Asia and killed forty-six people, became efficiently transmissible to humans and from person to person, it might cause a global pandemic affecting millions.

Although no one knows whether such a viral shift will occur, it would be prudent to pursue not simply an early warning system, but public education about contact with animals, research on possible vaccines, and organizing services to care for people who become ill. Perhaps the most effective preventive measure would be to create new job opportunities that make it unnecessary for people to rely on raising chickens and ducks to survive.

## 6.   Bioterrorism

An image of the world as an incubator of dreadful diseases that can cause epidemics gained currency with the spread of HIV infection in the 1980s, reinforced by popular books like "The Hot Zone" and movies like "Outbreak." When letters containing (non-contagious) anthrax killed five people soon after September 11, 2001, federal officials warned that terrorists might bring smallpox into the country next. Concern for infectious diseases "imported" from abroad transmogrified from a manageable medical problem into a terrifying world-wide conspiracy against Americans. Not only might viruses and parasites accidentally board a ship or airplane and fall out in America, but a terrorist might deliberately attack the country with biological weapons.

The combination of terrorism and disease has simultaneously focused much needed attention on public health and perversely narrowed public appreciation of public health largely to bioterrorism. The most positive response has been new federal funding to shore up the perennially neglected "public health infrastructure," the collection of public and private programs that study, prevent, and treat health problems that affect communities large and small. Less positive has been the emphasis on emergency preparedness to the detriment — some would say exclusion — of the less glamorous, ordinary tasks of public health practitioners, which may offer better protection against illness and death.

The country already has some experience with what today would be called bioterrorists — from United States residents who used viruses or bacteria to frighten and make people sick. Only five deaths resulted, all from the anthrax letters mailed in 2001, while each year, influenza kills twenty to thirty thousand Americans. The federal government is spending millions of dollars to prepare for a terrorist attack using smallpox or other biological weapons, but still has not developed a plan to assure an adequate annual supply of influenza vaccine.

## B.  SUMMARY

These six trends suggest that, despite current public attention to bioterrorism, the field of public health is in fact wide-ranging and even expanding. It reaches around the world because both risks to health and ways to protect health are increasingly global, requiring more coordinated international attention. This global reach, coupled with concerns about bioterrorism and renewed constraints on state budgets, places the federal government in the forefront of public health today. A national view of public health may encourage recognition of its importance and the many social determinants of health. Indeed, as public health is increasingly tied to medicine, with internal specialties crossing professional boundaries and public health professionals increasingly seeking individual health promotion instead of removing external threats to populations, it may be time to change our terminology. Instead of medicine and public health, the world sees a field of Health, writ large, with shared components of research, prevention, treatment, and care throughout.

* * *

# NOTES AND QUESTIONS

**1.** As all of these materials demonstrate, the term "public health" has several different meanings and connotations.

As used in the IOM report, it appears that "public health" is virtually anything that has to do with the health status of the American public. In this regard, there is little real difference between the terms "health" and "public health," other than the underlying assumption, reverently adhered to by most people who identify themselves as public health professionals, that they view "public health" in terms of the whole population and not just on an individual-by-individual basis. Other "public health" authorities make similar claims, referring to their thinking as "population-" or "community-based."

Is there real meaning here? What does it really mean to view a health problem in community-based, population-based, or public health terms? What does it add — or subtract — from the analysis of any particular problem? Is it a skill or discipline? Or is it better described as a perspective or goal?

Some public health authorities have attempted to refine the definition of public health more specifically, albeit somewhat more pedantically. *See, e.g.,* Roger Detels & Lester Breslou, *Current Scope and Concerns in Public Health,* I Oxford Textbook of Public Health, 3–20 (R. Detels et al., eds., 4th ed. 2002). For one good effort to sort all this out in a critical manner, see Mark Rothstein, *Rethinking the Meaning of Public Health,* 30 J.L. Med. & Ethics 144 (2002) (finding three different variations in contemporary efforts to broadly define public health and rejecting them all in favor of a more narrow, legalistic definition).

**2.** With all due respect to these more sophisticated definitions of public health, the most literal definition of the term "public health" may be the most useful. That is, the term "public health" can be used simply as a reference to the broad range of activities, primarily governmental ("public"), that attempt to maintain and protect "health." In this functional and descriptive view, public health is what the local or county health department does; it is the various activities of the state's department of public health (which may be one part of a larger department of health or independent of other agencies that also conduct activities that can be regarded as public health); and, at the federal level, public health is what is done by a number of agencies, most prominently the CDC, the commonly-used acronym for the Centers for Disease Control and Prevention (*see* sidebar, *infra*) within the Department of Health and Human Services (DHHS). (To be comprehensive, at the federal level one should also include the federal Public Health Service within the DHHS, as well as a number of other federal agencies both within DHHS and in other federal departments that conduct research, fund programs, and carry out direct-service activities that can be described as public health). This is, of course, somewhat of an oversimplification. Public health programs are often carried out by non-governmental (usually non-profit) private organizations, either independently or with governmental funding. Examples include disaster relief, domestic or international disease control initiatives, substance abuse programs, and the like.

For a good, general discussion of what local, state, and federal public health agencies typically do and how they are organized, see Berhard J. Turnock,

PUBLIC HEALTH: WHAT IT IS AND HOW IT WORKS 121–167 (1997); for a good attempt to categorize various models for organizing state public health agencies, see LAWRENCE O. GOSTIN & JAMES G. HODGE, STATE PUBLIC HEALTH LAW ASSESSMENT REPORT 19–30 (Turning Point 2002). For one good example of how the authority for public health activities can be distributed among state and local agencies, see the description of public health powers in the State of Washington in Chapter Two, Section B[2], Note 6, *infra*.

**3.** Whether public health is defined in terms of everything that affects our health or more narrowly in terms of government agencies and their activities, any use of the term "public health" carries with it another meaning: Whether inspired by "community-" or "population-based thinking," by the principles of good science, or simply by common sense, public health activities are usually designed to influence a whole range of the social, environmental, and other factors outlined in the IOM report that have some causal role in health-related problems — as distinguished from individualized medical care which typically attempts to remedy the resulting impact of such factors on each individual affected. The distinction is not complete or even wholly accurate. In fact, government public health programs often provide individual medical care (*e.g.*, clinics in some local health departments, state and local public hospitals, or the Indian Health Service); conversely, individual physicians and other medical care practitioners often attempt to prevent health problems and promote health in their communities as well as in each patient. But make no mistake about it: Most people who use the term "public health" to describe health-related activities do so in part as a reminder of what their activities are generally not: "medicine."

Public health is also *public* health and generally not *private* medicine. That is to say, in part we refer to public health to emphasize the population-based thinking and preventive orientation that characterizes public health practice; but we also do so to draw attention to the public — meaning governmental — nature of the great bulk of public health activities. American practitioners of medical care have struggled hard to maintain their private and autonomous nature. And while that struggle has not been completely successful, when government crosses the line from what government can do in the health arena — what we call public health — and enters the area of individual medical practice, for example, when public health departments provide clinics for poor or uninsured people, it is always a controversial and politically volatile step.

**4.** The distinction between what is called public health and what is called private medicine is much more than a parsing of terms or even a reminder of an underlying political battle. It has important implications for public policy. As demonstrated in many different ways in each of the excerpts in this chapter, public health activities — mass immunizations, improved water supplies and sanitation, and so on — have been responsible for many important improvements in the nation's health. As the Rosenberg excerpts recount, Americans saw tremendous advances in health through the late 19th and early 20th century in the United States, measured even in the crudest of terms. The role of medicine in achieving these visible advances cannot be denied, but that role must be viewed in the context of the other social and economic improvements, and in light of various *public health* initiatives.

Sanitation, clean water, and decent housing saved more lives than the provision of individual medical care.

Others have argued that much the same could be said of the decades that followed. Americans in the 20th century witnessed wave after wave of biomedical advances, but the role of these advances in improving the health of Americans should not be exaggerated or overshadow that of other, *public health* measures, *e.g.*, health education and promotion programs, seat belts and other mandatory safety laws, and efforts to maintain water and air quality.

There was even an active school of criticism in the 1970s that argued that our focus on medicine and our tendency to overlook the role played by other influences was inhibiting advances in health and even harming us in some ways. *See* THOMAS MCKEOWN, THE ROLE OF MEDICINE: DREAM, MIRAGE, OR NEMESIS? (1976); IVAN ILLYCH, LIMITS TO MEDICINE (5th ed. 1976); RICK CARLSON, THE END OF MEDICINE (1975).

One author tried to describe this as the emergence of a "new public health":

. . . The origins of the "new" public health movement are generally located by commentators in the 1970s, a time when the writings of critics calling into question the efficacy and social cost of medicine were attracting attention and when other social movements championing improved living conditions and human rights were under way. Proponents of the "new" public health . . . were also influential in constructing a vision of the "cultural crisis of modern medicine." As a result, public health reformers began to argue that resources should be directed away from curative technologies to the prevention of illness and disease.

The "new" public health is typically represented as a reaction against both the individualistic and victim-blaming approach of health education and the curative model of biomedicine. It is heralded as a return to the concern with environmental factors that first generated the public health movement of the 19th century. Proponents of the "new" public health argue that during the early to mid-20th century the public health movement lost its direction in narrowing the focus on the individual, by championing preventive medicine rather than community health-oriented strategies to improve population health, and by being disease-focused rather than health-focused. They routinely refer to the time between the original public health movement of the mid- to late 19th century and the "renaissance" of public health in the 1970s, when therapeutic medical services took over and the emphasis on "holistic" and "preventive" health was lost. . . . Proponents often refer back to the original public health movement of the 19th century as an exemplar for remodeling the "new" public health, recalling its imputed interest in environmental and improved living standards, rather than the emphasis on the individual. . . .

DEBORAH LUPTON, THE IMPERATIVE OF HEALTH: PUBLIC HEALTH AND THE REGULATED BODY 49–50 (1995).

**5.** Whether the advocates of the "new" public health were accurate or merely provocative, they were only the most eloquent of many voices from within and without the public health professions that were increasingly frustrated in the last several decades of the 20th century by the lack of attention — and resources — directed towards public health activities. The 1988 IOM report, THE FUTURE OF THE PUBLIC'S HEALTH, attempted to document and publicize those frustrations. As discussed in the prologue to the IOM excerpt, *supra*, that report critiqued the existing public health infrastructure and the nation's preparation for contemporary public health problems and found both lacking. Despite the progress that could be traced to public health efforts, the 1988 IOM report argued, public health had captured neither the attention of the American public nor the support of its pocketbook. Most Americans looked to private medicine, not public health, for the solution to their health problems. "Public health is in disarray" became an oft-repeated quotation and the basis for a call to action.

What followed was a certain amount of political smoke but little direct political fire. The CDC, with the help of various state and local public health officials and several health-related professional organizations, attempted to organize political efforts at both the state and federal levels to improve the status of the nation's public health infrastructure. One such effort was the "Healthy People 2000 initiative," sponsored by the Public Health Service, which attempted to define workable goals for improving public health programs and enhancing the health status of Americans.

By the end of the decade, however, most of these goals had not been met. Those same sponsors published a series of documents updating that effort under the titles HEALTHY PEOPLE 2010: UNDERSTANDING AND IMPROVING HEALTH, HEALTHY PEOPLE 2010, and TRACKING HEALTHY PEOPLE 2010 — tacitly admitting that most of their projected goals had not been met. These documents, while excessive and excessively bureaucratic, nonetheless provide a detailed assessment of the health status of Americans, a specification of our unmet health needs, and techniques for measuring progress towards improvements. All those documents can be accessed at www.healthy people.gov/Document (last visited February 2005).

Ironically, the renewed attention and resources that public health would receive in the first decade of the 21st century had less to do with the efforts of the CDC or the IOM or anyone within the ranks of the public health professions, and more to do with the public's reaction to the events of September 11, 2001. For a description and discussion, see Chapter Eight, *infra*.

**6.** For a more general description of the health status of Americans, see DEPARTMENT OF HEALTH & HUMAN SERVICES, HEALTH UNITED STATES 2005 (the annual summary of trends in health and health care in the United States); for data on individual states, see www.cdc.gov/nchs/fastats (last visited January 2006). For comparable data concerning other countries, see www.who.int/en/ (last visited March 2005).

From the foregoing data, some reason that many health-related problems are more likely to be resolved by public health techniques than by medicine, and that we should transfer some of our public investment in medical care to a growing investment in public health. That has both a good side and a bad side. For example, such reasoning could be used to justify cutbacks in programs such as Medicaid and Medicare (at least if some of the resulting savings are used for other health-related programs or, if nothing more, that they are spared from budget cutbacks). For an attempt to illustrate this point, a further recounting of the data, and an analysis of the implications for health spending, see J. Michael McGinnis, Pamela Williams-Russo & James R. Knickman, *The Case for More Active Policy Attention to Health Promotion*, 21 HEALTH AFF. 78 (2003).

**7.** At a somewhat more mundane level, "public health" is also a term used to describe various professional activities. There are schools and professional organizations of public health, just as there are agencies and departments that in part define their mission by reference to public health. Again, none of these lines of distinction is completely discrete. Medical schools teach preventive medicine to some of their future physicians, mirroring what is being taught by their colleagues in the schools of public health. Medical and health service researchers often apply the same techniques as their public health counterparts — and study similar if not identical problems.

There also are discrete areas of expertise that are typically, although not exclusively, used by public health professionals, most prominently epidemiology. Epidemiology is generally described as the study of the distribution of diseases or other health problems in a population and the attempt to ascertain their causes. Sometimes the term refers to the investigative work that typically follows an outbreak of an unknown disease or the sudden onset of a particular health problem — again, in a population. For a good description of epidemiology, epidemiologists, and what makes them different from other health-related researchers, see Alan Peterson & Deborah Lupton, *Epidemiology: Governing By Numbers*, in THE NEW PUBLIC HEALTH (1996). For a classic (even if somewhat out-dated) illustration of what epidemiologists do in the field, see BERTON ROUECHE, ELEVEN BLUE MEN, AND OTHER NARRATIVES OF MEDICAL DETECTION (1953). For definitions of terms that are frequently used in the analysis and discussion of epidemiological research, see JOHN M. LAST, DICTIONARY OF EPIDEMIOLOGY (4th ed. 2001). *See also* KERR L. WHITE, HEALING THE SCHISM: EPIDEMIOLOGY, MEDICINE, AND THE PUBLIC'S HEALTH (1991) (a good history of the development of the distinctive approach of epidemiology in studying public health problems and how epidemiology and its practitioners were often ignored in American medical education). Accessible texts on epidemiology include KENNETH J. ROTHMAN, EPIDEMIOLOGY — AN INTRODUCTION (2002); ANN ASCHENGRAU & GEORGE R. SEAGE, III, ESSENTIALS OF EPIDEMIOLOGY IN PUBLIC HEALTH (2003); RAJ BHOPAL, CONCEPTS OF EPIDEMIOLOGY. AN INTEGRATED INTRODUCTION TO THE IDEAS, THEORIES, PRINCIPLES, AND METHODS OF EPIDEMIOLOGY (2002).

# ORGANIZATIONAL CHART OF THE DEPARTMENT OF HEALTH & HUMAN SERVICES AS OF MARCH 2005

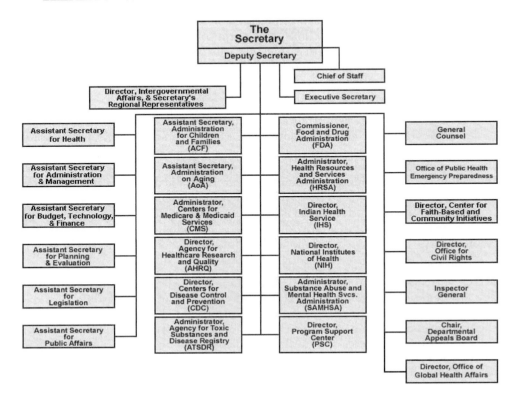

# SIDEBAR: THE HISTORY AND FUNCTIONS OF THE CDC

While there are numerous agencies within the federal government that carry on activities that could be legitimately called public health, the central institutional actor in the federal public health structure is the CDC, The Centers for Disease Control and Prevention.

The CDC is itself an agency within the Department of Health and Human Services that answers directly to the Secretary of the DHHS (and is no longer part of the separate Public Health Service).

First called the "Communicable Disease Center," then the "Center for Disease Control," then the "Centers for Disease Control," the CDC has morphed from a relatively obscure field surveillance agency to become the home of many of the research and data collection activities of the DHHS. The breadth of its mission is reflected in the names of some of its centers and sub-divisions within its organizational structure: National Center for Chronic Disease Prevention and Health (NCCDPHP), National Center for Environmental Health (NCEH), National Center for Health Statistics (NCHC), National Center for Infectious Diseases (NCID), National Institute for Occupational Safety and Health (NIOSH), and so on.

As of 2005, the CDC is an organization of over 5000 employees with facilities in a number of different cities and sharing offices with many state and local public health agencies. Its main facility in Atlanta houses nearly 2000 employees and is physically and organizationally attached to the campus of Emory University. In fact, CDC in Atlanta appears and functions much like a large university-based medical research center (except, of course, it has no students or patients).

The original Communicable Disease Center was organized in Atlanta, Georgia, on July 1, 1946 as a comparatively insignificant branch of the Public Health Service. Its predecessor had successfully kept the southeastern states free from malaria and typhus fever during World War II. CDC expanded its interests to include all communicable diseases and was designed to be the "servant" of the states, providing practical help whenever called. Distinguished scientists soon filled CDC's laboratories, and many states and foreign countries sent their public health staffs to Atlanta for training.

In 1949, CDC began the first-ever disease surveillance program, which confirmed that malaria, on which CDC spent the largest portion of its budget, had long since disappeared. Subsequently, disease surveillance became the cornerstone on which CDC's mission of service to the states was built and, in time, changed the practice of public health.

The outbreak of the Korean War in 1950 was the impetus for creating CDC's Epidemic Intelligence Service (EIS). The threat of biological warfare loomed, and the CDC leadership saw an opportunity to train epidemiologists who would guard against ordinary threats to public health while watching out for alien germs. The first class of EIS officers arrived in Atlanta for training in 1951 and pledged to go wherever they were called for the next 2 years. These "disease detectives" quickly gained fame for "shoe-leather epidemiology" through which they ferreted out the cause of disease outbreaks.

The survival of CDC as an institution was not at all certain in the 1950s. In 1947, Emory University gave land on Clifton Road for a headquarters, but construction did not begin for more than a decade. The PHS was so intent on research and the rapid growth of the National Institutes of Health that it showed little interest in what happened in Atlanta. Congress, despite the long delay in appropriating money for new buildings, was much more receptive than the PHS to CDC's pleas for support.

Two major health crises in the mid-1950s established CDC's credibility and ensured its survival. In 1955, when poliomyelitis appeared in children who had received the recently approved Salk vaccine, the national inoculation program was stopped (on CDC's recommendation). The cases were traced to contaminated vaccine from a laboratory in California; the problem was corrected, and the inoculation program was resumed. Two years later, surveillance was used again to trace the course of a massive influenza epidemic. From the data gathered in 1957 and subsequent years, the national guidelines for influenza vaccine were developed.

CDC grew by acquisition. The venereal disease program came to Atlanta in 1957 and with it the first Public Health Advisors, non-science college graduates destined to play an important role in making CDC's disease-control programs work. The tuberculosis program moved in 1960, followed by the immunization practices program and the MMWR (Morbidity and Mortality Weekly Report) in 1961. The Foreign Quarantine Service, one of the oldest and most prestigious units of PHS, came in 1967; many of its positions were soon switched to other uses as better ways of doing the work of quarantine, primarily through overseas surveillance, were developed. The long-established nutrition program also moved to CDC, as well as the National Institute for Occupational Safety and Health, and the work of already established units increased. Immunization tackled measles and rubella control; epidemiology added family planning and surveillance of chronic diseases. When CDC joined the international malaria-eradication program and accepted responsibility for protecting the earth from moon germs and vice versa, CDC's mission stretched overseas and into space.

CDC played a key role in one of the greatest triumphs of public health: the eradication of smallpox. In 1962 it established a smallpox surveillance unit, and a year later tested a newly developed jet gun and vaccine in the Pacific island nation of Tonga. After refining vaccination techniques in Brazil, CDC began work in Central and West Africa in 1966. When millions of people there had been vaccinated, CDC used surveillance to speed the work along. The World Health Organization used this "eradication escalation" technique elsewhere with such success that global eradication of smallpox was achieved by 1977. The United States spent only $32 million on the project, about the cost of keeping smallpox disease at bay for 2½ months.

CDC also achieved notable success at home tracking new and mysterious disease outbreaks. In the mid-1970s and early 1980s, it found the cause of Legionnaires disease and toxic-shock syndrome. A fatal disease, subsequently named acquired immunodeficiency syndrome (AIDS), was first mentioned in the June 5, 1981, issue of MMWR. Since then, MMWR has published numerous follow-up articles about AIDS, and one of the largest portions of CDC's budget and staff is assigned to address this disease.

Although CDC succeeded more often than it failed, it did not escape criticism. For example, television and press reports about the Tuskegee study on long-term effects of untreated syphilis in black men created a storm of protest in 1972. This study had been initiated by PHS and other organizations in 1932 and was transferred to CDC in 1957. Although the effectiveness of penicillin as a therapy for syphilis had been established during the late 1940s, participants in this study remained untreated until the study was brought to public attention. CDC also was criticized because of the 1976 effort to vaccinate the U.S. population against swine flu, the infamous killer of 1918-19. When some vaccinees developed Guillain-Barre syndrome, the campaign was stopped immediately; the epidemic never occurred.

    . . . .

The 1980s institutionalized what is considered to be a critically important scientific activity at CDC — the collaboration of laboratorians and epidemiologists. The decade began with the national epidemic of toxic-shock syndrome, documentation of the association with a particular brand of tampons, and the subsequent withdrawal of that brand from the market. CDC collaboration with the National Center for Health Statistics (NCHS) resulted in the removal of lead from gasoline, which in turn has markedly decreased this exposure in all segments of the population. The major public health event of the 1980s was the emergence of AIDS. CDC helped lead the response to this epidemic, including characterization of the syndrome and defining risk factors for disease.

CDC became involved in two very large epidemiologic studies during the 1980s. First, the Cancer and Steroid Hormone Study conducted in collaboration with the National Cancer Institute assessed the risks for breast, cervical, and ovarian cancers associated with both oral contraceptives and estrogen replacement therapy. Second, at the request of Congress, CDC undertook a series of studies of the health effects of service in Vietnam on veterans and their offspring, which led to a landmark contribution of the laboratory — the development of a serum test for dioxin able to measure the toxicant in parts per quadrillion. This decade also introduced scientifically based rapid assessment methods to disaster assistance and sentinel health event surveillance to occupational public health. Epi Info, a software system for the practice of applied epidemiology, was introduced and now has been translated into 12 languages for tens of thousands of users globally. Finally, during the 1980s, NCHS was moved to CDC, further enhancing CDC's information capabilities to meet national needs.

The 1990s . . . [were] characterized by continuing applications of CDC's classic field-oriented epidemiology, as well as by the development of new methodologies. For example, the disciplines of health economics and decision sciences were merged to create a new area of emphasis — prevention effectiveness — as an approach for making more rational choices for public health interventions. In 1993, the investigation of hantavirus pulmonary syndrome required a melding between field epidemiology and the need for sensitivity to and involvement of American Indians and their culture. Similarly, the response to global problems with Ebola virus and plague underscore[d] the importance of adapting these new methodologies. Other major CDC contributions to the world's health include[d] global polio eradication efforts and efforts to prevent neural tube defects. Finally, in October 1992, Congress changed CDC's official name to the Centers for Disease Control and Prevention, to recognize CDC's leadership role in prevention. . . . .

(adapted from CDC, *Historical Perspectives History of the CDC,* 45 MORBIDITY/MORTALITY WKLY REP. 526–530 (1996); *see also* ELIZABETH W. ETHERIDGE, SENTINEL FOR HEALTH: A HISTORY OF THE CDC (1992).)

# Chapter 2

# BASIC CONSTITUTIONAL PRINCIPLES APPLICABLE TO THE EXERCISE OF STATE AUTHORITY RELATING TO PUBLIC HEALTH

## A.  INTRODUCTION

This chapter is an introduction to the constitutional foundations of public health law. It reviews the basic constitutional principles describing the powers of the federal and, in particular, the state and local governments in matters concerning the public's health. In doing so, it also reviews principles concerning the distribution of power between the branches of government and among levels of government. Most fundamentally, this chapter outlines the basic issues that must be addressed in judicial, legislative, and administrative decision making that attempts to strike a balance between individual rights and the power of the government when it acts to protect the public's health.

Section B reviews a series of cases, both historical and contemporary, involving fairly traditional exercises of the states' police powers to protect the public's health and safety, ranging from mandatory vaccination to requirements for highway safety to prohibitions on the ownership or handling of potentially dangerous animals. In each case, the courts have to evaluate the importance of a perceived risk to public health against various claims of infringement on individual liberty, autonomy, or property interests. As illustrated by the "bookend" cases of *Jacobson* and *Lochner*, in most such cases, as typified by *Jacobson*, the courts defer to the judgment of local and state legislative bodies as to the proper balance between the public's and the individuals' interests. In a few cases, however, as demonstrated by *Lochner* and by some, though not all, more recent cases in which the individual's claim is based on religious beliefs, the courts more closely balance the competing concerns. As some of these cases also illustrate, the courts also have been somewhat reluctant to defer to legislative discretion where the government's claimed interest has more to do with protecting the individual from his/her own behavior, and less to do with protecting others (or somewhat more abstractly, the polity) from the individual's behavior.

Notwithstanding these exceptions, the state and federal courts have generally followed the lead of *Jacobson* in deferring to legislative discretion in virtually all matters where the state or federal law is directed towards eliminating a risk to a third party or to the public at large. Indeed, the principles of *Jacobson* have become the foundations of modern public health law.

Section C presents more contemporary public health cases that challenge state power to interfere with individual constitutional rights that did not exist at the time of *Jacobson*, including the right to privacy, and even with the practice of medicine in the context of the doctor-patient relationship. The state retains vast powers to protect individual health, but it reaches its limits when the state is attempting to force specific behaviors on individuals for the sake of their health. The state can, for example, require physicians to be licensed, but has much less authority to dictate actions physicians must, or must not, take with regard to their individual patients, and not just their pregnant patients.

The cases in Section D address questions that have presented more perplexing problems for modern courts. To what extent may government regulate the behavior of individuals where the underlying justification has less to do with some risk to public health or safety and is more clearly directed towards preventing conduct that is considered immoral or otherwise unacceptable? Here the distinction between risk to the individual and risk to the public at large is blurred, as the claimed justification for the government's regulation is that the individual's allegedly immoral behavior somehow harms the structure or climate of the community — in contrast to more tangible dimensions of its health.

## B. CONSTITUTIONAL PRINCIPLES: STATE REGULATION OF RISKS TO PUBLIC HEALTH AND SAFETY

### 1. Twentieth Century Foundations

### JACOBSON v. MASSACHUSETTS
197 U.S. 11 (1905)

\* \* \*

This case involves the validity, under the Constitution of the United States, of certain provisions in the statutes of Massachusetts relating to vaccination.

The Revised Laws of the Commonwealth, c. 75, § 137, provide that "the board of health of a city or town if, in its opinion, it is necessary for the public health or safety shall require and enforce the vaccination and revaccination of all the inhabitants thereof and shall provide them with the means of free vaccination. Whoever, being over twenty-one years of age and not under guardianship, refuses or neglects to comply with such requirement shall forfeit five dollars."

An exception is made in favor of "children who present a certificate, signed by a registered physician that they are unfit subjects for vaccination." § 139.

Proceeding under the above statutes, the Board of Health of the city of Cambridge, Massachusetts, on the twenty-seventh day of February, 1902, adopted the following regulation: "Whereas, smallpox has been prevalent to some extent in the city of Cambridge and still continues to increase; and whereas, it is necessary for the speedy extermination of the disease, that all persons not protected by vaccination should be vaccinated; and whereas, in the opinion of the board, the public health and safety require the vaccination or revaccination of all the inhabitants of Cambridge; be it ordered, that all the inhabitants of the city who have not been successfully vaccinated since March 1, 1897, be vaccinated or revaccinated."

Subsequently, the Board adopted an additional regulation empowering a named physician to enforce the vaccination of persons as directed by the Board at its special meeting of February 27.

The above regulations being in force, the plaintiff in error, Jacobson, was proceeded against by a criminal complaint in one of the inferior courts of Massachusetts. . . .

The defendant, having been arraigned, pleaded not guilty. The government put in evidence the above regulations adopted by the Board of Health and made proof tending to show that its chairman informed the defendant that by refusing to be vaccinated he would incur the penalty provided by the statute, and would be prosecuted therefor; that he offered to vaccinate the defendant without expense to him; and that the offer was declined and defendant refused to be vaccinated.

   . . . .

**Mr. Justice Harlan, after making the foregoing statement, delivered the opinion of the court.**

. . . [W]e assume for the purposes of the present inquiry that . . . [the statute's] provisions require, at least as a general rule, that adults not under guardianship and remaining within the limits of the city of Cambridge must submit to the regulation adopted by the Board of Health. Is the statute, so construed, therefore, inconsistent with the liberty which the Constitution of the United States secures to every person against deprivation by the State?

The authority of the State to enact this statute is to be referred to what is commonly called the police power — a power which the State did not surrender when becoming a member of the Union under the Constitution. Although this court has refrained from any attempt to define the limits of that power, yet it has distinctly recognized the authority of a State to enact quarantine laws and "health laws of every description;" indeed, all laws that relate to matters completely within its territory and which do not by their necessary operation affect the people of other States. According to settled principles the police power of a State must be held to embrace, at least, such reasonable regulations established directly by legislative enactment as will protect the public health and the public safety. It is equally true that the State may invest local bodies called into existence for purposes of local administration with authority in some appropriate way to safeguard the public health and the public safety. The mode or manner in which those results are to be accomplished is within the discretion of the State, subject, of course, so far as Federal power is concerned, only to the condition that no rule prescribed by a State, nor any regulation adopted by a local governmental agency acting under the sanction of state legislation, shall contravene the Constitution of the United States or infringe any right granted or secured by that instrument. . . .

We come, then, to inquire whether any right given, or secured by the Constitution, is invaded by the statute as interpreted by the state court. The defendant insists that his liberty is invaded when the State subjects him to fine or imprisonment for neglecting or refusing to submit to vaccination; that a compulsory vaccination law is unreasonable, arbitrary and oppressive, and, therefore, hostile to the inherent right of every freeman to care for his own body and health in such way as to him seems best; and that the execution of such a law against one who objects to vaccination, no matter for what reason, is nothing short of an assault upon his person. But the liberty secured by the Constitution of the United States to every person within its jurisdiction does not import an absolute right in each person to be, at all times and in all circumstances, wholly freed from restraint. There are manifold restraints to which every person is necessarily subject for the common good. On any other basis organized society could not exist with safety to its members. Society based on the rule that each one is a law unto himself would soon be confronted with disorder and anarchy. Real liberty for all could not exist under the operation of a principle which recognizes the right of each individual person to use his own, whether in respect of his person or his property, regardless of the injury that may be done to others. This court has more than once recognized it as a fundamental principle that "persons and property are subjected to all kinds of restraints and burdens, in order to secure the general comfort, health, and prosperity of the State. . . . In *Crowley v. Christensen,* 137 U.S. 86, 89, we said: "The possession and enjoyment of all rights are subject to such reasonable conditions as may be deemed by the governing authority of the country essential to the safety, health, peace, good order and morals of the community. Even liberty itself, the greatest of all rights, is not unrestricted license to act according to one's own will. It is only freedom from restraint under conditions essential to the equal enjoyment of the same right by others. It is then liberty regulated by law." . . . [A] fundamental principle of the social compact . . . [reflected in the Massachusetts Constitution of 1780 is that] the whole people covenants with each citizen, and each citizen with the whole people, that all shall be governed by certain laws for "the common good," and that government is instituted for "the common good, for the protection, safety, prosperity and happiness of the people, and not for the profit, honor or private interests of any one man. . . ."

Applying these principles to the present case, it is to be observed that the legislature of Massachusetts required the inhabitants of a city or town to be vaccinated only when, in the opinion of the Board of Health, that was necessary for the public health or the public safety. The authority to determine for all what ought to be done in such an emergency must have been lodged somewhere or in some body; and surely it was appropriate for the legislature to refer that question, in the first instance, to a Board of Health, composed of persons residing in the locality affected and appointed, presumably, because of their fitness to determine such questions. To invest such a body with authority over such matters was not an unusual nor an unreasonable or arbitrary requirement. Upon the principle of self-defense, of paramount necessity, a community has the right to protect itself against an epidemic of disease which threatens the safety of its members. It is to be observed that when the regulation in question was adopted, smallpox, according to the recitals in the regulation adopted by the Board of Health, was prevalent to some extent in the city of Cambridge and the disease was increasing. If such was the situation — and nothing is asserted or appears in the record to the contrary — if we are to attach any value whatever to the knowledge which, it is safe to affirm, is common to all civilized peoples touching smallpox and the methods most usually employed to eradicate that disease, it cannot be adjudged that the present regulation of the Board of Health was not necessary in order to protect the public health and secure the public safety. Smallpox being prevalent and increasing at Cambridge, the court would usurp the functions of another branch of government if it adjudged, as matter of law, that the mode adopted under the sanction of the State, to protect the people at large, was arbitrary and not justified by the necessities of the case. We say necessities of the case, because it might be that an acknowledged power of a local community to protect itself against an epidemic threatening the safety of all, might be exercised in particular circumstances and in reference to particular persons in such an arbitrary, unreasonable manner, or might go so far beyond what was reasonably required for the safety of the public, as to authorize or compel the courts to interfere for the protection of such persons. . . . There is, of course, a sphere within which the individual may assert the supremacy of his own will and rightfully dispute the authority of any human government, especially of any free government existing under a written constitution, to interfere with the exercise of that will. But it is equally true that in every well-ordered society charged with the duty of conserving the safety of its members the rights of the individual in respect of his liberty may at times, under the pressure of great dangers, be subjected to such restraint, to be enforced by reasonable regulations, as the safety of the general public may demand. . . .

[The Court here makes passing reference to "the liberty secured by the Fourteenth Amendment," in a discussion of the proper reach of liberty in a well-regulated society.]

Looking at the propositions embodied in the defendant's rejected offers of proof it is clear that they are more formidable by their number than by their inherent value. Those offers in the main seem to have had no purpose except to state the general theory of those of the medical profession who attach little or no value to vaccination as a means of preventing the spread of smallpox or who think that vaccination causes other diseases of the body. What everybody knows the court must know, and therefore the state court judicially knew, as this court knows, that an opposite theory accords with the common belief and is maintained by high medical authority. We must assume that when the statute in question was passed, the legislature of Massachusetts was not unaware of these opposing theories, and was compelled, of necessity, to choose between them. It was not compelled to commit a matter involving the public health and safety to the final decision of a court or jury. It is no part of the function of a court or a jury to determine which one of two modes was likely to be the most effective for the protection of the public against disease. That was for the legislative department to determine in the light of all the information it had or could obtain. It could not properly abdicate its function to guard the public health and safety. The state legislature proceeded upon the theory which recognized vaccination as at least an effective if not the best known way in which to meet and suppress the evils of a smallpox epidemic that imperiled an entire population. Upon what sound principles as to the relations existing between the different departments of government can the court review this action of the legislature? If there is any such power in the judiciary to review legislative action in respect of a matter affecting the general welfare, it can only be when that which the legislature has done comes within the rule that if a statute purporting to have been enacted to protect the public health, the public morals or the public safety, has no real or substantial relation to those objects, or is, beyond all question, a plain, palpable invasion of rights secured by the fundamental law, it is the duty of the courts to so adjudge, and thereby give effect to the Constitution.

Whatever may be thought of the expediency of this statute, it cannot be affirmed to be, beyond question, in palpable conflict with the Constitution. Nor, in view of the methods employed to stamp out the disease of smallpox, can anyone confidently assert that the means prescribed by the State to that end has no real or substantial relation to the protection of the public health and the public safety. . . .

[The Court here quotes from a recent New York State Court of Appeals opinion upholding the constitutionality of a law excluding all unvaccinated children from public schools.]

. . . It must be conceded that some laymen, both learned and unlearned, and some physicians of great skill and repute, do not believe that vaccination is a preventive of smallpox. The common belief, however, is that it has a decided tendency to prevent the spread of this fearful disease and to render it less dangerous to those who contract it. While not accepted by all, it is accepted by the mass of people, as well as by most members of the medical profession. It has been general in our State and in most civilized nations for generations. It is generally accepted in theory and generally applied in practice, both by the voluntary action of the people and in obedience to the command of law. Nearly every State of the Union has statutes to encourage, or directly or indirectly to require, vaccination, and this is true of most nations of Europe. . . . A common belief, like common knowledge, does not require evidence to establish its existence, but may be acted upon without proof by the legislature and the courts. . . . The fact that the belief is not universal is not controlling, for there is scarcely any belief that is accepted by everyone. The possibility that the belief may be wrong, and that science may yet show it to be wrong, is not conclusive; for the legislature has the right to pass laws which, according to the common belief of the people, are adapted to prevent the spread of contagious diseases. In a free country, where the government is by the people, through their chosen representatives, practical legislation admits of no other standard of action; for what the people believe is for the common welfare must be accepted as tending to promote the common welfare, whether it does in fact or not. Any other basis would conflict with the spirit of the Constitution, and would sanction measures opposed to a republican form of government. While we do not decide and cannot decide that vaccination is a preventive of smallpox, we take judicial notice of the fact that this is the common belief of the people of the State, and with this fact as a foundation we hold that the statute in question is a health law, enacted in a reasonable and proper exercise of the police power. . . .

   . . . .

The defendant offered to prove that vaccination "quite often" caused serious and permanent injury to the health of the person vaccinated; that the operation

"occasionally" resulted in death; that it was "impossible" to tell "in any particular case" what the results of vaccination would be or whether it would injure
the health or result in death; that "quite often" one's blood is in a certain condition of impurity when it is not prudent or safe to vaccinate him; that there
is no practical test by which to determine "with any degree of certainty"
whether one's blood is in such condition of impurity as to render vaccination
necessarily unsafe or dangerous; that vaccine matter is "quite often" impure
and dangerous to be used, but whether impure or not cannot be ascertained by
any known practical test; that the defendant refused to submit to vaccination
for the reason that he had, "when a child," been caused great and extreme suffering for a long period by a disease produced by vaccination; and that he had
witnessed a similar result of vaccination not only in the case of his son, but in
the cases of others.

These offers, in effect, invited the court and jury to go over the whole ground
gone over by the legislature when it enacted the statute in question. The legislature assumed that some children, by reason of their condition at the time,
might not be fit subjects of vaccination; and it is suggested — and we will not
say without reason — that such is the case with some adults. But the defendant did not offer to prove that, by reason of his then condition, he was in fact
not a fit subject of vaccination at the time he was informed of the requirement
of the regulation adopted by the Board of Health. It is entirely consistent with
his offer of proof that, after reaching full age, he had become, so far as medical skill could discover, and when informed of the regulation of the Board of
Health was, a fit subject of vaccination, and that the vaccine matter to be used
in his case was such as any medical practitioner of good standing would regard
as proper to be used. The matured opinions of medical men everywhere, and
the experience of mankind, as all must know, negative the suggestion that it
is not possible in any case to determine whether vaccination is safe. Was
defendant exempted from the operation of the statute simply because of his
dread of the same evil results experienced by him when a child and had
observed in the cases of his son and other children? Could he reasonably claim
such an exemption because "quite often" or "occasionally" injury had resulted
from vaccination, or because it was impossible, in the opinion of some, by any
practical test, to determine with absolute certainty whether a particular person could be safely vaccinated?

It seems to the court that an affirmative answer to these questions would
practically strip the legislative department of its function to care for the public health and the public safety when endangered by epidemics of disease.
Such an answer would mean that compulsory vaccination could not, in any
conceivable case, be legally enforced in a community, even at the command of
the legislature, however widespread the epidemic of smallpox, and however
deep and universal was the belief of the community and of its medical advis-
ers, that a system of general vaccination was vital to the safety of all.

We are not prepared to hold that a minority, residing or remaining in any
city or town where smallpox is prevalent, and enjoying the general protection
afforded by an organized local government, may thus defy the will of its constituted authorities, acting in good faith for all, under the legislative sanction
of the state. If such be the privilege of a minority then a like privilege would

belong to each individual of the community, and the spectacle would be presented of the welfare and safety of an entire population being subordinated to the notions of a single individual who chooses to remain a part of that population. We are unwilling to hold . . . [this] to be an element in the liberty secured by the Constitution of the United States. . . . The safety and health of the people of Massachusetts are, in the first instance, for the Commonwealth to guard and protect. They are matters that do not ordinarily concern the National Government. . . . [W]e do not perceive that this legislation has invaded any right secured by the Federal Constitution.

Before closing this opinion we deem it appropriate, in order to prevent misapprehension as to our views, to observe — perhaps to repeat a thought already sufficiently expressed — that the police power of a State, whether exercised by the legislature, or by a local body acting under its authority, may be exerted in such circumstances or by regulations so arbitrary and oppressive in particular cases as to justify the interference of the courts to prevent wrong and oppression. Extreme cases can be readily suggested. Ordinarily such cases are not safe guides in the administration of the law. It is easy, for instance, to suppose the case of an adult who is embraced by the mere words of the act, but yet to subject whom to vaccination in a particular condition of his health or body, would be cruel and inhuman in the last degree. We are not to be understood as holding that the statute was intended to be applied to such a case, or, if it was so intended, that the judiciary would not be competent to interfere and protect the health and life of the individual concerned. "All laws" this court has said, "should receive a sensible construction. General terms should be so limited in their application as not to lead to injustice, oppression or absurd consequence. It will always, therefore, be presumed that the legislature intended exceptions to its language which would avoid results of that character. The reason of the law in such cases should prevail over its letter." Until otherwise informed by the highest court of Massachusetts we are not inclined to hold that the statute establishes the absolute rule that an adult must be vaccinated if it be apparent or can be shown with reasonable certainty that he is not at the time a fit subject of vaccination or that vaccination, by reason of his then condition, would seriously impair his health or probably cause his death. No such case is here presented. It is the case of an adult who, for aught that appears, was himself in perfect health and a fit subject of vaccination, and yet, while remaining in the community, refused to obey the statute and the regulation adopted in execution of its provisions for the protection of the public health and the public safety, confessedly endangered by the presence of a dangerous disease.

. . . .

The judgment of the court below must be affirmed. . . .

[Justice Brewer and Justice Peckham dissented.]

———————

# NOTES AND QUESTIONS

*Jacobson* is widely regarded as the seminal decision in American public health law, largely because it upholds the constitutional validity of the state's curtailment of individual liberty in the interests of public health. Yet it is a rich case not only for its primary holding, but also because it illuminates many other characteristic features of public health law. The following notes explore some of these matters.

**1.** The court's opinion makes plain that the authority of a state to enact and enforce "health laws of every description" rests firmly within the "police power" that is an inherent artifact of the political sovereignty of each state, undiminished in this regard by its entry into the Union. These were non-controversial matters by 1905. *See generally* ERNST FREUND, THE POLICE POWER: PUBLIC POWER AND CONSTITUTIONAL RIGHTS (1904) (police power is "the power of promoting the public welfare by restraining and regulating the use of liberty and property . . .", *id.* at iii, 3; the "public welfare" referred to in the definition embraces "the primary social interests of safety [which includes health], order, and morals," which the Supreme Court "concedes on principle to the states. . . .", *id.* at 7). Professor Freund's lengthy 1904 treatise catalogs state exercises of the police power. The term has the same broad scope today, but in the intervening century legislatures have applied it even more widely.

**2.** Note the law's mechanism for triggering governmental action. The Massachusetts legislature did not directly require (though it surely could have) that persons in the state be vaccinated. Rather, the legislature empowered municipal boards of health to make that decision, if "in [the board's] . . . opinion" this was "necessary for the public health and safety. . . ." It was not until the Cambridge Board of Health adopted, and the authorities then attempted to enforce, the regulation calling for vaccination of Cambridge residents, that the coercive impact of law came into play.

This kind of delegation of formal legal power and discretion — common by the time *Jacobson* was decided and noted with approval by the Court — remains a key feature of public health law. Instead of making specific decisions about precisely what to do and when, legislatures at all levels often enact rather general laws that initiate a policymaking process, delegating to an administrative arm of government important policy choices, standard-setting authority, and other powers. These are sometimes the more difficult (one is tempted to say the "real") decisions that must be made in order to implement an effective law. Massachusetts' delegation from the state to city boards of health to decide whether and when to impose vaccination was "vertical." With at least equal frequency, legislative bodies delegate power and discretion "horizontally" to an executive-branch agency at the same level of government, to flesh out, implement, and enforce the law. For example, 100 years later, contemporary immunization statutes in many states broadly establish immunization as a condition of school attendance, but delegate to state health departments (sometimes in conjunction with state education agencies) the authority to determine and, over time, modify the specifics: which vaccines are required for school attendance, administration dosages and schedules, implementation of statutory exemptions, and other programmatic matters. The agencies thus "complete" and apply the law, through administrative rule-making or other mechanisms.

Imagine yourself a Massachusetts legislator in the early 1900s. Based on what you know from the case, why might the approach actually taken — conferring broad discretion about vaccinating citizens in municipal boards of health — appeal to you? What considerations, more generally, support legislative delegations of authority to administrative bodies for legal and programmatic implementation in complex regulatory matters? What are some of the drawbacks of this approach?

**3.** Observe the opinion's strong emphasis on the primacy of legislatures, and the limited role of courts, in establishing public health policy: the "legislature (not the court) is primarily the judge" of the "good and welfare of the commonwealth"; "the court would usurp" the legislative function if it ruled that vaccination was impermissible, since the legislature had already decided that it was proper. In short, it is for the democratic, elected branches, who are accountable to the people, to make the fundamental decisions about the community's welfare and values. Advocates of all viewpoints on pending legislation have the formal opportunity to make themselves heard, and (as the *Jacobson* Court observed) the pro- and anti-vaccine advocates were apparently heard here. It is not for a court to sit in judgment on the "expediency" of the resulting policy choice.

Finally, linking back to the discussion of the police power in note 1, *Jacobson* reflects a reality of the federalist structure of the American union: "The safety and the health of the people of . . . [a state] are, in the first instance, for that . . . [state] to guard and protect. They are matters that do not ordinarily concern the National Government . . ." (opinion, *supra*). Of course, as a practical matter, the continued expansion of federal involvement in the country's health under generous application of the enumerated federal constitutional powers has undermined this observation considerably in the past century, as was discussed in Chapter One. Nonetheless it remains true as a matter of formal constitutional doctrine.

**4.** By contemporary judicial standards, the precise constitutional framework under which the Court analyzed Jacobson's claim is a bit shadowy. Jacobson pressed two vague constitutional theories which the Court rejected out of hand: that the Massachusetts statute violated the Constitution's "Preamble," tending to defeat its "purposes"; and that it violated the "spirit" of the Constitution. A third theory was that the law "was in derogation of . . . the clauses [of the Fourteenth Amendment] . . . providing that no State shall make or enforce any law abridging the privileges or immunities of citizens of the United States, nor deprive any person of life, *liberty* or property *without due process of law. . . .*" [emphasis added].

Were you able to discern that the Court's analysis, in fact, focuses on part of this third theory — the proper reach of "liberty" in the 14th Amendment? In substance, the Court took seriously Jacobson's claim that this provision extended to freedom from compelled vaccination — even though, of course, no reference whatsoever can be found in the Constitution to medical dimensions of "liberty" (much less to "bodily integrity" or "vaccination"). It proceeded to balance that liberty against the counterweight of the state's interest in protecting public health and, further, to assess the "fit" between the state's interest and the chosen means of its expression. These are the hallmarks of what is now called "substantive due process" analysis under the 14th Amendment. Indeed, in a modern case, Chief Justice Rehnquist — not an advocate of a broad judicial interpretation of "liberty" — recognized (somewhat begrudgingly) that it "may be inferred" that the *Jacobson* Court viewed freedom from state-imposed medical treatment as a constitutionally-protected dimension of "liberty." *Cruzan v. Director, Missouri Department of Health*, 497 U.S. 261, 278 (1990) (also discussing more recent cases that have explicitly embraced 14th Amendment "liberty" — protection for refusing unwanted medical care. *Cruzan* is explored in Chapter Three, Section B[2], *infra*). In fact, it is difficult to read *Jacobson* as *not* recognizing the constitutional basis of such a claim — even though it was trumped, under the circumstances, by the state's overriding interest in public health.

As the Court recognized, legislatures routinely impose manifold intrusions upon individuals' liberty. You can readily identify dozens of examples that you encounter in your daily life. What is it about coerced medical treatment that arguably distinguishes it from many other such intrusions, and arguably lends special, even if here-unavailing, credence to a claim of constitutional protection?

**5.** The outcome of the case tells us that the Court found the polity's interest in having Jacobson vaccinated, against his preferences, was sufficiently great to outweigh his constitutionally-protected liberty interest. Can you determine, with confidence, the precise nature and content of the state's interest(s) on which the Court relied?

There are at least three possible interests a state might assert in having citizens vaccinated. (This note presents these interests in the specific context of vaccination, but they are of near-universal applicability in explorations of state "interests in public health" more generally.) One is protecting people against the consequences of their own failure to be vaccinated — whether based on ignorance, misunderstanding, poverty, recalcitrance, or *bona fide* intellectual opposition. This is what might be thought of as the most "paternalistic" of state interests. (If you prefer a softer word, try "beneficence.") Another is protecting others: the more people in a group who enjoy immunity from a contagious disease, the less chance an epidemic will develop and spread to any who are susceptible. In this view, restraining an individual's liberty by vaccinating him may be justified primarily on the basis of protecting others from harm — the classic rationale advanced by John Stuart Mill in his book *On Liberty*. A third is protecting or advancing the interests of the polity itself — "the state," or the collective, as an organized entity, as distinguished from the interests and preferences of individual members.

Consider the Court's opinion in light of each of these interests (or any others you might be able to think of). Which one(s) are visible in the opinion? Is the Court's presentation of them persuasive? What is your own view of the strength of these interests? Do you subscribe to the result in *Jacobson*, either for the reasons given by the Court (as you understand them), or for your own reasons? As you will see in progressing through these materials, courts frequently assert the state's "interest in public health" without actually exploring or explaining, with any great clarity, the underlying content of that interest in the particularized context of the case. Sometimes the nature and legitimacy of the state interest may appear self-evident to you. On the other hand, sometimes it may not seem so clear, or may not appear to withstand careful consideration. It is worth maintaining your critical judgment about such matters.

**6.** The case recognizes that there are constitutional limitations on state legislative power, even though finding none applicable here. (Consider *Lochner*, *infra*, in connection with these limits). First, the law cannot be "irrational," in the sense that no rational person could believe it capable of achieving its intended aim — here, preventing smallpox. For the Court, the existence of the medical debate over efficacy, taken up and reflected in the legislative deliberations, defeats any claim that the law is "irrational." The Court here is suggesting that the fact that a contested policy enjoys support among reasonable persons, acting reasonably, comes close to establishing *ipso facto* its "rationality." Second, the law cannot impose what is "beyond all question, a plain, palpable invasion of a Constitutional right," a formulation that imposes a high burden of proof and clarity on the party seeking to establish a law's constitutional flaw, a burden that was unmet by Jacobson here. Third, the Court suggests that any law that failed to accommodate persons for whom vaccination would create a grave health risk would be constitutionally infirm, and courts would stay its application to such persons, even absent an express textual exemption. (If the Court, and the Massachusetts high court, seem to have been a little quick to dismiss Jacobson's claim of potential medical unfitness, this may be because the claim was not really in issue: the Massachusetts court had ruled that forced immunization was not permissible under the law, and that the only sanction for noncompliance allowable was the statutory fine. *Commonwealth v. Pear*, 183 Mass. 242, 248, 66 N.E. 719, 722 (1903)). Fourth, the Court suggests the importance to its holding of the actual existence of the danger protected against — a threatened epidemic — which was both a condition the statute imposed on cities' exercise of the delegated power, and a duly-made finding by the Cambridge Board of Health. Absent the finding of such "necessity," there is reason to think that, at the time, mandatory vaccination might not have passed constitutional muster:

> Only the emergency of present danger can justify quarantine, isolation or removal to hospital and compulsory treatment, and it is at least doubtful whether vaccination can be made compulsory apart from such necessity, certainly not under a mere general delegation of authority to administrative bodies; but such general delegation is sufficient to cover the most ample powers in case of an emergency. . . .

FREUND, *supra*, Note 1, at 116. According to one account, the actual threat of an epidemic — the "necessity" — may not have been as great as the opinion implies. *See* Michael R. Albert, Kristen G. Ostheimer & Joel G. Breman, *The Last Small Epidemic in Boston and the Vaccination Controversy, 1901–1903*, 344 NEW ENG. J. MED. 375–79 (2001). It should not surprise us that the Court took Cambridge's finding at face value. Is it wise for courts to do so?

Today, we do not demand the threat of a pending epidemic to require child-hood immunizations for school, suggesting perhaps that the standard for "necessity" has relaxed considerably as the benefits and general safety of immunizations have become better-established.

Finally, of course, under the supremacy clause, a state law must fall where in conflict with a federal law enacted under Congress' enumerated constitutional powers.

**7.** The sanction authorized by the state statute for noncompliance with a Board of Health's vaccination order was a $5.00 forfeiture; the Massachusetts Supreme Judicial Court further "ordered that . . . Jacobson stand committed [jailed] until the fine was paid." 197 U.S. at 14. (Apparently Jacobson had not yet done so.) Thus, neither the formal provisions of law nor, so far as we can determine, government officials, permitted physically seizing Jacobson, restraining him by force, and vaccinating him against his will (although, according to one account, this is precisely what *did* happen, with the assistance of the police, to some homeless persons in Boston who objected to being vaccinated; Albert et al., *supra,* Note 6, at 376. Boston's small-pox ordinance forbade such conduct. *Id.* at 375. If true, this suggests something about the relevance of socioeconomic status to equal legal treatment). Do the sanctions imposed on Jacobson for noncompliance seem more, or less, draconian than vaccination itself would be?

The means of enforcing modern immunization law are analogous: In most states, immunizations are required for school attendance, but are not physically imposed upon the children of unwilling parents. Yet since school non-attendance is educationally and socially disadvantageous to children, may be stigmatizing and, more concretely, can be punished as truancy (unless a family opts for "home schooling"), there is surely coercion at play here. Do such indirect sanctions suggest a general societal unease with truly mandatory medical treatment, and a preference for coercion over frank physical force? Are you more or less comfortable with one approach than with the other? Why?

## LOCHNER v. NEW YORK
### 198 U.S. 45 (1905)

Peckham, Justice.

* * *

The indictment, it will be seen, charges that the plaintiff in error violated the one hundred and tenth section of article 8, chapter 415, of the Laws of 1897, known as the labor law of the State of New York, in that he wrongfully and unlawfully required and permitted an employee working for him to work more than sixty hours in one week. There is nothing in any of the opinions delivered in this case, either in the Supreme Court or the Court of Appeals of the State, which construes the section, in using the word "required," as referring to any physical force being used to obtain the labor of an employee. It is assumed that the word means nothing more than the requirement arising from voluntary contract for such labor in excess of the number of hours specified in the statute. . . . All the opinions assume that there is no real distinction, so far as this question is concerned, between the words "required" and "permitted." The mandate of the statute that "no employee shall be required or permitted to work," is the substantial equivalent of an enactment that "no employee shall contract or agree to work," more than ten hours per day, and as there is no provision for special emergencies the statute is mandatory in all cases. It is not an act merely fixing the number of hours which shall constitute a legal day's work, but an absolute prohibition upon the employer, permitting, under any circumstances, more than ten hours work to be done in his establishment. . . .

The statute necessarily interferes with the right of contract between the employer and employees, concerning the number of hours in which the latter may labor in the bakery of the employer. The general right to make a contract in relation to his business is part of the liberty of the individual protected by the Fourteenth Amendment of the Federal Constitution. Under that provision no State can deprive any person of life, liberty or property without due process of law. The right to purchase or to sell labor is part of the liberty protected by this amendment, unless there are circumstances which exclude the right. There are, however, certain powers, existing in the sovereignty of each State in the Union, somewhat vaguely termed police powers, the exact description and limitation of which have not been attempted by the courts. Those powers, broadly stated and without, at present, any attempt at a more specific limitation, relate to the safety, health, morals and general welfare of the public. Both property and liberty are held on such reasonable conditions as may be imposed by the governing power of the State in the exercise of those powers, and with such conditions the Fourteenth Amendment was not designed to interfere.

The State, therefore, has power to prevent the individual from making certain kinds of contracts, and in regard to them the Federal Constitution offers no protection. If the contract be one which the State, in the legitimate exercise of its police power, has the right to prohibit, it is not prevented from prohibiting it by the Fourteenth Amendment. Contracts in violation of a statute, either of the Federal or State government, or a contract to let one's property for immoral purposes, or to do any other unlawful act, could obtain no protection from the Federal Constitution, as coming under the liberty of person or free contract. Therefore, when the State, by its legislature, in the assumed exercise of its police powers, has passed an act which seriously limits the right to labor or the right of contract in regard to their means of livelihood between persons who are *sui juris* (both employer and employee), it becomes of great importance to determine which shall prevail — the right of the individual to labor for such time as he may choose, or the right of the State to prevent the individual from laboring or from entering into any contract to labor, beyond a certain time prescribed by the State.

. . . Among the later cases where the state law has been upheld by this court is that of *Holden v. Hardy,* 169 U.S. 366. A provision in the act of the legislature of Utah was there under consideration, the act limiting the employment of workmen in all underground mines or workings, to eight hours per day, "except in cases of emergency, where life or property is in imminent danger." It also limited the hours of labor in smelting and other institutions for the reduction or refining of ores or metals to eight hours per day, except in like cases of emergency. The act was held to be a valid exercise of the police powers of the State. A review of many of the cases on the subject, decided by this and other courts, is given in the opinion. It was held that the kind of employment, mining, smelting, etc., and the character of the employees in such kinds of labor, were such as to make it reasonable and proper for the State to interfere to prevent the employees from being constrained by the rules laid down by the proprietors in regard to labor. The following citation from the observations of the Supreme Court of Utah in that case was made by the judge writing the opinion of this court, and approved: "The law in question is confined to the protection of that class of people engaged in labor in underground mines, and in smelters and other works wherein ores are reduced and refined. This law applies only to the classes subjected by their employment to the peculiar conditions and effects attending underground mining and work in smelters, and other works for the reduction and refining of ores. Therefore it is not necessary to discuss or decide whether the legislature can fix the hours of labor in other employments."

It will be observed that, even with regard to that class of labor, the Utah statute provided for cases of emergency wherein the provision of the statute would not apply. The statute now before this court has no emergency clause in it; and, if the statute is valid, there are no circumstances and no emergencies under which the slightest violation of the provisions of the act would be innocent. . . .

The latest case decided by this court, involving the police power, is that of *Jacobson v. Massachusetts,* decided at this term. . . . It related to compulsory vaccination, and the law was held valid as a proper exercise of the police powers with reference to the public health. It was stated in the opinion that it was a case "of an adult who, for aught that appears, was himself in perfect health and a fit subject for vaccination, and yet, while remaining in the community, refused to obey the statute and the regulation adopted in execution of its provisions for the protection of the public health and the public safety, confessedly endangered by the presence of a dangerous disease." That case is also far from covering the one now before this court.

. . . .

It must, of course, be conceded that there is a limit to the valid exercise of the police power by the State. There is no dispute concerning this general proposition. Otherwise the Fourteenth Amendment would have no efficacy and the legislatures of the States would have unbounded power, and it would be enough to say that any piece of legislation was enacted to conserve the morals, the health or the safety of the people; such legislation would be valid, no matter how absolutely without foundation the claim might be. . . . In every case that comes before this court, therefore, where legislation of this character is concerned and where the protection of the Federal Constitution is sought, the question necessarily arises: Is this a fair, reasonable and appropriate exercise of the police power of the State, or is it an unreasonable, unnecessary and arbitrary interference with the right of the individual to his personal liberty or to enter into those contracts in relation to labor which may seem to him appropriate or necessary for the support of himself and his family? Of course the liberty of contract relating to labor includes both parties to it. The one has as much right to purchase as the other to sell labor.

This is not a question of substituting the judgment of the court for that of the legislature. If the act be within the power of the State it is valid, although the judgment of the court might be totally opposed to the enactment of such a law. But the question would still remain: Is it within the police power of the State? And that question must be answered by the court.

The question whether this act is valid as a labor law, pure and simple, may be dismissed in a few words. There is no reasonable ground for interfering with the liberty of person or the right of free contract, by determining the hours of labor, in the occupation of a baker. There is no contention that bakers as a class are not equal in intelligence and capacity to men in other trades or manual occupations, or that they are not able to assert their rights and care for themselves without the protecting arm of the State, interfering with their independence of judgment and of action. They are in no sense wards of the State. Viewed in the light of a purely labor law, with no reference whatever to the question of health, we think that a law like the one before us involves neither the safety, the morals nor the welfare of the public, and that the interest of the public is not in the slightest degree affected by such an act. The law must be upheld, if at all, as a law pertaining to the health of the individual engaged in the occupation of a baker. It does not affect any other portion of the public than those who are engaged in that occupation. Clean and wholesome bread does not depend upon whether the baker works but ten hours per day or only sixty hours a week. The limitation of the hours of labor does not come within the police power on that ground.

. . . .

This case has caused much diversity of opinion in the state courts. In the Supreme Court two of the five judges composing the Appellate Division dissented from the judgment upholding the statute. Although found in what is called a labor law of the State, the Court of Appeals has upheld the act as one relating to the public health — in other words, as a health law. One of the judges of the Court of Appeals, in upholding the law, stated that, in his opinion, the regulation in question could not be sustained unless they were able to say, from common knowledge, that working in a bakery and candy factory was an unhealthy employment. The judge held that, while the evidence was not uniform, it still led him to the conclusion that the occupation of a baker or confectioner was unhealthy and tended to result in diseases of the respiratory organs. Three of the judges dissented from that view, and they thought the occupation of a baker was not to such an extent unhealthy as to warrant the interference of the legislature with the liberty of the individual.

We think the limit of the police power has been reached and passed in this case. There is, in our judgment, no reasonable foundation for holding this to be necessary or appropriate as a health law to safeguard the public health or the health of the individuals who are following the trade of a baker. . . .

We think that there can be no fair doubt that the trade of a baker, in and of itself, is not an unhealthy one to that degree which would authorize the legislature to interfere with the right to labor, and with the right of free contract on the part of the individual, either as employer or employee. In looking through statistics regarding all trades and occupations, it may be true that the trade of a baker does not appear to be as healthy as some other trades, and is also vastly more healthy than still others. To the common understanding the trade of a baker has never been regarded as an unhealthy one. Very likely physicians would not recommend the exercise of that or of any other trade as a remedy for ill health. Some occupations are more healthy than others, but we think there are none which might not come under the power of the legislature to supervise and control the hours of working therein if the mere fact that the occupation is not absolutely and perfectly healthy is to confer the right upon the legislative department of the Government. It might be safely affirmed that almost all occupations affect the health. There must be more than the mere fact of the possible existence of some small amount of unhealthiness to warrant legislative interference with liberty. . . .

It is also urged, pursuing the same line of argument, that it is to the interest of the State that its population should be strong and robust, and therefore any legislation which may be said to tend to make people healthy must be valid as health laws, enacted under the police power. If this be a valid argument and a justification for this kind of legislation, it follows that the protection of the Federal Constitution from undue interference with liberty of person and freedom of contract is visionary, wherever the law is sought to be justified as a valid exercise of the police power. Scarcely any law but might find shelter under such assumptions, and conduct, properly so called, as well as contract, would come under the restrictive sway of the legislature. Not only the hours of employees, but the hours of the employers, could be regulated, and doctors, lawyers, scientists, all professional men, as well as athletes and artisans, could be forbidden to fatigue their brains and bodies by prolonged hours of exercise, lest the fighting strength of the State be impaired. . . .

It was further urged on the argument that restricting the hours of labor in the case of bakers was valid because it tended to cleanliness on the part of the workers, as a man was more apt to be cleanly when not overworked, and if cleanly then his "output" was also more likely to be so. What has already been said applies with equal force to this contention. We do not admit the reasoning to be sufficient to justify the claimed right of such interference. The State in that case would assume the position of a supervisor, or *pater familias,* over every act of the individual, and its right of governmental interference with his hours of labor, his hours of exercise, the character thereof, and the extent to which it shall be carried would be recognized and upheld. In our judgment it is not possible in fact to discover the connection between the number of hours a baker may work in the bakery and the healthful quality of the bread made by the workman. The connection, if any exists, is too shadowy and thin to build any argument for the interference of the legislature. If the man works ten hours a day it is all right, but if ten and a half or eleven his health is in danger and his bread may be unhealthful, and, therefore, he shall not be permitted to do it. This, we think, is unreasonable and entirely arbitrary. When assertions such as we have adverted to become necessary in order to give, if possible, a plausible foundation for the contention that the law is a "health law," it gives rise to at least a suspicion that there was some other motive dominating the legislature than the purpose to subserve the public health or welfare.

. . . .

[Justice Harlan, with Justice White and Justice Day, wrote a dissent.]

# NOTES AND QUESTIONS

**1.** Justice Peckham (who dissented in *Jacobson*) asserts in *Lochner* that the *Jacobson* case, decided earlier the same year, "is . . . far from covering the one now before this court," but offers no explanation for this conclusion. Do you agree? The *Lochner* Court also asserts that its decision "is not a question of substituting the judgment of the court for that of the legislature." Why does the Court make this rather defensive assertion? If the Court is *not* doing what it denies doing in this respect, what then *is* it doing?

Consider the various ways in which the conception of the proper role of courts seems radically different between the two cases. What factors seem most likely to explain the Court's deferential approach to state legislation in *Jacobson*, and its much more skeptical and demanding approach in *Lochner*?

**2.** *Jacobson* and *Lochner* could be regarded as the "bookend" cases of public health law. *Jacobson* is particularly significant for the reasons discussed in the notes following that case, and is referenced with approval in virtually all subsequent cases that attempt to define the scope of the state's power in matters relating to public health and in determining the courts' role in reviewing exercises of the states' discretion. *Lochner*, on the other hand, was overruled during the New Deal (*see West Coast Hotel Co. v. Parrish*, 300 U.S. 379 (1937) and has been generally rejected ever since. References to *Lochner* since the 1930s are generally confined to illustrations of what the courts should *not* do in reviewing state regulatory legislation: In particular, judges should not (the critique goes) "read into" general constitutional phrases like the "liberty" clause of the 14th Amendment their own personally-preferred values in order to enshrine those values against legislative erosion or regulation.

Note, however, that what modern courts criticize in *Lochner* is the Court's elaboration of a "constitutional right to contract" out of the general word "liberty." The underlying analysis in *Lochner* — what modern courts would generally describe as "judicial close scrutiny" of legislation — is, in fact, still applied by courts, but not to that discredited right. Rather, close scrutiny is sometimes applied in circumstances where an otherwise legitimate exercise of the states' police powers affects one (or more) of a small number of *other* constitutionally protected rights or interests that have achieved preferred judicial status. In this sense, *Lochner*'s legacy survives its own demise. Of course, the critical (and still controversial) question is which types of public health laws will be subject to such "close scrutiny." While special constitutional protection for economic "rights" of the kind recognized in *Lochner* has long since been abandoned, a few other values affected by some types of public health laws do enjoy comparatively privileged constitutional treatment; these are described in the cases and materials in Section C, *infra* (see *Roe* and *Casey*), and also in Chapter Three, Section B[1], Note 5, *infra,* and Section B[2] (although they are clearly exceptions to the more general rule). Are there any other circumstances under which a health-related law will be "closely scrutinized?"

**3.** Since *Lochner's* abandonment, most courts have followed the lead of the *Jacobson* decision and deferred to state legislative authority in matters relating to the public's health, at least where the state's interest is protecting third parties from some risk created by the affected individual. It has been frequently recognized that the state has the power — should it choose to use it — to examine and quarantine people suspected of carrying contagious diseases (In some unusual cases, involuntary treatment has even been imposed). See cases and materials in Chapter Three, *infra.* The state has the power to require medical examinations or vaccination as a condition of school attendance, compulsory examination of people getting married, or a license for people engaged in certain occupations where infection can be spread, such as food handler or hospital worker.

The state's police power also has been consistently interpreted to include the power to take such health-related measures as fluoridating the public water supply (*see* Note 5, Section B[2], *infra*), again under the rationale that the state police powers clearly include broad authority to protect the health, safety, and welfare of the public; and that when these interests are at stake, the legislatures should be given wide discretion by the courts to fashion appropriate means to protect them.

Prior to *Jacobson,* other early interpretations of the broad scope of the police powers and the wide latitude generally allowed by the courts to legislative discretion in defining and applying those powers include *Dent v. West Virginia,* 129 U.S. 114 (1889) (examining the scope of the states' discretion to regulate the practice of medical care); *Lawton v. Steele,* 152 U.S. 133 (1892) (outlining the power of the state to abate nuisances under the police powers); *Austin v. Tennessee,* 179 U.S. 343 (1900) (upholding Tennessee's limits on the sale of cigarettes); *Compagnie Francaise de Navigation a Vapeur v. State Board of Health,* 186 U.S. 380 (1902) (upholding the state power to quarantine interstate commercial goods to protect public). The courts also have generally upheld the state's power to require compliance with fire, safety, and sanitation laws, in both private and public buildings. *The New York City Friends of Ferrets* case, at Section B[2], *infra,* is a good contemporary illustration of the breadth of the police power and the constitutional analysis of its implementation.

**4.** As suggested in Note 3, *Jacobson* articulated a vision of radical deference to legislative judgments about public health policy. One question raised by this vision involves the nature and kind of evidentiary showing that a legislature has to make to satisfy the court that a "reasonable relationship" exists between the proposed state activity and the state's legitimate interest in the health, safety, or welfare of the public. *Jacobson* goes so far as to suggest that a "widespread public belief" in the need for a health measure may be sufficient justification, although the facts in *Jacobson* certainly make the case for Massachusetts' vaccination law much stronger (although perhaps not as strong as the Court believed). Despite this language, it is likely that a modern court would require more than a belief and probably some sort of scientifically derived basis for a legislative decision to undertake any program that requires compulsory vaccination or medical treatment or that would otherwise directly affect individual liberty in a substantial way. Nonetheless, a "reasonable relationship" is still far less than scientific proof — at least in most public health cases. *See, e.g., Buhl v. Hannigan,* 16 Cal. App. 4th 1612, 1620 Cal. Rptr. 2d 740, 743-744 (1993) (upholding a state motorcycle helmet law). Only in those relatively few areas where the courts "closely scrutinize" legislation (see Note 3, *supra*, and cross-references therein) do they demand anything comparable to scientific proof.

**5.** Shortly after *Lochner* was decided, the Supreme Court upheld an Oregon statute limiting the hours that laundresses could work to ten hours a day. *Muller v. Oregon*, 197 U.S. 45 (1905). The famous brief of Louis Brandeis helped convince the Justices that the law was warranted to protect public health — specifically health of women — as a matter of public interest:

> That woman's physical structure and the performance of maternal functions place her at a disadvantage in the struggle for subsistence is obvious. This is especially true when the burdens of motherhood are upon her. Even when they are not, by abundant testimony of the medical fraternity continuance for a long time on her feet at work, repeating this from day to day, tends to injurious effects upon the body, and as healthy mothers are essential to vigorous offspring, the physical well-being of woman becomes an object of public interest and care in order to preserve the strength and vigor of the race.

*Id.* at 421.

*Muller* was rightly praised for breaking through the Court's resistance to public health legislation that regulates industry. The ensuing deference to legislative choices gave medical and public health experts considerable influence in determining what counts as a matter of public interest and how it should be handled. Yet *Muller* also illustrates how such expertise sometimes depends more on the culture of the times than scientific certainty. A more disturbing example is seen in *Buck v. Bell, infra*, Chapter Three.

## 2. Contemporary Issues: Of Helmets, Seat Belts, Ferrets, Fluoridation

### ABATE OF GEORGIA v. GEORGIA
### 137. F. Supp. 2d 1349 (N.D. Ga. 2001)

Thrash, Judge.

\* \* \*

This is an action challenging the constitutionality of Georgia's motorcycle helmet law. It is brought pursuant to 42 U.S.C. § 1983 and is before the Court on Defendants' Motion to Dismiss. . . .

#### I. BACKGROUND

Plaintiff ABATE of Georgia, Inc. ("ABATE") brings this suit on behalf of itself and all others similarly situated. ABATE is an acronym for American Bikers Active Toward Education. Its main purposes are to promote motorcycling and the rights of motorcyclists. The named Defendants in this case are Roy E. Barnes, in his official capacity as Governor of Georgia, Commissioner Robert E. Hightower of the Georgia Department of Public Safety in his official and individual capacities, [and] the Georgia Board of Public Safety. . . .

The Georgia General Assembly has enacted a statute that requires all persons to wear "protective headgear" while operating or riding a motorcycle. At the time this action was filed, the statute, O.C.G.A. § 40-6-315, provided:

    (a) No person shall operate or ride upon a motorcycle unless he or she is wearing protective headgear which complies with standards established by the Board of Public Safety.

    (b) No person shall operate or ride upon a motorcycle if the motorcycle is not equipped with a windshield unless he or she is wearing an eye-protective device of a type approved by the Board of Public Safety.

    (c) This Code section shall not apply to persons riding within an enclosed cab or motorized cart. This Code section shall not apply to a person operating a three-wheeled motorcycle used only for agricultural purposes.

    (d) The Board of Public Safety is authorized to approve or disapprove protective headgear and eye-protective devices required in this Code section and to issue and enforce regulations establishing standards and specifications for the approval thereof. The Board of Public Safety shall publish lists of all protective headgear and eye-protective devices by name and type which have been approved by it.

O.C.G.A. § 40-6-315 (Supp. 1999).

The statute was amended in the 2000 session of the Georgia General Assembly to substitute the newly created Commissioner of Motor Vehicle Safety as the applicable regulatory authority. . . .

Pursuant to the authority granted by the statute, the Board of Public Safety has promulgated rules and regulations that establish standards for headgear and eye-protective devices. . . . These regulations define technical standards that acceptable headgear and eye-protective devices must satisfy. The regulations also require that manufacturers affix a permanent label showing that the equipment complies with the applicable standard. Helmets are held to the standards set by the United States Department of Transportation. . . . Compliance requirements for eye-protective devices are determined in accordance with those test methods . . . of the American Standards Institute Standard. . . . It is undisputed that the Board of Public Safety has not published lists of all protective headgear and eye-protective devices by name and type which have been approved by it.

    . . . First, Plaintiffs contend that the Board of Public Safety's failure to publish a list of approved headgear and eye protection devices violates Plaintiffs' rights under the First, Fifth and Fourteenth Amendments to the Constitution of the United States. Second, Plaintiffs contend that the requirements that motorcyclists wear headgear and eye-protective devices are unconstitutionally vague. Plaintiffs argue that the failure of the Board of Public Safety to publish lists of approved gear has prevented ABATE's members and others similarly situated from knowing what equipment satisfies the requirements of O.C.G.A. § 40-6-315. Consequently, Plaintiffs claim they have been issued citations for allegedly violating the statute resulting in points being placed on their driver's licenses, suspension of driving privileges, and other sanctions.

. . . .

Many states have enacted statutes that require motorcyclists to wear protective headgear. *See generally* Alan S. Wasserstrom, Annotation, *Validity of Traffic Regulation Requiring Motorists to Wear Helmets or Other Protective Gear,* 72 A.L.R. 5th 607, 607 (1999). Motorcycle helmet laws generally require motorcyclists to wear helmets or other protective devices that have been approved by a state agency. . . . The statutes "reflect a widespread effort to combat the rising death and injury toll of accidents that involve motorcyclists." Motorcyclists have mounted a variety of challenges to the constitutional validity of these statutes. ("This appeal presents us with the latest in a long line of challenges to the constitutionality of mandatory helmet laws."). Plaintiffs in this case challenge the constitutionality of Georgia's statute, O.C.G.A. § 40-6-315. Defendants respond that the suit should be dismissed for failure to state a claim upon which relief can be granted.

. . . Plaintiffs' argument underlying all [their constitutional] claims is that O.C.G.A. § 40-6-315 and the regulations promulgated pursuant to it are unconstitutionally vague: "[the] statutory requirements as mandated by the Georgia Legislature [and interpreted by the state regulations] cannot be intelligently applied by the citizens of the State of Georgia so as to make an intelligent and knowledgeable determination of what does or does not meet the statutory requirements necessary to be in compliance with the instant statute in question."

Plaintiffs do not state explicitly whether they are making a facial challenge, an as-applied challenge, or both. Consequently, construing the Second Amended Complaint in the light most favorable to Plaintiffs, the Court will presume that they are making both. A facial challenge to a statute asserts that the statute is unconstitutional on its face. In other words, the challenge asserts that the statute is unconstitutional generally and without reference to any particular set of facts. An as-applied challenge, in contrast, asserts that the statute is unconstitutional because of the manner in which it was applied in the particular case.

A "facial challenge to a legislative act is, of course, the most difficult challenge to mount successfully, since the challenger generally must establish that no set of circumstances exists under which the challenged statute would be valid." The fact that an act "might conceivably operate unconstitutionally under some set of circumstances is insufficient to render it wholly invalid" since the Supreme Court does not recognize "an 'overbreadth' doctrine outside the limited context of the First Amendment." In other words, where a law does not implicate First Amendment rights, it can be challenged for vagueness only "as applied," unless the enactment is "impermissibly vague in all its applications." . . .

In this case, Plaintiffs have alleged a First Amendment violation, but they fail to specify the nature of the alleged violation. Plaintiffs have cited no cases that operating or riding a motorcycle without a helmet is an exercise of their rights of free speech, freedom of religion or their right to peaceably assemble and petition the government for redress of grievances. The Court on its own research has found no such cases. Without any case support whatsoever, the Court refuses to broaden the First Amendment by concluding that it is implicated in the enforcement of motorcycle helmet laws. . . . There is no First Amendment right to ride a motorcycle wearing a baseball cap, a bandana, or bareheaded.

Plaintiffs also allege a due process violation on grounds that a motorcyclist cannot determine whether he is meeting the headgear requirements of the statute. This facial due process challenge, however, must fail because the statute clearly proscribes some conduct, such as riding a motorcycle without any protective head-covering whatsoever. An as-applied challenge also must fail because as-applied challenges are fact-specific. They cannot be brought on behalf of a class; they must be brought on a case-by-case basis. A court "will not sift through the entire class to determine whether the statute was constitutionally applied in each case.". . .

Additionally, there is no substantive due process privacy right implicated in this case. The Eleventh Circuit has explained in another motorcycle helmet case that "[t]here is little that could be termed private in the decision whether to wear safety equipment on the open road." There is no right to be let alone that is implicated in this case. Accordingly, if Plaintiffs' Second Amended Complaint can be construed as including a substantive due process privacy challenge to O.C.G.A. § 40-6-315, that due process challenge must fail also. Finally, the Court notes that the applicable regulations merely require Plaintiffs to check to see if their headgear has affixed to it the applicable U.S. Department of Transportation certification. Such a requirement does not seem vague at all. As a matter of fact, it seems a simple way to tell if one's headgear meets the statutory requirements.

Plaintiffs also allege a violation of their equal protection rights protected by the Fourteenth Amendment. Motorcycle riders, however, are not a protected class. Requiring a person who rides a motorcycle to wear a helmet serves a rational purpose. An occupant of an automobile who is wearing a seatbelt is likely to remain in the vehicle in an accident. In contrast, a motorcyclist involved in an accident is much more likely to end up on the pavement with the chance of a serious head injury. Failure to require motorcyclists to wear appropriate headgear may increase costs to the taxpaying public, and the Georgia General Assembly's desire to limit such costs constitutes a rational purpose for O.C.G.A. § 40-6-315. As Justice Powell, sitting by designation with the Eleventh Circuit explained in *Picou v. Gillum*:

> A motorcyclist without a helmet is more likely to suffer serious injury than one wearing the prescribed headgear. State and local governments provide police and ambulance services, and the injured cyclist may be hospitalized at public expense. If permanently disabled, the cyclist could require public assistance for many years. As Professor Tribe has expressed it, "[in] a society unwilling to abandon bleeding bodies on the highway, the motorcyclist or driver who endangers himself plainly imposes costs on others."

Motorcycle helmet laws are a permissible means of attempting to reduce this cost. "Legislatures and not courts have the primary responsibility for balancing conflicting interests in safety and individual autonomy." Plaintiffs' equal protection argument is without merit.

\* \* \*

# NEW YORK CITY FRIENDS OF FERRETS v. CITY OF NEW YORK
## 876 F. Supp. 529 (S.D.N.Y. 1995)

Schwartz, Judge.

\* \* \*

New York City Friends of Ferrets, an unincorporated association of individuals in New York City who own or wish to own ferrets as household pets, bring this action challenging the legality of the City of New York's (the "City") prohibition against the keeping of ferrets within the City limits and the requirement that in any case where a ferret is reported to have bitten a human being, the ferret be immediately surrendered to the New York City Department of Health ("DOH") and humanely destroyed in order to conduct a rabies examination.

Plaintiff seeks a judgment declaring that the City's regulation of ferret ownership denies plaintiff's members of liberty and property without due process of law and violates the Equal Protection Clause of the United States Constitution.

Webster's New World Dictionary of the American Language (College Ed.1968) defines a ferret as "a kind of weasel, easily tamed and used for hunting or killing of rabbits, rats. . . ." Two types of ferrets can be found in the United States: the black footed ferret (*Mustela nigripes*) and the domestic or common ferret (*Mustela putorius* or *Mustela putorious furo*). This action involves domestic ferrets and, hereinafter, the term "ferret" shall refer to common or domestic ferrets. Domestic ferrets have been bred in captivity, initially for the purposes of hunting, since the fourth century B.C., and have, more recently, become a popular household pet in the United States. . . .

The City moves to dismiss the Complaint. . . . We note that the parties have submitted affidavits and other evidence to the Court to be considered on the motion to dismiss. Such materials lie outside the four corners of the pleadings; accordingly, the court must either exclude the additional materials from our consideration and decide the motion based solely upon the complaint, or convert the motion to one for summary judgment. . . . The Court has determined to consider materials which the parties have submitted; therefore, we elect to convert this motion to dismiss into a motion for summary judgment, and interpret the expanded record accordingly.

Summary judgment is appropriate where "the pleadings, depositions, answers to interrogatories, and admissions on file, together with affidavits, if any, show that there is no genuine issue as to any material fact and that the moving party is entitled to a judgment as a matter of law." . . . The burden of proof, however, lies with the moving party and we must resolve all ambiguities and draw all inferences in favor of the party against whom summary judgment is sought. . . .

The Equal Protection Clause of the Fourteenth Amendment to the United States Constitution guarantees that classifications imposed by law will not be used to burden a group of people arbitrarily. As the challenged Municipal Code provisions regulating ferret ownership do not classify people based on "suspect" criteria, such as race or nationality, they are constitutionally permissible under equal protection analysis so long they bear a rational relationship to a legitimate state interest. Thus, "the Equal Protection Clause is satisfied so long as there is a plausible policy reason for the classification, . . . the legislative facts on which the classification is apparently based rationally may have been considered to be true by the governmental decisionmaker, . . . and the relationship of the classification to its goal is not so attenuated as to render the distinction arbitrary or irrational. . . ."

The courts, moreover, show great deference to legislatures' choices in creating classifications, even where those classifications seem imperfect. A law will not fail to pass constitutional muster under equal protection analysis merely because it contains classifications which are underinclusive — that is, which "do not include all who are similarly situated with respect to a rule, and thereby burden less than would be logical to achieve the intended government end." . . .

In its exercise of the power to protect its citizens — to wit its police power — the City is also limited by the constitutional requirement that the sovereign may not deprive citizens of property without due process of law [citation to *Jacobson*]. Where, as here, the exercise of police power does not affect fundamental rights, such as voting or freedom of speech, we apply the same rational basis analysis used under the constitutional guarantee of equal protection. Thus, deprivation of private property pursuant to an exercise of police power is constitutionally permissible where the challenged legislative enactment bears a rational relationship to legitimate legislative goal or purpose. . . .

In applying the rational basis analysis to a health and welfare regulation, such as the portions of the Health Code at issue here, courts apply a basic test of reasonableness; that is, a police power regulation is to be upheld if the requirements of the law have a rational connection with the promotion and protection of public safety. . . . Moreover, courts have noted that:

> [t]he exceedingly strong presumption of constitutionality applies not only to enactments of the Legislature but to ordinances of municipalities as well. While this presumption is rebuttable . . . only as a last resort should courts strike down legislation on the ground of unconstitutionality. The ordinance may not be arbitrary. It must be reasonably related to some manifest evil which, however, need only be reasonably apprehended. It is also presumed that the legislative body has investigated and found the existence of a situation showing or indicating the need for or desirability of the ordinance, and, if any state of facts [that can be proven or] assumed justifies the disputed measure, this court's power of inquiry ends. Thus, as to reasonableness, plaintiffs in

order to succeed have the burden of showing that "no reasonable basis at all" existed for the challenged provision of the ordinance.

. . . .

The City has submitted significant materials in support of its decision to classify ferrets as wild animals and to insist upon the immediate euthanasia and testing of any ferret reported to have bitten a human. This evidence includes the affidavits of [public health officials from around the country].

The City explains its decisions to classify ferrets as a species which is "wild, ferocious, fierce, dangerous or naturally inclined to do harm," to prohibit the keeping of ferrets in New York City, and to destroy and examine any ferret reported to have bitten a human being and suspected of having rabies as the product of several public health and safety concerns. First, the City contends that, despite their recent popularity as household pets, ferrets remain prone to vicious, unprovoked attacks on humans, particularly children and infants. In support of this assertion, the City has submitted various epidemiological studies and monographs. . . . [One of the researchers has also] received information on 452 ferret attacks from this period, with reports concentrated (425 episodes) in California and the neighboring states of Arizona and Oregon. . . .

The City has also submitted materials to illustrate the disturbing frequency among these documented ferret bitings of unprovoked attacks on infants and small children, characterized in some instances by a large number of bites covering the child's face and body. The California DHS *Pet European Ferrets* study catalogued among its data 63 unprovoked attacks on infants and small children less than three years of age. . . .

The City also furnishes evidentiary support for its second articulated public health concern underlying its decision to prohibit ownership of ferrets as pets and to euthanize and test immediately for rabies ferrets that bite humans, namely, that failure to take such measures risks an increase in the spread of rabies in the New York City area. As a threshold matter, the City points out that New York City is presently under a rabies alert and rabies has been declared endemic in the Metropolitan area. . . .

The City's motivating public health concern relating to ferrets and rabies centers on the lack of knowledge of the behavioral symptoms of the rabid ferret and the indeterminate viral shedding period in the animal. The clinical signs of rabies in dogs and cats are well-known. It has also been established, moreover, that the time from which a dog or cat has the rabies virus in its saliva (i.e., begins its viral shedding period) to the time that the animal will exhibit the clinical behavioral signs indicating rabies does not exceed ten days. . . . Accordingly, the World Health Organization and the Compendium of Animal Rabies Control . . . recommend that a healthy dog or cat that bites a person should be confined and observed for 10 days. If the dog or cat exhibits behavioral signs suggestive of rabies, the foregoing authorities recommend that the animal be humanely killed, its head removed, and the brain tissue examined for the rabies virus.

The viral shedding period in ferrets is unknown. In addition, the clinical behavioral signs of rabies in ferrets are not well established, and such data as exist suggest that the clinical signs of the disease may be less noticeable in ferrets than in dogs and cats. . . . Euthanasia and immediate testing remain the recommended course of action in biting incidents involving ferrets, the City points out, despite the approval by the United States Department of Agriculture of the IMRAB rabies vaccine for ferrets, because no vaccine is completely efficacious and the above discussed uncertainties regarding the etiology of rabies in ferrets persist.

The final public health risk posed by ownership of ferrets as pets, according to the City, is the potential for ferrets to escape and form feral populations, as have stray cats and dogs. Such a development may lead to the decimation of certain wildlife species as well as excessive competition with other wild natural predators. . . .

The City also emphasizes that the foregoing considerations have persuaded a number of states to prohibit or regulate the ownership of ferrets as pets in precisely the manner that the City has by means of its enactment of the Health Code regulations at issue here. . . .

Plaintiff offers two affidavits, those of Dr. Kent Marshall and Dr. Freddie Ann Hoffman in support of its position. We note as a threshold matter that certain issues confront this Court with respect to the disinterested, unbiased and expert status of these affiants. First, both suggest an actual or apparent conflict of interest. It is not disputed that Dr. Marshall maintains a veterinary practice in Wayne County, New York, site of Marshall Farms USA, Inc. — a large ferret breeding farm owned by Dr. Marshall's parents. Dr. Hoffman is the Vice-President of the American Ferret Association, Inc., an organization whose purpose is to promote the keeping of ferrets as pets. Even more significant, Dr. Hoffman submits no proof of her professional training or expertise in the veterinary issues at the core of this case. She is a board certified pediatrician specializing in the study of blood and tumors, and is presently employed by the U.S. Food and Drug Administration.

. . . .

A central tenet of plaintiff's constitutional claims is that pet ferrets pose no greater a danger to public health and safety — as measured by incidence of bites, severity of injury, and risk of rabies infection — than pet dogs. The City, however, offers unrefuted evidence in support of the proposition that comparisons between dogs and ferrets with respect to the foregoing public health parameter are inapposite. First, there is reason to suspect that ferret bites are underreported relative to dog bites because of the frequent public health policy requirement that pet ferrets be euthanized if they bite humans as well as the lack of the almost uniform public health requirement that dog bites be reported. Accordingly, any comparison of rate or frequency of bites as between dogs and ferrets is likely to be skewed in favor of ferrets. Second, the more recent experience of adoption of ferrets in somewhat more significant numbers as domestic pets — and the lack of sound estimates of the number of pet ferrets — as opposed to the longstanding and well documented presence of dogs in that role, renders statistical comparisons of biting and rabies incidents between the two species of limited usefulness.

. . . .

With respect to the pathogenesis of rabies in ferrets, plaintiff's own expert, Dr. Hoffman, has acknowledged in her writings on the subject of ferrets as pets that:

> The duration of viral shedding following exposure to rabies has not yet been adequately determined in ferrets. Therefore, no quarantine period can be recommended. As a result, once a ferret has bitten a person, local health authorities may require that the ferret be euthanized for rabies testing regardless of immunization status. For this reason, ferret advocates consider the evaluation of the viral shedding time in the context of a well — controlled study to be the single most important issue impacting on the health and welfare of the pet ferret today.

... Plaintiff submits no such study to this Court, nor furnishes evidence that any of the foregoing national animal public health organizations have been made aware that such data exists and is reliable. ... In short, plaintiff fails to dispute the City's evidence in connection with one of its most pressing articulated concerns in regulating ferret ownership — to wit, the uncertain viral shedding period in rabid ferrets — and makes no showing with respect to Dr. Hoffman's claims regarding the dangers posed by rabid ferrets.

Finally, plaintiff emphasizes that New York City does not regulate pit bull terriers, which have been shown to be dangerous in certain circumstances, and suggests that the absence of such regulation establishes a constitutional infirmity, under the Equal Protection Clause, of the Health Code regulations relating to ferrets. We disagree. ... [T]he Constitution does not prohibit underinclusive statutes *per se*. That the City has chosen, in the field of ownership of animals, to regulate ferrets and not pit bull terriers, simply embodies the permissible exercise of its discretion to address "[e]vils in the same field [which] may be of different dimensions and proportions, requiring different remedies ... The [City] may select one phase of one field and apply a remedy there, neglecting the others.". ... Plaintiff's arguments with respect to regulation of pit bulls, and, in fact, plaintiff's appeal to the regulation of dogs and cats in general, betray its fundamental misconception of constitutional equal protection and due process analysis as such analysis applies to public safety laws. The Constitution simply does not guarantee owners of ferrets regulatory status precisely equal to the status of owners of other animals, even potentially dangerous animals, but rather mandates only that the decision of the sovereign to regulate them, as well as the nature of that regulation, have a rational basis and not be undertaken and applied arbitrarily and capriciously. Here, the undisputed evidence ... establishes that the City's ban on ferrets and its summary euthanasia and testing of ferrets that bite humans has ample basis in public health concerns regarding the propensity of pet ferrets to bite, particularly infants and small children, and the uncertain pathogenesis of rabies in domestic ferrets; therefore, the City's regulation of ferret ownership cannot be deemed arbitrary or irrational.

* * *

# NOTES AND QUESTIONS

**1.** *ABATE of Georgia v. Georgia* raises some fairly novel theories, but the ultimate decision to uphold the Georgia law on the core issue — state power to compel helmet use — is only one example of what has been virtually a unanimous trend. Almost every state supreme court in each and every jurisdiction has been asked to consider the constitutionality of motorcycle helmet legislation, and all have come to the same conclusion: Such legislation is clearly within the state's police powers. *See, e.g., Benning v. Vermont,* 161 Vt. 472, 641 A.2d 757 (1994); *Buhl,* Section B[1], Note 4, *supra;* and the ALR annotation cited in ABATE, *supra.* No court has found that mandatory helmet laws involve or infringe on the type of important individual right that can require courts to more "jealously" guard individual conduct from attempts by the state to impose restrictions, such as the Court did in *Lochner.* To the contrary, the courts have generally adopted the low level of scrutiny applied in *Jacobson,* asking only whether mandatory helmet laws are a legitimate exercise of the state's police powers in the more limited sense, requiring only that the state show that such legislation is reasonably related to the public's health, safety, welfare, or morals. As one court described what it considered its proper, deferential role:

> The legislature [under the police powers] has the power to control and regulate the use of the highways. Moreover, if the relation between the statute and the public welfare is debatable, the legislative judgment must be accepted, because of the presumption of constitutionality afforded a statute.

*Adrian v. Poucher,* 398 Mich. 316, 317, 247 N.W.2d 798, 799 (1976). As in *Jacobson,* the fact that some oppose such legislation, and even argue that it (paradoxically) is actually counterproductive when it comes to safety (*e.g.,* by obscuring bikers' vision), does not change the judicial role: such arguments are for the legislature to debate and decide, and not for the courts to revisit or reverse: "Plaintiffs are not entitled to have the courts act as a super-legislature and retry legislative judgments based on evidence presented to the court . . . [t]he question before us is whether the link between safety for highway users and the helmet law is rational, not whether we agree [with the legislature] that the statute actually leads to safer highways." *Benning, supra,* 641 A.2d at 762.

Motorcycle enthusiasts did win one minor victory. *See Easyriders Freedom F.I.G.H.T. v. Hannigan,* 92 F.3d 1486 (9th Cir. 1996) (upholding the power of the state to enact such legislation generally, but overturning the conviction where the cyclist could not be expected to know that he was wearing a helmet that did not meet legal standards in that state).

What is interesting about these cases, and where the courts have been somewhat inconsistent, has been their reasoning concerning *why* legislative discretion should be given such broad deference in this context. In particular, the courts have not been able to decide whether helmet requirements should be characterized as an attempt to protect the health and safety of the public — meaning third parties affected by the cyclist or the passenger — or whether helmet laws are primarily attempts to protect the wearer from the risks he or she would otherwise choose to assume. As discussed earlier, although the courts generally have given the legislatures great discretion in fashioning "public health laws," meaning laws that protect other members of the public from one individual's conduct, some courts have at least suggested that truly paternalistic laws, those that protect the individual only from his or her own conduct, may not be so easily upheld. Some courts have reasoned that such legislation may fall within the reach of the police powers but should trigger a more demanding judicial review — as the *Lochner* Court reviewed the New York legislation — and therefore require the Court to review more closely the state's actual purposes, the effectiveness of the particular legislative scheme, and the actual impact on the individual's interest. On occasion, courts have gone farther and suggested that if the legislation is found to be truly paternalistic, it must be invalidated. As one judge argued (dissenting from his court's decision in *Poucher* to uphold the state's mandatory helmet law):

> The protection of an individual from himself is not among the proper functions of government.
>
> . . . [O]therwise there would be no restriction or limitation to this power, and the State could regulate an individual's life, his way of living, and even his way of thinking. The statute is not concerned with the preservation of public safety, health, order, morals, or welfare; and though the headgear requirement may be beneficent, nevertheless, it is unconstitutional because it attempts to infringe upon and stifle the fundamental personal right of liberty, under which each individual may act as he sees fit to preserve his own safety if he does not harm others in doing so. . . .
>
> The fact that the general public may consider it foolhardy to ride a motorcycle without a safety helmet is alone insufficient basis or justification for defining the nonuse of a helmet a criminal offense. I believe that our State Constitution affords one the privilege of making a fool of himself. . . .

398 Mich. at 322; 247 N.W.2d at 801 (C.J. Kavanagh, dissenting).

Somewhat understandably, most courts have labored to avoid addressing the question of the validity of truly paternalistic legislation. Instead they have attempted to find a public or third-party interest in helmet legislation and, therefore, they have limited their review to a more conservative judicial role. To do so, the courts have had to rely, at times, on some rather tortured judicial logic. Some courts have argued that third parties are affected by cyclists who ride without helmets because a serious motorcycle accident will cause a traffic hazard or cause harm to other motorists. Other courts have argued that protecting cyclists and their passengers from injury or death promotes society's interest in maintaining a strong and productive citizenry. One court went so far as to recognize the "well known fact" that cyclists ride near the center of the road and are therefore more likely to cross into oncoming traffic if injured. The majority of courts, however, have focused on what is perhaps the strongest argument to characterize mandatory helmet legislation as a "public health law:" that serious injuries resulting from a failure to wear protective helmets may result in an economic burden on the public as well as on the families of the victims. Given the costs to the public of motorcycle injuries, most courts regard helmet legislation as well within the state's discretion and a matter over which the judiciary will exercise limited review. See Chapter 6 for further exploration of paternalism in public health law.

**2.** As of June 2006, 20 states required all motorcycle riders to wear helmets and another 26 required helmets only for minors. Six states had repealed their mandatory motorcycle helmet laws, with several others poised to do so. A better financed lobby led by motorcycle associations argued that people should be trusted to make their own choices about risky products and behaviors, including same sex marriage and abortion. They also argued for making the roads safer for both cars and motorcycles. See Eileen McNamara, *Not Using Their Heads*, THE BOSTON GLOBE, June 18, 2006, at B1.

Debate may have been fueled by Ben Roethlisberger, the Pittsburgh Steeler's quarterback, who was seriously injured in the face and head when a car hit the motorcycle he was riding without a helmet. One reporter noted two paradoxes in public reaction to the absence of a helmet. "As a champion N.F.L. quarterback, Roethlisberger is a brilliant risk/benefit analyst, making split-second decisions about probabilities and consequences even as linemen try to bury him. So how could a savvy risk manager ride without a helmet, a low-reward, high-risk activity that exposes a team, a city and untold corporate interests to its consequences?" The second paradox noted was that "Roethlisberger became a football star and brought a championship to Pittsburgh by accepting physical risks that ordinary people would avoid. So how can these critics, who have benefited from his acceptance of physical risk, get all snippy that he took *this* one?" John Leland, *The Superstar Athlete Is Paid to Take Risks, Right*? N.Y. TIMES, June 18, 2006, at WK3 (emphasis in original). Paul Slovic noted that our past experience shapes our perception of a risk as manageable or too high. For example, if a rider has not had an accident after many miles on a motorcycle, he may not consider himself at risk for injury without a helmet. According to Leland's interview with Slovic, "Wearing a helmet is a cost, measured in comfort, and perhaps liberty, but provides a benefit only if there is a crash. After a number of safe rides, Dr. Slovic said, 'you feel you're rewarded for not wearing one and punished for wearing one.'" *Id.*

**3.** Mandatory seat belt legislation has generated far less litigation than the helmet legislation but the same judicial response. See, e.g., Atwater v. City of Lago Vista, 532 U.S. 318 (2001); State v. Hartog, 440 N.W.2d 852 (Iowa), cert. denied, 493 U.S. 1005 (1989). But as with the helmet cases, in these cases the courts have made efforts to characterize the underlying purpose of the legislation as protecting third parties from harm, not protecting the individual required to comply with the law.

There is one case involving highway safety in which the court both was unwilling to defer to legislative discretion and held, ultimately, that the state had exceeded its police powers. In 1989, the Minnesota Supreme Court reviewed the constitutionality of a state law that required all vehicles traveling on public roads to have specific warning devices. Members of the Amish community refused to attach such devices to their horse-drawn buggies, arguing that to do so would violate various Amish principles; nonetheless they were convicted on resulting criminal charges. The Minnesota Supreme Court ruled that the state law interfered with the freedom of the Amish to practice their religion as secured by the First Amendment to the U.S. Constitution. On appeal, the U.S. Supreme Court vacated the judgment of the state court, ruling that the state court had misinterpreted the demands of the First Amendment. On rehearing, the state court found that the state law interfered with the freedom of religion protected by the state constitution, and, once again, invalidated the prosecution. In doing so on state constitutional grounds, the state effectively prevented any subsequent appeal to the U.S. Supreme Court. *State v. Hershberger*, 462 N.W.2d 393 (Minn. 1990). A few other state courts have interpreted their constitutions similarly. *See State v. Miller*, 549 N.W.2d 235, 202 Wis. 2d 56 (1996). *Cf.* discussion of *Smith,* Section B[3], *infra.*

**4.** *New York City Friends of Ferrets* is another good, prototypical illustration of the manner in which most courts will review public health legislation and defer to legislative judgment concerning the importance of various risks and the proper remedial response. It also is a good illustration of another dimension of constitutional analysis: the extent to which the principles of equal protection limit the ability of the government to discriminate in exercising otherwise valid public health measures. In the traditional language of equal protection analysis, except where certain "suspect classifications" are made or where some "fundamental interests" are affected by the governmental classification (such as the free exercise of religion, as discussed in Section B[3], *infra*), both the state and the federal legislatures are free to distinguish between categories of risks and various public health problems, so long as they have some rational basis for doing so. To be rational, a classification need not attack the most serious problem first or all problems of comparable merit. For a general discussion, see *New York City Transit Authority v. Beazer,* 440 U.S. 568 (1979); *Williamson v. Lee Optical*, 348 U.S. 483 (1955).

As illustrated in the *Ferret* decision, if the city chooses to regulate ferret bites and not dog or cat bites, it needs only some rational basis for believing that ferret bites are a problem and that banning their ownership or even requiring their destruction is an appropriate means for responding to the problem. The fact that some people think that the problem is less important or that some critics question whether the severe measures adopted by the city are really necessary is irrelevant to the court. Such choices are left to legislative discretion and limited only by political, not constitutional constraints. If anything, the review of the evidence for and against regulating the ownership of ferrets undertaken by the court in *New York City Friends of Ferrets* is somewhat more extensive than the highly deferential judicial attitude reflected in most public health cases — so long as *Jacobson* is followed and the rationality standard is applied. Note that in this regard, the equal protection analysis of the substantive right affected by an exercise of the police power mirrors the substantive due process analysis of that power.

**5.** Perhaps the most intriguing illustration of both the breadth of the constitutional authority of the state governments in matters relating to public health as well as the political parameters within which that authority may be exercised involves state and local efforts to fluoridate drinking water. In some ways, such efforts test the outer limits of government authority. Fluoridating water is primarily an effort to prevent dental caries. Dental caries can be related to other health conditions, can cause pain and discomfort, and may even make eating and drinking more difficult, but they are clearly not a life-threatening condition or even something that, in relative terms, threatens overall health status. Moreover, fluoridation of water supply is largely an effort to protect individual people from their own bad decisions. Dental caries are not communicable. Fluoridation protects children from the neglectful decisions of their parents, but there is no child neglect in the traditional sense. Fluoridation of water, even more so than mandatory helmet legislation, is largely a paternalistic effort, not a protection of third parties. Nonetheless, virtually all courts that have been asked to consider whether such efforts fall within the broad reach of the states' police powers have upheld the constitutionality of fluoridation of water. *See, e.g., Quiles v. City of Boynton Beach*, 802 So. 2d 397 (Fla. App. 2001); *Young v. Board of Health of Somerville*, 61 N.J. 76, 293 A.2d 164 (1972).

For a rather provocative attack on these decisions and an effort to document the claims that fluoridation is ineffective in preventing dental caries and causes cancer and other health problems, see John Remington Graham & Pierre Morian, *Highlights in North American Litigation During the Twentieth Century on Artificial Fluoridation of Public Water Supplies*, 14 J. LAND USE & ENV'T L. 195 (1999). For a more traditional view of the benefits of fluoridation, see CDC, *Achievements in Public Health 1900–1999: Fluoridation of Drinking Water to Prevent Dental Caries*, 48 MORBIDITY/MORTALITY WKLY REP. 933-940 (1999).

Contrast this view of the scope of state authority — pure paternalism — with the view in FREUND, THE POLICE POWER, Section B[1], Note 1, *supra*, at 59. Is there even a contrast? Does it make a difference if you can identify a sub-group of individuals, *e.g.*, minors, who need to be protected?

**6.** Many legal disputes over the legitimacy of various public health programs focus not on the broad constitutional parameters within which the government must operate, but whether the particular measures under consideration have been authorized by state or, in some cases, city or county legislative bodies. A good illustration can be found in *Spokane County Health Dist. v. Brockett*, 120 Wash. 2d 140, 839 P.2d 324 (1992). In the jurisdiction of Washington, the state legislature has given local health departments both general authority and additional specific statutory mandates. The state supreme court has on several occasions alluded to a provision of the Washington State Constitution which appears to grant authority directly to the county health departments — apart from any statutory authority that they may have been given by the state legislature (although this portion of the *Brockett* decision is clearly *dictum* and not the basis for the court's holding). As a result, in many cases, the legality of any public health measure taken at the local level may require some parsing of the various statutory schemes, and often raises interesting questions of administrative law and statutory preemption. But at least in Washington and, perhaps in other jurisdictions with similarly written state constitutons, there is also the possibility that a local jurisdictions may be acting under its own (state) constitutional authority, apart from any state authorizing legislation. For a good (and relevant) example, see *Parkland Light & Water Co. v. Tacoma-Pierce County Bd. of Health*, 151 Wash. 2d 428, 90 P.2d 37 (2004) (holding that the local health department could not require the fluoridation the water

supply because of a conflict with a statewide statute giving local water authorities discretionary authority to fluoridate the water).

**7.** For good general references on state public health programs, what they
do, and their underlying legal structure, see PUBLIC HEALTH LAW WORK GROUP,
HEALTH OFFICER PRACTICE GUIDE FOR COMMUNICABLE DISEASE CONTROL IN
CALIFORNIA (2005), found at www.dhs.ca.gov/ps/dcdc/ (last visited February
2006).

## 3.  Religion and Public Health

Many people have strongly-held beliefs about the proper roles of religion,
medical care and government in their health and spiritual well-being.
Accordingly, state activities to protect public health are sometimes met by
religiously-based objections to particular programs or requirements. This section explores the constitutional tensions that arise in this context, and the
ongoing search for accommodation in a pluralistic society.

### STATE EX REL. SWANN v. PACK
527 S.W.2d 99 (Tenn. 1975),
*cert. denied*, 424 U.S. 954 (1976)

Henry, Justice.

* * *

We granted certiorari in this case to determine whether the State of
Tennessee may enjoin a religious group from handling snakes as a part of its
religious service and in accordance with its Articles of Faith, on the basis of
such action constituting a public nuisance.

. . . .

To place this controversy in proper perspective, we note the pleadings and
trial proceedings.

On April 14, 1973, the District Attorney General of the Second Judicial
Circuit filed his petition in the Circuit Court at Newport charging that
respondents Pack and certain designated Elders, including Albert Ball, had
been handling snakes as a part of their church service "for the last two years";
that this was one of the rituals of the church to test the faith and sincerity of
belief of church members; that Pastor Pack "has become anointed," along with
other members of the church and has "advanced" to using deadly drugs, to
wit, strychnine; that at a church service on April 7, 1973 snakes were handled
and an "Indian boy was bitten and his arm became swollen"; that two named
church members drank strychnine and died as a result; that, at the funeral
of one of these, Pastor Pack, and others, handled snakes; and that Pastor
Pack has proclaimed his intentions to continue these practices. The prayer
was for an injunction enjoining respondents "from handling, displaying, or
exhibiting poisonous snakes or taking or using strychnine or other poisonous

medicines." In the alternative, and upon failure of the named defendants to cease and desist, petitioner prayed that the church be padlocked as a public nuisance.

By order entered April 21, 1973, the trial court found these facts to be true; that § 39-2208 had been violated and ordered that the defendants be (e)njoined from handling poisonous snakes or using deadly poisons in any church service . . . until further orders of the Court.[1]

. . . .

Moreover the record reflects that . . . the trial judge added, in his own hand-writing, the following: "However, any person who wishes to swallow strychnine or other poison may do so if he does not make it available to any other persons."

The further result of this order was that defendants could not practice snake handling, from which death *might* ensue[2] but could drink strychnine, a highly poisonous drug.

The record reflects no explanation for this incongruity.

Thereafter, the District Attorney General filed a second petition alleging stepped up activity at the Holiness Church. On July 1, 1973, "a national convention for the snake handlers' cult of the United States" was held and "many dangerous and poisonous snakes were displayed" and one of the handlers had been bitten and was in a Chattanooga hospital recuperating [footnote omitted]. Services were conducted on July 3 and July 7, 1973, and again snakes were handled. All this led the District Attorney General to conclude and charge that Cocke County was in imminent danger and likely to "become the snake handling capital of the world."

In response to this citation, respondents were held in contempt, fined and sentenced, but sentences were suspended in each case, "until the said defendant handles poisonous snakes at said church. . . ."

Up to this point defendants had not been represented by counsel.

By order entered August 18, 1973 respondents were jailed in default of payment of the fines theretofore imposed and directed to appear on August 25, 1973 to show cause why they should not be required to serve the sentences.

. . . .

---

[1] Section 39-2208 reads as follows:

*Handling snakes so as to endanger life – Penalty.* — It shall be unlawful for any person, or persons, to display, exhibit, handle or use any poisonous or dangerous snake or reptile in such a manner as to endanger the life or health of any person.

Any person violating the provisions of this section shall be guilty of a misdemeanor and punished by a fine of not less than fifty dollars ($50.00) nor more than one hundred and fifty dollars ($150), or by confinement in jail not exceeding six (6) months, or by both such fine and imprisonment, in the discretion of the court.

[2] The most common question that arises regarding ritual snake handling is the surprisingly small number of fatalities. L.M. Klauner, "the undoubted authority on the rattlesnake," writes that the fatalities from this cause (rattlesnake bite) for the entire United States, with a population of over 160 million, seldom exceed 30 per year. Of every 100 people bitten by rattlesnakes, only about 3 will die. W. LaBarre, *They Shall Take Up Serpents,* pp. 13–14 (University of Minnesota Press 1962). . . .

It was stipulated that various witnesses would testify that they had never seen anyone other than designated representatives of this particular church handle snakes; that they never saw any person who was either a parishioner or a nonmember present at the church services who had ever been placed in immediate danger.

It was further stipulated that an anthropologist would testify that snake handling is a legitimate part of their religious service; that she had never seen anyone endangered by handling snakes; that proper precautions were always taken; and that handling snakes is a legitimate and historic part of the church service. Two other witnesses would verify this testimony.

It was further stipulated that the "Indian boy," bitten at one of the services, was thirty years old.

It was further stipulated that the Holiness Church of God in Jesus Name is located about a half mile from the nearest paved road, and at the end of a dead-end, dirt, private, mountain road and on property owned by the church.

   . . . .

By final decree the trial judge made the injunction permanent, directing that defendants "be perpetually enjoined from handling, displaying or exhibiting dangerous and poisonous snakes at the said Holiness Church of God in Jesus Name. . . ." [As explained in Section VIII of the opinion, the state court of appeals modified and upheld the injunction.]

II

The history and development of the Holiness Church is relevant.

   . . . .

To say that this is not a conventional movement would be a masterpiece of understatement. Its beliefs and practices are, to say the least, unconventional and out of harmony with contemporary customs, mores and notions of morality. They oppose drinking (to include carbonated beverages, tea and coffee), smoking, dancing, the use of cosmetics, jewelry or other adornment. They regard the use of medicine as a sure sign of lack of faith in God's ability to cure the sick and look upon medical doctors as being for the use of those who do not trust God. When greeting each other, the men use the "holy kiss," a mouth-to-mouth osculation "accompanied by a vigorous, if not passionate hug." The "holy kiss" is not exchanged between members of the opposite sexes.

But it is their belief in handling serpents that has catapulted them into the limelight and has produced their legal difficulties.

There is some apparent confusion with respect to their purpose in the use of serpents as a central practice in their religious beliefs. *Harden,* et al. *v. State,* 188 Tenn. 17, 216 S.W.2d 708 (1948), treated snake handling as being "the test and proof of the sincerity of their belief." In this record it is asserted that the use of serpents is designed as a test of the faith and sincerity of church members. Our research indicates that this is not precisely correct. Their basic reason is compliance with the scripture as they interpret it, and as required by their Articles of Faith. But the practice of snake handling is not a test of faith, nor proof of godliness. Its sole purpose is to "confirm the word." In the words of Alfred Ball, a defendant to this suit:

We don't take up serpents, handle fire or drink strychnine to test the faith of the people at all. That's not the point of it. . . . These are signs that God said would follow the believers. And, these signs are to confirm the Word of God, and that's the only purpose for them. . . . They're not to test the faith of the person doing it. They're not to test whether he's a good person. It's simply and only to confirm the Word of God. That's all God intended the signs for, and that's the only reason we do them.

. . . .

Whether the practice is to "test the faith," is not relevant to this controversy. We only make the distinction in the interest of an accurate and comprehensive statement of the beliefs of this religious group and its admittedly unusual ritual.

. . . .

Lastly, it should be pointed out that snakes are only handled when the member or handler has become "anointed." As we understand this phenomenon and the emotional reaction it produces, it is something akin to saying that a member doesn't handle snakes until the "spirit moves him." Unquestionably this is an emotional stimulus produced by extreme faith and generating great courage. Perhaps the whole belief in "anointment" can best be summed up by the defendant, Liston Pack:

It comes from inside. . . . If you've got the Holy Ghost in you, it'll come out and nothing can hurt you. Faith brings contact with God and then you're anointed. It is not tempting God. You can't tempt God by doing what He says do. You can have faith, but if you never feel the anointing, you had better leave the serpent alone.

Such is the nature of the religious group with which we deal.

. . . There is, however, no requirement under our State or Federal Constitution that any religious group be conventional or that it be numerically strong in order that its activities be protected. Nor is there any requirement that its practices be in accord with prevailing views.

The First Amendment to the Constitution of the United States requires in clear terms that:

Congress shall make no law respecting an establishment of religion, or prohibiting the free exercise thereof. . . .

Article 1, Section 3 of the Constitution of Tennessee contains a substantially stronger guaranty of religious freedoms. It provides:

That all men have a natural and indefeasible right to worship Almighty God according to the dictates of their own conscience; that no man can of right be compelled to attend, erect, or support any place of worship, or to maintain any minister against his consent; that no human authority can, in any case whatever, control or interfere with the rights of conscience; and that no preference shall ever be given, by law, to any religious establishment or mode of worship.

A "mode of worship," even of a religious group wherein the handling of serpents is central to its Articles of Faith, is constitutionally protected under the Constitution of Tennessee and of the United States.

. . . .

Under our constitutions, a citizen may be a devout Christian, a dedicated Jew or a consummate infidel — or he may be a member of the Holiness Church of God in Jesus Name. The government must view all citizens and all religious beliefs with absolute and uncompromising neutrality. The day this Country ceases to countenance irreligion or unusual or bizarre religions, it will cease to be free for all religions. We must prefer none and disparage none.

We, therefore, hold that the Holiness Church of God in Jesus Name is a constitutionally protected religious group.

This is not to say, however, that this or any other religious group has an absolute and unbridled right to pursue any practice of its own choosing. The right to believe is absolute; the right to act is subject to reasonable regulation designed to protect a compelling state interest. This belief-action dichotomy has been the subject of numerous decisions of the Supreme Court of the United States.

IV

. . . .

> They may believe without fear of any punishment that it is right to handle poisonous snakes while conducting religious services. But the right to practice that belief "is limited by other recognized powers, equally precious to mankind." One of those equally as precious rights is that of society's protection from a practice, religious or otherwise, which is dangerous to life and health.

[Citation to *Harden, supra.*]

There cannot be any question that the [trial court] acted upon acceptable legal principles and precedents in declaring the Tennessee Snake Handler's Act constitutional in the face of an attack based upon the Freedom of Religion Clauses of the state and federal constitutions. This is not, however, to say that its application would necessarily be constitutional under all circumstances as is hereinafter pointed out. *Harden* simply holds that the statute does not violate the freedom of religion guarantees of the federal or state constitutions and that . . . "[the defendants] had handled snakes in such a manner as to endanger the life or health of any person." Neighboring states having similar statutes have uniformly upheld and applied them.

. . . .

[In 1972, the U.S. Supreme Court held in *Wisconsin v. Yoder*] that permitting the Amish to educate their children, after they have completed the eighth grade, in their own way and in deference to their established religious views, the statutory requirement to the contrary notwithstanding, would not impair the health of the children, nor result in their inability to be self-supporting or to discharge the duties and responsibilities of citizenship, nor in any way materially detract from the welfare of society. Therefore, the Court held that the state's interest was not so compelling as to overrule the freedom of the Amish to pursue their established religious practice.

Respondent urges upon us that the "belief-action" dichotomy was expressly rejected by the Court in *Yoder.* . . . What the Court actually rejected was the "idea that religiously grounded conduct is always outside the protection of the Free Exercise Clause." The consistent holding of the courts has been that belief is *always* protected, but that conduct or action is subject to regulation in the manner and to the extent hereinabove set forth.

The opinion of the [Tennessee] Court of Appeals [in this case] . . . reasons that subsequent decisions of the Supreme Court of the United States "have removed the theoretical underpinnings on which [*Harden,* an earlier Tennessee decision] was based." The opinion recites: "The *Harden* decision was premised on the subsequently rejected belief-action dichotomy in free exercise cases, requiring merely a rational relationship between restrictions on religious conduct and the state interest served by the restrictions."

We respectfully differ with our brothers of the Court of Appeals. . . .

We read nothing in *Yoder* that would fault the analytic approach of the *Harden* Court or cause us to reject its reasoning or results.

We hold that under the First Amendment to the Constitution of the United States and under the substantially stronger provisions of Article 1, Section 3 of the Constitution of Tennessee, a religious practice may be limited, curtailed or restrained to the point of outright prohibition, where it involves a clear and present danger to the interests of society; but the action of the state must be reasonable and reasonably dictated by the needs and demands of society as determined by the nature of the activity as balanced against societal interests. Essentially, therefore, the problem becomes one of a balancing of interests between religious freedom and the preservation of the health, safety and morals of society. The scales must be weighed in favor of religious freedom, and yet the balance is delicate.

The right to the free exercise of religion is not absolute and unconditional. Nor is its sweep susceptible of discrete and concrete compartmentalization. It is perforce, of necessity, a vague and nebulous notion, defying the certainties of definition and the niceties of description. At some point the freedom of the individual must wane and the power, duty and interest of the state becomes compelling and dominant.

Certain guidelines do, however, emerge under both constitutions. Free exercise of religion does not include the right to violate statutory law. It does not include the right to commit or maintain a nuisance. The fact that one acts from the promptings of religious beliefs does not immunize against lawless conduct. But, again, the scales are always weighted in favor of free exercise and the state's interest must be compelling; it must be substantial; the danger must be clear and present and so grave as to endanger paramount public interests.

We decide this controversy in the light of these objectives. In doing so we have not lost sight of the fact that snake handling is central to respondents' faith. We recognize that to forbid snake handling is to remove the theological heart of the Holiness Church and this has prompted this Court to investigate and research this matter with meticulous care and to announce its decision through an unusually extensive opinion.

V

We agree with the Court of Appeals that Tennessee's snake handling statute (§ 39-2208 T.C.A.) is not controlling. However, it cannot be ignored. It proscribes, to some extent, the conduct with which we deal. The trial judge based his judgment, in part, upon its violation and, in a very real sense, it represents a part of the public policy of our state, as declared by the legislature.

This statute is not as comprehensive or as conclusive as is generally believed. Nor is it a model of clarity. In material particulars it makes it unlawful "(t)o display, exhibit, handle or use any poisonous or dangerous snake or reptile *in such manner as to endanger the life or health of any person.*"

At a glance, it is self-evident that it does not forbid snake handling *per se*. It condemns the *manner* and not the *fact* of snake handling. Conversely it permits snake handling if done in a careful and prudent manner or, in the statutory terminology, under any circumstances or in any manner which does not endanger the life or health of any person.

Obviously, it was not intended to prevent zoologists or herpetologists from handling snakes or reptiles as a part of their professional pursuits, nor to preclude handling by those who do so as a hobby, nor those who are engaged in scientific or medical pursuits requiring the handling of snakes.

It is equally obvious that the phrase "any person" must mean any other person. If the Legislature had not so intended it would have placed a period at the end of the word reptile, leaving language which made it unlawful "to display, exhibit, handle or use any poisonous snake or reptile." Not having done this one must logically assume that the Legislature was concerned with the *manner* and not the *fact* of snake handling, leaving the zoologist, the herpetologist or anyone else to their own devices subject only to the admonition that their handling must not be done "in such manner as to endanger the life or health of any (other) person." But this is from a standpoint of criminal violations.

Convictions under this statute involve proof of two elements: (1) that poisonous or dangerous snakes or reptiles were handled and (2) in such manner as to endanger the life or health of any other person. . . .

. . . .

Under this record, showing as it does, the handling of snakes in a crowded church sanctuary, with virtually no safeguards, with children roaming about unattended, with the handlers so enraptured and entranced that they are in a virtual state of hysteria and acting under the compulsion of "anointment," we would be derelict in our duty if we did not hold that respondents and their confederates have combined and conspired to commit a public nuisance and plan to continue to do so. The human misery and loss of life at their "Homecoming" of April 7, 1970 is proof positive.

Our research confirms the general pattern.

Tennessee has the right to guard against the unnecessary creation of widows and orphans. Our state and nation have an interest in having a strong, healthy, robust, taxpaying citizenry capable of self-support and of bearing arms and adding to the resources and reserves of manpower. We, therefore, have a substantial and compelling state interest in the face of a clear and present danger so grave as to endanger paramount public interests.

It has been held that a state may compel polio shots, *McCartney v. Austin*, 57 Misc. 2d 525, 293 N.Y.S.2d 188 (Sup. Ct. 1968); may regulate child labor, *Prince v. Massachusetts*, 321 U.S. 158, 64 S. Ct. 438, 88 L. Ed. 645 (1944); may require compulsory chest x-rays, State ex rel. *Holcomb v. Armstrong,* 39 Wash. 2d 860, 239 P.2d 545 (1955); may decree compulsory water fluoridation, *Kraus v. City of Cleveland,* 163 Ohio St. 559, 127 N.E.2d 609 (1955); may mandate vaccinations as a condition of school attendance, *Wright v. Dewitt School District,* 238 Ark. 906, 385 S.W.2d 644 (1965); and may compel medical care to a dying patient, *Application of President and Directors of Georgetown College, Inc.,* 118 U.S. App. D.C. 80, 331 F.2d 1000 (1964).

. . . [W]e hold that those who publicly handle snakes in the presence of other persons and those who are present aiding and abetting are guilty of creating and maintaining a public nuisance. Yes, the state has a right to protect a person from himself and to demand that he protect his own life.

. . . .

## VIII

The trial judge enjoined the respondents from handling poisonous snakes or using deadly poisons in any church service . . . but authorized the consumption of strychnine. He erred. The Court of Appeals modified the injunction so as to enjoin respondents from handling, displaying or exhibiting dangerous and poisonous snakes in such manner as will endanger the life or health of persons who do not consent to exposure to such danger. There is no reason . . . for applying a "consenting adult" criterion.

On remand the trial judge will enter an injunction perpetually enjoining and restraining all parties respondent from handling, displaying or exhibiting dangerous and poisonous snakes or from consuming strychnine or any other poisonous substances, within the confines of the State of Tennessee.

At this time it is view of this Court that no useful purpose would be served by punishing respondents for contempt of court.

. . . We gave consideration to limiting the prohibition to handling snakes in the presence of children, but rejected this approach because it conflicts with the parental right and duty to direct the religious training of his children. We considered the adoption of a "consenting adult" standard but, again, this practice is too fraught with danger to permit its pursuit in the frenzied atmosphere of an emotional church service, regardless of age or consent. We considered restricting attendance to members only, but this would destroy the evangelical mission of the church. We considered permitting only the handlers themselves to be present, but this frustrates the purpose of confirming the faith to non-believers and separates the pastor and leaders from the congregation. We could find no rational basis for limiting or restricting the practice, and could conceive of no alternative plan or procedure which would be palatable to the membership or permissible from a standpoint of compelling state interest. The very considerations which impel us to outright prohibition would preclude fragmentation of the religious services or the pursuit of this practice on a limited basis.

\* \* \*

# EMPLOYMENT DIVISION v. SMITH
## 494 U.S. 872 (1990)

Scalia, Justice.

\* \* \*

This case requires us to decide whether the Free Exercise Clause of the First Amendment permits the State of Oregon to include religiously inspired peyote use within the reach of its general criminal prohibition on use of that drug, and thus permits the State to deny unemployment benefits to persons dismissed from their jobs because of such religiously inspired use.

I

Oregon law prohibits the knowing or intentional possession of a "controlled substance" unless the substance has been prescribed by a medical practitioner. The law defines "controlled substance" as a drug classified in Schedules I through V of the Federal Controlled Substances Act. Persons who violate this provision by possessing a controlled substance listed on Schedule I are "guilty of a Class B felony." As compiled by the State Board of Pharmacy under its statutory authority, see § 475.035, Schedule I contains the drug peyote, a hallucinogen derived from the plant *Lophophora williamsii Lemaire. . . .*

Respondents Alfred Smith and Galen Black (hereinafter respondents) were fired from their jobs with a private drug rehabilitation organization because they ingested peyote for sacramental purposes at a ceremony of the Native American Church, of which both are members. When respondents applied to petitioner Employment Division (hereinafter petitioner) for unemployment compensation, they were determined to be ineligible for benefits because they had been discharged for work-related "misconduct." The Oregon Court of Appeals reversed that determination, holding that the denial of benefits violated the respondents' free exercise rights under the First Amendment. [The Oregon Supreme Court agreed.]

. . . .

II

A.

The Free Exercise Clause of the First Amendment, which has been made applicable to the States by incorporation into the Fourteenth Amendment . . . provides that "Congress shall make no law respecting an establishment of religion, or *prohibiting the free exercise thereof. . . .*" U.S. Const., Amdt. 1 (emphasis added). The free exercise of religion means, first and foremost, the right to believe and profess whatever religious doctrine one desires. Thus, the First

Amendment obviously excludes all "governmental regulation of religious *beliefs* as such." The government may not compel affirmation of religious belief, punish the expression of religious doctrines it believes to be false, impose special disabilities on the basis of religious views or religious status, or lend its power to one or the other side in controversies over religious authority or dogma. . . .

But the "exercise of religion" often involves not only belief and profession but the performance of (or abstention from) physical acts: assembling with others for a worship service, participating in sacramental use of bread and wine, proselytizing, abstaining from certain foods or certain modes of transportation. It would be true, we think (though no case of ours has involved the point), that a State would be "prohibiting the free exercise [of religion]" if it sought to ban such acts or abstentions only when they are engaged in them for religious reasons, or only because of the religious belief that they display. . . .

Respondents in the present case, however, seek to carry the meaning of "prohibiting the free exercise [of religion]" one large step further. They contend that their religious motivation for using peyote places them beyond the reach of criminal law that is not specifically directed at their religious practice, and that is concededly constitutional as applied to those who use the drug for other reasons. They assert, in other words, that "prohibiting the free exercise [of religion]" includes requiring any individual to observe a generally applicable law that requires (or forbids) the performance of an act that his religious belief forbids (or requires). . . .

. . . We have never held that an individual's religious beliefs excuse him from compliance with an otherwise valid law prohibiting conduct that the State is free to regulate. . . . We first had occasion to assert that principle in *Reynolds v. United States,* 98 U.S. 145, 25 L. Ed. 244 (1879), where we rejected the claim that criminal laws against polygamy could not be constitutionally applied to those whose religion commanded the practice. "Laws," we said, "are made for the government of actions, and while they cannot interfere with mere religious belief and opinions, they may with practices. . . ."

Subsequent decisions have consistently held that the right of free exercise does not relieve an individual of the obligation to comply with a "valid and neutral law of general applicability on the ground that the law proscribes (or prescribes) conduct that his religion prescribes (or proscribes)." In *Prince v. Massachusetts,* 321 U.S. 158, 88 L. Ed. 645, 64 S. Ct. 438 (1944), we held that a mother could be prosecuted under the child labor laws for using her children to dispense literature in the streets, her religious motivation notwithstanding. In *Braunfeld v. Brown,* 366 U.S. 599, 6 L. Ed. 2d 563, 81 S. Ct. 1144 (1961) (plurality opinion), we upheld Sunday-closing laws against the claim that they burdened the religious practices of persons whose religions compelled them to refrain from work on other days. In *Gillette v. United States,* 401 U.S. 437, 461, 28 L. Ed. 2d 168, 91 S. Ct. 828 (1971), we sustained the military Selective Service System against the claim that it violated free exercise by conscripting persons who opposed a particular war on religious grounds.

Our most recent decision involving a neutral, generally applicable regulatory law that compelled activity forbidden by an individual's religion was

*United States v. Lee,* 455 U.S., at 258–261, 71 L. Ed. 2d 127, 102 S. Ct. 1051. There, an Amish employer, on behalf of himself and his employees, sought exemption from collection and payment of Social Security taxes on the ground that the Amish faith prohibited participation in governmental support programs. We rejected the claim that an exemption was constitutionally required. There would be no way to distinguish the Amish believer's objection to Social Security taxes from the religious objections that others might have to the collection or use of other taxes. . . .

The only decisions in which we have held that the First Amendment bars application of a neutral, generally applicable law to religiously motivated action have involved not the Free Exercise Clause alone, but the Free Exercise Clause in conjunction with other constitutional protections, such as freedom of speech and of the press.

. . . .

The present case does not present such a hybrid situation, but a free exercise claim unconnected with any communicative activity or parental right. Respondents urge us to hold, quite simply, that when otherwise prohibitable conduct is accompanied by religious convictions, not only the convictions but the conduct itself must be free from governmental regulation. We have never held that, and decline to do so now. There being no contention that Oregon's drug law represents an attempt to regulate religious beliefs, the communication of religious beliefs, or the raising of one's children in those beliefs, the rule to which we have adhered ever since *Reynolds* plainly controls. . . .

### B.

Respondents argue that even though exemption from generally applicable criminal laws need not automatically be extended to religiously motivated actors, at least the claim for a religious exemption must be evaluated under the balancing test set forth in *Sherbert v. Verner,* 374 U.S. 398, 10 L. Ed. 2d 965, 83 S. Ct. 1790 (1963). Under the *Sherbert* test, governmental actions that substantially burden a religious practice must be justified by a compelling governmental interest. Applying that test we have, on three occasions, invalidated state unemployment compensation rules that conditioned the availability of benefits upon an applicant's willingness to work under conditions forbidden by his religion. . . . In recent years we have abstained from applying the *Sherbert* test. . . .

. . . The *Sherbert* test, it must be recalled, was developed in a context that lent itself to individualized governmental assessment of the reasons for the relevant conduct. As a plurality of the Court noted in *Roy,* a distinctive feature of unemployment compensation programs is that their eligibility criteria invite consideration of the particular circumstances behind an applicant's unemployment. . . .

Whether or not the decisions are that limited, they at least have nothing to do with an across-the-board criminal prohibition on a particular form of conduct. Although, as noted earlier, we have sometimes used the *Sherbert* test to analyze free exercise challenges to such laws, we have never applied the test to invalidate one. We conclude today that the sounder approach, and the approach in accord with the vast majority of our precedents, is to hold the test inapplicable to such challenges. The government's ability to enforce generally applicable prohibitions of socially harmful conduct, like its ability to carry out other aspects of public policy, "cannot depend on measuring the effects of a governmental action on a religious objector's spiritual development." . . .

Values that are protected against government interference through enshrinement in the Bill of Rights are not thereby banished from the political process. Just as a society that believes in the negative protection accorded to the press by the First Amendment is likely to enact laws that affirmatively foster the dissemination of the printed word, so also a society that believes in the negative protection accorded to religious belief can be expected to be solicitous of that value in its legislation as well. It is therefore not surprising that a number of States have made an exception to their drug laws for sacramental peyote use. But to say that a nondiscriminatory religious-practice exemption is permitted, or even that it is desirable, is not to say that it is constitutionally required, and that the appropriate occasions for its creation can be discerned by the courts. It may fairly be said that leaving accommodation to the political process will place at a relative disadvantage those religious practices that are not widely engaged in; but that unavoidable consequence of democratic government must be preferred to a system in which each conscience is a law unto itself or in which judges weigh the social importance of all laws against the centrality of all religious beliefs.

Because respondents' ingestion of peyote was prohibited under Oregon law, and because that prohibition is constitutional, Oregon may, consistent with the Free Exercise Clause, deny respondents unemployment compensation when their dismissal results from use of the drug. The decision of the Oregon Supreme Court is accordingly reversed.

\* \* \*

# LEPAGE v. STATE
## 18 P.3d 1177 (Wyoming 2001)

Kite, Justice.

\* \* \*

### Issues

Appellant Susan LePage presents the following issue: Did the Wyoming Department of Health act arbitrarily and capriciously or otherwise abuse its discretion and legal authority in denying the claimed religious exemption of Appellant? Appellee State of Wyoming, Department of Health phrases the issues as follows: Was the Department of Health's final decision to deny the Appellant's request for a religious exemption in accordance with the law? Was the Department of Health's denial of Appellant's request for a religious exemption constitutional and supported by substantial evidence?

Facts

On March 25, 1999, Mrs. LePage requested a religious exemption from the hepatitis B vaccination pursuant to § 21-4-309(a) on behalf of her daughter. Mrs. LePage outlined her concerns regarding the hepatitis B vaccination in a four-page letter. The State Health Officer for the Department of Health delayed a decision pending receipt of further information to assure that faith served as the basis for the request. In particular, the State Health Officer asked Mrs. LePage to define her beliefs as being religious-based and to explain how she acted upon her faith in a consistent manner. Mrs. LePage responded with a second letter, which restated her concerns. On June 10, 1999, Mrs. LePage's request for exemption was denied, and she was informed that, if her daughter was not immunized, she would be unable to attend school.

Mrs. LePage's initial letter began: "We, the parents . . . are petitioning for religious exemption of the Hepatitis B vaccine. Because of the strong religious beliefs of our family, we do not believe our daughter will engage in behavior that involve[s] exposure to blood or body fluids. We believe that the instituting of mandatory Hepatitis B vaccines is the direct result of our children growing up in a declining moral culture."

Mrs. LePage requested a hearing, and the matter was referred to the Office of Administrative Hearings (OAH). A hearing was held on August 5, 1999, at which time Mrs. LePage stated she had recently concluded that all vaccines were not "[G]od[']s will for our lives." The OAH rendered its decision and determined that Mrs. LePage had failed to provide evidence to justify the religious exemption. The Department of Health issued an amended final decision on September 28, 1999, which specifically found that Mrs. LePage's objection was based on personal, moral, or philosophical beliefs rather than on a principle of religion or a truly held religious conviction. Mrs. LePage appealed from the decision, and the district court certified the case to this court. . . .

[According to the court, the trial evidence shows that LePage did have her children vaccinated against other diseases in the past. It also shows that when LePage initially requested the religious exemption, it was based on her personal belief that the mandatory vaccination condoned immoral behavior which was contrary to how she raised her children. According to the court: "Both of her letters and the attachments provide information which showed that LePage's objection, while religiously based, was in fact philosophical. . . . The first time LePage expressed a truly religious based objection to the hepatitis B vaccine was at the hearing. [The defendants claimed] that the agency does not question that LePage is a devoutly religious individual and that she spent extensive time praying, fasting and reading the Bible. [Nor does it] question the fact that LePage now believes that all vaccinations are contrary to the word of her God and that she believes she sinned when having her children vaccinated in the past."

## Standard of Review

When a case is certified to this court, we examine the administrative agency's decision as if we were the reviewing court of the first instance. The issue presented in this case requires us to interpret [the state's law]. . . . This court affirms an agency's conclusions of law when they are in accordance with the law. When an agency has not invoked and properly applied the correct rule of law, we correct the agency's errors.

## Discussion

The United States Supreme Court held in *Jacobson v. Massachusetts* that a state has the authority to enact a mandatory immunization program through the exercise of its police power. Moreover, § 35-4-101 grants the Department of Health the power to prescribe rules and regulations for the management and control of communicable diseases. The question presented in this case requires us to interpret the language of § 21-4-309(a) which provides for mandatory immunization of Wyoming school children. That statute provides in pertinent part: "(a) Any person attending, full or part time, any public or private school, kindergarten through twelfth grade, shall within thirty (30) days after the date of school entry, provide to the appropriate school official written documentary proof of immunization. . . . Waivers shall be authorized by the state or county health officer upon submission of written evidence of religious objection or medical contraindication to the administration of any vaccine."

Mrs. LePage asserts the clear language of the exemption statute confirms that the issuance of a religious exemption is not a discretionary function but is a ministerial duty on the part of the Department of Health. Therefore, the Department of Health exceeded its authority by requiring more than an initial written objection which by statute appears to be sufficient to obtain a waiver. Conversely, the Department of Health argues that Wyoming's immunization waiver allows only for religious objections as opposed to personal or philosophical objections. Therefore, the Department of Health must review the asserted objection and determine whether it is based on sincerely held religious beliefs. The Department of Health determined that Mrs. LePage's religious waiver request was based on concerns regarding the health and safety risks of the vaccination as well as the mode of transmission of the hepatitis B virus. According to the Department of Health, Mrs. LePage failed to establish that the requested waiver was based on sincerely held religious beliefs which would entitle her to a waiver.

In interpreting statutes, we primarily determine the legislature's intent from the words used in the statute. . . . First, we must determine . . . "if the statute is ambiguous by looking at the plain and ordinary meaning of the words contained therein." A "statute is unambiguous if its wording is such that reasonable persons are able to agree as to its meaning with consistency and predictability." "[W]hether an ambiguity exists in a statute is a matter of law to be determined by the court." However, "[s]trict adherence to our Wyoming constitution demands that the judicial branch of government recognize that it is without discretion, nor does it have any latitude, to apply statutes contrary to legislative intent once that intent has been ascertained."

The principal language in the statute which delineates the requirement to obtain a waiver provides: "Waivers shall be authorized." This court has observed that, when the word "shall" is employed, it is usually legally accepted as mandatory. Where a statute uses the mandatory language "shall," a court must obey the statute as a court has no right to make the law contrary to what is prescribed by the legislature.

The choice of the word "shall" intimates an absence of discretion by the Department of Health and is sufficiently definitive of the mandatory rule intended by the legislature. Similarly, the statutory language lacks any mention of an inquiry by the state into the sincerity of religious beliefs. As a result, the Department of Health exceeded its legislative authority when it conducted a further inquiry into the sincerity of Mrs. LePage's religious beliefs.

. . . As a creature of the legislature, an administrative agency has only the powers granted to it by statute, and the justification for the exercise of any authority by the agency must be found within the applicable statute. A statute will be strictly construed when determining the authority granted to an agency. . . . In other words, reasonable doubt of the existence of a power must be resolved against the exercise thereof. . . . The statute provides mandatory language, and the Department of Health may not circumvent the legislature's clear limitation of its powers or expand its power beyond its statutory authority. There is no justification found within the statute for the Department of Health to institute a religious inquiry. As a result, the decision to do so is not in accordance with the law.

Furthermore, construing the statute as the Department of Health suggests raises questions concerning the extent to which the government should be involved in the religious lives of its citizens. Should an individual be forced to present evidence of his/her religious beliefs to be scrutinized by a governmental employee? If parents have not consistently expressed those religious beliefs over time, should they be denied an exemption? Can parents have beliefs that are both philosophical and religious without disqualifying their exemption request? Should the government require a certain level of sincerity as a benchmark before an exemption can be granted? If the legislature chose to address these types of questions with further legislation, such legislation would call into question the constitutional prohibition against governmental interference with the free exercise of religion under Article 1, section 18 of the Wyoming Constitution. However, those issues need not be addressed in this case because the statute does not provide the authority for such inquiry.

. . . .

We recognize the genuine concern that there could be increased requests for exemption and a potential for improper evasion of immunization. The state certainly has a valid interest in protecting public school children from unwarranted exposure to infectious diseases. However, we have been presented with no evidence that the number of religious exemption waiver requests are excessive and are confident in our presumption that parents act in the best interest of their children's physical, as well as their spiritual, health. Again, if problems regarding the health of Wyoming's school children develop because this self-executing statutory exemption is being abused, it is the legislature's responsibility to act within the constraints of the Wyoming and United States Constitutions.

* * *

# NOTES AND QUESTIONS

**1.** There are a few situations in which more rigorous judicial scrutiny of public health legislation has been justified by the law's impact on family autonomy, religious practices, or other individual, constitutionally protected rights. For present purposes, legislation affecting the practice of religion is probably the most illustrative example. In such circumstances, the courts may undertake to weigh independently the merits and impact of the legislation on the asserted constitutional interests, much as the *Lochner* did, rather than defer to legislative judgment as in *Jacobson*. In some cases, such as was demonstrated in *State v. Hershberger*, discussed in Section B[2], Note 3, *supra*, the legislation is invalidated; in others, the courts independently weigh the merits of the legislation yet ultimately uphold the state legislation.

*Swann v. Pack* is a good illustration, albeit one with a somewhat offbeat set of facts. Note first of all that, analogous to the helmet and seat belt decisions, the Tennessee court struggled — not very successfully — to characterize the legislation as designed exclusively for the protection of third parties. Three paragraphs after observing that the criminal statute was "not a model of clarity," the court declared it "obvious" that the law's prohibition against handling poisonous reptiles must apply exclusively to endangerment of persons "other" than the practitioner himself. Consider the statutory language yourself. Is the court's reading "obvious," rather than debatable or even strained? Perhaps the court, without explanation, was implementing the frequently-invoked principle that courts should "strictly" interpret ambiguous criminal statutes, to avoid unfairness and lack of notice to defendants about what conduct is proscribed. Whatever the reason, the court's interpretation of the statute makes it unnecessary for it to address openly a tough question: whether the state may use the *criminal* law to prohibit a religious practice on the ground that it is hazardous to the practitioner himself.

But the proper meaning of the criminal statute does not seem to be the actual issue in the case. No criminal charges were actually filed in *Swann*. Rather, the issue concerns application of the *equitable* remedy of injunction. And in this context, the court does not appear to be so hesitant: It orders entry of a permanent injunction against the contested hazardous practices. In explanation, the court *embraces* the permissibility of barring religiously-based practices in the interest of protecting the *practitioners themselves* against the hazards: "Yes, the state has a right to protect a person from himself and to demand that he protect his own life."

Why is the court so eager to avoid possible *criminal* punishment of persons who engage in religious rituals hazardous to themselves, while at the same time willing to impose an equally-"paternalistic" *civil* injunction against performance of the same rituals? Is the court applying close scrutiny? Do you agree with the court's disposition of the case?

However you view the outcome and reasoning of the *Swann* decision, not all laws that have some effect on religion or religious activities will be given this sort of careful (albeit still somewhat unclear) judicial consideration. This is the significance of the *Smith* decision.

The implications of *Smith* are hard to appreciate outside of the context of the earlier decisions in *Sherbert v. Verner*, 374 U.S. 398 (1963), *Wisconsin v. Yoder*, 406 U.S. 205 (1972) and other decisions in which the Supreme Court appeared to "closely scrutinize" state laws that had an effect on the practice of religion, even where those laws were laws of "general applicability." In *Smith*, a slim majority of the Court attempted — somewhat unsuccessfully — to distinguish these earlier cases on their facts and claim that *Smith* was a factually different case, one involving a law of general applicability. But the laws in *Sherbert* (denying benefits to people who voluntarily refused employment) and *Yoder* (requiring all people to send their children to school until the age of sixteen) were apparently laws of "general applicability" as well: neither targeted religiously motivated conduct. Nonetheless, the *Smith* majority found these earlier cases distinguishable. For a further discussion of these earlier cases and the distinction made in *Smith,* see *City of Boerne v. Flores*, 521 U.S. 507 (1997).

Barring a reversal of *Smith*, what the majority of the Court holds is that a law of general applicability that neither singles out religious activities nor is intended to regulate religious activities does not affect — in the constitutional sense — those activities. (Consider: Do you think the law in *Swann* was such a law?) As a consequence, a reviewing court need only find that the law is rationally related to some legitimate state interest; close scrutiny appears to have been abandoned for laws that are characterized this way. Thus, even where a public health law of general applicability affects, in any real or practical sense, the practice of religion, it does not affect it in the constitutional sense of implicating the First Amendment's heightened protection of the exercise of religion. As a consequence, that law need only be a rational exercise of the states' authority. Whether *Smith* applies to other rights protected by the First Amendment or, for that matter, to other constitutional rights, is not clear from *Smith* or any of the Court's subsequent decisions. Nonetheless, the case's holding illustrates an important corollary to states' basic public health authority, underscoring legislative power to regulate broadly and emphasizing the limited role of the courts in reviewing exercises of that power.

**2.** *LePage* raises nearly the mirror-image problem to that of *Smith*: Can the state constitutionally choose to *exempt* some individuals, on the basis of their religious beliefs, from otherwise-valid public health laws? The answer is not entirely straightforward. Note, at the outset, that the court does not doubt the state's right to require immunization as a condition for attending public school. Nor is there reason to think it would take more than a cursory look at the underlying justifications for the law, instead deferring to legislative discretion much in the manner of *Jacobson* and its progeny. So the focus is on the religious basis for exemption.

In *Prince v. Massachusetts,* 321 U.S. 158 (1944), the Court rejected a free exercise defense raised by a woman who claimed she could not constitutionally be prosecuted under child labor laws for having used her children to distribute religious pamphlets. The Court observed: "The [First Amendment] right to practice religion freely does not include liberty *to expose the community or the child to communicable disease or the latter to ill health or death.*" 321 U.S. at 166-67 (emphasis added). This language suggests that the states' interest in the health of the community in general, and in children as particular objects of government protection, outweighs religiously-based objections to compliance. In fact, as we have seen, in *Smith,* Justice Scalia invokes *Prince* as authority for the idea that a "valid and neutral law of general applicability" is not rendered unconstitutional because of its secondary impact on religious freedom. Finally, there is case law that is precisely on point. *See, e.g., Boone v. Boozman,* 217 F. Supp. 2d, 938, 952–55 (E.D. Ark. 2002) (applying *Smith* analysis to conclude that compulsory school immunization law lacking any religious exemption was a law of general applicability that did not merit heightened scrutiny and upholding the law against free exercise challenge). Accordingly, while all but two states do allow for exemption on religious grounds, these are properly understood as discretionary policy accommodations, rather than constitutional necessities.

But as *LePage* suggests, the exercise of that legislative largesse toward religious objectors to immunization can itself raise difficult federal and/or state constitutional issues. The *LePage* court in effect required the state to treat the mere fact of *claiming* a "religious" exemption as establishing, *per se,* its legitimacy. The court barred further state inquiry into the basis of the claim. What reasons, both statutory and constitutional, does the *LePage* court give for making this choice? By contrast, many other state courts have insisted (sometimes on the basis of more demanding statutory language) that the claimant prove, for example, that the objector sincerely adheres to a particular religious denomination whose articulated doctrine demonstrably rejects immunization. What arguments might support this more searching form of inquiry? Consider the hazards in both extremes.

Finally, in those states that provide exemptions only to "established" religions — presumably in order to limit opportunity for disingenuous invocation of the exemption — "non-traditional" believers may be ineligible. Accordingly, in some cases they have attacked the exemption on grounds that it favors one religion (or group of religions) over another, in violation of either the establishment (*see, e.g., Boone v. Boozman, supra,* 217 F. Supp. at 945–52) or equal protection clauses. In some of these cases, plaintiffs have prevailed.

In light of such complexities, one might think that avoiding religious exemptions entirely would be the "safest" (and surely the constitutionally simplest) legislative course to follow. The fact that these legislative exemptions are so widely adopted attests to the influence of religion in American political life, and to the felt civic need for its ongoing accommodation.

About 20 states have enacted broader exemptions based on personal philosophy or beliefs about immunization. *See, e.g.,* ARIZ. REV. STAT. § 15-873 (parents authorized to refuse immunization of child based on "personal beliefs," provided parent is informed about risks and benefits of immunization as well as risks of non-immunization) and § 15-873.C. (non-immunized children excluded from school during disease-outbreak periods). Such provisions are broad enough to *include* religiously-based objections, but they largely avoid the complexities of *specifically*-religious exemptions, outlined above. What hazards, if any, do they generate? If you were a legislator, what approach would you favor in this area?

Finally, to complete our review of legislative exemptions, all 50 states recognize exemptions for those who are shown to be medically unfit to receive immunizations. Indeed, *Jacobson* told us in *dictum* that such an exemption is constitutionally necessary, and under proper circumstances the exemption would be implied even were it not included in the law's text.

The immunization requirements of each state can be found in Sabin Vaccine Institute, *Immunization Requirements by State, available at* www.sabin.org/PDF/Immunization_schedule_2005.pdf (last visited January 2007) and in Centers for Disease Control, *2001-2002 State Immunization Requirements, available at* www.immunize.org/laws/izlaws01-02.pdf (last visited January 2007). The latter document, although current only through 2002, also identifies each state's medical, religious, or philosophical exemptions, as discussed in this Note. For a more current summary of those exemptions in all states, see The National Network for Immunization Information, *Common Questions About School Immunization Laws, available at* www.immunization info.org/assets/files/PDFs/4_SCH.pdf (last visited Jan. 7, 2007); Jody Ruskamp-Hatz and Elizabeth Hackney, *Exemptions for Childhood Immunizations*, 14(30) Nat'l Conf. of State Legislatures Legisbrief (June/July 2006).

In leaving this section, it should not be overlooked that, in any of these kinds of cases, a state's constitution may provide for more protection for religion, privacy, or any other individual interest than is reflected in federal constitutional rulings like *Smith*.

## C.  CONSTITUTIONAL PRINCIPLES: THE RIGHT TO PRIVACY

### ROE v. WADE
#### 410 U.S. 113 (1973)

Blackmun, Justice.

* * *

This Texas federal appeal presents constitutional challenges to state criminal abortion legislation. The Texas statutes under attack here are typical of those that have been in effect in many States for approximately a century. We forthwith acknowledge our awareness of the sensitive and emotional nature of the abortion controversy, of the vigorous opposing views, even among physicians, and of the deep and seemingly absolute convictions that the subject inspires. One's philosophy, one's experiences, one's exposure to the raw edges of human existence, one's religious training, one's attitudes toward life and family and their values, and the moral standards one establishes and seeks to observe, are all likely to influence and to color one's thinking and conclusions about abortion.

Our task, of course, is to resolve the issue by constitutional measurement, free of emotion and of predilection. We seek earnestly to do this, and, because we do, we have inquired into, and in this opinion place some emphasis upon, medical and medical-legal history and what that history reveals about man's attitudes toward the abortion procedure over the centuries.

## I

The Texas statutes that concern us here . . . make it a crime to "procure an abortion," as therein defined, or to attempt one, except with respect to "an abortion procured or attempted by medical advice for the purpose of saving the life of the mother." Similar statutes are in existence in a majority of the States.

## II

Jane Roe, a single woman who was residing in Dallas County, Texas, instituted this federal action in March 1970 against the District Attorney of the county. She sought a declaratory judgment that the Texas criminal abortion statutes were unconstitutional on their face, and an injunction restraining the defendant from enforcing the statutes.

Roe alleged that she was unmarried and pregnant; that she wished to terminate her pregnancy by an abortion "performed by a competent, licensed physician, under safe, clinical conditions"; that she was unable to get a "legal" abortion in Texas because her life did not appear to be threatened by the continuation of her pregnancy; and that she could not afford to travel to another jurisdiction in order to secure a legal abortion under safe conditions. She claimed that the Texas statutes were unconstitutionally vague and that they abridged her right of personal privacy, protected by the First, Fourth, Fifth, Ninth, and Fourteenth Amendments. By an amendment to her complaint Roe purported to sue "on behalf of herself and all other women" similarly situated.

The appellee notes, however, that the record does not disclose that Roe was pregnant at the time of the District Court hearing on May 22, 1970, or on the following June 17 when the court's opinion and judgment were filed. And he suggests that Roe's case must now be moot because she and all other members of her class are no longer subject to any 1970 pregnancy.

But when, as here, pregnancy is a significant fact in the litigation, the normal 266-day human gestation period is so short that the pregnancy will come to term before the usual appellate process is complete. If that termination makes a case moot, pregnancy litigation seldom will survive much beyond the trial stage, and appellate review will be effectively denied. Our law should not be that rigid. Pregnancy often comes more than once to the same woman, and in the general population, if man is to survive, it will always be with us. Pregnancy provides a classic justification for a conclusion of nonmootness. It truly could be "capable of repetition, yet evading review."

We, therefore, agree with the District Court that Jane Roe had standing to undertake this litigation, that she presented a justiciable controversy, and that the termination of her 1970 pregnancy has not rendered her case moot.

V

The principal thrust of appellant's attack on the Texas statutes is that they improperly invade a right, said to be possessed by the pregnant woman, to choose to terminate her pregnancy. Appellant would discover this right in the concept of personal "liberty" embodied in the Fourteenth Amendment's Due Process Clause; or in personal, marital, familial, and sexual privacy said to be protected by the Bill of Rights or its penumbras, see *Griswold v. Connecticut,* 381 U.S. 479 (1965); *Eisenstadt v. Baird,* 405 U.S. 438 (1972); or among those rights reserved to the people by the Ninth Amendment, *Griswold v. Connecticut,* 381 U.S., at 486 (Goldberg, J., concurring). Before addressing this claim, we feel it desirable briefly to survey, in several aspects, the history of abortion, for such insight as that history may afford us, and then to examine the state purposes and interests behind the criminal abortion laws.

VI

It perhaps is not generally appreciated that the restrictive criminal abortion laws in effect in a majority of States today are of relatively recent vintage. Those laws, generally proscribing abortion or its attempt at any time during pregnancy except when necessary to preserve the pregnant woman's life, are not of ancient or even of common-law origin. Instead, they derive from statutory changes effected, for the most part, in the latter half of the 19th century.

1. *Ancient attitudes.* These are not capable of precise determination. We are told that at the time of the Persian Empire abortifacients were known and that criminal abortions were severely punished. We are also told, however, that abortion was practiced in Greek times as well as in the Roman Era, and that "it was resorted to without scruple." The Ephesian, Soranos, often described as the greatest of the ancient gynecologists, appears to have been generally opposed to Rome's prevailing free-abortion practices. He found it necessary to think first of the life of the mother, and he resorted to abortion when, upon this standard, he felt the procedure advisable. Greek and Roman law afforded little protection to the unborn. If abortion was prosecuted in some places, it seems to have been based on a concept of a violation of the father's right to his offspring.

2. *The Hippocratic Oath.* What then of the famous Oath that has stood so long as the ethical guide of the medical profession and that bears the name of the great Greek (460(?)-377(?) B.C.), who has been described as the Father of Medicine, the "wisest and the greatest practitioner of his art," and the "most important and most complete medical personality of antiquity," who dominated the medical schools of his time, and who typified the sum of the medical knowledge of the past? The Oath varies somewhat according to the particular translation, but in any translation the content is clear: "I will give no deadly medicine to anyone if asked, nor suggest any such counsel; and in like manner I will not give to a woman a pessary to produce abortion."

Although the Oath is not mentioned in any of the principal briefs in this case, it represents the apex of the development of strict ethical concepts in medicine, and its influence endures to this day. Why did not the authority of Hippocrates dissuade abortion practice in his time and that of Rome? The late Dr. Edelstein provides us with a theory: The Oath was not uncontested even in Hippocrates' day; only the Pythagorean school of philosophers frowned upon the related act of suicide. Most Greek thinkers, on the other hand, commended abortion, at least prior to viability. For the Pythagoreans, however, it was a matter of dogma. For them the embryo was animate from the moment of conception, and abortion meant destruction of a living being. The abortion clause of the Oath, therefore, "echoes Pythagorean doctrines," and "in no other stratum of Greek opinion were such views held or proposed in the same spirit of uncompromising austerity."

Dr. Edelstein then concludes that the Oath originated in a group representing only a small segment of Greek opinion and that it certainly was not accepted by all ancient physicians. He points out that medical writings down to Galen (A.D. 130-200) "give evidence of the violation of almost every one of its injunctions." But with the end of antiquity a decided change took place. Resistance against suicide and against abortion became common. The Oath came to be popular. The emerging teachings of Christianity were in agreement with the Pythagorean ethic. The Oath "became the nucleus of all medical ethics" and "was applauded as the embodiment of truth." Thus, suggests Dr. Edelstein, it is "a Pythagorean manifesto and not the expression of an absolute standard of medical conduct."

This, it seems to us, is a satisfactory and acceptable explanation of the Hippocratic Oath's apparent rigidity. It enables us to understand, in historical context, a long-accepted and revered statement of medical ethics.

3. *The common law.* It is undisputed that at common law, abortion performed before "quickening" — the first recognizable movement of the fetus *in utero*, appearing usually from the 16th to the 18th week of pregnancy — was not an indictable offense. The absence of a common-law crime for pre-quickening abortion appears to have developed from a confluence of earlier philosophical, theological, and civil and canon law concepts of when life begins. These disciplines variously approached the question in terms of the point at which the embryo or fetus became "formed" or recognizably human, or in terms of when a "person" came into being, that is, infused with a "soul" or "animated." A loose consensus evolved in early English law that these events occurred at some point between conception and live birth. This was "mediate animation." Although Christian theology and the canon law came to fix the point of animation at 40 days for a male and 80 days for a female, a view that persisted until the 19th century, there was otherwise little agreement about the precise time of formation or animation. There was agreement, however, that prior to this point the fetus was to be regarded as part of the mother, and its destruction, therefore, was not homicide. Due to continued uncertainty about the precise time when animation occurred, to the lack of any empirical basis for the 40-80-day view, and perhaps to Aquinas' definition of movement as one of the two first principles of life, Bracton focused upon quickening as

the critical point. The significance of quickening was echoed by later common-law scholars and found its way into the received common law in this country.

Whether abortion of a quick fetus was a felony at common law, or even a lesser crime, is still disputed. Bracton, writing early in the 13th century, thought it homicide. But the later and predominant view, following the great common-law scholars, has been that it was, at most, a lesser offense. In a frequently cited passage, Coke took the position that abortion of a woman "quick with child" is "a great misprision, and no murder." Blackstone followed, saying that while abortion after quickening had once been considered manslaughter (though not murder), "modern law" took a less severe view. A recent review of the common-law precedents argues, however, that those precedents contradict Coke and that even post-quickening abortion was never established as a common-law crime. This is of some importance because while most American courts ruled, in holding or *dictum*, that abortion of an unquickened fetus was not criminal under their received common law, others followed Coke in stating that abortion of a quick fetus was a "misprision," a term they translated to mean "misdemeanor." That their reliance on Coke on this aspect of the law was uncritical and, apparently in all the reported cases, *dictum* (due probably to the paucity of common-law prosecutions for post-quickening abortion), makes it now appear doubtful that abortion was ever firmly established as a common-law crime even with respect to the destruction of a quick fetus.

4. *The English statutory law.* England's first criminal abortion statute, Lord Ellenborough's Act, came in 1803. It made abortion of a quick fetus, § 1, a capital crime, but in § 2 it provided lesser penalties for the felony of abortion before quickening, and thus preserved the "quickening" distinction. In 1929, the Infant Life (Preservation) Act, came into being. Its emphasis was upon the destruction of "the life of a child capable of being born alive." It made a willful act performed with the necessary intent a felony. It contained a proviso that one was not to be found guilty of the offense "unless it is proved that the act which caused the death of the child was not done in good faith for the purpose only of preserving the life of the mother."

Recently, Parliament enacted a new abortion law. This is the Abortion Act of 1967. The Act permits a licensed physician to perform an abortion where two other licensed physicians agree (a) "that the continuance of the pregnancy would involve risk to the life of the pregnant woman, or of injury to the physical or mental health of the pregnant woman or any existing children of her family, greater than if the pregnancy were terminated," or (b) "that there is a substantial risk that if the child were born it would suffer from such physical or mental abnormalities as to be seriously handicapped."

5. *The American law.* In this country, the law in effect in all but a few States until mid-19th century was the pre-existing English common law. Connecticut, the first State to enact abortion legislation, adopted in 1821 that part of Lord Ellenborough's Act that related to a woman "quick with child." The death penalty was not imposed. Abortion before quickening was made a crime in that State only in 1860. In 1828, New York enacted legislation that, in two respects, was to serve as a model for early anti-abortion statutes. First, while barring destruction of an unquickened fetus as well as a quick fetus, it made the

former only a misdemeanor, but the latter second-degree manslaughter. Second, it incorporated a concept of therapeutic abortion by providing that an abortion was excused if it "shall have been necessary to preserve the life of such mother, or shall have been advised by two physicians to be necessary for such purpose." By 1840, when Texas had received the common law, only eight American States had statutes dealing with abortion. It was not until after the War Between the States that legislation began generally to replace the common law. Most of these initial statutes dealt severely with abortion after quickening but were lenient with it before quickening. Most punished attempts equally with completed abortions. While many statutes included the exception for an abortion thought by one or more physicians to be necessary to save the mother's life, that provision soon disappeared and the typical law required that the procedure actually be necessary for that purpose.

Gradually, in the middle and late 19th century the quickening distinction disappeared from the statutory law of most States and the degree of the offense and the penalties were increased. By the end of the 1950's, a large majority of the jurisdictions banned abortion, however and whenever performed, unless done to save or preserve the life of the mother. The exceptions, Alabama and the District of Columbia, permitted abortion to preserve the mother's health. Three States permitted abortions that were not "unlawfully" performed or that were not "without lawful justification," leaving interpretation of those standards to the courts. In the past several years, however, a trend toward liberalization of abortion statutes has resulted in adoption, by about one-third of the States, of less stringent laws

It is thus apparent that at common law, at the time of the adoption of our Constitution, and throughout the major portion of the 19th century, abortion was viewed with less disfavor than under most American statutes currently in effect. Phrasing it another way, a woman enjoyed a substantially broader right to terminate a pregnancy than she does in most States today. At least with respect to the early stage of pregnancy, and very possibly without such a limitation, the opportunity to make this choice was present in this country well into the 19th century. Even later, the law continued for some time to treat less punitively an abortion procured in early pregnancy.

*6. The position of the American Medical Association.* The anti-abortion mood prevalent in this country in the late 19th century was shared by the medical profession. Indeed, the attitude of the profession may have played a significant role in the enactment of stringent criminal abortion legislation during that period.

An AMA Committee on Criminal Abortion was appointed in May 1857. It presented its report, 12 Trans. of the Am. Med. Assn. 73–78 (1859), to the Twelfth Annual Meeting. That report observed that the Committee had been appointed to investigate criminal abortion "with a view to its general suppression." It deplored abortion and its frequency and it listed three causes of "this general demoralization":

> The first of these causes is a wide-spread popular ignorance of the true character of the crime — a belief, even among mothers themselves, that the foetus is not alive till after the period of quickening.

The second of the agents alluded to is the fact that the professionals themselves are frequently supposed careless of foetal life. . . .

The third reason of the frightful extent of this crime is found in the grave defects of our laws, both common and statute, as regards the independent and actual existence of the child before birth, as a living being. These errors, which are sufficient in most instances to prevent conviction, are based, and only based, upon mistaken and exploded medical dogmas. With strange inconsistency, the law fully acknowledges the foetus *in utero* and its inherent rights, for civil purposes; while personally and as criminally affected, it fails to recognize it, and to its life as yet denies all protection.

The Committee then offered, and the Association adopted, resolutions protesting "against such unwarrantable destruction of human life," calling upon state legislatures to revise their abortion laws, and requesting the cooperation of state medical societies "in pressing the subject."

In 1871 a long and vivid report was submitted by the Committee on Criminal Abortion. It ended with the observation, "We had to deal with human life. In a matter of less importance we could entertain no compromise. An honest judge on the bench would call things by their proper names. We could do no less." 22 Trans. of the Am. Med. Assn. 258 (1871). It proffered resolutions, adopted by the Association, *id.*, at 38-39, recommending, among other things, that it "be unlawful and unprofessional for any physician to induce abortion or premature labor, without the concurrent opinion of at least one respectable consulting physician, and then always with a view to the safety of the child — if that be possible," and calling "the attention of the clergy of all denominations to the perverted views of morality entertained by a large class of females — aye, and men also, on this important question."

Except for periodic condemnation of the criminal abortionist, no further formal AMA action took place until 1967. In that year, the Committee on Human Reproduction urged the adoption of a stated policy of opposition to induced abortion, except when there is "documented medical evidence" of a threat to the health or life of the mother, or that the child "may be born with incapacitating physical deformity or mental deficiency," or that a pregnancy "resulting from legally established statutory or forcible rape or incest may constitute a threat to the mental or physical health of the patient," two other physicians "chosen because of their recognized professional competence have examined the patient and have concurred in writing," and the procedure "is performed in a hospital accredited by the Joint Commission on Accreditation of Hospitals." The providing of medical information by physicians to state legislatures in their consideration of legislation regarding therapeutic abortion was "to be considered consistent with the principles of ethics of the American Medical Association." This recommendation was adopted by the House of Delegates. Proceedings of the AMA House of Delegates 40–51 (June 1967).

In 1970, after the introduction of a variety of proposed resolutions, and of a report from its Board of Trustees, a reference committee noted "polarization of the medical profession on this controversial issue"; division among those who had testified; a difference of opinion among AMA councils and committees; "the remarkable shift in testimony" in six months, felt to be influenced "by the rapid changes in state laws and by the judicial decisions which tend to make abortion more freely available"; and a feeling "that this trend will continue." On June 25, 1970, the House of Delegates adopted preambles and most of the resolutions proposed by the reference committee. The preambles emphasized "the best interests of the patient," "sound clinical judgment," and "informed patient consent," in contrast to "mere acquiescence to the patient's demand." The resolutions asserted that abortion is a medical procedure that should be performed by a licensed physician in an accredited hospital only after consultation with two other physicians and in conformity with state law, and that no party to the procedure should be required to violate personally held moral principles. Proceedings of the AMA House of Delegates 220 (June 1970). The AMA Judicial Council rendered a complementary opinion.

7. *The position of the American Public Health Association.* In October 1970, the Executive Board of the APHA adopted Standards for Abortion Services. These were five in number:

a. Rapid and simple abortion referral must be readily available through state and local public health departments, medical societies, or other nonprofit organizations.

b. An important function of counseling should be to simplify and expedite the provision of abortion services; it should not delay the obtaining of these services.

c. Psychiatric consultation should not be mandatory. As in the case of other specialized medical services, psychiatric consultation should be sought for definite indications and not on a routine basis.

d. A wide range of individuals from appropriately trained, sympathetic volunteers to highly skilled physicians may qualify as abortion counselors.

e. Contraception and/or sterilization should be discussed with each abortion patient.

Recommended Standards for Abortion Services, 61 Am. J. Pub. Health 396 (1971).

It was said that "a well-equipped hospital" offers more protection "to cope with unforeseen difficulties than an office or clinic without such resources. . . . The factor of gestational age is of overriding importance." Thus, it was recommended that abortions in the second trimester and early abortions in the presence of existing medical complications be performed in hospitals as inpatient procedures. For pregnancies in the first trimester, abortion in the hospital with or without overnight stay "is probably the safest practice." An abortion in an extramural facility, however, is an acceptable alternative "provided arrangements exist in advance to admit patients promptly if unforeseen complications develop." Standards for an abortion facility were listed. It was said that at present abortions should be performed by physicians or osteopaths who are licensed to practice and who have "adequate training."

## VII

Three reasons have been advanced to explain historically the enactment of criminal abortion laws in the 19th century and to justify their continued existence.

It has been argued occasionally that these laws were the product of a Victorian social concern to discourage illicit sexual conduct. Texas, however, does not advance this justification in the present case, and it appears that no court or commentator has taken the argument seriously. The appellants and *amici* contend, moreover, that this is not a proper state purpose at all and suggest that, if it were, the Texas statutes are overbroad in protecting it since the law fails to distinguish between married and unwed mothers.

A second reason is concerned with abortion as a medical procedure. When most criminal abortion laws were first enacted, the procedure was a hazardous one for the woman. This was particularly true prior to the development of antisepsis. Antiseptic techniques, of course, were based on discoveries by Lister, Pasteur, and others first announced in 1867, but were not generally accepted and employed until about the turn of the century. Abortion mortality was high. Even after 1900, and perhaps until as late as the development of antibiotics in the 1940's, standard modern techniques such as dilation and curettage were not nearly so safe as they are today. Thus, it has been argued that a State's real concern in enacting a criminal abortion law was to protect the pregnant woman, that is, to restrain her from submitting to a procedure that placed her life in serious jeopardy

Modern medical techniques have altered this situation. Appellants and various *amici* refer to medical data indicating that abortion in early pregnancy, that is, prior to the end of the first trimester, although not without its risk, is now relatively safe. Mortality rates for women undergoing early abortions, where the procedure is legal, appear to be as low as or lower than the rates for normal childbirth. Consequently, any interest of the State in protecting the woman from an inherently hazardous procedure, except when it would be equally dangerous for her to forgo it, has largely disappeared. Of course, important state interests in the areas of health and medical standards do remain. The State has a legitimate interest in seeing to it that abortion, like any other medical procedure, is performed under circumstances that insure maximum safety for the patient. This interest obviously extends at least to the performing physician and his staff, to the facilities involved, to the availability of after-care, and to adequate provision for any complication or emergency that might arise. The prevalence of high mortality rates at illegal "abortion mills" strengthens, rather than weakens, the State's interest in regulating the conditions under which abortions are performed. Moreover, the risk to the woman increases as her pregnancy continues. Thus, the State retains a definite interest in protecting the woman's own health and safety when an abortion is proposed at a late stage of pregnancy.

The third reason is the State's interest — some phrase it in terms of duty — in protecting prenatal life. Some of the argument for this justification rests on the theory that a new human life is present from the moment of conception. The State's interest and general obligation to protect life then extends, it is argued, to prenatal life. Only when the life of the pregnant mother herself is at stake, balanced against the life she carries within her, should the interest of the embryo or fetus not prevail. Logically, of course, a legitimate state interest in this area need not stand or fall on acceptance of the belief that life begins at conception or at some other point prior to live birth. In assessing the

State's interest, recognition may be given to the less rigid claim that as long as at least potential life is involved, the State may assert interests beyond the protection of the pregnant woman alone.

Parties challenging state abortion laws have sharply disputed in some courts the contention that a purpose of these laws, when enacted, was to protect prenatal life. Pointing to the absence of legislative history to support the contention, they claim that most state laws were designed solely to protect the woman. Because medical advances have lessened this concern, at least with respect to abortion in early pregnancy, they argue that with respect to such abortions the laws can no longer be justified by any state interest. There is some scholarly support for this view of original purpose. The few state courts called upon to interpret their laws in the late 19th and early 20th centuries did focus on the State's interest in protecting the woman's health rather than in preserving the embryo and fetus. Proponents of this view point out that in many States, including Texas, by statute or judicial interpretation, the pregnant woman herself could not be prosecuted for self-abortion or for cooperating in an abortion performed upon her by another. They claim that adoption of the "quickening" distinction through received common law and state statutes tacitly recognizes the greater health hazards inherent in late abortion and impliedly repudiates the theory that life begins at conception.

It is with these interests, and the weight to be attached to them, that this case is concerned.

### VIII

The Constitution does not explicitly mention any right of privacy. In a line of decisions, however, going back perhaps as far as *Union Pacific R. Co. v. Botsford*, 141 U.S. 250, 251 (1891), the Court has recognized that a right of personal privacy, or a guarantee of certain areas or zones of privacy, does exist under the Constitution. In varying contexts, the Court or individual Justices have, indeed, found at least the roots of that right in the First Amendment, *Stanley v. Georgia*, 394 U.S. 557, 564 (1969); in the Fourth and Fifth Amendments, *Terry v. Ohio*, 392 U.S. 1, 8-9 (1968); in the penumbras of the Bill of Rights, *Griswold v. Connecticut*, 381 U.S., at 484-485; in the Ninth Amendment, *id.*, at 486 (Goldberg, J., concurring); or in the concept of liberty guaranteed by the first section of the Fourteenth Amendment, see *Meyer v. Nebraska*, 262 U.S. 390, 399 (1923). These decisions make it clear that only personal rights that can be deemed "fundamental" or "implicit in the concept of ordered liberty," *Palko v. Connecticut*, 302 U.S. 319, 325 (1937), are included in this guarantee of personal privacy. They also make it clear that the right has some extension to activities relating to marriage, *Loving v. Virginia*, 388 U.S. 1, 12 (1967); procreation, *Skinner v. Oklahoma*, 316 U.S. 535, 541-542 (1942); contraception, *Eisenstadt v. Baird*, 405 U.S., at 453-454; *id.*, at 460, 463-465 (White, J., concurring in result); family relationships, *Prince v. Massachusetts*, 321 U.S. 158, 166 (1944); and child rearing and education, *Pierce v. Society of Sisters*, 268 U.S. 510, 535 (1925), *Meyer v. Nebraska, supra*.

This right of privacy, whether it be founded in the Fourteenth Amendment's concept of personal liberty and restrictions upon state action, as we feel it is, or, as the District Court determined, in the Ninth Amendment's reservation of rights to the people, is broad enough to encompass a woman's decision whether or not to terminate her pregnancy. The detriment that the State would impose upon the pregnant woman by denying this choice altogether is apparent. Specific and direct harm medically diagnosable even in early pregnancy may be involved. Maternity, or additional offspring, may force upon the woman a distressful life and future. Psychological harm may be imminent. Mental and physical health may be taxed by child care. There is also the distress, for all concerned, associated with the unwanted child, and there is the problem of bringing a child into a family already unable, psychologically and otherwise, to care for it. In other cases, as in this one, the additional difficulties and continuing stigma of unwed motherhood may be involved. All these are factors the woman and her responsible physician necessarily will consider in consultation.

On the basis of elements such as these, appellant and some *amici* argue that the woman's right is absolute and that she is entitled to terminate her pregnancy at whatever time, in whatever way, and for whatever reason she alone chooses. With this we do not agree. Appellant's arguments that Texas either has no valid interest at all in regulating the abortion decision, or no interest strong enough to support any limitation upon the woman's sole determination, are unpersuasive. The Court's decisions recognizing a right of privacy also acknowledge that some state regulation in areas protected by that right is appropriate. As noted above, a State may properly assert important interests in safeguarding health, in maintaining medical standards, and in protecting potential life. At some point in pregnancy, these respective interests become sufficiently compelling to sustain regulation of the factors that govern the abortion decision. The privacy right involved, therefore, cannot be said to be absolute. In fact, it is not clear to us that the claim asserted by some *amici* that one has an unlimited right to do with one's body as one pleases bears a close relationship to the right of privacy previously articulated in the Court's decisions. The Court has refused to recognize an unlimited right of this kind in the past. *Jacobson v. Massachusetts*, 197 U.S. 11 (1905) (vaccination); *Buck v. Bell*, 274 U.S. 200 (1927) (sterilization).

We, therefore, conclude that the right of personal privacy includes the abortion decision, but that this right is not unqualified and must be considered against important state interests in regulation.

We note that those federal and state courts that have recently considered abortion law challenges have reached the same conclusion. A majority, in addition to the District Court in the present case, have held state laws unconstitutional, at least in part, because of vagueness or because of overbreadth and abridgment of rights. Others have sustained state statutes.

Although the results are divided, most of these courts have agreed that the right of privacy, however based, is broad enough to cover the abortion decision; that the right, nonetheless, is not absolute and is subject to some limitations; and that at some point the state interests as to protection of health, medical standards, and prenatal life, become dominant. We agree with this approach.

Where certain "fundamental rights" are involved, the Court has held that regulation limiting these rights may be justified only by a "compelling state interest," and that legislative enactments must be narrowly drawn to express only the legitimate state interests at stake.

## IX

The District Court held that the appellee failed to meet his burden of demonstrating that the Texas statute's infringement upon Roe's rights was necessary to support a compelling state interest, and that, although the appellee presented "several compelling justifications for state presence in the area of abortions," the statutes outstripped these justifications and swept "far beyond any areas of compelling state interest." Appellant and appellee both contest that holding. Appellant, as has been indicated, claims an absolute right that bars any state imposition of criminal penalties in the area. Appellee argues that the State's determination to recognize and protect prenatal life from and after conception constitutes a compelling state interest. As noted above, we do not agree fully with either formulation.

A. The appellee and certain *amici* argue that the fetus is a "person" within the language and meaning of the Fourteenth Amendment. In support of this, they outline at length and in detail the well-known facts of fetal development. If this suggestion of personhood is established, the appellant's case, of course, collapses, for the fetus' right to life would then be guaranteed specifically by the Amendment. The appellant conceded as much on reargument. On the other hand, the appellee conceded on reargument that no case could be cited that holds that a fetus is a person within the meaning of the Fourteenth Amendment.

The Constitution does not define "person" in so many words. Section 1 of the Fourteenth Amendment contains three references to "person." The first, in defining "citizens," speaks of "persons born or naturalized in the United States." The word also appears both in the Due Process Clause and in the Equal Protection Clause. "Person" is used in other places in the Constitution. But in nearly all these instances, the use of the word is such that it has application only postnatally. None indicates, with any assurance, that it has any possible pre-natal application.[1]

All this, together with our observation, *supra*, that throughout the major portion of the 19th century prevailing legal abortion practices were far freer than they are today, persuades us that the word "person," as used in the Fourteenth Amendment, does not include the unborn. This is in accord with

---

[1] When Texas urges that a fetus is entitled to Fourteenth Amendment protection as a person, it faces a dilemma. Neither in Texas nor in any other State are all abortions prohibited. Despite broad proscription, an exception always exists. The exception contained in Art. 1196, for an abortion procured or attempted by medical advice for the purpose of saving the life of the mother, is typical. But if the fetus is a person who is not to be deprived of life without due process of law, and if the mother's condition is the sole determinant, does not the Texas exception appear to be out of line with the Amendment's command?

Further, the penalty for criminal abortion specified by Art. 1195 is significantly less than the maximum penalty for murder prescribed by Art. 1257 of the Texas Penal Code. If the fetus is a person, may the penalties be different?

the results reached in those few cases where the issue has been squarely presented.

This conclusion, however, does not of itself fully answer the contentions raised by Texas, and we pass on to other considerations.

B. The pregnant woman cannot be isolated in her privacy. She carries an embryo and, later, a fetus, if one accepts the medical definitions of the developing young in the human uterus. The situation therefore is inherently different from marital intimacy, or bedroom possession of obscene material, or marriage, or procreation, or education, with which *Eisenstadt* and *Griswold*, *Stanley*, *Loving*, Skinner, and *Pierce* and *Meyer* were respectively concerned. As we have intimated above, it is reasonable and appropriate for a State to decide that at some point in time another interest, that of health of the mother or that of potential human life, becomes significantly involved. The woman's privacy is no longer sole and any right of privacy she possesses must be measured accordingly.

Texas urges that, apart from the Fourteenth Amendment, life begins at conception and is present throughout pregnancy, and that, therefore, the State has a compelling interest in protecting that life from and after conception. We need not resolve the difficult question of when life begins. When those trained in the respective disciplines of medicine, philosophy, and theology are unable to arrive at any consensus, the judiciary, at this point in the development of man's knowledge, is not in a position to speculate as to the answer.

It should be sufficient to note briefly the wide divergence of thinking on this most sensitive and difficult question. There has always been strong support for the view that life does not begin until live birth. This was the belief of the Stoics. It appears to be the predominant, though not the unanimous, attitude of the Jewish faith. It may be taken to represent also the position of a large segment of the Protestant community, insofar as that can be ascertained; organized groups that have taken a formal position on the abortion issue have generally regarded abortion as a matter for the conscience of the individual and her family. As we have noted, the common law found greater significance in quickening. Physicians and their scientific colleagues have regarded that event with less interest and have tended to focus either upon conception, upon live birth, or upon the interim point at which the fetus becomes "viable," that is, potentially able to live outside the mother's womb, albeit with artificial aid. Viability is usually placed at about seven months (28 weeks) but may occur earlier, even at 24 weeks. The Aristotelian theory of "mediate animation," that held sway throughout the Middle Ages and the Renaissance in Europe, continued to be official Roman Catholic dogma until the 19th century, despite opposition to this "ensoulment" theory from those in the Church who would recognize the existence of life from the moment of conception. The latter is now, of course, the official belief of the Catholic Church. As one brief *amicus* discloses, this is a view strongly held by many non-Catholics as well, and by many physicians. Substantial problems for precise definition of this view are posed, however, by new embryological data that purport to indicate that conception is a "process" over time, rather than an event, and by new medical techniques such as menstrual extraction, the "morning-after" pill, implantation of embryos, artificial insemination, and even artificial wombs.

In areas other than criminal abortion, the law has been reluctant to endorse any theory that life, as we recognize it, begins before live birth or to accord legal rights to the unborn except in narrowly defined situations and except when the rights are contingent upon live birth. For example, the traditional rule of tort law denied recovery for prenatal injuries even though the child was born alive. That rule has been changed in almost every jurisdiction. In most States, recovery is said to be permitted only if the fetus was viable, or at least quick, when the injuries were sustained, though few courts have squarely so held. In a recent development, generally opposed by the commentators, some States permit the parents of a stillborn child to maintain an action for wrongful death because of prenatal injuries. Such an action, however, would appear to be one to vindicate the parents' interest and is thus consistent with the view that the fetus, at most, represents only the potentiality of life. Similarly, unborn children have been recognized as acquiring rights or interests by way of inheritance or other devolution of property, and have been represented by guardians *ad litem*. Perfection of the interests involved, again, has generally been contingent upon live birth. In short, the unborn have never been recognized in the law as persons in the whole sense.

## X

In view of all this, we do not agree that, by adopting one theory of life, Texas may override the rights of the pregnant woman that are at stake. We repeat, however, that the State does have an important and legitimate interest in preserving and protecting the health of the pregnant woman, whether she be a resident of the State or a nonresident who seeks medical consultation and treatment there, and that it has still another important and legitimate interest in protecting the potentiality of human life. These interests are separate and distinct. Each grows in substantiality as the woman approaches term and, at a point during pregnancy, each becomes "compelling."

With respect to the State's important and legitimate interest in the health of the mother, the "compelling" point, in the light of present medical knowledge, is at approximately the end of the first trimester. This is so because of the now-established medical fact that until the end of the first trimester mortality in abortion may be less than mortality in normal childbirth. It follows that, from and after this point, a State may regulate the abortion procedure to the extent that the regulation reasonably relates to the preservation and protection of maternal health. Examples of permissible state regulation in this area are requirements as to the qualifications of the person who is to perform the abortion; as to the licensure of that person; as to the facility in which the procedure is to be performed, that is, whether it must be a hospital or may be a clinic or some other place of less-than-hospital status; as to the licensing of the facility; and the like.

This means, on the other hand, that, for the period of pregnancy prior to this "compelling" point, the attending physician, in consultation with his patient, is free to determine, without regulation by the State, that, in his medical judgment, the patient's pregnancy should be terminated. If that decision is reached, the judgment may be effectuated by an abortion free of interference by the State.

With respect to the State's important and legitimate interest in potential life, the "compelling" point is at viability. This is so because the fetus then presumably has the capability of meaningful life outside the mother's womb. State regulation protective of fetal life after viability thus has both logical and biological justifications. If the State is interested in protecting fetal life after viability, it may go so far as to proscribe abortion during that period, except when it is necessary to preserve the life or health of the mother.

Measured against these standards, the Texas Penal Code, in restricting legal abortions to those "procured or attempted by medical advice for the purpose of saving the life of the mother," sweeps too broadly. The statute makes no distinction between abortions performed early in pregnancy and those performed later, and it limits to a single reason, "saving" the mother's life, the legal justification for the procedure. The statute, therefore, cannot survive the constitutional attack made upon it here.

## XI

To summarize and to repeat:

1. A state criminal abortion statute of the current Texas type, that excepts from criminality only a lifesaving procedure on behalf of the mother, without regard to pregnancy stage and without recognition of the other interests involved, is violative of the Due Process Clause of the Fourteenth Amendment

(a) For the stage prior to approximately the end of the first trimester, the abortion decision and its effectuation must be left to the medical judgment of the pregnant woman's attending physician.

(b) For the stage subsequent to approximately the end of the first trimester, the State, in promoting its interest in the health of the mother, may, if it chooses, regulate the abortion procedure in ways that are reasonably related to maternal health.

(c) For the stage subsequent to viability, the State in promoting its interest in the potentiality of human life may, if it chooses, regulate, and even proscribe, abortion except where it is necessary, in appropriate medical judgment, for the preservation of the life or health of the mother.

2. The State may define the term "physician," as it has been employed in the preceding paragraphs of this Part XI of this opinion, to mean only a physician currently licensed by the State, and may proscribe any abortion by a person who is not a physician as so defined.

This holding, we feel, is consistent with the relative weights of the respective interests involved, with the lessons and examples of medical and legal history, with the lenity of the common law, and with the demands of the profound problems of the present day. The decision leaves the State free to place increasing restrictions on abortion as the period of pregnancy lengthens, so long as those restrictions are tailored to the recognized state interests. The decision vindicates the right of the physician to administer medical treatment according to his professional judgment up to the points where important state interests provide compelling justifications for intervention. Up to those points, the abortion decision in all its aspects is inherently, and primarily, a medical decision, and basic responsibility for it must rest with the physician.

Our conclusion that Art. 1196 is unconstitutional means, of course, that the Texas abortion statutes, as a unit, must fall.

\* \* \*

# DOE v. BOLTON
## 410 U.S 179 (1973)

Blackmun, Justice.

\* \* \*

[The primary issue in this case is whether the state could require concurrence of a review committee or even of a second physician in the abortion decision.]

IV A. *Roe v. Wade, supra,* sets forth our conclusion that a pregnant woman does not have an absolute constitutional right to an abortion on her demand. What is said there is applicable here and need not be repeated. . . .

The appellants recognize that a century ago medical knowledge was not so advanced as it is today, that the techniques of antisepsis were not known, and that any abortion procedure was dangerous for the woman. To restrict the legality of the abortion to the situation where it was deemed necessary, in medical judgment, for the preservation of the woman's life was only a natural conclusion in the exercise of the legislative judgment of that time. A State is not to be reproached, however, for a past judgmental determination made in the light of then-existing medical knowledge. It is perhaps unfair to argue, as the appellants do, that because the early focus was on the preservation of the woman's life, the State's present professed interest in the protection of embryonic and fetal life is to be downgraded. That argument denies the State the right to readjust its views and emphases in the light of the advanced knowledge and techniques of the day. . . .

We agree with the District Court, 319 F. Supp., at 1058, that the medical judgment may be exercised in the light of all factors — physical, emotional, psychological, familial, and the woman's age — relevant to the well-being of the patient. All these factors may relate to health. This allows the attending physician the room he needs to make his best medical judgment. And it is room that operates for the benefit, not the disadvantage, of the pregnant woman.

This is not to say that Georgia may not or should not, from and after the end of the first trimester, adopt standards for licensing all facilities where abortions may be performed so long as those standards are legitimately related to the objective the State seeks to accomplish. The appellants contend that such a relationship would be lacking even in a lesser requirement that an abortion be performed in a licensed hospital, as opposed to a facility, such as a clinic, that may be required by the State to possess all the staffing and services necessary to perform an abortion safely (including those adequate to handle serious complications or other emergency, or arrangements with a nearby hospital to provide such services). Appellants and various *amici* have presented us with a mass of data purporting to demonstrate that some facilities other than hospitals are entirely adequate to perform abortions if they possess these qualifications. The State, on the other hand, has not presented persuasive data to show that only hospitals meet its acknowledged interest in insuring the quality of the operation and the full protection of the patient. We feel compelled to agree with appellants that the State must show more than it has in order to prove that only the full resources of a licensed hospital, rather than those of some other appropriately licensed institution, satisfy these health interests. We hold that the hospital requirement of the Georgia law, because it fails to exclude the first trimester of pregnancy, see *Roe* v. *Wade, ante,* at 163, is also invalid. In so holding we naturally express no opinion on the medical judgment involved in any particular case, that is, whether the patient's situation is such that an abortion should be performed in a hospital, rather than in some other facility.

2. *Committee approval.* The second aspect of the appellants' procedural attack relates to the hospital abortion committee. . . .

Appellants attack the discretion the statute leaves to the committee. The most concrete argument they advance is their suggestion that it is still a badge of infamy "in many minds" to bear an illegitimate child, and that the Georgia system enables the committee members' personal views as to extramarital sex relations, and punishment therefor, to govern their decisions. This approach obviously is one founded on suspicion and one that discloses a lack of confidence in the integrity of physicians. To say that physicians will be guided in their hospital committee decisions by their predilections on extramarital sex unduly narrows the issue to pregnancy outside marriage. (Doe's own situation did not involve extramarital sex and its product.) The appellants' suggestion is necessarily somewhat degrading to the conscientious physician, particularly the obstetrician, whose professional activity is concerned with the physical and mental welfare, the woes, the emotions, and the concern of his female patients. He, perhaps more than anyone else, is knowledgeable in this area of patient care, and he is aware of human frailty, so-called "error," and needs. The good physician — despite the presence of rascals in the medical profession, as in all others, we trust that most physicians are "good" — will have sympathy and understanding for the pregnant patient that probably are not exceeded by those who participate in other areas of professional counseling.

It is perhaps worth noting that the abortion committee has a function of its own. It is a committee of the hospital and it is composed of members of the institution's medical staff. The membership usually is a changing one. In this way, its work burden is shared and is more readily accepted. The committee's function is protective. It enables the hospital appropriately to be advised that its posture and activities are in accord with legal requirements. It is to be remembered that the hospital is an entity and that it, too, has legal rights and legal obligations.

Saying all this, however, does not settle the issue of the constitutional propriety of the committee requirement. Viewing the Georgia statute as a whole, we see no constitutionally justifiable pertinence in the structure for the advance approval by the abortion committee. With regard to the protection of potential life, the medical judgment is already completed prior to the committee stage, and review by a committee once removed from diagnosis is basically redundant. We are not cited to any other surgical procedure made subject to committee approval as a matter of state criminal law. The woman's right to receive medical care in accordance with her licensed physician's best judgment and the physician's right to administer it are substantially limited by this statutorily imposed overview. . . .

We conclude that the interposition of the hospital abortion committee is unduly restrictive of the patient's rights and needs that, at this point, have already been medically delineated and substantiated by her personal physician. To ask more serves neither the hospital nor the State.

3. *Two-doctor concurrence.* . . .

. . . the required confirmation by two Georgia-licensed physicians in addition to the recommendation of the pregnant woman's own consultant [remains] (making under the statute, a total of six physicians involved, including the three on the hospital's abortion committee).We conclude that this provision, too, must fall.

The statute's emphasis, as has been repetitively noted, is on the attending physician's "best clinical judgment that an abortion is necessary." That should be sufficient. The reasons for the presence of the confirmation step in the statute are perhaps apparent, but they are insufficient to withstand constitutional challenge. Again, no other voluntary medical or surgical procedure for which Georgia requires confirmation by two other physicians has been cited to us. If a physician is licensed by the State, he is recognized by the State as capable of exercising acceptable clinical judgment. If he fails in this, professional censure and deprivation of his license are available remedies. Required acquiescence by co-practitioners has no rational connection with a patient's needs and unduly infringes on the physician's right to practice. The attending physician will know when a consultation is advisable — the doubtful situation, the need for assurance when the medical decision is a delicate one, and the like. Physicians have followed this routine historically and know its usefulness and benefit for all concerned. It is still true today that "reliance must be placed upon the assurance given by his license, issued by an authority competent to judge in that respect, that he [the physician] possesses the requisite qualifications. . . ."

\* \* \*

# NOTES AND QUESTIONS

**1.** Abortion has long been, and remains, the most politicized medical procedure in the United States. It has been the subject of more state and federal legislation than all other medical procedures combined. The U.S. Supreme Court, which almost never hears cases about medical procedures, has regularly heard cases over the past 30 years concerning the constitutionality of various state laws designed to limit abortion. Nonetheless, it is probably not an overstatement to say that *Roe v. Wade* is the most important health-related case of all time. This is not just because it struck down all of the state abortion statutes that existed at the time. It is also because it applied the constitutional "right of privacy" in a way that could potentially protect individual decision-making from state interference in a variety of contexts (such as the right to refuse medical treatment). The Court also adds two new dimensions to "public health" cases: the protection of individual rights, and the protection of the practice of medicine. This means, for example, that state public health rules will have to be consistent not only with the constitutional rights of individuals, they will also have to take into account basic rules of medical practice, including medical ethics and medical licensing.

In this regard, *Doe v. Bolton* is an underappreciated case, concentrating as it does on the right of a licensed physician to practice medicine without interference from the state in requiring him or her to present a treatment plan to a committee, or even to another physician, for concurrence. Justice Blackmun, who often said the best years of his life were working as general counsel to the Mayo Clinic, strongly believed that the law should support physicians in their practice of medicine, not hinder it. In his view, expressed in both of these decisions, state licensing of physicians was sufficient for the protection of the public; after that, the doctor-patient relationship should suffice. It has even been suggested that *Roe v. Wade* and *Doe v. Bolton* together can be read as suggesting that there is a constitutional "right to privacy" that attaches to the doctor-patient relationship itself. Do you agree? *See* George J. Annas, Leonard H. Glantz & Wendy K. Mariner, *The Right of Privacy Protects the Doctor-Patient Relationship*, 263 JAMA 858 (1990); and *see generally* Symposium, *Justice Harry Blackmun: The Supreme Court and the Limits of Medical Privacy*, 13 AM. J.L. & MED. 153 (1987); and LINDA GREENHOUSE, BECOMING JUSTICE BLACKMUN: HARRY BLACKMUN'S SUPREME COURT JOURNEY (2005).

**2.** Note that *Roe* cites both *Jacobson* (Section B[1], *supra*) and *Buck v. Bell* (*see* Chapter 3, Section B[2], *infra*) for the proposition that rights are not absolute. What is the relevance of this citation, especially to the compulsory sterilization case of *Buck*? There are many issues that *Roe* and *Doe* left unresolved. For example, could a state require parental consent (in the case of a minor) or spousal consent (in the case of a married woman) to abortion? These and other issues are resolved in *Planned Parenthood of Central Missouri v. Danforth,* 428 U.S. 52 (1976), which was the first abortion case decided by the Supreme Court after *Roe*. *Roe,* although it was decided by a 7 to 2 majority, nonetheless continued to be viewed as the most controversial decision of the Court ever, primarily because of its viability line and its exception for a woman's health that continued even after viability. Thus when the Court had an opportunity to review the entire opinion anew in the case of *Planned Parenthood v. Casey,* 505 U.S. 833 (1992) many thought the Court would overturn *Roe*. Instead it re-inforced it, although it adopted a new test for pre-viability regulations (the so-called "undue burden" test), and reverted to calling the abortion decision an aspect of "liberty" rather than "privacy." Some comments from the three Justice "joint opinion" (Souter, Kennedy, and O'Connor) merit attention:

> Liberty finds no refuge in a jurisprudence of doubt. Yet 19 years
> after our holding that the Constitution protects a woman's right to

terminate her pregnancy in its early stages, *Roe v. Wade*, 410 U.S. 113 (1973), that definition of liberty is still questioned. . . .

After considering the fundamental constitutional questions resolved by Roe, principles of institutional integrity, and the rule of *stare decisis*, we are led to conclude this: the essential holding of *Roe v. Wade* should be retained and once again reaffirmed.

It must be stated at the outset and with clarity that *Roe*'s essential holding, the holding we reaffirm, has three parts. First is a recognition of the right of the woman to choose to have an abortion before viability and to obtain it without undue interference from the State. Before viability, the State's interests are not strong enough to support a prohibition of abortion or the imposition of a substantial obstacle to the woman's effective right to elect the procedure. Second is a confirmation of the State's power to restrict abortions after fetal viability, if the law contains exceptions for pregnancies which endanger a woman's life or health. And third is the principle that the State has legitimate interests from the outset of the pregnancy in protecting the health of the woman and the life of the fetus that may become a child. These principles do not contradict one another; and we adhere to each.

## II

. . . .

The inescapable fact is that adjudication of substantive due process claims may call upon the Court in interpreting the Constitution to exercise that same capacity which by tradition courts always have exercised: reasoned judgment. . . .

Our obligation is to define the liberty of all, not to mandate our own moral code. . . .

. . .

Our law affords constitutional protection to personal decisions relating to marriage, procreation, contraception, family relationships, child rearing, and education. Our cases recognize "the right of the individual, married or single, to be free from unwarranted governmental intrusion into matters so fundamentally affecting a person as the decision whether to bear or beget a child." *Eisenstadt v. Baird.* Our precedents "have respected the private realm of family life which the state cannot enter. These matters, involving the most intimate and personal choices a person may make in a lifetime, choices central to personal dignity and autonomy, are central to the liberty protected by the Fourteenth Amendment. At the heart of liberty is the right to define one's own concept of existence, of meaning, of the universe, and of the mystery of human life. Beliefs about these matters could not define the attributes of personhood were they formed under compulsion of the State.

These considerations begin our analysis of the woman's interest in terminating her pregnancy but cannot end it, for this reason: though the abortion decision may originate within the zone of conscience and belief, it is more than a philosophic exercise. Abortion is a unique act. It is an act fraught with consequences for others: for the woman who must live with the implications of her decision; for the persons who perform and assist in the procedure; for the spouse, family, and society which must confront the knowledge that these procedures exist, procedures some deem nothing short of an act of violence against innocent human life; and, depending on one's beliefs, for the life or potential life that is aborted. Though abortion is conduct, it does not follow that the State is entitled to proscribe it in all instances. That is because the liberty of the woman is at stake in a sense unique to the human condition and so unique to the law. The mother who carries a child to full term is subject to anxieties, to physical constraints, to pain that only she must bear. . . . Her suffering is too intimate and personal for the State to insist, without more, upon its own vision of the woman's role, however dominant that vision has been in the course of our history and our culture. The destiny of the woman must be shaped to a large extent on her own conception of her spiritual imperatives and her place in society.

It should be recognized, moreover, that in some critical respects the abortion decision is of the same character as the decision to use contraception, to which *Griswold v. Connecticut, Eisenstadt v. Baird,* and *Carey v. Population Services International,* afford constitutional protection. We have no doubt as to the correctness of those decisions. They support the reasoning in *Roe* relating to the woman's liberty because they involve personal decisions concerning not only the meaning of procreation but also human responsibility and respect for it. The same concerns are present when the woman confronts the reality that, perhaps despite her attempts to avoid it, she has become pregnant.

    . . .

IV

. . . We conclude that the basic decision in *Roe* was based on a constitutional analysis which we cannot now repudiate. The woman's liberty is not so unlimited, however, that from the outset the State cannot show its concern for the life of the unborn, and at a later point in fetal development the State's interest in life has sufficient force so that the right of the woman to terminate the pregnancy can be restricted.

That brings us, of course, to the point where much criticism has been directed at *Roe*, a criticism that always inheres when the Court draws a specific rule from what in the Constitution is but a general standard. We conclude, however, that the urgent claims of the woman to retain the ultimate control over her destiny and her body, claims implicit in the meaning of liberty, require us to perform that function. Liberty must not be extinguished for want of a line that is clear. And it falls to us to give some real substance to the woman's liberty to determine whether to carry her pregnancy to full term.

We conclude the line should be drawn at viability, so that before that time the woman has a right to choose to terminate her pregnancy. We adhere to this principle for two reasons. First, as we have said, is the doctrine of *stare decisis*. Any judicial act of line-drawing may seem somewhat arbitrary, but *Roe* was a reasoned statement, elaborated with great care. We have twice reaffirmed it in the face of great opposition. . . .

The second reason is that the concept of viability, as we noted in *Roe*, is the time at which there is a realistic possibility of maintaining and nourishing a life outside the womb, so that the independent existence of the second life can in reason and all fairness be the object of state protection that now overrides the rights of the woman . . .

The woman's right to terminate her pregnancy before viability is the most central principle of *Roe v. Wade*. It is a rule of law and a component of liberty we cannot renounce.

. . .

Though the woman has a right to choose to terminate or continue her pregnancy before viability. . . . States are free to enact laws to provide a reasonable framework for a woman to make a decision that has such profound and lasting meaning. This, too, we find consistent with *Roe*'s central premises, and indeed the inevitable consequence of our holding that the State has an interest in protecting the life of the unborn. . . .

. . .

. . . Before viability, *Roe* and subsequent cases treat all governmental attempts to influence a woman's decision on behalf of the potential life within her as unwarranted. This treatment is, in our judgment, incompatible with the recognition that there is a substantial state interest in potential life throughout pregnancy.

The very notion that the State has a substantial interest in potential life leads to the conclusion that not all regulations must be deemed unwarranted. Not all burdens on the right to decide whether to terminate a pregnancy will be undue. In our view, the undue burden standard is the appropriate means of reconciling the State's interest with the woman's constitutionally protected liberty.

A finding of an undue burden is a shorthand for the conclusion that a state regulation has the purpose or effect of placing a substantial obstacle in the path of a woman seeking an abortion of a nonviable fetus. A statute with this purpose is invalid because the means chosen by the State to further the interest in potential life must be calculated to inform the woman's free choice, not hinder it. And a statute which, while furthering the interest in potential life or some other valid state interest, has the effect of placing a substantial obstacle in the path of a woman's choice cannot be considered a permissible means of serving its legitimate ends. . . . Regulations designed to foster the health of a woman seeking an abortion are valid if they do not constitute an undue burden.

505 U.S. at 844–78.

**3.** It was only a matter of time before the Court would hear a case on the constitutionality of laws restricting so-called partial-birth abortion. When the Court heard a challenge to Nebraska's law, statutes relating to partial-birth abortion had been enacted in 30 states, and two bills banning such abortions had been passed by Congress. All the appeals courts except one, the Seventh Circuit Court of Appeals, had found these laws unconstitutional, and the opinion of that court rested on an extremely narrow interpretation of the law. The controversies surrounding partial-birth abortion are over how to describe the procedure and whether physicians ever need to use it to protect the health of a pregnant woman. The Supreme Court confronted these issues in the case of *Stenberg v. Carhart*, 530 U.S. 914 (2000).

The Nebraska law provides that "no partial birth abortion shall be performed in this state, unless such procedure is necessary to save the life of the mother whose life is endangered by a physical disorder, physical illness, or physical injury, including a life-endangering physical condition caused by or arising from the pregnancy itself." Like the federal acts twice passed by Congress and vetoed by President Bill Clinton, the Nebraska law defined partial-birth abortion as "an abortion in which the person performing the abortion partially delivers vaginally a living unborn child before killing the unborn child and completing the delivery." The law further defines the phrase "partially delivers vaginally a living unborn child before killing the unborn child" to mean "deliberately and intentionally delivering into the vagina a living unborn child, or a substantial portion thereof, for the purpose of performing a procedure that the person performing such procedure knows will kill the unborn child and does kill the unborn child." Violation of the law is a felony that carries a prison term of up to 20 years, a fine of up to $25,000, and automatic revocation of a medical license.

Dr. Leroy Carhart, a Nebraska physician who performs abortions, sued in federal court to have the law declared unconstitutional. By a 5 to 4 vote the Court agreed. Their opinion is best understood as a direct application to the Nebraska law of the principles articulated in the decisions in *Roe* and *Casey*. *Roe* made it clear that the state could not favor the life of the fetus over the life or health of the pregnant woman. The Court in *Casey* affirmed the core holding of *Roe*, that states cannot outlaw abortion before the time of fetal viability and can do so thereafter only if the woman's life and health are protected. States were permitted, however, to regulate abortions so long as any restriction did not impose an "undue burden" on the pregnant woman's liberty interest in terminating her pregnancy. The Nebraska ban applies throughout pregnancy and has no exception to preserve a woman's health. Because it is a criminal statute, the legislature had to be very clear about what exactly the statute prohibited. In order to determine exactly what was and was not prohibited, Justice Breyer, like the trial court judge, devoted nearly the entirety of his opinion to describing various abortion procedures and comparing them with the language of the Nebraska law.

On the basis of information from medical textbooks and the position taken by the American College of Obstetricians and Gynecologists, Breyer concluded that "intact D&E and D&X [dilation and extraction] are sufficiently similar for us [the Court] to use the terms interchangeably." There are no accurate statistics available on the number of dilation-and-extraction abortions performed in the United States, and Breyer cited estimates ranging from 640 to 5000 cases per year. He found that such abortions are performed for a variety of reasons, including reducing the danger caused by the passage of sharp bone fragments through the cervix, minimizing the number of surgical instruments used (and thereby decreasing the likelihood of uterine perforation), reducing the likelihood of infection, and helping to ensure the removal of all fetal tissue. Dilation and extraction is also the preferred method for fetuses with hydrocephaly and anomalies incompatible with fetal survival. Regarding the necessity of a health exception, Breyer asked if the ban would in fact adversely affect the health of pregnant women who want to terminate their pregnancies. Breyer concluded that it would, on the basis of the belief of "significant medical authority" that "in some circumstances, D&X would be the safest procedure."

Justice Thomas disagreed that the state cannot second-guess physicians who believe use of a particular abortion method is necessary to preserve a woman's health. He argued that the majority opinion "eviscerates *Casey's* undue burden standard and imposes unfettered abortion on demand." In his view, the resolution of differences among physicians regarding the safety of abortion procedures should be left to the state legislatures. The dissenters, in short, did not believe that physicians can be trusted to make good-faith decisions about the health of their patients.

Ultimately, the central question regarding abortion remains who should make the decision: the state or women and their physicians together. The answer of the Supreme Court, as articulated in *Roe* and its companion case, *Doe*, and now strongly reinforced in *Stenberg*, is that the decision belongs to the woman and her physician together. In this respect, the Court has been remarkably consistent in all the abortion cases it has heard. *See, e.g.*, George J. Annas, *"Partial Birth Abortion" and the Supreme Court*, 344 N. ENG. J. MED. 174 (2001). In 2003 Congress passed a bill substantially identical to the Nebraska bill and President Bush signed it. The Court is scheduled to review its constitutionality in its 2007 term.

# D.  CONSTITUTIONAL PRINCIPLES: STATE REGULATION OF "IMMORAL" BEHAVIOR

The constitutional principles explored thus far in this chapter apply to government promotion of the health and safety of the public, primarily in connection with the risk of physical (and sometimes mental) harms. Health and safety, of course, are not the only interests that states protect under the police power: Many laws are designed to advance and protect property and other economic interests, regulate business and industry, address various kinds of inequalities, and countless other matters. See FREUND, THE POLICE POWER, Section B[1], Note 1, *supra*. Generally, however, all such examples share a common attribute: The particular harm sought to be prevented is a concrete and tangible (even if not always a physical) one. And in the field of public health law, the regulation of those risks that *are* primarily physical remains the leading example.

The states' police power, however, has generally been understood as including, as well, the (somewhat hazier) authority to regulate "morals." In this area the harms sought to be prevented may often be less concrete and demonstrable, and more speculative or contested, than in the areas described above. In contrast to Sections A and B of this Chapter, the question raised by the cases in this section is whether the same basic constitutional principles are or should be applied any differently when the powers of the government are justified, either tacitly or explicitly, primarily by moral objections to certain kinds of activities.

## LAWRENCE v. TEXAS
### 539 U.S. 558 (2003)

Kennedy, Justice.

\* \* \*

Liberty protects the person from unwarranted government intrusions into a dwelling or other private places. In our tradition the State is not omnipresent in the home. And there are other spheres of our lives and existence, outside the home, where the State should not be a dominant presence. Freedom extends beyond spatial bounds. Liberty presumes an autonomy of self that includes freedom of thought, belief, expression, and certain intimate conduct. The instant case involves liberty of the person both in its spatial and in its more transcendent dimensions.

. . . .

In Houston, Texas, officers of the Harris County Police Department were dispatched to a private residence in response to a reported weapons disturbance. They entered an apartment where one of the petitioners, John Geddes Lawrence, resided. The right of the police to enter does not seem to have been questioned. The officers observed Lawrence and another man, Tyron Garner, engaging in a sexual act. The two petitioners were arrested, held in custody overnight, and charged and convicted before a Justice of the Peace.

The complaints described their crime as "deviate sexual intercourse, namely anal sex, with a member of the same sex (man)." The applicable state law . . . provides: "A person commits an offense if he engages in deviate sexual intercourse with another individual of the same sex." The statute defines "[d]eviate sexual intercourse" as follows: "(A) any contact between any part of the genitals of one person and the mouth or anus of another person; or "(B) the penetration of the genitals or the anus of another person with an object."

The petitioners . . . challenged the statute as a violation of the Equal Protection Clause of the Fourteenth Amendment and of a like provision of the Texas Constitution. Those contentions were rejected. The petitioners, having entered a plea of *nolo contendere,* were each fined $200 and assessed court costs of $141.25.

The Court of Appeals for the Texas Fourteenth District considered the petitioners' federal constitutional arguments [to be controlled by *Bowers v. Hardwick*] . . .

We granted certiorari to consider three questions:

1. Whether petitioners' criminal convictions under the Texas 'Homosexual Conduct' law — which criminalizes sexual intimacy by same-sex couples, but not identical behavior by different-sex couples — violate the Fourteenth Amendment guarantee of equal protection of the laws.

2. Whether petitioners' criminal convictions for adult consensual sexual intimacy in the home violate their vital interests in liberty and privacy protected by the Due Process Clause of the Fourteenth Amendment.

3. Whether [*Bowers*] should be overruled.

In *Griswold* the Court invalidated a state law prohibiting the use of drugs or devices of contraception and counseling or aiding and abetting the use of contraceptives. The Court described the protected interest as a right to privacy and placed emphasis on the marriage relation and the protected space of the marital bedroom. . . . After *Griswold* it was established that the right to make certain decisions regarding sexual conduct extends beyond the marital relationship. [citing *Eisenstadt v. Baird*]

The opinions in *Griswold* and *Eisenstadt* were part of the background for the decision in *Roe v. Wade* . . .

. . . .

The Court began its substantive discussion in *Bowers* as follows: "The issue presented is whether the Federal Constitution confers a fundamental right upon homosexuals to engage in sodomy and hence invalidates the laws of the many States that still make such conduct illegal and have done so for a very long time." That statement, we now conclude, discloses the Court's own failure to appreciate the extent of the liberty at stake. To say that the issue in *Bowers* was simply the right to engage in certain sexual conduct demeans the claim the individual put forward, just as it would demean a married couple were it to be said marriage is simply about the right to have sexual intercourse. . . . The statutes do seek to control a personal relationship that, whether or not entitled to formal recognition in the law, is within the liberty of persons to choose without being punished as criminals.

This, as a general rule, should counsel against attempts by the State, or a court, to define the meaning of the relationship or to set its boundaries absent injury to a person or abuse of an institution the law protects. It suffices for us to acknowledge that adults may choose to enter upon this relationship in the confines of their homes and their own private lives and still retain their dignity as free persons. When sexuality finds overt expression in intimate conduct with another person, the conduct can be but one element in a personal bond that is more enduring. The liberty protected by the Constitution allows homosexual persons the right to make this choice.

[The Court then critiques the summary of prior state and common laws that governed sodomy, as set out in *Bowers*.]

In summary, the historical grounds relied upon in *Bowers* are more complex than the majority opinion and the concurring opinion by Chief Justice Burger indicate. Their historical premises are not without doubt and, at the very least, are overstated.

It must be acknowledged . . . that for centuries there have been powerful voices to condemn homosexual conduct as immoral. The condemnation has been shaped by religious beliefs, conceptions of right and acceptable behavior, and respect for the traditional family. For many persons these are not trivial concerns but profound and deep convictions accepted as ethical and moral principles to which they aspire and which thus determine the course of their lives. These considerations do not answer the question before us, however. The issue is whether the majority may use the power of the State to enforce these views on the whole society through operation of the criminal law. "Our obligation is to define the liberty of all, not to mandate our own moral code."

   . . . .

In our own constitutional system the deficiencies in *Bowers* became even more apparent in the years following its announcement. The 25 States with laws prohibiting the relevant conduct referenced in the *Bowers* decision are reduced now to 13, of which 4 enforce their laws only against homosexual conduct. In those States where sodomy is still proscribed, whether for same-sex or heterosexual conduct, there is a pattern of nonenforcement with respect to consenting adults acting in private. . . .

   . . . .

As an alternative argument in this case, counsel for the petitioners and some *amici* contend that *Romer* provides the basis for declaring the Texas statute invalid under the Equal Protection Clause. [In *Romer v. Evans*, 517 U.S. 620 (1996), the Court held that a state constitutional amendment attempting to prevent the enactment of any law protecting homosexuals from discrimination was a violation of the federal Constitution because it lacked any legitimate purpose.] That is a tenable argument, but we conclude the instant case requires us to address whether *Bowers* itself has continuing validity. Were we to hold the statute invalid under the Equal Protection Clause some might question whether a prohibition would be valid if drawn differently, say, to prohibit the conduct both between same-sex and different-sex participants.

Equality of treatment and the due process right to demand respect for conduct protected by the substantive guarantee of liberty are linked in important respects, and a decision on the latter point advances both interests. If protected conduct is made criminal and the law which does so remains unexamined for its substantive validity, its stigma might remain even if it were not enforceable as drawn for equal protection reasons. When homosexual conduct is made criminal by the law of the State, that declaration in and of itself is an invitation to subject homosexual persons to discrimination both in the public and in the private spheres. . . .

   . . . .

The rationale of *Bowers* does not withstand careful analysis. In his dissenting opinion in *Bowers,* Justice Stevens came to these conclusions:

> Our prior cases make two propositions abundantly clear. First, the fact that the governing majority in a State has traditionally viewed a particular practice as immoral is not a sufficient reason for upholding a law prohibiting the practice; neither history nor tradition could save a law prohibiting miscegenation from constitutional attack. Second, individual decisions by married persons, concerning the intimacies of their physical relationship, even when not intended to produce off-spring, are a form of "liberty" protected by the Due Process Clause of the Fourteenth Amendment. Moreover this protection extends to intimate choices by unmarried as well as married persons. . . .

Justice Stevens' analysis, in our view, should have been controlling in *Bowers* and should control here.

*Bowers* was not correct when it was decided, and it is not correct today. It ought not to remain binding precedent. *Bowers v. Hardwick* should be and now is overruled.

. . . .

The present case does not involve minors. It does not involve persons who might be injured or coerced or who are situated in relationships where consent might not easily be refused. It does not involve public conduct or prostitution. It does not involve whether the government must give formal recognition to any relationship that homosexual persons seek to enter. The case does involve two adults who, with full and mutual consent from each other, engaged in sexual practices common to a homosexual lifestyle. The petitioners are entitled to respect for their private lives. The State cannot demean their existence or control their destiny by making their private sexual conduct a crime. Their right to liberty under the Due Process Clause gives them the full right to engage in their conduct without intervention of the government. . . . The Texas statute furthers no legitimate state interest which can justify its intrusion into the personal and private life of the individual.

Had those who drew and ratified the Due Process Clauses of the Fifth Amendment or the Fourteenth Amendment known the components of liberty in its manifold possibilities, they might have been more specific. They did not presume to have this insight. They knew times can blind us to certain truths and later generations can see that laws once thought necessary and proper in fact serve only to oppress. As the Constitution endures, persons in every generation can invoke its principles in their own search for greater freedom.

The judgment of the Court of Appeals . . . is reversed, and the case is remanded for further proceedings not inconsistent with this opinion.

* * *

# WILLIAMS v. ALABAMA
## 378 F. 3d 1232 (11th Cir. 2004)

Birch, Judge.

\* \* \*

Alabama's Anti-Obscenity Enforcement Act prohibits, among other things, the commercial distribution of "any device designed or marketed as useful primarily for the stimulation of human genital organs for any thing of pecuniary value." Ala. Code § 13A-12-200.2 (Supp. 2003). The Alabama statute proscribes a relatively narrow bandwidth of activity. It prohibits only the sale — but not the use, possession, or gratuitous distribution — of sexual devices (in fact, the users involved in this litigation acknowledge that they already possess multiple sex toys). The law does not affect the distribution of a number of other sexual products such as ribbed condoms or virility drugs. Nor does it prohibit Alabama residents from purchasing sexual devices out of state and bringing them back into Alabama. Moreover, the statute permits the sale of ordinary vibrators and body massagers that, although useful as sexual aids, are not "designed or marketed . . . primarily" for that particular purpose. Finally, the statute exempts sales of sexual devices "for a *bona fide* medical, scientific, educational, legislative, judicial, or law enforcement purpose." This case, which is now before us on appeal for the second time, involves a challenge to the constitutionality of the Alabama statute. The ACLU, on behalf of various individual users and vendors of sexual devices, initially filed suit seeking to enjoin the statute . . .

. . . [T]he district court . . . scrutinize[d] the statute under rational basis review. Concluding that the statute lacked any rational basis, the district court permanently enjoined its enforcement . . . We reversed the district court's conclusion that the statute lacked a rational basis and held that the promotion and preservation of public morality provided a rational basis. . . . We then remanded the action to the district court for further consideration of the *as-applied* fundamental-rights challenge.

On remand, the district court again struck down the statute. [T]he district court held that the statute unconstitutionally burdened the right to use sexual devices within private adult, consensual sexual relationships. After a lengthy discussion of the history of sex in America, the district court announced a fundamental right to "sexual privacy," which, although unrecognized under any existing Supreme Court precedent, the district court found to be deeply rooted in the history and traditions of our nation. . . .

Alabama now appeals that decision. The only question on this appeal is whether the statute, as applied to the involved users and vendors, violates any fundamental right protected under the Constitution. . . .

## II. Discussion

Our *de novo* review begins with a discussion of the asserted right. Here, we reaffirm our conclusion that no Supreme Court precedents, including the recent decision in *Lawrence v. Texas*, 539 U.S. 558 (2003), are decisive on the question of the existence of such a right. Because the ACLU is asking us to recognize a new fundamental right, we then apply the analysis required by *Washington v. Glucksberg*, 521 U.S. 702 (1997). . . .

## A. Asserted Right

. . . According to the ACLU, the State of Alabama, through its prohibition on the commercial distribution of sex toys *qua* sex toys, has intruded into the most intimate of places — the bedrooms of its citizens — and the lawful sexual conduct that occurs therein. While the statute's reach does not directly proscribe the sexual conduct in question, it places — without justification — a substantial and undue burden on the ability of the plaintiffs to obtain devices regulated by the statute. By restricting sales of these devices to plaintiffs, Alabama has acted in violation of the fundamental rights of privacy and personal autonomy that protect an individual's lawful sexual practices guaranteed by the First, Fourth, Fifth, Ninth, and Fourteenth Amendments of the United States Constitution.

The ACLU invokes "privacy" and "personal autonomy" as if such phrases were constitutional talismans. In the abstract, however, there is no fundamental right to either. Undoubtedly, many fundamental rights currently recognized under Supreme Court precedent touch on matters of personal autonomy and privacy. However, "[t]hat many of the rights and liberties protected by the Due Process Clause sound in personal autonomy does not warrant the sweeping conclusion that any and all important, intimate, and personal decisions are so protected."[ ] Such rights have been denominated "fundamental" not simply because they implicate deeply personal and private considerations, but because they have been identified as "deeply rooted in this Nation's history and tradition and implicit in the concept of ordered liberty, such that neither liberty nor justice would exist if they were sacrificed." [Citations to *Glucksberg* omitted.]

Nor, contrary to the ACLU's assertion, have the Supreme Court's substantive-due-process precedents recognized a free-standing "right to sexual privacy." . . .

The Supreme Court's most recent opportunity to recognize a fundamental right to sexual privacy came in *Lawrence v. Texas*, where petitioners and *amici* expressly invited the court to do so. That the *Lawrence* Court had declined the invitation was this court's conclusion in our recent decision in *Lofton v. Sec'y of Dept. of Children and Family Servs.*, 358 F.3d 804, 815-16 (11th Cir. 2004). In *Lofton* [w]e concluded that, although *Lawrence* clearly established the unconstitutionality of criminal prohibitions on consensual adult sodomy, "it is a strained and ultimately incorrect reading of *Lawrence* to interpret it to announce a new fundamental right" — whether to homosexual sodomy specifically or, more broadly, to all forms of sexual intimacy. We noted in particular that the *Lawrence* opinion did not employ fundamental-rights analysis and that it ultimately applied rational-basis review, rather than strict scrutiny, to the challenged statute.

. . . .

In short, we decline to extrapolate from *Lawrence* and its *dicta* a right to sexual privacy triggering strict scrutiny. To do so would be to impose a fundamental-rights interpretation on a decision that rested on rational-basis grounds, that never engaged in *Glucksberg* analysis, and that never invoked strict scrutiny. Moreover, it would be answering questions that the *Lawrence* Court appears to have left for another day. Of course, the Court may in due course expand *Lawrence*'s precedent in the direction anticipated by the dissent. But for us preemptively to take that step would exceed our mandate as a lower court.

## B.   *Glucksberg* Analysis

First, in analyzing a request for recognition of a new fundamental right, or extension of an existing one, we "must begin with a careful description of the asserted right." Second, and most critically, we must determine whether this asserted right, carefully described, is one of "those fundamental rights and liberties which are, objectively, deeply rooted in this Nation's history and tradition, and implicit in the concept of ordered liberty, such that neither liberty nor justice would exist if they were sacrificed."

## 1.   Careful Description

As we noted in *Williams II*, the district court's initial opinion "narrowly framed the analysis as the question whether the concept of a constitutionally protected right to privacy protects an individual's liberty to use sexual devices when engaging in lawful, private, sexual activity." On appeal, we affirmed this formulation. . . .

As [now] formulated by the district court, the [fundamental] right [to "sexual privacy"] potentially encompasses a great universe of sexual activities, including many that historically have been, and continue to be, prohibited. At oral arguments, the ACLU contended that "no responsible counsel" would challenge prohibitions such as those against pederasty and adult incest under a "right to sexual privacy" theory. However, mere faith in the responsibility of the bar scarcely provides a legally cognizable, or constitutionally significant, limiting principle in applying the right in future cases.

The sole limitation provided by the district court's ruling was that the right would extend only to *consenting adults*. The consenting-adult formula, of course, is a corollary to John Stuart Mill's celebrated "harm principle," which would allow the state to proscribe only conduct that causes identifiable harm to another. Regardless of its force as a policy argument, however, it does not translate *ipse dixit* into a constitutionally cognizable standard.

If we were to accept the invitation to recognize a right to sexual intimacy, this right would theoretically encompass such activities as prostitution, obscenity, and adult incest — even if we were to limit the right to consenting adults. This in turn would require us to subject all infringements on such activities to strict scrutiny. In short, by framing our inquiry so broadly as to look for a general right to sexual intimacy, we would be answering many questions not before us on the present facts.

One of "the cardinal rules" of constitutional jurisprudence is that the scope of the asserted right — and thus the parameters of the inquiry — must be dictated "by the precise facts" of the immediate case.

In *Glucksberg*, the lower court and the petitioners had variously characterized the asserted right as "a liberty interest in determining the time and manner of one's death," "a liberty to choose how to die and a right to control one's final days," and the "liberty of competent, terminally ill adults to make end-of-life decisions free of undue government interference." The Court rejected these characterizations as overbroad, noting its "tradition of carefully formulating the interest at stake in substantive-due-process cases." Then, looking to the specific statute under challenge — a ban on assisted suicide — the Court recast the asserted right as "a right to commit suicide which itself includes a right to assistance in doing so," or as "a right to commit suicide with another's assistance."

We begin by observing that the broad rights to "privacy" and "sexual privacy" invoked by the ACLU are not at issue. The statute invades the privacy of Alabama residents in their bedrooms no more than does any statute restricting the availability of commercial products for use in private quarters as sexual enhancements. Instead, the challenged Alabama statute bans the commercial distribution of sexual devices. At a minimum, therefore, the putative right at issue is the right to sell and purchase sexual devices.

It is more than that, however. For purposes of constitutional analysis, restrictions on the ability to purchase an item are tantamount to restrictions on the use of that item. Thus it was that the *Glucksberg* Court analyzed a ban on *providing* suicide assistance as a burden on the right to *receive* suicide assistance. Similarly, prohibitions on the *sale* of contraceptives have been analyzed as burdens on the *use* of contraceptives. . . . Because a prohibition on the distribution of sexual devices would burden an individual's ability to use the devices, our analysis must be framed not simply in terms of whether the Constitution protects a right to *sell* and *buy* sexual devices, but whether it protects a right to *use* such devices.

## 2. "History and Tradition" and "Implicit in the Concept of Ordered Liberty"

With this "careful description" in mind, we turn now to the second prong of the fundamental-rights inquiry. The crucial inquiry under this prong is whether the right to use sexual devices when engaging in lawful, private sexual activity is (1) "objectively, deeply rooted in this Nation's history and tradition" and (2) "implicit in the concept of ordered liberty, such that neither liberty nor justice would exist if [it] were sacrificed." . . .

We find that the district court, in reaching this conclusion, erred on four levels. The first error relates back to the district court's over-broad framing of the asserted right in question. Having framed the relevant right as a generalized "right to sexual privacy," the district court's history and tradition analysis consisted largely of an irrelevant exploration of the history of sex in America. Second, we find that this analysis placed too much weight on contemporary practice and attitudes with respect to sexual conduct and sexual devices. Third, rather than look for a history and tradition of *protection* of the asserted right, the district court asked whether there was a history and tradition of state *non-interference* with the right. Finally, we find that the district court's uncritical reliance on certain expert declarations in interpreting the historical record was flawed and that its reliance on certain putative "concessions" was unfounded.

. . . .

In short, nothing in *Glucksberg* indicates that an absence of historical *prohibition* is tantamount, for purposes of fundamental-rights analysis, to an historical record of *protection* under the law. Not only does the record before us fail to evidence such a deeply rooted right, but it suggests that, to the extent that sex toys historically have attracted the attention of the law, it has been in the context of proscription, not protection.

The chief example of this proscription is the "Comstock Laws," federal and state legislation adopted in the late 1800s. The federal Comstock Act of 1873 was a criminal statute directed at "the suppression of Trade in and Circulation of obscene Literature and Articles of immoral Use." The Act prohibited importation of and use of the mails for transporting, among other things, "every article or thing intended or adapted for any indecent or immoral use." Various states also enacted similar statutes prohibiting the sale of such articles.

Even if these prohibitions on sexual devices were not widespread or vigorously enforced, their mere existence significantly undermines the argument that sexual devices historically have been free from state interference. In light of these realities, the negative inference drawn by the district court — that the scarcity of explicit reference to sexual devices in statutory schemes and reported cases reflects a "deliberate non-interference," — is too speculative a basis for constitutionalizing a hitherto unrecognized right.

\* \* \*

Barkett, Circuit Judge, dissenting.

The majority's decision rests on the erroneous foundation that there is no substantive due process right to adult consensual sexual intimacy in the home and erroneously assumes that the promotion of public morality provides a rational basis to criminally burden such private intimate activity. These premises directly conflict with the Supreme Court's holding in *Lawrence v. Texas*, 539 U.S. 558 (2003).

This case is not, as the majority's demeaning and dismissive analysis suggests, about sex or about sexual devices. It is about the tradition of American citizens from the inception of our democracy to value the constitutionally protected right to be left alone in the privacy of their bedrooms and personal relationships. As Justice Brandeis stated in the now famous words of his dissent in *Olmstead v. United States*, 277 U.S. 438 (1928), when "[t]he makers of our Constitution undertook to secure conditions favorable to the pursuit of happiness . . . [t]hey conferred, as against the government, the right to be let alone — the most comprehensive of rights and the right most valued by civilized men." [*Olmstead* upheld a criminal conviction based on evidence derived from a wiretap of a personal telephone call.]

The majority claims that *Lawrence* failed to recognize the substantive due process right of consenting adults to engage in private sexual conduct. Conceding that *Lawrence* must have done something, the majority acknowledges that *Lawrence* "established the unconstitutionality of criminal prohibitions on consensual adult sodomy." The majority refuses, however, to acknowledge why the Court in *Lawrence* held that criminal prohibitions on consensual sodomy are unconstitutional. This failure underlies the majority's flawed conclusion in this case.

. . . *Lawrence* held that a state may not criminalize sodomy because of the existence of the very right to private sexual intimacy that the majority refuses to acknowledge. *Lawrence* reiterated that its prior fundamental rights cases protected individual choices "concerning the intimacies of [a] physical relationship." Because of this precedent, the *Lawrence* Court overruled *Bowers*, concluding that *Bowers* had "misapprehended the claim of liberty there presented" as involving a particular sexual act rather than the broader right of adult sexual privacy. Instead of heeding the Supreme Court's instruction regarding *Bowers'* error, the majority repeats it, ignoring *Lawrence*'s teachings about how to correctly frame a liberty interest affecting sexual privacy.

Compounding this error, the majority also ignores *Lawrence's* holding that although history and tradition may be used as a "starting point," they are not the "ending point" of a substantive due process inquiry. In cases solely involving adult consensual sexual privacy, the Court has never required that there be a long-standing history of affirmative legal protection of specific conduct before a right can be recognized under the Due Process Clause. To the contrary, because of the fundamental nature of this liberty interest, this right has been protected by the Court despite historical, legislative restrictions on private sexual conduct. Applying the analytical framework of *Lawrence* compels the conclusion that the Due Process Clause protects a right to sexual privacy that encompasses the use of sexual devices.

Finally, even under the majority's own constrained and erroneous interpretation of *Lawrence*, we are, at a bare minimum, obliged to revisit this Court's previous conclusion in *Williams II*, that Alabama's law survives the most basic level of review, that of rational basis. . . .

There is no question that *Lawrence* was decided on substantive due process grounds. The doctrine of substantive due process requires, first, that every law must address in a relevant way only a legitimate governmental purpose. In other words, no law may be arbitrary and capricious but rather must address a permissible state interest in a way that is rationally related to that interest. As a consequence, any law challenged as violating a substantive due process right must survive rational-basis review.

. . . .

The majority neglects to address whether Alabama's statute has a rational basis even though Alabama relies upon the same justification for criminalizing private sexual activity rejected by *Lawrence* — public morality. In

*Lawrence*, Texas had explicitly relied upon public morality as a rational basis for its sodomy law. In *Williams II*, this Court previously upheld Alabama's law on rational basis grounds, relying on the now defunct *Bowers* to conclude that public morality provides a legitimate state interest. . . . Obviously, now that *Bowers* has been overruled, this proposition is no longer good law and we must, accordingly, revisit our holding in *Williams II*. Yet despite the *Lawrence* Court's rejection of public morality as a legitimate state interest that can justify criminalizing private consensual sexual conduct, the majority, although acknowledging that the district court will have to do so, never once addresses how our holding in *Williams II* can remain good law.

\* \* \*

# GOODRIDGE v. DEPARTMENT OF PUBLIC HEALTH
### 440 Mass. 309, 798 N.E.2d 941 (2003)

Marshall, Chief Justice.

\* \* \*

Marriage is a vital social institution. The exclusive commitment of two individuals to each other nurtures love and mutual support; it brings stability to our society. For those who choose to marry, and for their children, marriage provides an abundance of legal, financial, and social benefits. In return it imposes weighty legal, financial, and social obligations. The question before us is whether, consistent with the Massachusetts Constitution, the Commonwealth may deny the protections, benefits, and obligations conferred by civil marriage to two individuals of the same sex who wish to marry. . . .

. . . Many people hold deep-seated religious, moral, and ethical convictions that marriage should be limited to the union of one man and one woman, and that homosexual conduct is immoral. Many hold equally strong religious, moral, and ethical convictions that same-sex couples are entitled to be married, and that homosexual persons should be treated no differently than their heterosexual neighbors. Neither view answers the question before us. Our concern is with the Massachusetts Constitution as a charter of governance for every person properly within its reach. "Our obligation is to define the liberty of all, not to mandate our own moral code." [citing *Lawrence*]

Whether the Commonwealth may use its formidable regulatory authority to bar same-sex couples from civil marriage is a question not previously addressed by a Massachusetts appellate court. It is a question the United States Supreme Court left open as a matter of Federal law in *Lawrence,* where it was not an issue. There, the Court affirmed that the core concept of common human dignity protected by the Fourteenth Amendment to the United States Constitution precludes government intrusion into the deeply personal realms of consensual adult expressions of intimacy and one's choice of an intimate partner. The Court also reaffirmed the central role that decisions whether to marry or have children bear in shaping one's identity. The Massachusetts Constitution is, if anything, more protective of individual liberty and equality than the Federal Constitution; it may demand broader protection for fundamental rights; and it is less tolerant of government intrusion into the protected spheres of private life. [See discussion of the Massachusetts Constitution, *infra* in this opinion.]

Barred access to the protections, benefits, and obligations of civil marriage, a person who enters into an intimate, exclusive union with another of the same sex is arbitrarily deprived of membership in one of our community's most rewarding and cherished institutions. That exclusion is incompatible with the constitutional principles of respect for individual autonomy and equality under law.

## I

The plaintiffs are fourteen individuals from five Massachusetts counties. . . .

The plaintiffs include business executives, lawyers, an investment banker, educators, therapists, and a computer engineer. Many are active in church, community, and school groups. They have employed such legal means as are available to them — for example, joint adoption, powers of attorney, and joint ownership of real property — to secure aspects of their relationships. Each plaintiff attests a desire to marry his or her partner in order to affirm publicly their commitment to each other and to secure the legal protections and benefits afforded to married couples and their children.

The Department of Public Health (department) is charged by statute with safeguarding public health. Among its responsibilities, the department oversees the registry of vital records and statistics (registry), which "enforce[s] all laws" relative to the issuance of marriage licenses and the keeping of marriage records, and which promulgates policies and procedures for the issuance of marriage licenses by city and town clerks and registers. . . .

In March and April, 2001, each of the plaintiff couples attempted to obtain a marriage license from a city or town clerk's office. [T]hey completed notices of intention to marry on forms provided by the registry . . . together with the required health forms and marriage license fees. In each case, the clerk either refused to accept the notice of intention to marry or denied a marriage license to the couple on the ground that Massachusetts does not recognize same-sex marriage. . . .

On April 11, 2001, the plaintiffs filed suit in the Superior Court against the department and the commissioner seeking a judgment that "the exclusion of the [p]laintiff couples and other qualified same-sex couples from access to marriage licenses, and the legal and social status of civil marriage, as well as the protections, benefits and obligations of marriage, violates Massachusetts law." The plaintiffs alleged violation of [various provisions of the Massachusetts Constitution]. The department, represented by the Attorney General, admitted to a policy and practice of denying marriage licenses to same-sex couples. It denied that its actions violated any law. . . .

. . . .

After the complaint was dismissed and summary judgment entered for the defendants, the plaintiffs appealed. Both parties requested direct appellate review, which we granted.

II

Although the plaintiffs refer in passing to "the marriage statutes," they focus, quite properly, on G.L. c. 207, the marriage licensing statute, which controls entry into civil marriage. . . .

. . . [F]or all the joy and solemnity that normally attend a marriage, G.L. c. 207, governing entrance to marriage, is a licensing law. The plaintiffs argue that because nothing in that licensing law specifically prohibits marriages between persons of the same sex, we may interpret the statute to permit "qualified same sex couples" to obtain marriage licenses, thereby avoiding the question whether the law is constitutional. This claim lacks merit.

We interpret statutes to carry out the Legislature's intent, determined by the words of a statute interpreted according to "the ordinary and approved usage of the language." [The statute's] definition of marriage, as both the department and the Superior Court judge point out, derives from the common law. . . . Far from being ambiguous, [the statute] confirms the General Court's intent to hew to the term's common-law and quotidian meaning concerning the genders of the marriage partners.

The intended scope of G.L. c. 207 is also evident in its consanguinity provisions. . . . The only reasonable explanation is that the Legislature did not intend that same-sex couples be licensed to marry. . . .

III

The larger question is whether, as the department claims, government action that bars same-sex couples from civil marriage constitutes a legitimate exercise of the State's authority to regulate conduct, or whether, as the plaintiffs claim, this categorical marriage exclusion violates the Massachusetts Constitution. We have recognized the long-standing statutory understanding, derived from the common law, that "marriage" means the lawful union of a woman and a man. But that history cannot and does not foreclose the constitutional question.

The plaintiffs' claim that the marriage restriction violates the Massachusetts Constitution can be analyzed in two ways. Does it offend the Constitution's guarantees of equality before the law? Or do the liberty and due process provisions of the Massachusetts Constitution secure the plaintiffs' right to marry their chosen partner? In matters implicating marriage, family life, and the upbringing of children, the two constitutional concepts frequently overlap, as they do here. . . . Much of what we say concerning one standard applies to the other.

We begin by considering the nature of civil marriage itself. Simply put, the government creates civil marriage. In Massachusetts, civil marriage is, and since pre-Colonial days has been, precisely what its name implies: a wholly secular institution. . . . No religious ceremony has ever been required to validate a Massachusetts marriage.

. . . .

Civil marriage is created and regulated through exercise of the police power. . . . "Police power" (now more commonly termed the State's regulatory authority) is an old-fashioned term for the Commonwealth's lawmaking authority, as bounded by the liberty and equality guarantees of the Massachusetts Constitution. . . . In broad terms, it is the Legislature's power to enact rules to regulate conduct, to the extent that such laws are "necessary to secure the health, safety, good order, comfort, or general welfare of the community."

Without question, civil marriage enhances the "welfare of the community." It is a "social institution of the highest importance." Civil marriage anchors an ordered society by encouraging stable relationships over transient ones. It is central to the way the Commonwealth identifies individuals, provides for the orderly distribution of property, ensures that children and adults are cared for and supported whenever possible from private rather than public funds, and tracks important epidemiological and demographic data.

Marriage also bestows enormous private and social advantages on those who choose to marry. Civil marriage is at once a deeply personal commitment to another human being and a highly public celebration of the ideals of mutuality, companionship, intimacy, fidelity, and family. . . . Because it fulfils yearnings for security, safe haven, and connection that express our common humanity, civil marriage is an esteemed institution, and the decision whether and whom to marry is among life's momentous acts of self-definition.

Tangible as well as intangible benefits flow from marriage. . . .

The benefits accessible only by way of a marriage license are enormous, touching nearly every aspect of life and death. The department states that "hundreds of statutes" are related to marriage and to marital benefits. . . .

Exclusive marital benefits that are not directly tied to property rights include the presumptions of legitimacy and parentage of children born to a married couple and evidentiary rights, such as the prohibition against spouses testifying against one another about their private conversations, applicable in both civil and criminal cases. Other statutory benefits of a personal nature available only to married individuals include qualification for bereavement or medical leave to care for individuals related by blood or marriage; an automatic "family member" preference to make medical decisions for an incompetent or disabled spouse who does not have a contrary health care proxy. . . .

Where a married couple has children, their children are also directly or indirectly, but no less auspiciously, the recipients of the special legal and economic protections obtained by civil marriage[,] [n]otwithstanding the Commonwealth's strong public policy to abolish legal distinctions between marital and nonmarital children in providing for the support and care of minors. . . .

It is undoubtedly for these concrete reasons, as well as for its intimately personal significance, that civil marriage has long been termed a "civil right.". . . The United States Supreme Court has described the right to marry as "of fundamental importance for all individuals" and as "part of the fundamental 'right of privacy' implicit in the Fourteenth Amendment's Due Process Clause.". . .

Without the right to marry — or more properly, the right to choose to marry — one is excluded from the full range of human experience and denied full protection of the laws for one's "avowed commitment to an intimate and lasting human relationship."

Unquestionably, the regulatory power of the Commonwealth over civil marriage is broad, as is the Commonwealth's discretion to award public benefits. Individuals who have the choice to marry each other and nevertheless choose not to may properly be denied the legal benefits of marriage. But that same logic cannot hold for a qualified individual who would marry if she or he only could.

. . . .

The Massachusetts Constitution protects matters of personal liberty against government incursion as zealously, and often more so, than does the Federal Constitution, even where both Constitutions employ essentially the same language. That the Massachusetts Constitution is in some instances more protective of individual liberty interests than is the Federal Constitution is not surprising. Fundamental to the vigor of our Federal system of government is that "state courts are absolutely free to interpret state constitutional provisions to accord greater protection to individual rights than do similar provisions of the United States Constitution."

The individual liberty and equality safeguards of the Massachusetts Constitution protect both "freedom from" unwarranted government intrusion into protected spheres of life and "freedom to" partake in benefits created by the State for the common good. Both freedoms are involved here. Whether and whom to marry, how to express sexual intimacy, and whether and how to establish a family — these are among the most basic of every individual's liberty and due process rights. And central to personal freedom and security is the assurance that the laws will apply equally to persons in similar situations. . . .

The Massachusetts Constitution requires, at a minimum, that the exercise of the State's regulatory authority not be "arbitrary or capricious." Under both the equality and liberty guarantees, regulatory authority must, at very least, serve "a legitimate purpose in a rational way"; a statute must "bear a reasonable relation to a permissible legislative objective." . . .

The plaintiffs challenge the marriage statute on both equal protection and due process grounds. With respect to each such claim, we must first determine the appropriate standard of review. Where a statute implicates a fundamental right or uses a suspect classification, we employ "strict judicial scrutiny." For all other statutes, we employ the "'rational basis' test." For due process claims, rational basis analysis requires that statutes "bear[ ] a real and substantial relation to the public health, safety, morals, or some other phase of the general welfare." For equal protection challenges, the rational basis test requires that "an impartial lawmaker could logically believe that the classification would serve a legitimate public purpose that transcends the harm to the members of the disadvantaged class."

. . . For the reasons we explain below, we conclude that the marriage ban does not meet the rational basis test for either due process or equal protection.

Because the statute does not survive rational basis review, we do not consider the plaintiffs' arguments that this case merits strict judicial scrutiny.

The department posits three legislative rationales for prohibiting same-sex couples from marrying: (1) providing a "favorable setting for procreation"; (2) ensuring the optimal setting for child rearing, which the department defines as "a two-parent family with one parent of each sex"; and (3) preserving scarce State and private financial resources. We consider each in turn.

The judge in the Superior Court endorsed the first rationale, holding that "the state's interest in regulating marriage is based on the traditional concept that marriage's primary purpose is procreation." This is incorrect. Our laws of civil marriage do not privilege procreative heterosexual intercourse between married people above every other form of adult intimacy and every other means of creating a family. General Laws c. 207 contains no requirement that the applicants for a marriage license attest to their ability or intention to conceive children by coitus. Fertility is not a condition of marriage, nor is it grounds for divorce. People who have never consummated their marriage, and never plan to, may be and stay married. . . .

Moreover, the Commonwealth affirmatively facilitates bringing children into a family regardless of whether the intended parent is married or unmarried, whether the child is adopted or born into a family, whether assistive technology was used to conceive the child, and whether the parent or her partner is heterosexual, homosexual, or bisexual. If procreation were a necessary component of civil marriage, our statutes would draw a tighter circle around the permissible bounds of nonmarital child bearing and the creation of families by noncoital means. . . .

The "marriage is procreation" argument singles out the one unbridgeable difference between same-sex and opposite-sex couples, and transforms that difference into the essence of legal marriage. . . . In so doing, the State's action confers an official stamp of approval on the destructive stereotype that same-sex relationships are inherently unstable and inferior to opposite-sex relationships and are not worthy of respect.

The department's first stated rationale, equating marriage with unassisted heterosexual procreation, shades imperceptibly into its second: that confining marriage to opposite-sex couples ensures that children are raised in the "optimal" setting. Protecting the welfare of children is a paramount State policy. Restricting marriage to opposite-sex couples, however, cannot plausibly further this policy. "The demographic changes of the past century make it difficult to speak of an average American family. The composition of families varies greatly from household to household." Moreover, we have repudiated the common-law power of the State to provide varying levels of protection to children based on the circumstances of birth. The "best interests of the child" standard does not turn on a parent's sexual orientation or marital status. . . .

The department has offered no evidence that forbidding marriage to people of the same sex will increase the number of couples choosing to enter into opposite-sex marriages in order to have and raise children. There is thus no rational relationship between the marriage statute and the Commonwealth's proffered goal of protecting the "optimal" child rearing unit. Moreover, the department readily concedes that people in same-sex couples may be "excellent" parents. . . . While establishing the parentage of children as soon as possible is crucial to the safety and welfare of children, same-sex couples must undergo the sometimes lengthy and intrusive process of second-parent adoption to establish their joint parentage. While the enhanced income provided by marital benefits is an important source of security and stability for married couples and their children, those benefits are denied to families headed by same-sex couples. While the laws of divorce provide clear and reasonably predictable guidelines for child support, child custody, and property division on dissolution of a marriage, same-sex couples who dissolve their relationships find themselves and their children in the highly unpredictable terrain of equity jurisdiction. Given the wide range of public benefits reserved only for married couples, we do not credit the department's contention that the absence of access to civil marriage amounts to little more than an inconvenience to same-sex couples and their children. . . .

No one disputes that the plaintiff couples are families, that many are parents, and that the children they are raising, like all children, need and should have the fullest opportunity to grow up in a secure, protected family unit. Similarly, no one disputes that, under the rubric of marriage, the State provides a cornucopia of substantial benefits to married parents and their children.

In this case, we are confronted with an entire, sizeable class of parents raising children who have absolutely no access to civil marriage and its protections because they are forbidden from procuring a marriage license. It cannot be rational under our laws, and indeed it is not permitted, to penalize children by depriving them of State benefits because the State disapproves of their parents' sexual orientation.

The third rationale advanced by the department is that limiting marriage to opposite-sex couples furthers the Legislature's interest in conserving scarce State and private financial resources. The marriage restriction is rational, it argues, because the General Court logically could assume that same-sex couples are more financially independent than married couples and thus less needy of public marital benefits, such as tax advantages, or private marital benefits, such as employer-financed health plans that include spouses in their coverage.

An absolute statutory ban on same-sex marriage bears no rational relationship to the goal of economy. First, the department's conclusory generalization — that same-sex couples are less financially dependent on each other than opposite-sex couples — ignores that many same-sex couples, such as many of the plaintiffs in this case, have children and other dependents (here, aged parents) in their care. . . . Second, Massachusetts marriage laws do not condition receipt of public and private financial benefits to married individuals on a demonstration of financial dependence on each other; the benefits are available to married couples regardless of whether they mingle their finances or actually depend on each other for support.

The department suggests additional rationales for prohibiting same-sex couples from marrying. . . . It argues that broadening civil marriage to include same-sex couples will trivialize or destroy the institution of marriage as it has historically been fashioned. Certainly our decision today marks a significant change in the definition of marriage as it has been inherited from the common law, and understood by many societies for centuries. But it does not disturb the fundamental value of marriage in our society.

Here, the plaintiffs seek only to be married, not to undermine the institution of civil marriage. They do not want marriage abolished. They do not attack the binary nature of marriage, the consanguinity provisions, or any of the other gate-keeping provisions of the marriage licensing law. Recognizing the right of an individual to marry a person of the same sex will not diminish the validity or dignity of opposite-sex marriage, any more than recognizing the right of an individual to marry a person of a different race devalues the marriage of a person who marries someone of her own race. . . .

It has been argued that, due to the State's strong interest in the institution of marriage as a stabilizing social structure, only the Legislature can control and define its boundaries. Accordingly, our elected representatives legitimately may choose to exclude same-sex couples from civil marriage in order to assure all citizens of the Commonwealth that (1) the benefits of our marriage laws are available explicitly to create and support a family setting that is, in the Legislature's view, optimal for child rearing, and (2) the State does not endorse gay and lesbian parenthood as the equivalent of being raised by one's married biological parents. These arguments miss the point. The Massachusetts Constitution requires that legislation meet certain criteria and not extend beyond certain limits. It is the function of courts to determine whether these criteria are met and whether these limits are exceeded. In most instances, these limits are defined by whether a rational basis exists to conclude that legislation will bring about a rational result. . . . We owe great deference to the Legislature to decide social and policy issues, but it is the traditional and settled role of courts to decide constitutional issues.

The history of constitutional law "is the story of the extension of constitutional rights and protections to people once ignored or excluded." As a public institution and a right of fundamental importance, civil marriage is an evolving paradigm. . . . Alarms about the imminent erosion of the "natural" order of marriage were sounded over the demise of anti-miscegenation laws, the expansion of the rights of married women, and the introduction of "no-fault" divorce. Marriage has survived all of these transformations, and we have no doubt that marriage will continue to be a vibrant and revered institution.

We also reject the argument suggested by the department, and elaborated by some amici, that expanding the institution of civil marriage in Massachusetts to include same-sex couples will lead to interstate conflict. We would not presume to dictate how another State should respond to today's decision. But neither should considerations of comity prevent us from according Massachusetts residents the full measure of protection available under the Massachusetts Constitution. . . .

Several *amici* suggest that prohibiting marriage by same-sex couples reflects community consensus that homosexual conduct is immoral. Yet Massachusetts has a strong affirmative policy of preventing discrimination on the basis of sexual orientation.

The department has had more than ample opportunity to articulate a constitutionally adequate justification for limiting civil marriage to opposite-sex unions. It has failed to do so. The department has offered purported justifications for the civil marriage restriction that are starkly at odds with the comprehensive network of vigorous, gender-neutral laws promoting stable families and the best interests of children. It has failed to identify any relevant characteristic that would justify shutting the door to civil marriage to a person who wishes to marry someone of the same sex.

The marriage ban works a deep and scarring hardship on a very real segment of the community for no rational reason. The absence of any reasonable relationship between, on the one hand, an absolute disqualification of same-sex couples who wish to enter into civil marriage and, on the other, protection of public health, safety, or general welfare, suggests that the marriage restriction is rooted in persistent prejudices against persons who are (or who are believed to be) homosexual. "The Constitution cannot control such prejudices but neither can it tolerate them. Private biases may be outside the reach of the law, but the law cannot, directly or indirectly, give them effect."

. . . .

We construe civil marriage to mean the voluntary union of two persons as spouses, to the exclusion of all others. This reformulation redresses the plaintiffs' constitutional injury and furthers the aim of marriage to promote stable, exclusive relationships. It advances the two legitimate State interests the department has identified: providing a stable setting for child rearing and conserving State resources. It leaves intact the Legislature's broad discretion to regulate marriage.

. . . We declare that barring an individual from the protections, benefits, and obligations of civil marriage solely because that person would marry a person of the same sex violates the Massachusetts Constitution. We vacate the summary judgment for the department. We remand this case to the Superior Court for entry of judgment consistent with this opinion. . . .

\* \* \*

# NOTES AND QUESTIONS

1. In *Lawrence,* Justices Kennedy, Breyer, Stevens, and Souter, with a separate concurring opinion of Justice O'Connor, did what the Supreme Court has seldom done: It explicitly reconsidered a fairly recent decision, *Bowers v. Hardwick,* 478 U.S. 186 (1986), and held that it was "not correct when it was decided and it is not correct today." *Lawrence* considered a Texas statute (similar to the Georgia statute considered in *Bowers*) making it a crime for two persons of the same sex to engage in intimate sexual conduct. Reviewing the arguments that had been made in *Bowers,* Kennedy's opinion critiqued the conclusion in *Bowers* that there had been a long tradition of allowing the states to regulate or prohibit homosexual conduct and the *Bowers* Court's conclusion that that conduct was not protected by the Constitution. In Kennedy's view, the history of regulation of sexual conduct was more equivocal and many

of the laws cited by the *Bowers* opinion were largely a result of 19th century political trends. Most importantly, as the excerpt above demonstrates, the majority opinion held that *Bowers* had "demeaned" the constitutional significance of the privacy interest affected by such laws, by characterizing it as right to "engage in certain kinds of sexual conduct" rather than as a right to be free of criminally-sanctioned state control of a personal relationship, even if that relationship was not entitled to "formal legal recognition" (by which Kennedy presumably meant some form of civil validation of a homosexual partnership).

The Court then went on to compare the private activities of homosexuals to the conduct protected in *Planned Parenthood of Southeastern Pa. v. Casey*, 505 U.S. 833 (1992), and the other abortion cases and — while not using the term "fundamental interest" — clearly indicated that the private sexual conduct of homosexuals was entitled to the same degree of judicial protection as that in its previous right to privacy cases:

> . . . The case does involve two adults who, with full and mutual consent from each other, engaged in sexual practices common to a homosexual lifestyle. The petitioners are entitled to respect for their private lives. The State cannot demean their existence or control their destiny by making their private sexual conduct a crime. Their right to liberty under the Due Process Clause gives them the full right to engage in their conduct without intervention of the government. . . . The Texas statute furthers no legitimate state interest which can justify its intrusion into the personal and private life of the individual.

539 U.S. at 578.

Significantly, the Court considered whether a state may act to regulate or even prohibit homosexual conduct in order to protect minors, those who might be injured or coerced, or those who have not given their consent, or to prohibit public displays or prostitution, just as the state can regulate contraceptives or abortions where certain compelling or legitimate interests can properly be served. In such circumstances, the Court seems to contemplate, there may be "injury to a person or abuse of an institution the law protects" that is lacking in the case before it, which by contrast generates no such harm. Such governmental purposes, however, can be achieved only by legislation that survives close scrutiny, or the "undue burden" test, or whatever language is used to describe the restrictions applied by the Court to legislation that affects interests entitled to especially strong Constitutional protection — a limitation on government power that is far more substantial and demanding than that articulated in *Bowers*. Not surprisingly, the majority opinion found that the state's claimed interests were insufficient to justify the burden on the individuals' constitutional rights to engage in (consensual, private) sexual behavior.

*Lawrence* sheds some light on the question posed at the outset of this section: the extent of the states' ability to regulate individual conduct to achieve moral purposes. At least where that individual conduct involves strongly-protected constitutional interests, any state effort to do so will be subject to the kind of judicial scrutiny the *Lawrence* Court applied in evaluating and rejecting the Texas statute. What *Lawrence* did not address, however, is whether a state's interest is sufficient to justify its prevention of other kinds of activities — *e.g.*, gambling or tattooing — that are considered immoral by some members of the public, but do *not* involve the exercise of constitutionally protected interests. Regulation or prohibition of activities of this kind is subject to a "rationality" or some other lower standard of review. As discussed in Section A of this Chapter, the classic statement of the police powers, frequently repeated in public health cases, is that the states can do anything that is reasonably related to the "health, safety, welfare, or morals" of the public; most courts seek to find and invoke some health-, safety-, or welfare-related purpose for public health legislation. Nonetheless, in cases like *Bowers* where the state regulation is admitted to be morality-based, the courts have acknowledged that morality can be a proper state purpose. *Lawrence* did not reject that part of *Bowers*. But other specific illustrations are hard to come by. Indeed, most potential controversies over the government's authority to regulate morality involve sexual activity and many of these, though not all, are arguably within constitutional protections, especially after *Lawrence*.

**2.** Early definitions of the state's police power included protecting the public's safety, health, welfare, good order, and morality. Laws prohibiting acts considered immoral or disruptive of good order were common in the 18th and 19th centuries, such as laws prohibiting blasphemy, indecent attire and operating a business on the Sabbath, laws prohibiting marriage between races or within certain bounds of consanguinity, or laws prohibiting contraception, abortion, sodomy, and tobacco use. Many such laws provoked controversy. In some cases, advances in scientific knowledge undercut the early rationale for a law, while in others, political or economic objections forced their repeal or limitation. In still others, legal challenges based on constitutional protections of individual liberty succeeded in removing laws prohibiting interracial marriage, contraception, abortion and consensual sodomy, regardless of public opinion. Today, in practice, purely moral justifications are rarely put forth as the sole reason to justify legislation. In the past few decades, for example, Sunday closing laws were upheld as offering a day of rest for workers, rather than a day of worship. Since *Lawrence* was decided in 2003, the question is whether, by itself, morality or any particular moral theory remains a legitimate goal of the state sufficient to override personal freedoms, or whether the law must necessarily serve an independent reason of public safety, health, or welfare.

**3.** *Utah v. Green*, P.3d 820 (Utah 2004), raises some of these same issues, although, again, it does not provide definitive answers. Green, an "avowed polygamist," participated in simultaneous conjugal-type relationships with multiple women. These women all used Green's surname and bore children who also use the Green surname. Some of the women entered into licensed marriages with Green. The remaining women participated in unlicensed ceremonies, after which they considered themselves married to Green. Green avoided being in more than one licensed marriage at a time by terminating each licensed marriage by divorce prior to obtaining a license for a new marriage. Green then continued his relationships with each of the women he divorced as if no divorce had occurred. Green appeared on various television shows with the women, consistently referring to the women as his wives, and the women likewise acknowledged spousal relationships. In these television appearances, Green acknowledged that his conduct was potentially punishable under Utah criminal statutes.

Utah charged Green with bigamy. A jury found him guilty on four counts. Green appealed claiming that (1) Utah's bigamy statute violated his federal constitutional right to free exercise of religion; (2) Utah's bigamy statute was unconstitutionally vague in light of Green's conduct; and (3) the State's use of Utah's unsolemnized marriage statute to establish a legal marriage to some of his wives was unconstitutional. The state supreme court rejected all of his claims. With respect to his Free Exercise claim, the court reasoned:

> . . . We conclude that Utah's bigamy statute is rationally related to several legitimate government ends. First, this state has an interest in regulating marriage. As stated in *Reynolds* [a 19th Century U.S. Supreme Court case upholding Utah's criminalization of bigamy in its state constitution], marriage may be viewed as a type of "civil contract": "Upon it society may be said to be built, and out of its fruits spring social relations and social obligations and duties, with which government is necessarily required to deal." . . .

> The State of Utah's interest in regulating marriage has resulted in a network of laws, many of which are premised upon the concept of monogamy. . . .

> Beyond the State's interest in regulating marriage as an important social unit, or in maintaining its network of laws, Utah's bigamy statute serves additional legitimate government ends. Specifically, prohibiting bigamy implicates the State's interest in preventing the perpetration of marriage fraud, as well as its interest in preventing the misuse of government benefits associated with marital status.

> Most importantly, Utah's bigamy statute serves the State's interest in protecting vulnerable individuals from exploitation and abuse. The practice of polygamy, in particular, often coincides with crimes targeting women and children. Crimes not unusually attendant to the practice of polygamy include incest, sexual assault, statutory rape, and failure to pay child support. Moreover, the closed nature of polygamous communities makes obtaining evidence of and prosecuting these crimes challenging. ("Given the highly private nature of sexual abuse and the self-imposed isolation of polygamous communities, prosecution may well prove impossible. This wall of silence may present a compelling justification for criminalizing the act of polygamy, prosecuting offenders, and effectively breaking down the wall that provides a favorable environment in which crimes of physical and sexual abuse can thrive.")

> All of the foregoing interests are legitimate, if not compelling, interests of the State, and Utah's bigamy statute is rationally related to the furthering of those interests. We therefore hold that Utah's bigamy statute does not violate the Free Exercise Clause of the First Amendment of the United States Constitution. . . .

99 P.3d at 829-30.

Note that Green based his primary constitutional claim on his Free Exercise rights. Suppose he had argued that he was exercising his right to privacy, as defined by *Lawrence*. Would this make any difference to either the analysis or the outcome in this case? Should it? Note also that the court goes to considerable length to find some state interest that protects some third party, *e.g.*, exploited women or children, and avoids considering whether the state could object to the practice of polygamy simply because it is regarded as immoral or otherwise inappropriate. If the state had defended the law solely on that ground, which level of review — "close scrutiny" (or its equivalent), or "rationality" — would be properly applicable? Would the state interest be sufficient to survive either level of review? Both levels?

**4.** As we saw in *Williams v. Alabama, supra* this section, the circuit court's majority opinion both distinguished *Lawrence* and implied that it was incorrectly decided. Consequently, it held that the Alabama statute criminalizing the sale of "sex toys" involved activities that did not merit heightened constitutional protection and, therefore, the law was subject to a rationality standard. Moreover, under a rationality standard, the state could merely argue that it had a moral objection to the sale (and, presumably, use) of sex toys: ". . . the promotion and preservation of public morality provided a rational basis" for the criminal proscription.

This is hardly an accurate reading of *Lawrence*, as the dissent points out. But it does allow the court to address and decide the oft-avoided question: Can the state regulate or prohibit an activity, at least one that is not specially protected by the state or federal constitutions, merely because the state legislature finds it immoral?

Assume for purposes of argument that the *Williams* court is correct about the state's discretion to regulate non-protected activities to achieve moral purposes. What limits would there be on legislative discretion? More to the point for present purposes, what would be the implications for various public health programs? Is it enough, for example, that we find obesity "repulsive" or smoking "stupid"? Is it possible that public health officials should applaud such a broad reading of government power? Can you think of circumstances under which those same officials should fear such a reading of the law?

**5.** *Goodridge* is a fascinating case for a number of reasons, not the least of which is the fact that the Massachusetts Supreme Court does in *Goodridge* what all state supreme courts can, but seldom do: It reaches into its own state constitution to build a constitutional foundation for its decision. What reasons do state courts have for taking this approach? One, of course, is clear: Such a decision cannot be overturned by any federal court, even the Supreme Court (except on "supremacy clause" grounds, which would not be available absent a contrary and prohibitive federal rule, either statutory or constitutional). What other reasons might there be? If the Massachusetts (or any other state or federal) court had instead analyzed state-law prohibitions on gay marriage on the basis of federal constitutional doctrine, how might application of *Lawrence* affect that analysis? Do you think the court's characterization of *Lawrence* as turning on "the core concept of common human dignity" is accurate?

The Massachusetts Court also does what some courts do when faced with potentially far-reaching questions of constitutional law: It finds a way to decide the case without deciding some of the more controversial questions that the case had apparently posed. In this case, the court holds that it need not decide whether the Massachusetts marriage laws warrant close judicial scrutiny, because in the court's view, the Massachusetts law does not even satisfy the "rationality" standard. In doing so, the court avoids the need to specify exactly which individual rights are affected by the Massachusetts law or commenting on any other laws that might affect such rights.

In a related vein, the court also seems to remain somewhat vague as to whether its analysis and conclusion are based on state-law notions of equal protection, due process, or both.

Consider whether you find the court's description of its methodology persuasive. Although the court purports to apply "rationality" review, is it really doing so? Note the skepticism with which the court greets several of the bases for the law articulated by the state. Does this track the kind of "rationality" review we have seen in earlier cases? It may help to know that, under "rationality" review, a law usually needn't be "perfect" in achieving its goals in order to be upheld. For example, the state's second asserted interest — ensuring the "optimal" setting for child-rearing, and viewing this as fostered by a heterosexual marital couple — is not a "perfect" justification for the law, simply because — even assuming, *arguendo*, that it were generally true — there are surely circumstances in which it will turn out *not* to be true, and in which less traditional families will do better for children's welfare. But why is it, as a constitutional matter, irrational? Under close scrutiny, of course, the imperfect fit may properly be viewed as unnecessarily restrictive. But under deferential scrutiny, such failings don't necessarily transform a law into an "irrational" policy enactment.

Further, isn't the court, in substance, requiring the state to justify its interests to the court — in effect, saying to the state, "show me" — rather than simply *presuming* the constitutional sufficiency of the state's interests and their fit with the chosen means, and requiring the *plaintiff* to affirmatively establish why no reasonable person could attach credence thereto? If this is an accurate description of what the court is doing, then it can be seen as an (unarticulated) burden-shifting that, more typically, is done only under "close" scrutiny, and then forthrightly.

*Goodridge* only briefly touches on the argument that the state may justify its statutory limits on same-sex measures as an effort to protect the morals of the public. Interestingly, in this connection it invokes a definition of the "police power" that includes most of the familiar elements — "the health, safety, good order, comfort, or general welfare of the community" — but omits "morals," another commonly-cited element. However, in the part of the opinion discussing the level of scrutiny, it does mention "morals." It dismisses the argument as inconsistent with the state's many efforts to protect homosexuals from discrimination. Does this make sense? Is it possible — more to the point, is it "rational" — for a state to oppose discrimination against homosexuals but still deny them licenses to marry? If Massachusetts were to repeal its discrimination laws, would it then be constitutionally permissible to disallow same-sex marriage on moral grounds? If notions of morality can be the rational basis for state action such as this, what other activities could be regulated or prohibited? Is there anything that could *not* be?

As a practical matter, these questions are most likely to be addressed in the context of laws attempting to regulate sexual behavior, to discriminate on the basis of sexual orientation, or in related issues in which the underlying motivation is difficult to disguise. In most other matters, especially those that fall within the broader limits of public health problems, the primary purpose of such efforts — or at least the purpose that will be publicly touted — will more likely be tied to some health, safety, or welfare justification, matters with which the courts will be more familiar — and comfortable.

Finally, note the procedural dimensions of the case, which came to the high court on review of a trial court's grant of summary judgment to the state. There had been no trial — and there would be none, since the high court not only reversed that judgment, but remanded the case "for entry of judgment consistent with this opinion." This, of course, foreclosed further fact-finding and exploration of matters that might well have been illuminating.

# Chapter 3

# CONTAGIOUS DISEASES: QUARANTINE AND OTHER LIBERTY-RESTRICTING RESPONSES

## A.  INTRODUCTION

This chapter begins with a series of case studies involving the use of compulsory confinement and other forms of coercion to control the spread of infectious disease. We start with an examination of governmentally-imposed restrictions on liberty in connection with active tuberculosis (in Section B), devoting a separate subsection to the general right of individuals to refuse unwanted medical treatment. We turn next to HIV/AIDS (in Section C) and then consider measures that may be necessary and appropriate in response to new diseases such as SARS (Section D) or the "bird flu" (influenza, Section E). Organizing the materials on this basis, we believe, is more likely to illuminate the difficulties of adapting available governmental interventions to the particular threat than would be achieved by separate discussions of each kind of governmental intervention. The final section of the chapter (Section F) anticipates how the states and the federal government will react if and when the nation is required to respond to some large-scale, rapidly moving disease outbreak, arising either from a bioterrorist event or a naturally-spreading epidemic. This subject is dealt with here in the context of government compulsory action, but is taken up as a case study for all types of public health preparation and responses for new epidemics and terrorist attacks in chapter 8 as a way to integrate the entire text.

Two sets of thematic issues are developed in the case studies and the exploration of emergency responses: (1) the importance of understanding the nature and etiology of the disease, particularly the manner and speed with which it is spread and its morbidity and mortality, in evaluating the appropriateness and effectiveness of any use of isolation or quarantine; (2) the implications of applying due process and other constitutional principles in the individually-oriented manner that has characterized judicial application of these constitutional constraints on government action in the past. These themes bracket the range of possible public health responses: On the one hand, modern therapeutic techniques may allow for the control of the spread of disease with minimal supervision of people who are potentially contagious; on the other, SARS, the bird flu, or some other as yet unidentified biological threat may require the type of draconian responses that most Americans have never witnessed in their lifetime. Indeed, there are serious questions as to whether the nation's public health infrastructure, its legal system (as it operated traditionally), and even its basic means for maintaining social order are sufficiently prepared for some of the worst-case scenarios that must at least be considered if not anticipated.

# SIDEBAR: A NOTE ON TERMINOLOGY

The terminology used in reference to contagious diseases is sometimes imprecise, but some distinctions can be important. The following summary attempts to clarify commonly used terms.

***Infectious, Contagious, and Communicable Diseases.*** Many diseases are infectious, but not all of these are contagious. An *infectious* disease is any disease that can be transmitted *to* a human being by means of a virus, bacterium or parasite, which infects the person. A *contagious* disease is an infectious disease that can be transmitted *from* one person *to* another. Many statutes use the term "communicable" as a synonym for contagious, to emphasize person-to-person transmissibility and, by implication, to distinguish other kinds of infectious diseases.

***Quarantine and Isolation.*** The terms quarantine and isolation are sometimes used interchangeably in common parlance, and indeed both are aimed at preventing transmission of contagious disease. Statutes and judicial opinions often use quarantine as a generic term for both. Scholars and researchers often distinguish between the two, however.

Generally, isolation means keeping a patient *known* to have a contagious disease separate (isolated) from other people — usually in a room in hospital or other medical facility — in order to prevent transmission. Isolation is now part of standard medical procedure for anyone with a serious contagious disease in the hospital, and is typically accepted voluntarily by patients as part of their treatment. When patients do not accept voluntary isolation, *compulsory* isolation (confinement) may be sought; this requires judicial approval. The circumstances in which it is appropriate are limited, requiring (1) a serious contagious disease that (2) can be spread through casual contact, and (3) the transmission of which cannot readily be prevented voluntarily — either because the patient is unwilling or unable to avoid the risks of infecting others, or because he actually seeks to do so.

Quarantine, a broader intervention, describes steps that restrict the movement or activities of well persons who may have been *exposed* to contagious disease and may thus present the risk of transmitting it further; it may include sealing off ships, houses, or geographic areas thought to harbor such a disease. Quarantine typically keeps a person wherever she may be at the time the restriction is imposed, which will often (but not necessarily) be at home.

***Outbreaks, Epidemics, and Pandemics.*** An *outbreak* of disease is a sudden increase in the number of cases of a disease beyond what is normally expected, ordinarily in a particular locality. An *epidemic* is a broader outbreak in a larger geographic area. However, some epidemiologists treat any outbreak as equivalent to an epidemic. A *pandemic* is an epidemic that spreads to several countries. How many cases of any specific disease can be expected under normal circumstances varies from country to country. In many countries, especially in the developing world, certain diseases (such as malaria) remain constantly in the population and are called *endemic*.

> MICHAEL GREGG, ed., FIELD EPIDEMIOLOGY (2002). In the United States, diseases like malaria, poliomyelitis, measles, rabies, or plague are normally so rare that any increase in the number of cases warrants an investigation to find and eliminate the cause.

## B. CASE STUDY: TUBERCULOSIS

The materials in Subsection 1 focus on tuberculosis. In doing so, they introduce a number of legal doctrines that arise in a broad range of other public health problems as well; for that reason they are lengthier than most of the other sections of this chapter. Subsection 2 explores the distinctive right to refuse medical care, which similarly can arise in (but is not unique to) tuberculosis control.

As you read later sections of this chapter, think about the cross-cutting issues first explored here.

### 1.　Contagion, Confinement, Class, and the Constitution

### GREENE v. EDWARDS
#### 164 W. Va. 326, 263 S.E.2d 661 (1980)

PER CURIAM:

* * *

William Arthur Greene, the relator in this original habeas corpus proceeding, is involuntarily confined in Pinecrest Hospital under an order of the Circuit Court of McDowell County entered pursuant to the terms of the West Virginia Tuberculosis Control Act, W. Va. Code, 26-5A-1, *et seq.* He alleges, among other points, that the Tuberculosis Control Act does not afford procedural due process because: (1) it fails to guarantee the alleged tubercular person the right to counsel; (2) it fails to insure that he may cross-examine, confront and present witnesses; and (3) it fails to require that he be committed only upon clear, cogent and convincing proof. We agree.

A petition alleging that Mr. Greene was suffering from active communicable tuberculosis was filed with the Circuit Court of McDowell County on October 3, 1979. After receiving the petition, the court, in accordance with the terms of . . . [the state law] fixed a hearing in the matter for October 10, 1979. The court also caused a copy of the petition and a notice of the hearing to be served upon Mr. Greene. The papers served did not notify Mr. Greene that he was entitled to be represented by counsel at the hearing.

After commencement of the October 10, 1979 hearing, the court, upon learning that Mr. Greene was not represented, appointed an attorney for him. The court then, without taking a recess so that the relator and his attorney could consult privately, proceeded to take evidence and to order Mr. Greene's commitment.

Section 26-5A-5, the statute under which the commitment proceedings in this case were conducted, provides in part:

> If such practicing physician, public health officer, or chief medical officer having under observation or care any person who is suffering from tuberculosis in a communicable stage is of the opinion that the environmental conditions of such person are not suitable for proper isolation or control by any type of local quarantine as prescribed by the state health department, and that such person is unable or unwilling to conduct himself and to live in such a manner as not to expose members of his family or household or other persons with whom he may be associated to danger of infection, he shall report the facts to the department of health which shall forthwith investigate or have investigated the circumstances alleged. If it shall find that any such person's physical condition is a health menace to others, the department of health shall petition the circuit court of the county in which such person resides, or the judge thereof in vacation, alleging that such person is afflicted with communicable tuberculosis and that such person's physical condition is a health menace to others, and requesting an order of the court committing such person to one of the state tuberculosis institutions. Upon receiving the petition, the court shall fix a date for hearing thereof and notice of such petition and the time and place for hearing thereof shall be served personally, at least seven days before the hearing, upon the person who is afflicted with tuberculosis and alleged to be dangerous to the health of others. If, upon such hearing, it shall appear that the complaint of the department of health is well founded, that such person is afflicted with communicable tuberculosis, and that such person is a source of danger to others, the court shall commit the individual to an institution maintained for the care and treatment of persons afflicted with tuberculosis. . . .

It is evident from an examination of this statute that its purpose is to prevent a person suffering from active communicable tuberculosis from becoming a danger to others. A like rationale underlies our statute governing the involuntary commitment of a mentally ill person. . . .

In *Hawks v. Lazaro*, we examined the procedural safeguards which must be extended to persons charged under our statute governing the involuntary hospitalization of the mentally ill. We noted that Article 3, Section 10 of the West Virginia Constitution and the Fifth Amendment to the United States Constitution provide that no person shall be deprived of life, liberty, or property without due process of law; we stated: "This Court recognized in [an earlier case] that, 'liberty, full and complete liberty, is a right of the very highest nature. It stands next in order to life itself. The Constitution guarantees and safeguards it. An adjudication of insanity is a partial deprivation of it.'"

We concluded that due process required that persons charged under [the state civil commitment law] must be afforded: (1) an adequate written notice detailing the grounds and underlying facts on which commitment is sought; (2) the right to counsel; (3) the right to be present, cross-examine, confront and present witnesses; (4) the standard of proof to warrant commitment to be by clear, cogent and convincing evidence; and (5) the right to a verbatim transcript of the proceeding for purposes of appeal. . . .

Because the Tuberculosis Control Act and the Act for the Involuntary Hospitalization of the Mentally Ill have like rationales, and because involuntary commitment for having communicable tuberculosis impinges upon the right to "liberty, full and complete liberty" no less than involuntary commitment for being mentally ill, we conclude that the procedural safeguards set forth in *Hawks v. Lazaro, supra,* must, and do, extend to persons charged under Section 26-5A-5. . . .

We noted in [*Hawks*] that where counsel is to be appointed in proceedings for the involuntary hospitalization of the mentally ill, the law contemplates representation of the individual by the appointed guardian in the most zealous, adversary fashion consistent with the Code of Professional Responsibility. Since this decision, we have concluded that appointment of counsel immediately prior to a trial in a criminal case is impermissible since it denies the defendant effective assistance of counsel. It is obvious that timely appointment and reasonable opportunity for adequate preparation are prerequisites for fulfillment of appointed counsel's constitutionally assigned role in representing persons charged with having communicable tuberculosis.

In the case before us, counsel was not appointed for Mr. Greene until after the commencement of the commitment hearing. Under the circumstances, counsel could not have been properly prepared to defend Mr. Greene. For this reason, the relator's writ must be awarded and he must be accorded a new hearing.

. . . .

For the reasons stated above, the writ of habeas corpus is awarded, and the relator is ordered discharged, but such discharge is hereby delayed for a period of thirty days during which time the State may entertain further proceedings to be conducted in accordance with the principles expressed herein.

\* \* \*

# CITY OF NEWARK v. J.S.
279 N.J. Super. 178, 652 A.2d 265 (1993)

Goldman, J.

\* \* \*

The defendant, J.S., is a 40-year-old African-American male suffering from TB and HIV disease. Hospital authorities requested that Newark intervene when J.S. sought to leave the hospital against medical advice. J.S. was found dressed in street clothes, sitting in the hospital lobby. Once he wandered to the pediatrics ward. He had a prior history of disappearances and of releases against medical advice, only to return via the emergency room when his health deteriorated. Allegedly, J.S. failed to follow proper infection control guidelines or take proper medication when in the hospital and failed to complete treatment regimens following his release. In March of 1993 J.S. had been discharged and deposited in a taxicab, which was given the address of a shelter to which he was to be driven. J.S. was given an appointment at a TB clinic a bus trip away from the shelter. J.S.'s Supplemental Security Income check was being delivered to another hospital, so he had no money. He did not keep his TB clinic appointment and was labeled as "non-compliant."

A sputum sample confirmed that J.S. had *active* TB. TB is a communicable disease caused by a bacteria or bacilli complex, *mycobacterium (M.) tuberculosis*. One of the oldest diseases known to affect humans, it was once known as consumption or the great "white plague" because it killed so many people. Human infection with *M. tuberculosis* was a leading cause of death until antituberculous drugs were introduced in the 1940s. While it can affect other parts of the body, such as lymph nodes, bones, joints, genital organs, kidneys, and skin, it most often attacks the lungs. It is transmitted by a person with what is called *active* TB by airborne droplets projected by coughing or sneezing. When the organism is inhaled into the lungs of another, TB infection can result. Usually this happens only after close and prolonged contact with a person with *active* TB. Most of those who become infected do not manifest any symptoms because the body mounts an appropriate immune response to bring the infection under control; however, those infected display a positive tuberculin skin test. The infection (sometimes called *latent* TB) can continue for a lifetime, and infected persons remain at risk for developing *active* TB if their immune systems become impaired.

Typical symptoms of *active* TB include fatigue, loss of weight and appetite, weakness, chest pain, night sweats, fever, and persistent cough. Sputum is often streaked with blood; sometimes massive hemorrhages occur if TB destroys enough lung tissue. Fluid may collect in the pleural cavity. Gradual deterioration occurs. If *active* TB is not treated, death is common.

Only persons with *active* TB are contagious. That active state is usually easily treated through drugs. Typically a short medication protocol will induce a remission and allow a return to daily activities with safety. A failure to continue with medication may lead to a relapse and the development of MDR-TB (multiple drug resistant TB), a condition in which the TB bacilli do not respond to at least two (isoniazid and rifampin) of the primary treatments, so that the active state is not easily cured and contagiousness continues for longer periods.

Death often results because it takes time to grow cultures and to determine the drugs to which the organism is sensitive. By the time that discovery is made, it may be too late, particularly for a person whose immune system has been compromised by a co-morbidity such as HIV disease. For that reason a wide range of drugs, currently four or five, is tried initially while the cultures are grown and sensitivities detected, particularly if MDR-TB is suspected. Once sensitivities are discovered, medication can be adjusted so that ineffective drugs are eliminated and at least two effective drugs are always used. Medical treatment protocols have been established by the United States Centers for Disease Control and Prevention (CDC) and the American Thoracic Society. These protocols are being used for J.S. as they are for all patients under the supervision of New Jersey's Tuberculosis Control Program.

*Active* TB of the lungs is considered contagious and requires immediate medical treatment, involving taking several drugs. Usually, after only a few days of treatment, infectiousness is reduced markedly. After two to four weeks of treatment, most people are no longer contagious and cannot transmit TB to others even if they cough or sneeze while living in close quarters. Usually exposure over a prolonged time is required, and less than thirty per cent (30%) of family members living closely with an infected person and unprotected by prophylactic drugs will become infected by the patient with *active* TB. On the other hand, transmission has been known to occur with as little as a single two-hour exposure to coughing, sneezing, etc., of a person with *active* TB. To cure TB, however, continued therapy for six to twelve months may be required. Failure to complete the entire course of therapy risks a relapse and the development of MDR-TB.

MDR-TB results when only some TB bacilli are destroyed and the surviving bacilli develop a resistance to standard drugs and thus become more difficult to destroy. This resistance may involve several drugs and directly results from a patient's failure to complete therapy. There have been no reports of TDR-TB (totally drug resistant TB) in New Jersey, so J.S. can be cured if effective drugs are found in time.

TB is more serious in persons with impaired immune systems, which can result from poor health, chronic abuse of alcohol or drugs, old age, chemotherapy for cancer, or HIV infection. Such persons are more likely to develop *active* TB if they already harbor the TB bacilli. By way of example, ninety per cent of persons with *latent* TB (these persons are neither sick nor contagious) and with an intact immune system will never develop *active* TB during their entire lives. On the other hand persons with HIV disease with *latent* TB will develop *active* TB at the rate of eight per cent per year.

The human immunodeficiency virus is the cause of acquired immune deficiency syndrome (AIDS). HIV infection weakens the body's natural ability to fight disease. As the immune system deteriorates, those infected with HIV may become clinically ill with many serious illnesses. These are called opportunistic diseases and include pneumonia, some forms of cancer, fungal and parasitic diseases, certain viral diseases, direct damage to the nervous system, and TB. Persons infected with HIV are at much greater risk of developing active TB if they have latent TB. Once a person with HIV disease develops one of these opportunistic diseases, that person is classified as having AIDS.

New Jersey's statutory scheme for dealing with TB dates from 1912 when the predecessor to N.J.S.A. 30:9-57 was first adopted. Only minor amendments have been made since 1917. [That statute now provides:]

> A person with communicable tuberculosis who fails to obey the rules or regulations promulgated . . . by the State Department of Health for the care of tubercular persons and for the prevention of the spread of tuberculosis, or who is an actual menace to the community or to members of his household, may be committed to a hospital or institution, designated by the State Commissioner of Health with the approval of the Commissioner of Human Services for the care and custody of such person or persons by the Superior Court, upon proof of service upon him of the rules and regulations and proof of violation thereafter, or upon proof by the health officer of the municipality in which the person resides, or by the State Commissioner of Health or

his authorized representative, that he is suffering from tuberculosis, and is an actual menace to the community, or to members of his household. Two days' notice of the time and place of hearing shall in all cases be served upon the person to be committed. Proof of such service shall be made at the hearing. The court may also make such order for the payment for care and treatment as may be proper. The superintendent or person in charge of said hospital or institution to which such person has been committed shall detain said person until the State Commissioner of Health shall be satisfied that the person has recovered to the extent that he will not be a menace to the community or to members of his household or that the person will so conduct himself that he will not constitute such a menace.

[The foregoing statutory text appears in a footnote in the original opinion.]

This law allows me to enter an order committing a person to a hospital if he or she is "suffering from" TB and "is an actual menace to the community." Notice of the hearing is required and was provided. Neither the statute nor the implementing regulation provides any guidance on the procedures to follow when such applications are made, nor what standards are to be used in issuing such orders. There is no case law in New Jersey providing guidance on these and many other related issues.

The regulatory schemes in other jurisdictions vary widely. There are older schemes like that in New Jersey which provide little or no guidance. There are those that provide detailed procedural details to guarantee due process while still allowing detention, isolation, quarantine, or confinement in the most extreme cases.

. . . .

Newark's attempt to protect the health of its citizenry is an archetypical expression of police power. [Citation to *Jacobson v. Massachusetts.*] The claim of "disease" in a domestic setting has the same kind of power as the claim of "national security" in matters relating to foreign policy. Both claims are very powerful arguments for executive action. Both claims are among those least likely to be questioned by any other branch of government and therefore subject to abuse. The potential abuse is of special concern when the other interest involved is the confinement of a human being who has committed no crime except to be sick.

[As the Supreme Court has explained], [t]he Fourteenth Amendment requires "that deprivation of life, liberty or property by adjudication be preceded by notice and opportunity for hearing appropriate to the nature of the case." The parameters of due process require an analysis of both the individual and governmental interests involved and the consequences and avoidability of the risks of error and abuse. Here the clash of competing interests is at its peak. Hardly any state interest is higher than protecting its citizenry from disease. Hardly any individual interest is higher than the liberty interest of being free from confinement. The consequences of error and abuse are grave for both the state and the individual.

The United States Supreme Court has recognized that "civil commitment for any purpose constitutes a significant deprivation of liberty that requires due process protection." [Citation to *Addington v. Texas.*] A person has the right to notice, counsel, and must be afforded the opportunity to present opposing evidence and argument, and to cross examine witnesses. . . . Illness alone cannot be the basis for confinement. [Citation to *O'Connor v. Donaldson.*] To justify confinement it must be shown that the person is likely to pose a danger to self or to others. The proofs must show that there is a "substantial risk of dangerous conduct within the foreseeable future." These proofs must be shown by clear and convincing evidence. The terms of confinement must minimize the infringements on liberty and enhance autonomy. Periodic reviews are required. Lesser forms of restraint must be used when they would suffice to fulfill the government interests.

. . . [A] court must satisfy itself that there were no less restrictive alternatives available to the "drastic curtailment" of rights inherent in the civil confinement of a person. . . .

Even though the governmental purpose be legitimate and substantial, that purpose cannot be pursued by means that broadly stifle fundamental personal liberties when the end can be more narrowly achieved. The breadth of legislative abridgement must be viewed in the light of less drastic means for achieving the same basic purpose.

[The court then discusses *Greene*, included *supra* in these materials.]

[The New Jersey statute] provides a comprehensive set of procedures and standards reflecting modern ideas of mental health treatment and modern concepts of constitutional law.

Some provisions establish procedures to enhance fairness and to reduce the risks of error and abuse. Persons whose confinement is sought must be provided counsel. Such persons are entitled to adequate notice of the hearing and discovery before the hearing. The hearing must be held expeditiously to avoid unnecessary confinement. The hearing must be held *in camera* if requested to protect privacy interests. Prior to the hearing an independent examination paid for by the committing authority must be provided upon request. The person sought to be confined has the right to be present, to cross-examine witnesses and to present testimony. The hearing must be on the record. Evidence must be under oath. Periodic court reviews are mandated. All proofs must be shown by clear and convincing evidence.

There are additional requirements. Illness alone cannot be a basis for involuntary commitment. Persons may not be confined merely because they present a risk of future conduct which is socially undesirable. A court must find that the risk of infliction of serious bodily injury upon another is probable in the reasonably foreseeable future. History, actual conduct, and recent behaviors must be considered. Dangerous conduct is not the same as criminal conduct. Dangerous conduct involves not merely violations of social norms but significant injury to persons or substantial destruction of property. The evaluation of the risk involves considering the likelihood of dangerous conduct, the seriousness of the harm that would ensue if such conduct took place, and its probability within the reasonably foreseeable future. A person's past conduct is important evidence of future conduct. If a person is only dangerous with regard to certain individuals, the likelihood of contact with such individuals must be taken into account.

. . . [M]any commentators have suggested that the most apt analogy for commitments for medical reasons is the model of civil commitments for mental illness. This was the analogy seized upon by the West Virginia Supreme Court in *Greene*. Professor George J. Annas recently similarly referred to the problem of TB:

> The closest legal analogy is provided by court cases that have reviewed the constitutionality of state statutes permitting the involuntary commitment of mental patients on the basis that they have a disease that causes them to be dangerous.

. . .

. . . The constitutional concept of due process is designed to prevent irrational discrimination by ensuring a forum that can hear opposing perspectives and by insisting that distinctions are rationally based. "The decisive consideration where personal liberty is involved is that each individual's fate must be adjudged on the facts of his own case, not on the general characteristics of a "class" to which he may be assigned." [Citation omitted.]

. . .

Thus, it becomes possible to reconcile public health concerns, constitutional requirements, [and] civil liberties . . . simultaneously. Good public health practice considers human rights so there is no conflict. Since coercion is a difficult and expensive means to enforce behaviors, voluntary compliance is the public health goal. Compliance is more likely when authorities demonstrate sensitivity to human rights. . . .

That these interests are reconcilable does not mean that any one case will be easy to reconcile. Any individualized balancing process is a challenge. But it does mean that the principles by which that process is governed can be made clear and without conflict or contradiction. Moreover, to the extent that current laws regarding the commitment of those with TB are so ancient that they fail to meet modern standards of due process . . . it is the responsibility of our courts to ensure that there are procedures to ensure the rights of individuals whose proposed confinement invokes the judicial process. There is no need to declare the New Jersey TB control statute unconstitutional so long as it is interpreted to be consistent with the Constitution. . . . It must be remembered that this statute was first enacted in 1912, yet it had provisions requiring notice and a judicial hearing. The statute required proof that the person be "an actual menace to the community or to members of his household." The Legislature intended to permit the confinement of someone with TB but only under circumstances consistent with due process. Many of the rights we now recognize were unheard of in 1912. . . . Therefore I construe N.J.S.A. 30:9-57 so as to include those rights necessitated by contemporary standards of due process. . . .

The first step of the individualized analysis required here is to define precisely what Newark seeks. During the active phase of TB, isolation of J.S., as opposed to confinement or imprisonment, is what is required. If J.S. lived in a college dormitory with other roommates, different quarters would have to be found for him. If J.S. lived in a private home and could be given a private bedroom or others in the household could be given prophylactic antibiotic therapy, confinement to his own home might be appropriate. J.S. is homeless, and a shelter where he would risk infecting others, including those with impaired immune systems, would probably be the worst place for him to stay. Because *active* TB can be serious and can be potentially contagious by repeated contact, there are few options for the homeless with *active* TB. As Professor Annas said:

> Although these safeguards [constitutional rights] may seem impressive, in fact the only issues likely to concern a judge in a tuberculosis commitment proceeding are two factual ones: Does the person have active tuberculosis, and does the person present a danger of spreading it to others? Since it is unlikely that any case will be brought by public health officials when the diagnosis is in doubt, the primary issues will be the danger the patient presents to others and the existence of less restrictive alternatives to confinement that might protect the public equally well.

I find that the answers to the questions posed by Professor Annas have been provided by Newark and have been established by clear and convincing evidence. There is no question but that J.S. has active TB. There is no question but that he poses a risk to others who may be in contact with him, particularly in close quarters. Because he is homeless, there is no suggestion of any other place he could stay that would be less restrictive than a hospital.

The hearing I conducted was designed to comport to all the requirements of due process and with all the requirements of a commitment hearing under [state law].

I find that J.S. presents a significant risk to others unless isolated. Hospital confinement is the least restrictive mode of isolation proposed to me. The only request at this time is that J.S. be confined until he has shown three negative sputum tests demonstrating that his TB is no longer active. This is narrow, limited, and very reasonable, but because the time period for treatment is indefinite, I will initially set an initial court review to be held in three weeks. . . . unless J.S. has earlier been determined to have gone into remission from active TB. In that event J.S. will be released immediately unless Newark seeks confinement for another reason.

. . . Newark will have the burden of proving the need for further confinement; however, unless there is a change in condition, I will consider the evidence presented . . . along with whatever updates may be necessary. . . . If there is no change, then the current order will likely continue. Obviously J.S. will also have the opportunity to present evidence; however, discovery shall be provided by each side to the other and to me at least one week in advance of the hearing date.

In the interim I will utilize the well-established procedures New Jersey has in place for civil commitments of the mentally ill. Although some procedures may not apply to the confinement of those with contagious diseases like TB, until and unless a more specific law is enacted, the only available and constitutional mechanism is to use these tested mental health statutes, court rules, and the case law thereunder. . . .

Newark also wanted J.S. ordered to provide sputum samples and take his medication as prescribed. The testimony was that a forced sputum sample requires a bronchoscopy, a procedure involving sedation and requiring separate informed consent because of its risks. No facts were shown to justify such a diagnostic procedure where it might cause harm to J.S. As to continued treatment, testimony showed that the medications were quite toxic, dangerous, and some required painful intramuscular administration. J.S. is being asked to take many pills causing numerous side effects, including nausea and pain. The efficacy of the drugs will be unknown until receipt of sensitivity reports.

These facts cannot justify a remedy as broad as Newark seeks. J.S. has the right to refuse treatment even if this is medically unwise. . . . He must remain isolated until he is no longer contagious. Contagiousness cannot be assessed unless he gives sputum samples. While he can refuse to provide sputum samples and refuse bronchoscopy, his release from isolation may be delayed, as he will be unable to satisfy the conditions of release. The same is true with his refusal to take medication. If he refuses, he may not get better. If J.S. continues to suffer from active TB, he will be unable to satisfy the conditions of release.

On the other hand if J.S. cooperates with his caregivers, provides sputum samples, and takes his medication willingly, then upon his improvement, Newark will have a difficult time proving that he needs confinement because he is not cooperative. His in-hospital conduct will go a long way towards demonstrating his ability to follow medical therapy once released and will be considered if after his active TB is cured, J.S.'s confinement is sought because his alleged failure to follow continued therapy will make him a future risk. I would then have to consider an order . . . which would simply require J.S. to take his medication.

* * *

## NOTES AND QUESTIONS

### The Nature and Prevalence of Tuberculosis

**1.** Tuberculosis (TB), which is caused by the bacterium *Mycobacterium tuberculosis,* is the paradigmatic contagious disease because it is transmitted through the air by droplets (most often from coughing or sneezing) without anyone's knowledge. It is a serious disease — often disabling, sometimes fatal, and readily spread (at least to those in close and prolonged contact with a person who has an "active" case, which is the only time it can be transmitted). TB is not easily prevented let alone eradicated. As acknowledged in J.S. and described in the article by Rosen in the first chapter of this text, TB has been around for a long time and it is likely to be with us for the foreseeable future.

One reason why preventing or treating TB is problematic is its peculiar etiology. Most people who contract the disease don't know they have it. Roughly 10 percent of those who are infected with TB develop "active" cases and, as a consequence, become contagious. If treated quickly and with the proper regimen of drugs, the infection can essentially always be eliminated, and after two weeks of treatment patients are generally no longer contagious. But because the initial treatment can cause the disease to go into remission, people with "active" TB can assume that they are cured in a short period of time when, in fact, they need to continue drug therapy for four to six months. To make matters worse, people who end their therapy prematurely may not only relapse, but may develop multi-drug resistant TB — which is harder to eliminate, requires considerably lengthier treatment, and, of course, can be transmitted in that form to others. (Incomplete treatment of an individual case, in essence, tends to eliminate the "weaker" germs and to favor replication by and transmission of those which have developed some resistance to the medications — a problem both for the recovery of the individual and, ultimately, for the health of all human populations). *See generally* Joia S. Mukherjee et al., *Programmes and Principles in Treatment of Multidrug-resistant Tuberculosis*, 363 THE LANCET 474 (Feb. 7, 2004). For discussion of the treatment complexities that accompany MDR-TB, see Notes 8–10, *infra*.

According to the CDC, in 2003 there were nearly 15,000 cases of tuberculosis reported in the United States, a "case rate" of 5.1 per hundred thousand in the population. There were approximately 800 deaths as a direct result. This was, in relative terms, good news; it represented a 45 percent decrease from the case rate in 1992, a tribute to improved public education, better and more sophisticated drugs, and, presumably, the success of public health authorities in locating, isolating, and treating people with TB — occasionally over their objection. *See* Note 8, *infra*.

The prevalence of tuberculosis in the United States is not evenly distributed. While everyone is susceptible — as one authority put it, "we all breathe the same air" — over 50 percent of the cases in 2003 occurred in people who were foreign-born. The rates also were higher in minority populations, and among the homeless, people in prisons and other institutions, and in people with weakened immune systems. For more details and updates on the prevalence and distribution of TB, see www.cdc/gov/nchstp/tb (last visited February 2005).

**2.** From an international perspective, TB is a public problem of much greater magnitude. Indeed, in many underdeveloped countries TB can be properly regarded as an epidemic. According to data published by the World Health organization (WHO), TB is the second leading killer of adults in the world, accounting for nearly two million deaths each year. Almost two *billion* people, about one third of the world's population, are infected with TB. For updates and additional information, see www.niaid.nih.gov/ (last visited February 2005); www.who.int/mediacentre/factsheets/ (last visited February 2005).

Whatever we do in the United States and whatever our success in preventing and treating cases of TB domestically, these efforts should not overlook the much larger and more intractable problem TB represents for the rest of the world, especially in underdeveloped countries. One thing is clear, however: As we have learned in the United States, the problem will not be resolved simply by providing better medical care, even if that were possible. Other broader, public health techniques (sanitation, improved housing, improved standards of living) will have to be employed to combat the social and environmental conditions that allow TB to flourish. TB will remain a world-wide problem so long as the social and environmental conditions that facilitate the spread of diseases like TB persist.

These observations, unfortunately, are not unique to the problem of TB. The same can be said about many other public health problems in underdeveloped countries. Indeed, TB has often been cited as the stereotypical example of a disease that is as much a social problem as it is a medical or even health problem. See, *e.g.*, the classic history of TB by RENE DUBOS & JEAN DUBOS, THE WHITE PLAGUE (1952) (arguing that, even as antibiotics were making headway against the disease, TB was a problem that would persist so long as poor housing, malnutrition, and poverty were widespread). For some commentary on the seriousness of the world-wide problem and some bio-medical techniques for addressing it, see Patricia C. Kuszler, *Balancing the Barriers, Exploiting and Creating Incentives to Promote Development of New Tuberculosis Treatments*, 71 WASH. L. REV. 919, 938–967 (1996).

**3.** The distinction between the magnitude of the problem of TB in the United States and that in underdeveloped countries is only temporal. Prior to the discovery of various antibiotic treatments, the rates of TB in the United States and throughout the rest of the world were essentially at levels that remain today in some underdeveloped countries. At the turn of the 20th century, TB was the leading cause of death in the Western hemisphere countries. Even in 1950, TB was the leading cause of death in the United States for people between the ages of 15 and 30. Understandably, TB control and prevention efforts and public health programs were virtually synonymous terms, leading to various public education campaigns, massive screening programs in many communities (chest X-rays to identify "tubercoles," tumors filled with TB bacilli, were considered the preferred diagnostic technique until the 1960s), and, in some parts of the country, rather aggressive efforts to locate and isolate people who were diagnosed with TB. While some of these efforts were voluntary, others were unapologetically not, especially those that focused on low income and homeless populations. For one well-written, illustrative account of this era in TB control and prevention, see BARRON H. LERNER, CONTAGION AND CONFINEMENT: CONTROLLING TUBERCULOSIS ALONG THE SKID ROAD (1998) (describing the programs of forcible detention of people in Seattle, Washington — mostly homeless — in the 1950s and 1960s as the "most aggressive" in the country).

### Key Constitutional Issues in Government Control of "Dangerous" Individuals

The following notes explore constitutional doctrines implicated when government seeks to curtail the liberty of persons it believes may pose danger to others. As the TB cases so vividly suggest, one form of individual "dangerousness" can arise from contagious disease. But, as we will see, other forms of dangerousness exist, and provoke similar public health policy responses.

In the 1980s and 1990s there was a marked increase in the rates of TB in the United States, due in large part to the increased incidence of multiple drug resistant forms of the disease (MDR-TB) discussed in Note 1, the so-called "new tuberculosis." In this context many local and state public health authorities began considering anew the use of mandatory treatment and confinement, especially for people thought to be unlikely or reluctant to comply fully with modern treatment regimens on their own.

But by then the legal landscape in which these old public health interventions originated had changed significantly. Modern concepts of procedural and substantive due process relating to individual rights flowered in the 1960s (although originating earlier) and expanded subsequently. In contemporary cases like *Greene* and *J.S.*, the courts are asked to apply these doctrines to statutory schemes and public health techniques that were developed decades before, at a time when individual rights enjoyed both less political solicitude and less judicial protection. The following set of notes explores these and related issues.

**4.** Both Mr. Greene and J.S. claim that they were confined without due process of law in violation of their rights to liberty under the 14th Amendment. This note and the next explore the doctrine underlying these claims.

The 14th Amendment forbids states to "deprive any person of life, liberty, or property without due process of law." (The 5th Amendment imposes the same constraint on the federal government). This language contemplates, at least, that government must follow fair procedures in its pursuit of the named "deprivations." You should recognize, here, a policy assumption that is widespread in the law: the view that sound *procedures* (which we can endeavor to apply rigorously and conscientiously irrespective of what we think we know about "the facts") will increase the likelihood of accurate *outcomes* (which are often difficult or impossible to know in advance). Appropriate procedural safeguards should increase the likelihood of good results — convicting the guilty (and not the innocent), civilly confining those who will not take medications that prevent spread of dangerous infection of others (and not those who *will* do so), and the like.

Determining whether there has been a violation of a person's right to procedural due process requires answering three questions: has there been [at the hands of government] (1) a "deprivation"? (2) of "life, liberty, or property"? (3) without "due process of law"? ERWIN CHEMERINSKY, CONSTITUTIONAL LAW: PRINCIPLES AND POLICIES 422 (1997). Despite complexities in other areas, when government health authorities civilly confine a person in the interests of public health, the answer to the first two questions is plainly "yes". In this circumstance the state "deprives" a person of her "liberty" in the classic sense of limiting physical freedom. Thus, most often, the critical question in public health is the third: Did the state follow a constitutionally-adequate *process* in pursuing and implementing this liberty deprivation?

The main question, accordingly, will usually be "What 'process' is constitutionally 'due'?" At one extreme, the most stringent procedural safeguards are those that must be employed for criminal prosecutions, when government seeks to punish a person by incarceration. A number of these arise from the text of the Bill of Rights: protection of individual privacy and freedom from self-incrimination; avoidance of double-jeopardy; prompt processing of the case; a public trial; an impartial jury; fair notice of charges and an opportunity to mount a defense; right to confront and cross-examine witnesses; compulsory process of favorable witnesses and evidence; assistance of a lawyer; non-excessive bail; avoidance of excessive or cruel punishment. Accompanying the foregoing are other required safeguards: "fundamental fairness" (including impartial determination of guilt or innocence and respect for individual dignity); proof of guilt beyond a reasonable doubt; and properly-implemented sentencing within legislatively-prescribed limits. JOHN E. NOWAK & RONALD D. ROTUNDA, CONSTITUTIONAL LAW 592–94 (6th ed. 2000). Additional elements of criminal due process are a decision based on the record, with stated reasons; a right to pre-trial discovery; and a transcript of the proceedings. *Id.* at 583–84.

In other contexts, however, such as *civil* deprivations of liberty (or property) for public health and other reasons, the judicial answer to the question "What 'process' is constitutionally 'due'"? is simultaneously sensible and unsatisfying: "It depends." At a minimum, and regardless of circumstances, due process requires notice to the person of the charges he faces (or, in our context, notice of the issues concerning his health status or behavior that are to be determined, and the consequences for him of the outcome); the opportunity for a meaningful hearing; and an impartial decision maker. CHEMERINSKY, *supra*, at 450. Yet these are general, not specific, requirements that might be met in various ways. *Id.* The most concrete guidance offered by the Supreme Court is comparably general. In *Mathews v. Eldridge*, 424 U.S. 319 (1976), the Court instructed courts to evaluate three factors in order to determine what procedures must accompany governmental deprivations of liberty or property:

> First, the private interest that will be affected by the official action; second, the risk of an erroneous deprivation of such interest through the procedures used, and the probative value, if any, of additional or substitute procedural safeguards; and finally, the Government's interest, including the function involved and the fiscal and administrative burdens that the additional or substitute procedural requirement would entail. This test . . . can be praised because it focuses a court's attention on what seem to be the right questions. It seems clearly correct that the nature of the proceeding should be a function of the [nature of the liberty or property] interest involved, the degree to which the procedure will make a difference, and the cost to the government. An expensive trial-type hearing would be out of place for a minor interest in a situation where there is little likelihood of a factual dispute. But an adversarial hearing is essential, despite its expense, if there is a fundamental right at stake [*see* Note 5, *infra*], such as the right of parents to the custody of their children.

> Yet, *Mathews* also can be criticized for failing to provide any real guidance as to how courts should balance the competing interests. The reality is that courts have enormous discretion in evaluating each of the three factors and especially how to balance them. . . .

CHEMERINSKY, *supra*, at 452; *see also* NOWAK & ROTUNDA, *supra*, at 589.

Before proceeding further, ask yourself how civil confinement to prevent contagious disease transmission is similar to, and how it is different from, imprisonment for violation of the criminal law. Consider the implications of your judgment for determining what "process" is "due" in the former circumstance.

In *Greene*, the court's focus is almost entirely on the proper application of the foregoing principles of procedural due process to the West Virginia statute. In undertaking this task, the court does what most modern courts have done since *Mathews v. Eldridge*: treat the requirements of procedural due process as general principles of procedural fairness, not as a laundry list of specific requirements. The *Greene* court, noting the parallels between the civil commitment of the mentally ill and the involuntary confinement of people with TB, applies its holding in a prior civil commitment decision to "read into" the West Virginia TB statute the procedural requirements of notice, counsel, an adversarial hearing, and a standard of proof of "clear, cogent and convincing evidence." Similarly, in *J.S.*, the court "read into" the New Jersey statute — enacted (like many) some time ago — considerably more elaborate procedures than its text contained, deeming them constitutionally necessary. (What alternatives might the court have had? Which approach makes more sense to you?) While following the *Mathews* approach, both courts also appear to be applying the procedural due process principles of their own *state* constitutions as well, a not uncommon practice in public health-related cases.

Give some thought to the stakes of the flexible *Mathews* balancing test in the specific context of public health. Consider first the particular kind of liberty deprivation at stake — *e.g.*, civil institutionalization, home-based isolation, mandated direct observation of drug-administration, etc. How much weight should be attached to each? How much weight should be given to the (sometimes-competing) goal of public protection? How much weight to the importance of avoiding two types of mistakes — unnecessary deprivations of liberty on one hand, and avoidable public exposure to risk of disease on the other? What procedures seem most likely to achieve the goals you think most important?

**5.** *Substantive* due process, although based on the same constitutional language as procedural due process, asks quite a different question. A substantive due process claim challenges the state's power to enact and enforce a particular law at all. Instead of focusing on procedural fairness, here courts undertake a "substantive" inquiry: Does the government have an adequate reason for infringing on the asserted interest in life, liberty, or property, in the particular manner that the law in question allows or requires it to do? This, of course, implicates the constitutional permissibility of the *content* of the law itself, not the *procedures* employed to enforce it. And, as we saw in Chapter Two, it can place the court in the position of balancing the comparative importance, or "weight," of the asserted state and individual interests.

The judicial answer to a substantive due process question usually turns on the level of scrutiny applied. Under "rational basis" review, which is applied to a very broad range of economic and other regulatory legislation, the state policy will generally prevail provided that it is "rationally related" to a "legitimate government purpose." The idea here — though not the language or the particular kind of liberty-interest being infringed — echoes *Jacobson*. Under "strict scrutiny," which is applied to a limited range of certain kinds of liberty interests (generally known as "fundamental rights"), the government will prevail only if it can show that "the law is necessary to achieve a compelling government purpose." Here, the idea — though, again, not the language or the particular kind of liberty interest being infringed — echoes *Lochner*. And, as in *Lochner*, the court will take a comparably aggressive role in balancing the competing interests for itself, rather than giving strong deference to the balance struck by the legislature (*see* Chapter Two, *infra*). Generally speaking, the "liberty" interests that currently enjoy the heightened protection of "fundamental" status under the 14th Amendment due process clause include certain kinds of family autonomy (the right to marry, the right to custody of one's children and to control their upbringing), reproductive autonomy (the rights to procreate and to acquire and use contraceptives, to abortion), travel, voting, and access to courts. CHEMERINSKY, *supra*, at 638–746.

Unlike its procedural counterpart, substantive due process has long been controversial. Some argue that it strains the very words of the 14th amendment to find "substantive" limitations on the ends that government may constitutionally pursue in language that seems, on its face, to be exclusively "procedural." Others assert that using this language to protect rights that are not explicitly mentioned in the Constitution, but are instead elaborated out of a phrase as vague as "liberty" — and are thus "created" by judges — is frankly illegitimate. *See* CHEMERINSKY, *supra*, at 421. (Some rights the Supreme Court has deemed "fundamental" *are* rooted in constitutional text, and according them heightened protection is far less controversial than doing so for rights elaborated out of the word "liberty" in the 14th Amendment alone). Perhaps most importantly, critics proclaim that the doctrine simply enables particular judges at particular historical moments to "constitutionalize" their own preferred values — with the antidemocratic consequence that regulation of such matters is then "off limits" to the legislative branch. In this view, the late-20th century constitutional protection of personal decision making about abortion and reproduction is no less arbitrary and unprincipled than the early-20th century constitutional protection of "business liberty" reflected in *Lochner* and later abandoned (*see* Chapter Two). Defenders of substantive due process find it an unavoidable or appropriate element of determining the bounds of government power, with ample precedent in case law.

Properly presented and framed, the substantive due process question in the principal TB cases would begin with the question whether a patient with active TB has a constitutionally-protected "liberty" interest under the 14th Amendment in avoiding civil confinement, to which the answer will surely be "yes." Indeed it is likely that this most-basic kind of "liberty" would be seen as a "fundamental," or particularly strong, individual interest, triggering "close" judicial scrutiny. (In *Buck v. Bell*, Section B[2], *infra*, the analogous question would be whether a patient has a constitutionally protected liberty interest in avoiding compulsory sterilization — also surely "yes"). The key question in the TB cases would then become whether the state may *nonetheless* permissibly confine that patient under the circumstances presented. Addressing this question systematically (which courts do not always do) would entail carefully identifying the precise state interest — preventing the infection of other persons with a harmful, contagious disease. Courts have generally viewed this interest as extremely strong — probably "compelling" in traditional constitutional parlance. Thus, in weighing the infringement on the TB patient's liberty against the asserted state interest in confining him, the court would likely find the state interest sufficient to justify the liberty-infringement. However, a final aspect of close (or "strict" or "heightened") scrutiny would probably also inquire whether confinement was the "least restrictive alternative" available for protecting the public's health under all the circumstances. If, for example, it were shown that, short of institutionalization, the patient was capable of isolating himself and taking his medication until he was rendered non-infectious, the court might yet prohibit the patient's confinement and order some alternative arrangement (or, perhaps more likely, order the authorities to settle upon and implement such an arrangement, if it is within their power to do so).

**6.** As many courts have observed, including those in *Greene* and *J.S.*, there are obvious parallels between state and local government efforts to involuntarily confine people with tuberculosis or other infectious diseases and the civil commitment of the mentally ill. Thus the extent to which the courts have permitted civil commitment in this related context provides some guidance as to what the state and federal courts should do in cases involving the involuntary commitment of people with contagious diseases.

In the most general terms, the courts have had little trouble upholding the power of the state to involuntarily confine the mentally ill (and, in many states, the mentally retarded). Until the 1960s, there was rarely any judicial supervision of these proceedings whatsoever. Since then, however, the Supreme Court has insisted that the constitutional requirements of procedural due process impose some important limits on the states' discretion in civil commitment, although nothing as demanding as the procedures that are required in the criminal process. As in other areas where a governmental action affects important individual or economic interests, the states are required to include the basic elements of procedural fairness. *See generally Mathews v. Eldridge, supra.* Nonetheless, the discretion allowed each state has been defined rather broadly. *See, e.g., Addington v. Texas*, 441 U.S. 418 (1979); *Heller v. Doe*, 509 U.S. 312 (1993). Most of the more recent decisions of the Supreme Court imply that the states (and local government) will be given wide discretion in determining the circumstances and length of confinement of the mentally ill.

The Supreme Court also has recognized that the due process clauses of the 5th and 14th Amendments impose substantive limits on the states' discretion to impose civil commitment. What those limits are, even in general terms, has not been clearly articulated. Thus, for example, some lower courts have held that states may civilly commit the mentally ill or mentally retarded, but only where minimally adequate treatment is provided. *See Wyatt v. Aderholdt*, 503 F.2d 1305 (5th Cir. 1974) (recognizing a "right to treatment" for involuntarily confined mentally ill). Few other courts have even considered this issue. The Supreme Court has never directly addressed the "right to treatment" argument, at least for people for whom treatment was withheld or denied. In *Jackson v. Indiana*, 406 U.S. 715 (1972), the Court held that there must be a reasonable connection between the state's underlying justification

for committing Jackson and the nature and length of his commitment, implying that the Court might consider a "right to treatment" claim if Indiana
argued that its purpose was to provide him with treatment. In
*O'Connor v. Donaldson*, 422 U.S. 563 (1975), the Court took one small step
toward the "right to treatment" argument, holding a state cannot civilly commit a mentally ill person who is not dangerous or unable to care for himself
where no treatment was made available, although it did not address the question of whether Donaldson could have been committed solely for purposes of
treating him even if he were not dangerous or unable to care for himself. *See
also Youngberg v. Romeo*, 457 U.S. 307 (1982) (recognizing a limited "right to
habilitation" for the mentally retarded). In general, however, the Supreme
Court has indicated that the states have very broad discretion in determining
the nature, terms, and length of any civil commitment.

In *Jones v. United States*, 463 U.S. 354 (1990), although the Court did not
openly retreat from standards it had articulated in earlier holdings, it emphasized the discretion that it would allow the states in civil commitment. Jones
was civilly committed after he was found not guilty by reason of insanity without a separate finding that he was mentally ill and dangerous at the time of
his commitment. The Court found that the findings of insanity (at the time of
the crime) and dangerousness implicit in his insanity defense were sufficiently
probative to allow for his civil commitment without additional post-conviction
procedures, although the Court noted that Jones would be entitled to release
when he was no longer dangerous or mentally ill.

In *Foucha v. Louisiana*, 504 U.S. 71 (1992), the Court reaffirmed that latter
qualification of the states' power and invalidated the extension of Foucha's
original commitment, following his successful not guilty by reason of insanity
plea. After four years of civil commitment, Foucha's doctors found that he was
no longer mentally ill although they still believed he was dangerous and had
an anti-social personality. The Court held that without at *current* finding of
mental illness, there is not constitutional basis for extending his civil commitment. At the least, the Court held, Foucha was entitled to constitutionally adequate procedures to establish the grounds for his commitment, as discussed in
*Jackson*. Most importantly, the Court essentially set out a two-pronged substantive standard for civil commitment: "The State may . . . confine a mentally
ill person if it shows by 'clear and convincing evidence that the individual is
mentally ill and dangerous.'"

A more difficult question is whether the state may involuntarily confine
mentally ill persons who are not dangerous to others but either harm themselves or are not capable of taking care of themselves. Most state civil commitment laws authorize confinement for such conditions, often generally
categorized as "dangerous to self." Although the Supreme Court has not
addressed the question directly, in *O'Connor, supra*, the Court mentions both
the state's legitimate interest in helping those in need and its discomfort with
a broad principle that would force help on all those who reject it:

> May the State confine the mentally ill merely to ensure them a liv-
> ing standard superior to that they enjoy in the private community?
> That the State has a proper interest in providing care and assistance
> to the unfortunate goes without saying. But the mere presence of

mental illness does not disqualify a person from preferring his home to the comforts of an institution. Moreover, while the State may arguably confine a person to save him from harm, incarceration is rarely if ever a necessary condition for raising the living standards of those capable of surviving safely in freedom, on their own or with the help of family or friends.

422 U.S. at 575.

**7.** Like civil commitment, a related line of cases involving "sexual predators" may illuminate the constitutional dimensions of civilly confining those with contagious disease. Consider *Kansas v. Hendricks*, 521 U.S. 346 (1997), a case in which the Supreme Court upheld a statute that provides for the civil commitment of sexual predators who have been convicted of sexually violent crimes, or have been found not guilty of such crimes by reason of insanity. Like civil commitment statutes previously upheld by the Court, the Kansas law requires that the individual be found to be dangerous. The Kansas law, like other similar state laws, was enacted largely in the belief that civil commitment laws might not apply to sexual predators, because they do not necessarily have a "mental illness" as that term is understood by the medical profession and used in civil commitment proceedings. Instead, the Kansas legislature's innovation (and the basis of Hendricks' challenge) was to replace "mental illness" with "mental abnormality," which it defined as a "volitional capacity which predisposes the person to commit sexually violent offenses in a degree constituting such person a menace to the health and safety of others." This formulation, according to a majority of the Court, satisfied the requirements of substantive due process. Some additional element beyond dangerousness is necessary to justify non-criminal confinement, but the Court emphasized that it did not require "any particular nomenclature" to describe that element as long as it affected the person's ability to control behavior:

> A finding of dangerousness, standing alone, is ordinarily not a sufficient ground upon which to justify indefinite involuntary commitment. We have sustained civil commitment statutes when they have coupled proof of dangerousness with the proof of some additional factor, such as "mental illness" or "mental abnormality." These added statutory requirements serve to limit involuntary civil confinement to those who suffer from a volitional impairment rendering them dangerous beyond their control.

521 U.S. at 358.

Hendricks also argued that the Kansas law was in reality criminal (in part because of its assertedly "punitive" nature) rather than civil, and that as such it violated the constitutional prohibitions against double jeopardy and *ex post facto* laws. In rejecting these claims, the majority also considered some of the issues that had been raised in the "right to treatment" cases discussed supra. According to Justice Thomas, there is no constitutional bar to the civil commitment of those for whom no treatment is available but who pose a danger to others: "A State could hardly be seen as furthering a 'punitive' purpose by involuntarily confining persons afflicted with an untreatable, highly contagious disease." [Citing reference to cases in which people with contagious diseases have been civilly confined.] Moreover, even if Hendricks's condition were treatable — the Court found the lower courts' findings unclear on this issue — the majority seemed little concerned with whether Hendricks was actually receiving treatment. In a dissenting opinion, however, Justice Breyer found that the issue was critical, arguing that "whether the [Due Process] clause requires Kansas to provide treatment that it concedes is potentially available to a person who it concedes is treatable is the basic substantive due process question." The dissent went on to answer the question, arguing that without treatment Hendricks's civil commitment would violate substantive due process requirements (and also would make the commitment punitive and, as a result, an *ex post facto* law).

In a subsequent decision, *Kansas v. Crane*, 534 U.S. 407 (2002), the Supreme Court qualified its decision in *Hendricks*. In *Crane*, Kansas applied the same statute at issue in *Hendricks* to involuntarily commit a person who was clearly dangerous, but for whom there had been no showing that he could not control his dangerous behavior. The state argued that Hendricks did not require such a showing in all cases. Justice Breyer, writing for a majority of the Court, responded:

> . . . *Hendricks* set forth no requirement of total or complete lack of control. *Hendricks* referred to the Kansas Act as requiring a "mental abnormality" or "personality disorder" that makes it "difficult, if not impossible [to control the dangerous behavior]." The word "difficult" indicates that the lack of control to which this Court referred was not absolute. Indeed . . . an absolutist approach is unworkable. Moreover, most severely ill people — even those commonly termed "psychopaths" — retain some ability to control their behavior. Insistence upon absolute lack of control would risk barring the civil commitment of highly dangerous persons suffering severe mental abnormalities.
>
> We do not agree with the State, however, insofar as it seeks to claim that the Constitution permits commitment of the type of dangerous sexual offender considered in *Hendricks* without any lack-of-control determination. *Hendricks* underscored the constitutional importance of distinguishing a dangerous sexual offender subject to civil commitment "from other dangerous persons who are perhaps more properly dealt with exclusively through criminal proceedings." That distinction is necessary lest "civil commitment" become a "mechanism for retribution or general deterrence" — functions properly those of criminal law, not civil commitment. . . .
>
> In recognizing that fact, we did not give to the phrase "lack of control" a particularly narrow or technical meaning. And we recognize that in cases where lack of control is at issue, "inability to control behavior" will not be demonstrable with mathematical precision. It is enough to say that there must be proof of serious difficulty in controlling behavior. And this, when viewed in light of such features of the case as the nature of the psychiatric diagnosis, and the severity of the mental abnormality itself, must be sufficient to distinguish the dangerous sexual offender whose serious mental illness, abnormality, or

disorder subjects him to civil commitment from the dangerous but typical recidivist convicted in an ordinary criminal case. . . .

534 U.S. at 411–12.

Subsequent to *Crane*, the Supreme Court decided another case from the
same jurisdiction, again refining the scope of the state's discretion to confine
sexual predators. *McKune v. Lile*, 536 U.S. 24 (2002) (Kansas requirement
that sex offender participate in "admission of responsibility" program does not
violate his 5th amendment right to remain silent).

Note that the TB statutes in *Greene* and *J.S.* apply to people who are dangerous and who, for one reason or another, refuse to take voluntary efforts to
protect others. There is no requirement of a finding of mental abnormality or
"lack of control," and old statutes often only refer to dangerousness. Like the
New Jersey court, judges often interpret such language in light of the cases
involving involuntary commitment of the mentally ill, and read the dangerousness requirement in the public health context as referring either to inability
or unwillingness of the patient to prevent transmission of the disease to
others.

## Contemporary Complications: The "New" TB and Its Treatment

**8.** The problem of incomplete treatment and its relationship to the development of multi-drug resistant TB (described in note 1, *supra*) is one reason why,
during the 1990s, some jurisdictions experimented with "directly observed
therapy" (DOT). Under DOT, health care workers actually supervise patients
believed more likely to be noncompliant — often targeting homeless persons —
in taking and completing their daily dose of medications. This is in fact what
happened in the *J.S.* case, as the judge noted in a final footnote: "At the
November 30, 1993 review hearing Newark presented additional expert testimony and J.S.'s updated medical records showing the situation unchanged.
But thereafter, J.S. began to take his medication faithfully and his active TB
was arrested. On January 10, 1994, J.S. was released from confinement pursuant to a consent order in which he agreed to DOT and agreed to being committed again if he failed to take his medicine. This consent order was approved
in open court in J.S.'s presence as there was no longer any need for isolation
once he no longer suffered from active TB." It is of note that the original hearing was conducted by speaker phone — the judge in his chambers, and the
patient and his caregivers in his hospital room. A proceeding conducted in
this manner can alone convince a judge that the patient is contagious and
dangerous.

**9.** Hongkham Souvannarath became a visible example of a modern tuberculosis patient when she was involuntarily jailed in California, allegedly for failing to comply with a TB treatment regimen. Fresno County paid $1.2 million
to settle her 1999 federal lawsuit, which claimed violation of her rights under
the U.S. Constitution and California state law. She also brought a state action,
in which a California appeals court ordered the county to cease using the jail
to detain patients with TB. *Souvannarath v. Hadden*, 95 Cal. App. 4th 1115,
116 Cal. Rptr. 2d 7 (5th Dist. Cal. 2002). The California Appellate Court noted
that fewer than 20 people had been detained in Fresno County for TB since
1995. The federal lawsuit and the events leading to her confinement suggest

that confinement may not be necessary (and patients need not become either recalcitrant or dangerous) if appropriate services are made available to patients in need. The relevant facts are not reported in the court decision, but are described in a case study by Public Health Institute, TB and the Law Project, *Souvannarath Case Study* (2003), *available at* www.phlaw.org. *See also* John Roemer, *Reclaiming a Soul*, DAILY JOURNAL (Apr. 30, 2001).

Ms. Souvannarath, a refugee from Laos who came to the United States in 1984, was diagnosed with MDR-TB in California in 1998. She obtained TB treatment from a county clinic for several months, but experienced side effects and understood little of either the disease or its treatment. She spoke very little English and the clinic's translator spoke little Laotian. Ultimately, Souvannarath decided to live with a son in Ohio who could better care for her, but he was delayed in picking her up for the move. The clinic gave Souvannarath a small supply of medications to last until she could enter a pre-arranged Ohio clinic's program, but she ran out of medications before her son arrived. Feeling fine without taking medications, Souvannarath did not seek more. The clinic discovered she had not arrived in Ohio and had her served with an order in English to appear at the clinic. When she did not appear, the county health officer issued a detention order. She was arrested at gun point by two police officers and a communicable disease specialist and confined in the county jail. When she cried that she was afraid of dying, a non-Laotian translator thought she was threatening suicide, so she was confined in a safety cell for 3 days. She remained in jail, where only one guard could attempt translation, for ten months, until she was provided with an attorney and a hearing. The court released her subject to electronic monitoring in May 1999. At a review hearing in July 1999, she was released unconditionally.

Ms. Souvannarath's case suggests several points at which the county clinic could have ensured continued treatment and prevented incarceration. Initially, a translator who could explain the disease, treatment, its length, benefits and side effects might have persuaded Ms. Souvannarath to seek additional medications when she ran out, even though the drugs made her feel worse. If clinic staff had developed a more trusting relationship with Ms. Souvannarath, she might have been more receptive to their requests that she continue taking the medication. Even if all that failed, an order authorizing clinic staff to come to her house and watch her take her medications (directly observed therapy or DOT) would have avoided incarcerating her. The clinic, perhaps the entire TB program, may have had insufficient funds to accomplish these tasks. (The state health department reportedly lobbied against the law prohibiting housing TB patients in jails in order to gain "flexibility in placing TB patients in the event jail beds are the only available beds for the [TB] program." *See Souvannarath v. Hadden*, 95 Cal. App. 4th 1115, 1127 (2002).) But patients should not be punished simply because their clinic is underfunded. Indeed, it appears that Ms. Souvannarath would never have been considered uncooperative, much less a danger, had the clinic had enough staff and funding to continue the care she willingly accepted originally.

**10.** What does it take for a person who is homeless to "comply" with medical treatment recommendations? J.S. was given an appointment to get treatment at a clinic that was "a bus ride away" from a shelter. How likely is it that a person without any income will be able to get to clinic appointments? When people do not show up for their appointments, they may be labeled "non-compliant patients," as J.S. was. What is the cause of non-compliance? Does it matter for purposes of satisfying the dangerousness standard?

In *City of Newark*, Judge Goldman relies heavily on the writings of public health law professors, including Larry Gostin (*Controlling the Resurgent Tuberculosis Epidemic: A 50-State Survey of TB Statutes and Proposals for Reform*, 296 JAMA 255 (1993)), and George J. Annas (*Control of Tuberculosis: The Law and the Public's Health*, 328 NEW ENG. J. MED. 585 (1993)). In that article Annas also writes:

> . . . [T]he burden of involuntary confinement will fall most heavily on the homeless and those who live in crowded, inadequate housing, because they have no place to "confine themselves" during treatment for active tuberculosis. Since the rationale for involuntary commitment is danger to others based on the contagiousness of the patient's disease, under existing state statutes (written before multidrug-resistant tuberculosis was identified as dangerous to the public) patients have a right to be released when their tuberculosis is no longer communicable and they are therefore no longer a danger to others. The possibility of acquiring and spreading multidrug-resistant tuberculosis poses a particularly difficult problem. Even though not currently a danger to others, the patient whose tuberculosis is inactive but not yet cured might be a danger in the future if a treatment regimen that will ultimately cure the patient is not followed and if, instead, the patient takes drugs in such a way as to transform tuberculosis into a multidrug-resistant variety, which later becomes active and communicable. Because clear and convincing evidence is required to prove dangerousness, the fact that a person might be a risk to others in the future is insufficient reason alone, under current laws, for confinement until cure.

Does the existence of multidrug-resistant tuberculosis mean that state laws regarding tuberculosis should be changed to permit confinement until cure? The answer depends on the actual danger the patients pose to the public and the relative effectiveness of less restrictive treatment alternatives. In the context of antidiscrimination laws, the Supreme Court has made it clear that more than just the fear of danger is required to exclude a person with tuberculosis from the workplace. In *School Board of Nassau County v. Arline*, 480 U.S. 273 (1987), the Court adopted the position of the American Medical Association as to what factual medical inquiries a court should make in determining the degree of danger posed by a tuberculosis carrier who taught schoolchildren and sought reinstatement in her job after she was fired because she had tuberculosis. Its requirements were that the following be ascertained:

> (a) the nature of the risk (how the disease is transmitted), (b) the duration of the risk (how long the carrier is infectious), (c) the severity of the risk (what is the potential harm to third parties)

and (d) the probabilities the disease will be transmitted and will cause varying degrees of harm. *Id.*

The Court continued, "In making these findings, courts normally should defer to the reasonable medical judgments of public health officials." *Id.* When the teacher had active tuberculosis, there was no question that she could be excluded from the classroom.

Exclusion from crowded environments is obviously less restrictive than confinement. Nonetheless, if a state legislature concluded after hearing evidence from public health officials that such confinement was required to protect the public's health because there was no effective, less restrictive alternative available, a statute should be passed permitting confinement until cure. The hearings before the legislature could also provide useful education for the public about the epidemic and its control, as well as the opportunity to discuss alternative treatment strategies. Thereafter, if an individual patient were given a timely hearing, legal representation, and other due-process protections and if involuntary confinement were resorted to only when there is clear and convincing evidence that outpatient treatment could not effectively protect the public from that particular patient, confinement until cure would probably be found constitutional. This could be justified, even though confinement of a psychotic patient who did not consistently take medication might not be, because the time of confinement would be limited and relatively short.

Obviously, interventions short of confinement, such as periodic checkups or monitoring, or even the routine administration of therapy under direct observation, are much to be preferred. Moreover, a "technological fix" such as a slow-release implant would eliminate the need for confinement until cure altogether. It is also appropriate to use monetary and other inducements to encourage compliance with outpatient therapy, since the effective treatment of tuberculosis benefits the entire community. In no event, however, should a confined person be physically forced to take medications against his or her will, although confinement might be continued indefinitely as long as the patient continued to be a danger to the public.

Current discussion is properly focusing not on confinement but on less restrictive interventions such as routine and universal use of directly observed therapy.[9,10] This "methadone maintenance" model of delivery is not now the standard of care, and a survey of state laws found only three states (Maine, Michigan, and Minnesota) that explicitly provide for such monitoring of treatment by state officials.[19] Although the data are incomplete, it appears that from 1976 through 1990, more than 80 percent of all patients with tuberculosis in the United States completed

---

[9] Mahon W., Jones M., McGovern T.M., et al., *Developing a system for TB prevention and care in New York City.* New York: *The AIDS in Prison Project, Correctional Association of New York,* September 1992.

[10] Califano J.A., *Three-headed dog from hell.* WASHINGTON POST, December 21, 1992:A21.

[19] Gostin L.O., *Controlling the resurgent tuberculosis epidemic*: 50-state survey of TB statutes and proposals for reform. JAMA 1993; 269:255–261.

12 continuous months of drug therapy.[5] The completion rate is much lower for New York, but it still involves a majority. There is an understandable egalitarian desire to try to treat everyone in the same way by subjecting everyone to directly observed therapy. There is, however, insufficient justification for requiring this annoying and inconvenient method of treatment for patients who are virtually certain to take their antituberculosis medications and thus pose no risk to the public health. This is not a case in which there is a conflict between public health and civil rights. It is simply common sense. As Dubos and Dubos rightly observe, measures to prevent the spread of tuberculosis generally do not require legal compulsion, because they "have acquired the compelling strength of common sense."[1]

Requiring all persons to take therapy under direct observation because it is necessary for some is wasteful, inefficient, and gratuitously annoying, and it undercuts the legitimate desire to individualize treatment and to use the least restrictive and intrusive public health interventions. Moreover, in many if not most cases, reasonable discharge planning (including the provision of housing for the homeless) and counseling will greatly improve voluntary compliance. Of course, it can be difficult to predict some patients' degree of compliance accurately, and individualized case-management strategies and monitoring will be necessary.[12,20]

Directly observed therapy remains clearly preferable to involuntary confinement, however, and diligent and imaginative efforts to deliver therapy on an outpatient basis should be made before involuntary confinement is contemplated. Both these legal interventions, however, concentrate on the victims of social neglect, rather than on the neglect itself. This focus is understandable, since poverty is a much more difficult problem to address than the treatment of tuberculosis, but the history of the disease shows that success in controlling tuberculosis depends much more on the general standard of living than on specific medical or legal interventions.

\* \* \*

Cases of involuntary commitment for a contagious disease reported in the past two decades often involved persons with tuberculosis, coinciding with a resurgence of tuberculosis in the United States between about 1988 and 1992. Most reported cases are clustered around New York City. *See, e.g., New York v. Antoinette*, 165 Misc. 2d 1014, 630 N.Y.S.2d 1008 (Sup. Ct. Queens Cty, 1995). In addition, most cases seeking involuntary confinement targeted recent

---

[5] Goble M., Iseman, M.D., Madsen L.A., Waite D., Ackerson L., Horsburgh C.R., Jr., *Treatment of 171 patients with Pulmonary Tuberculosis resistant to isoniazid and rifampin.* N. ENG. J. MED. 1993; 328:527–532.

[1] Dubos R., Dubos J., *The white plague: tuberculosis, man, and society.* Boston: Little, Brown, 1952.

[12] Recommendations of the Massachusetts Commission for the Elimination of Tuberculosis. Boston: Massachusetts Department of Public Health, December 8, 1992.

[20] Patient compliance with medical regimens. In: Wingson R., Scotch N.A., Sorenson J., Swazey J.P., *In sickness and in health: social dimensions of medical care.* St. Louis: C.V. Mosby, 1981:142–57.]

immigrants from countries where tuberculosis is prevalent, and people who were homeless or living in shelters, jail or prison, where tuberculosis can easily spread among people living in close quarters. Some also suffered from mental illness that impeded their ability to follow treatment regimens, or also had HIV, which increases the likelihood of active TB and complicates treatment. Others spoke little English and found the health care system difficult to navigate. Most were poor.

The response to rising rates of tuberculosis varied across the country. Some states tried to rebuild tuberculosis treatment programs that had lost financial support in preceding years. The Institute of Medicine noted that such programs declined when the federal government ended its categorical financing of TB treatment, and concluded that "without question the major reason for the resurgence of tuberculosis was the deterioration of the public health infrastructure essential for the control of tuberculosis." INSTITUTE OF MEDICINE, ENDING NEGLECT: THE ELIMINATION OF TUBERCULOSIS IN THE UNITED STATES 2 (May 2000). Others argued that the increase in cases was the result of mistakes in economic and public health policy in the preceding decade, which reduced services and increased the proportion of the population living in poverty, in prisons or in homeless shelters, all conditions that facilitated the spread of TB. *See, e.g.,* Andrew A. Skolnick, *Some Experts Suggest the Nation's 'War on Drugs' Is Helping Tuberculosis State a Deadly Comeback,* 268 JAMA 3177 (1992); FRANK RYAN, THE FORGOTTEN PLAGUE: HOW THE BATTLE AGAINST TUBERCULOSIS WAS WON — AND LOST (1993). New York was particularly hard hit, losing treatment programs and experiencing an especially large rise in TB. Unable to provide enough clinics, New York relied heavily on involuntary isolation and directly observed therapy (DOT). (New York abandoned its isolation and quarantine statute in 1959, but adopted a reinvigorated version in response to the rise in tuberculosis in the late 1980s, and expanded it further after the terrorist attack of September 11, 2001.) HIV advocacy groups claimed that New York substituted isolation for treatment. In contrast, Massachusetts, which had preserved its treatment programs, managed to bring tuberculosis under control more rapidly than New York. Massachusetts provided more personal services, including having public health nurses bring medicines to patients, whether at work or in a shelter, instead of forcing patients to come to a clinic during working hours. The incidence of tuberculosis began to decline again in 1993, with most states claiming that their approach succeeded, even when the approaches were quite different.

**11.** The State of Washington has a statute that delegates broad, general public health power and which reads: "[The State Board of Health] shall have supreme authority in matters of quarantine, and shall provide by rule and regulation procedures for the imposition and use of isolation and quarantine." *See* WASH. REV. CODE ch.70–070. State law also gives broad powers over matters relating to public health to local health departments. WASH. REV. CODE §§ 70.05.060 & 70.05.070. The Washington State Constitution grants broad powers to local health officials concerning local public health matters: "Any county, city, town or township may make and enforce within its limits all such local police, sanitary and other regulations as are not in conflict with general laws." Wash. Const. art. XI, § 11. The Washington Supreme Court has addressed this grant of authority and noted: "This is a direct delegation of the police power as ample within its limits as that possessed by the legislature itself. It requires no legislative sanction for its exercise so long as the subject-matter is local, and the regulation reasonable and consistent with the general laws." *Spokane County Health Dep't v. Brockett*, 120 Wash. 2d 140, 148, 839 P.2d 324 (1992). Finally, the governor of the state also has both statutory and implied powers (i.e., powers beyond those specified in legislation) to act in response to public health emergencies. *See, e.g., Cougar Business Owners Ass'n v. Washington*, 97 Wash. 2d 466, 647 P.2d 481 (1982) (discussing the authority of the governor to impose quarantine on certain areas affected by the Mt. St. Helen's explosion.)

With regard to involuntary confinement, Washington also has a specific statute governing confinement and treatment of people with TB, WASH. REV. CODE § 70.28 *et seq.*; another governing people with sexually transmitted diseases (STDs), WASH. REV. CODE § 70.24.005–107; and a statute providing for the civil commitment of the mentally ill. For a detailed discussion of each and their legislative history, see Lisa A. Vincler & Deborah L. Gordon, *Legislative Reform of Washington's Tuberculosis Law: The Tension Between Due Process and Protecting Public Health*, 71 WASH. L. REV. 989 (1996).

Obviously any action by the state or local health departments in Washington State has to comply with any applicable statute, and each of these statutes has to comply with the dictates of procedural and substantive due process and, for that matter, other requirements of the state and federal constitutions. Just as obviously, there may be a series of preemption and conflict problems (*e.g.*, determining whether a specific state law has overridden the general authority of the local health departments.) This in itself outlines a complicated research problem. But note the breadth of the general power delegated to the state health department and the even broader powers delegated to the local health departments by the state's statutes and its constitution. What are the limits on these truly extraordinary delegations of authority to state and, in some cases, local public health officials? On the one hand, this allows for a maximum of discretion at the agency and local level; on the other, it provides for the greatest risk of abuse. Which is better: To allow the legislature to decide what and how the agencies of the state and local government can act in each particular matter, or to allow state or local officials virtually unlimited discretion in matters relating to public health?

Note also that to the extent the state legislature has provided specific statutory schemes for dealing with such matters as TB and STIs, the state or local health departments may not be able to exceed the limits of those specific statutes in dealing with TB or STIs, although they have much flexible discretion with regard to other public health problems for which the legislature has not enacted specific legislation. Does this make sense? To what extent is the state poised to deal with future public health problems?

## 2. Coercion and the Right to Refuse Treatment

## CRUZAN v. DIRECTOR, MISSOURI DEPARTMENT OF HEALTH
### 497 U.S. 261 (1990)

Rehnquist, Chief Justice.

\* \* \*

On the night of January 11, 1983, Nancy Cruzan lost control of her car as she traveled down Elm Road in Jasper County, Missouri. The vehicle overturned, and Cruzan was discovered lying face down in a ditch without detectable respiratory or cardiac function. Paramedics were able to restore her breathing and heartbeat at the accident site, and she was transported to a hospital in an unconscious state. An attending neurosurgeon diagnosed her as having sustained probable cerebral contusions compounded by significant anoxia (lack of oxygen). The Missouri trial court in this case found that permanent brain damage generally results after 6 minutes in an anoxic state; it was estimated that Cruzan was deprived of oxygen from 12 to 14 minutes. She remained in a coma for approximately three weeks and then progressed to an unconscious state in which she was able to orally ingest some nutrition. In order to ease feeding and further the recovery, surgeons implanted a gastrostomy feeding and hydration tube in Cruzan with the consent of her then husband. Subsequent rehabilitative efforts proved unavailing. She now lies in a Missouri state hospital in what is commonly referred to as a persistent vegetative state: generally, a condition in which a person exhibits motor reflexes but evinces no indications of significant cognitive function. The State of Missouri is bearing the cost of her care.

After it had become apparent that Nancy Cruzan had virtually no chance of regaining her mental faculties, her parents asked hospital employees to terminate the artificial nutrition and hydration procedures. All agree that such a removal would cause her death. The employees refused to honor the request without court approval. The parents then sought and received authorization from the state trial court for termination. The court found that a person in Nancy's condition had a fundamental right under the State and Federal Constitutions to refuse or direct the withdrawal of "death prolonging procedures." The court also found that Nancy's "expressed thoughts at age twenty-five in somewhat serious conversation with a housemate friend that if sick or injured she would not wish to continue her life unless she could live at least halfway normally suggests that given her present condition she would not wish to continue on with her nutrition and hydration." The Supreme Court of Missouri reversed by a divided vote.

At common law, even the touching of one person by another without consent and without legal justification was a battery. Before the turn of the century, this Court observed that "no right is held more sacred, or is more carefully guarded, by the common law, than the right of every individual to the possession and control of his own person, free from all restraint or interference of others, unless by clear and unquestionable authority of law." *Union Pacific R.*

*Co. v. Botsford,* 141 U.S. 250, 251, 35 L. Ed. 734, 11 S. Ct. 1000 (1891). This notion of bodily integrity has been embodied in the requirement that informed consent is generally required for medical treatment. Justice Cardozo, while on the Court of Appeals of New York, aptly described this doctrine: "Every human being of adult years and sound mind has a right to determine what shall be done with his own body; and a surgeon who performs an operation without his patient's consent commits an assault, for which he is liable in damages." *Schloendorff v. Society of New York Hospital,* 211 N.Y. 125, 129–130, 105 N.E. 92, 93 (1914). The informed consent doctrine has become firmly entrenched in American tort law.

The logical corollary of the doctrine of informed consent is that the patient generally possesses the right not to consent, that is, to refuse treatment. Until about 15 years ago and the seminal decision in *In re Quinlan,* 70 N.J. 10, 355 A.2d 647, *cert. denied sub nom. Garger v. New Jersey,* 429 U.S. 922, 50 L. Ed. 2d 289, 97 S. Ct. 319 (1976), the number of right-to-refuse-treatment decisions was relatively few. Most of the earlier cases involved patients who refused medical treatment forbidden by their religious beliefs, thus implicating First Amendment rights as well as common-law rights of self-determination. More recently, however, with the advance of medical technology capable of sustaining life well past the point where natural forces would have brought certain death in earlier times, cases involving the right to refuse life-sustaining treatment have burgeoned. . . .

As these cases demonstrate, the common-law doctrine of informed consent is viewed as generally encompassing the right of a competent individual to refuse medical treatment. Beyond that, these cases demonstrate both similarity and diversity in their approaches to decision of what all agree is a perplexing question with unusually strong moral and ethical overtones. State courts have available to them for decision a number of sources — state constitutions, statutes, and common law — which are not available to us. In this Court, the question is simply and starkly whether the United States Constitution prohibits Missouri from choosing the rule of decision which it did. This is the first case in which we have been squarely presented with the issue whether the United States Constitution grants what is in common parlance referred to as a "right to die." . . .

The Fourteenth Amendment provides that no State shall "deprive any person of life, liberty, or property, without due process of law." The principle that a competent person has a constitutionally protected liberty interest in refusing unwanted medical treatment may be inferred from our prior decisions. In *Jacobson v. Massachusetts,* 197 U.S. 11, 24–30, 49 L. Ed. 643, 25 S. Ct. 358 (1905), for instance, the Court balanced an individual's liberty interest in declining an unwanted smallpox vaccine against the State's interest in preventing disease. Decisions prior to the incorporation of the Fourth Amendment into the Fourteenth Amendment analyzed searches and seizures involving the body under the Due Process Clause and were thought to implicate substantial liberty interests. *See, e.g., Breithaupt v. Abram,* 352 U.S. 432, 439, 1 L. Ed. 2d 448, 77 S. Ct. 408 (1957) ("As against the right of an individual that his person be held inviolable . . . must be set the interests of society . . .").

Just this Term, in the course of holding that a State's procedures for administering antipsychotic medication to prisoners were sufficient to satisfy due process concerns, we recognized that prisoners possess "a significant liberty interest in avoiding the unwanted administration of antipsychotic drugs under the Due Process Clause of the Fourteenth Amendment." *Washington v. Harper,* 494 U.S. 210, 221–222, 108 L. Ed. 2d 178, 110 S. Ct. 1028 (1990); ("The forcible injection of medication into a nonconsenting person's body represents a substantial interference with that person's liberty"). Still other cases support the recognition of a general liberty interest in refusing medical treatment. *Vitek v. Jones,* 445 U.S. 480, 494, 63 L. Ed. 2d 552, 100 S. Ct. 1254 (1980) (transfer to mental hospital coupled with mandatory behavior modification treatment implicated liberty interests); *Parham v. J. R.,* 442 U.S. 584, 600, 61 L. Ed. 2d 101, 99 S. Ct. 2493 (1979) ("[A] child, in common with adults, has a substantial liberty interest in not being confined unnecessarily for medical treatment"). But determining that a person has a "liberty interest" under the Due Process Clause does not end the inquiry; "whether respondent's constitutional rights have been violated must be determined by balancing his liberty interests against the relevant state interests." *Youngberg v. Romeo,* 457 U.S. 307, 321, 73 L. Ed. 2d 28, 102 S. Ct. 2452 (1982).

Petitioners insist that under the general holdings of our cases, the forced administration of life-sustaining medical treatment, and even of artificially delivered food and water essential to life, would implicate a competent person's liberty interest. Although we think the logic of the cases discussed above would embrace such a liberty interest, the dramatic consequences involved in refusal of such treatment would inform the inquiry as to whether the deprivation of that interest is constitutionally permissible. But for purposes of this case, we assume that the United States Constitution would grant a competent person a constitutionally protected right to refuse lifesaving hydration and nutrition.

Petitioners go on to assert that an incompetent person should possess the same right in this respect as is possessed by a competent person. They rely primarily on our decisions in *Parham v. J. R., supra,* and *Youngberg v. Romeo, supra.* In *Parham,* we held that a mentally disturbed minor child had a liberty interest in "not being confined unnecessarily for medical treatment," 442 U.S. at 600, but we certainly did not intimate that such a minor child, after commitment, would have a liberty interest in refusing treatment. In *Youngberg,* we held that a seriously retarded adult had a liberty interest in safety and freedom from bodily restraint, 457 U.S. at 320. *Youngberg,* however, did not deal with decisions to administer or withhold medical treatment.

The difficulty with petitioners' claim is that in a sense it begs the question: An incompetent person is not able to make an informed and voluntary choice to exercise a hypothetical right to refuse treatment or any other right. Such a "right" must be exercised for her, if at all, by some sort of surrogate. Here, Missouri has in effect recognized that under certain circumstances a surrogate may act for the patient in electing to have hydration and nutrition withdrawn in such a way as to cause death, but it has established a procedural safeguard to assure that the action of the surrogate conforms as best it may to the wishes expressed by the patient while competent. Missouri requires that evidence of the incompetent's wishes as to the withdrawal of treatment be proved by clear and convincing evidence. The question, then, is whether the United States Constitution forbids the establishment of this procedural requirement by the State. We hold that it does not.

Whether or not Missouri's clear and convincing evidence requirement comports with the United States Constitution depends in part on what interests the State may properly seek to protect in this situation. Missouri relies on its interest in the protection and preservation of human life, and there can be no gainsaying this interest. As a general matter, the States — indeed, all civilized nations — demonstrate their commitment to life by treating homicide as a serious crime. Moreover, the majority of States in this country have laws imposing criminal penalties on one who assists another to commit suicide. We do not think a State is required to remain neutral in the face of an informed and voluntary decision by a physically able adult to starve to death. . . .

But in the context presented here, a State has more particular interests at stake. The choice between life and death is a deeply personal decision of obvious and overwhelming finality. We believe Missouri may legitimately seek to safeguard the personal element of this choice through the imposition of heightened evidentiary requirements.

No doubt is engendered by anything in this record but that Nancy Cruzan's mother and father are loving and caring parents. If the State were required by the United States Constitution to repose a right of "substituted judgment" with anyone, the Cruzans would surely qualify. But we do not think the Due Process Clause requires the State to repose judgment on these matters with anyone but the patient herself. . . . the State may choose to defer only to those wishes, rather than confide the decision to close family members.

. . .

The judgment of the Supreme Court of Missouri is *Affirmed*.

. . .

O'Connor, Justice, concurring.

I agree that a protected liberty interest in refusing unwanted medical treatment may be inferred from our prior decisions, and that the refusal of artificially delivered food and water is encompassed within that liberty interest. . . .

I write separately to emphasize that the Court does not today decide the issue whether a State must also give effect to the decisions of a surrogate decisionmaker. In my view, such a duty may well be constitutionally required to protect the patient's liberty interest in refusing medical treatment. . . . Today's decision, holding only that the Constitution permits a State to require clear and convincing evidence of Nancy Cruzan's desire to have artificial hydration and nutrition withdrawn, does not preclude a future determination that the Constitution requires the States to implement the decisions of a patient's duly appointed surrogate.

. . . .

Brennan, Justice, with Justices Marshall and Blackmun, dissenting.

The starting point for our legal analysis must be whether a competent person has a constitutional right to avoid unwanted medical care. Earlier this Term, this Court held that the Due Process Clause of the Fourteenth Amendment confers a significant liberty interest in avoiding unwanted medical treatment. *Washington v. Harper,* 494 U.S. 210, 221–222, 108 L. Ed. 2d 178, 110 S. Ct. 1028 (1990). Today, the Court concedes that our prior decisions "support the recognition of a general liberty interest in refusing medical treatment." *See* 497 U.S. at 278. . . .

But if a competent person has a liberty interest to be free of unwanted medical treatment, as both the majority and Justice O'Connor concede, it must be fundamental. "We are dealing here with [a decision] which involves one of the basic civil rights of man." *Skinner v. Oklahoma ex rel. Williamson,* 316 U.S. 535, 541, 86 L. Ed. 1655, 62 S. Ct. 1110 (1942) (invalidating a statute authorizing sterilization of certain felons). Whatever other liberties protected by the Due Process Clause are fundamental, "those liberties that are 'deeply rooted in this Nation's history and tradition'" are among them. *Bowers v. Hardwick,* 478 U.S. 186, 192, 106 S. Ct. 2841, 92 L. Ed. 2d 140 (1986).

The right to be free from medical attention without consent, to determine what shall be done with one's own body, *is* deeply rooted in this Nation's traditions, as the majority acknowledges. *See* 497 U.S. at 270. This right has long been "firmly entrenched in American tort law" and is securely grounded in the earliest common law. *Ante,* at 269. *See also Mills v. Rogers,* 457 U.S. 291, 294, n.4, 73 L. Ed. 2d 16, 102 S. Ct. 2442 (1982) ("The right to refuse any medical treatment emerged from the doctrines of trespass and battery, which were applied to unauthorized touchings by a physician"). "Anglo-American law starts with the premise of thorough-going self determination. It follows that each man is considered to be master of his own body, and he may, if he be of sound mind, expressly prohibit the performance of lifesaving surgery, or other medical treatment." *Natanson v. Kline,* 186 Kan. 393, 406–407, 350 P.2d 1093, 1104 (1960). "The inviolability of the person" has been held as "sacred" and "carefully guarded" as any common-law right. *Union Pacific R. Co. v. Botsford,* 141 U.S. 250, 251–252, 35 L. Ed. 734, 11 S. Ct. 1000 (1891). Thus, freedom from unwanted medical attention is unquestionably among those principles "so rooted in the traditions and conscience of our people as to be ranked as fundamental." *Snyder v. Massachusetts,* 291 U.S. 97, 105, 78 L. Ed. 674, 54 S. Ct. 330 (1934). . . .

That there may be serious consequences involved in refusal of the medical treatment at issue here does not vitiate the right under our common-law tradition of medical self-determination. It is "a well-established rule of general law . . . that it is the patient, not the physician, who ultimately decides if treatment — any treatment — is to be given at all. . . . The rule has never been qualified in its application by either the nature or purpose of the treatment, or the gravity of the consequences of acceding to or foregoing it." *Tune v. Walter Reed Army Medical Hospital,* 602 F. Supp. 1452, 1455 (DC 1985). *See also Downer v. Veilleux,* 322 A.2d 82, 91 (Me. 1974) ("The rationale of this rule lies in the fact that every competent adult has the right to forego treatment, or even cure, if it entails what for him are intolerable consequences or risks, however unwise his sense of values may be to others"). I respectfully dissent.

\* \* \*

# BUCK v. BELL
## 274 U.S. 200 (1927)

Holmes, Justice.

\* \* \*

This is a writ of error to review a judgment of the Supreme Court of Appeals of the State of Virginia, affirming a judgment of the Circuit Court of Amherst County, by which the defendant in error, the superintendent of the State Colony for Epileptics and Feeble Minded, was ordered to perform the operation of salpingectomy upon Carrie Buck, the plaintiff in error, for the purpose of making her sterile. 143 Va. 310. The case comes here upon the contention that the statute authorizing the judgment is void under the Fourteenth Amendment as denying to the plaintiff in error due process of law and the equal protection of the laws.

Carrie Buck is a feeble minded white woman who was committed to the State Colony above mentioned in due form. She is the daughter of a feeble minded mother in the same institution, and the mother of an illegitimate feeble minded child. She was eighteen years old at the time of the trial of her case in the Circuit Court, in the latter part of 1924. An Act of Virginia, approved March 20, 1924, recites that the health of the patient and the welfare of society may be promoted in certain cases by the sterilization of mental defectives, under careful safeguard, &c.; that the sterilization may be effected in males by vasectomy and in females by salpingectomy, without serious pain or substantial danger to life; that the Commonwealth is supporting in various institutions many defective persons who if now discharged would become a menace but if incapable of procreating might be discharged with safety and become self-supporting with benefit to themselves and to society; and that experience has shown that heredity plays an important part in the transmission of insanity, imbecility, etc. The statute then enacts that whenever the superintendent of certain institutions including the above named State Colony shall be of opinion that it is for the best interests of the patients and of society that an inmate under his care should be sexually sterilized, he may have the operation performed upon any patient afflicted with hereditary forms of insanity, imbecility, &c., on complying with the very careful provisions by which the act protects the patients from possible abuse.

The superintendent first presents a petition to the special board of directors of his hospital or colony, stating the facts and the grounds for his opinion, verified by affidavit. Notice of the petition and of the time and place of the hearing in the institution is to be served upon the inmate, and also upon his guardian, and if there is no guardian the superintendent is to apply to the Circuit Court of the County to appoint one. If the inmate is a minor notice also is to be given to his parents if any with a copy of the petition. The board is to see to it that the inmate may attend the hearings if desired by him or his guardian.

The evidence is all to be reduced to writing, and after the board has made its order for or against the operation, the superintendent, or the inmate, or his guardian, may appeal to the Circuit Court of the County. The Circuit Court may consider the record of the board and the evidence before it and such other admissible evidence as may be offered, and may affirm, revise, or reverse the order of the board and enter such order as it deems just. Finally any party may apply to the Supreme Court of Appeals, which, if it grants the appeal, is to hear the case upon the record of the trial in the Circuit Court and may enter such order as it thinks the Circuit Court should have entered. There can be no doubt that so far as procedure is concerned the rights of the patient are most carefully considered, and as every step in this case was taken in scrupulous compliance with the statute and after months of observation, there is no doubt that in that respect the plaintiff in error has had due process of law.

The attack is not upon the procedure but upon the substantive law. It seems to be contended that in no circumstances could such an order be justified. It certainly is contended that the order cannot be justified upon the existing grounds. The judgment finds the facts that have been recited and that Carrie Buck "is the probable potential parent of socially inadequate offspring, likewise afflicted, that she may be sexually sterilized without detriment to her general health and that her welfare and that of society will be promoted by her sterilization," and thereupon makes the order. In view of the general declarations of the legislature and the specific findings of the Court, obviously we cannot say as matter of law that the grounds do not exist, and if they exist they justify the result. We have seen more than once that the public welfare may call upon the best citizens for their lives. It would be strange if it could not call upon those who already sap the strength of the State for these lesser sacrifices, often not felt to be such by those concerned, in order to prevent our being swamped with incompetence. It is better for all the world, if instead of waiting to execute degenerate offspring for crime, or to let them starve for their imbecility, society can prevent those who are manifestly unfit from continuing their kind. The principle that sustains compulsory vaccination is broad enough to cover cutting the Fallopian tubes. *Jacobson v. Massachusetts,* 197 U.S. 11. Three generations of imbeciles are enough.

But, it is said, however it might be if this reasoning were applied generally, it fails when it is confined to the small number who are in the institutions named and is not applied to the multitudes outside. It is the usual last resort of constitutional arguments to point out shortcomings of this sort. But the answer is that the law does all that is needed when it does all that it can, indicates a policy, applies it to all within the lines, and seeks to bring within the lines all similarly situated so far and so fast as its means allow. Of course so far as the operations enable those who otherwise must be kept confined to be returned to the world, and thus open the asylum to others, the equality aimed at will be more nearly reached.

Judgment affirmed.

Mr. Justice Butler dissents.

# NOTES AND QUESTIONS

**1.** *Cruzan* and *Buck* are incompatible. Both deal with incompetent patients and both cite *Jacobson* as authority. *Buck* cited *Jacobson* as support for a very general principle that public welfare was sufficient to justify involuntary sterilization. In doing so the decision extended the police power's reach from imposing a monetary penalty for refusing vaccination to forcing surgery on a young woman against her will and depriving her of future offspring. The Court did not require the state to demonstrate that sterilization was necessary and not arbitrary or oppressive. This suggests that the Court did not view *Jacobson* as requiring any substantive standard of necessity or reasonableness that would prevent what today would be considered an indefensible assault. The Court did not even consider that Carrie Buck might have any right to personal liberty. With the Court's imprimatur of involuntary sterilization laws, more than 60,000 Americans, mostly poor women, were sterilized by 1978. It was also used by the Nazis to help justify their own sterilization program, and was cited by the defense at the Nuremberg Trials. Of course, it is no longer either good law or good genetics. For an excellent history of *Buck v. Bell*, see Paul Lombardo, *Three Generations, No Imbeciles: New Light on* Buck v. Bell, 60 N.Y.U. L. Rev. 30 (1985); Paul Lombardo, *Taking Eugenics Seriously: Three Generations of ??? Are Enough?*, 30 Fla. St. U. L. Rev. 191 (2003).

**2.** As both the majority and minority in *Cruzan* make clear, the right to refuse treatment has always been taken seriously by the common law, and now also has strong support from constitutional doctrine as well. The majority's opinion can suggest no case involving treatment against the will of a free living competent person other than *Jacobson,* and that case does not stand for such a proposition. Instead they point to cases involving children and mentally-impaired prisoners. There is no suggestion that treatment could ever be forced on a competent adult for the adult's own good, including saving the adult's life, by any of the justices. This is a difficult case for the majority only because Nancy Cruzan is incapable of expressing her own wishes. That controversy remains regarding what treatment to compel an incompetent person to undergo, over either the wishes of their next-of-kin, or contrary to what it is believed the person would want done, is well-illustrated by the interference by the U.S. Congress, the Legislature and Governor of Florida, and the President of the United States in the decision of Michael Schiavo, upheld by every court that reviewed it, that it would be his wife's decision not to continue tube-feeding if she was in a permanent vegetative state. *See, e.g.,* George J. Annas, *"I Want to Live": Medicine Betrayed by Ideology in the Political Debate Over Terri Schiavo,* 35 Stetson L. Rev. 49 (2005); Norman L. Cantor, *The Relation Between Autonomy-Based Rights and Profoundly Mentally Disabled Persons,* 13 Annals of Health L. 37 (2004).

## C.   CASE STUDY: HIV/AIDS

### CITY OF NEW YORK v. NEW SAINT MARK'S BATHS
130 Misc. 2d 911; 497 N.Y.S.2d 979 (1986)

\* \* \*

This action by the health authorities of the City of New York is taken against defendant the New St. Mark's Baths (St. Mark's) as a step to limit the spread of the disease known as AIDS (Acquired Immune Deficiency Syndrome). The parties are in agreement with respect to the deadly character of this disease and the dire threat that its spread, now in epidemic proportions, poses to the health and well-being of the community. Both sides cite as authoritative the publication AIDS, 100 Questions and Answers, issued by the New York State Department of Health which is concededly based on the latest and most authoritative scientific findings. Thus, there is no disagreement that the rate of incidence of new cases of AIDS in New York State is approaching 200 a month; effective treatment is wholly lacking, and approximately 50% of all persons diagnosed with AIDS have died. The death rate for this disease increases to nearly 85% two years after diagnosis. The same percentage of AIDS patients suffer from special forms of pneumonia or cancer which are untreatable, and about 30% of these patients show symptoms of brain disease or severe damage to the spinal cord.

Immediately relevant to this litigation are the scientific facts with respect to AIDS risk groups. During the five years in which the disease has been identified and studied, 73% of AIDS victims have consisted of sexually active homosexual and bisexual men with multiple partners. AIDS is not easily transmittable through casual body contact or transmission through air, water or food. Direct blood-to-blood or semen-to-blood contact is necessary to transmit the virus. Cases of AIDS among homosexual and bisexual males are associated with promiscuous sexual contact, anal intercourse and other sexual practices which may result in semen-to-blood or blood-to-blood contact.

According to medical evidence submitted by *defendants*: "The riskiest conduct is thought to be that which allows the introduction of semen into the blood stream. Because anal intercourse may result in a tearing of internal tissues, that activity is considered high-risk for transmission."

Fellatio is also a high risk activity. As stated by the organizer of the AIDS Institute of the New York State Department of Health: "Any direct contact with the semen of an infected person may increase the risk of AIDS transmission. The deposition of semen in areas likely to contain abrasions, open sores, and cuts and concurrent inflammatory processes which could result in the presence of susceptible lymphocytes increase the risk of AIDS transmission. Because the mouth represents such an area (the epithelial tissue in the mouth is more susceptible to injury than the epithelial tissue in the vagina), fellatio presents a high risk for the transmission of AIDS."

## PRIOR PROCEEDINGS

On October 25, 1985 the State Public Health Council, with the approval of the intervening New York State Commissioner of Health, adopted an emergency resolution adding a new regulation to the State Sanitary Code. This added regulation, State Sanitary Code (10 NYCRR) § 24.2, specifically authorized local officials, such as the City plaintiffs (City) here, to close any facilities "in which high risk sexual activity takes place." More specifically, in *10 NYCRR 24-2.2*, the regulation provided: "Prohibited Facilities: No establishment shall make facilities available for the purpose of sexual activities in which high risk sexual activity takes place. Such facilities shall constitute a public nuisance dangerous to the public health."

In *10 NYCRR 24-2.1*, the regulation furnished definitions:

a. 'Establishment' shall mean any place in which entry, membership, goods or services are purchased.

b. 'High Risk Sexual Activity' shall mean anal intercourse and fellatio.

The Public Health Council based this regulation on the Commissioner's "findings" that: "Establishments including certain bars, clubs and bathhouses which are used as places for engaging in high risk sexual activities contribute to the propagation and spread of such AIDS-associated retro-viruses . . . . Appropriate public health intervention to discontinue such exposure at such establishments is essential to interrupting the epidemic among the people of the State of New York."

Thereafter, on or about December 9, 1985, the City commenced this action by order to show cause for an injunction closing the New St. Mark's Baths (St. Mark's) as a public nuisance citing the health risks at St. Mark's as defined in the State regulation. On December 19, 1985, following the issuance of a temporary restraining order defendants served papers in opposition to the City's motion for a preliminary injunction and cross-moved to dismiss the complaint for failure to state a cause of action. Defendants challenged the State regulation on the grounds that it was an invasion of defendants' patrons' rights to privacy and freedom of association under the United States Constitution.

Also on December 19, 1985, Paul Corrigan, Charles Dempsey, John Doe and Tom Roe, sought an order to intervene as party defendants. The proposed intervenors-defendants (intervenors) are described as "frequent patrons of the New St. Mark's Baths." The intervenors have also opposed the City's motion for a preliminary injunction. Intervenors also argue that the State regulation violates intervenors' rights to privacy and freedom of association.

On December 20, 1985, the Public Health Council promulgated *10 NYCRR 24-2.2* as a permanent regulation. The "findings" of the Public Health Council, as they relate to "high risk sexual activity," were similar to the "findings" of the Council in October. The regulation was approved by the Commissioner of Health and became effective on December 23, 1985.

On December 24, 1985, the State Commissioner of Health and the Attorney-General moved to intervene as plaintiffs to defend the validity of the State regulation.

This action is brought pursuant to the Nuisance Abatement Law. Under that law the City is empowered to enjoin public nuisances. . . .

## CONSTITUTIONAL CONSIDERATIONS

The City has submitted ample supporting proof that high risk sexual activity has been taking place at St. Mark's on a continuous and regular basis. Following numerous on-site visits by City inspectors, over 14 separate days, these investigators have submitted affidavits describing 49 acts of high risk sexual activity (consisting of 41 acts of fellatio involving 70 persons and 8 acts of anal intercourse involving 16 persons). This evidence of high risk sexual activity, all occurring either in public areas of St. Mark's or in enclosed cubicles left visible to the observer without intrusion therein, demonstrates the inadequacy of self-regulatory procedures by the St. Mark's attendant staff, and the futility of any less intrusive solution to the problem other than closure.

With a demonstrated death rate from AIDS during the first six months of 1985 of 1248. . . , plaintiffs and the intervening State officers have demonstrated a compelling State interest in acting to preserve the health of the population (*Jacobson v. Massachusetts,* 197 U.S. 11, 25–27. . .) Where such a compelling State interest is demonstrated even the constitutional rights of privacy and free association must give way provided, as here, it is also shown that the remedy adopted is the least intrusive reasonably available. Furthermore, it is by no means clear that defendants' rights will, in actuality, be adversely affected in a constitutionally recognized sense by closure of St. Mark's. The privacy protection of sexual activity conducted in a private home does not extend to commercial establishments simply because they provide an opportunity for intimate behavior or sexual release . . . . As stated in *Stratton v. Drumm* (445 F. Supp. 1305, 1309 [D. Conn. 1978]): "privacy and freedom of association . . . rights do not extend to commercial ventures."

The private intervenors, of course, are not commercial ventures. However, the closure of this bath house does not extinguish their opportunities for unrestricted association in establishments which avoid creating a serious risk to the public health.

Also, State police power has been upheld over claims of 1st Amendment rights of association where the nature of the assemblage is not for the advancement of beliefs and ideas but predominantly either for entertainment or gratification, involving a heterosexual "swinging club"; involving a skating rink; "the associational activities of the Elks and Moose are purely social and not political and therefore do not come within the core protection of the right to associate". A tangential impact upon association or expression is insufficient to obstruct the exercise of the State's police power to protect public health and safety.

To be sure, defendants and the intervening patrons challenge the soundness of the scientific judgments upon which the Health Council regulation is based, citing, *inter alia*, the observation of the City's former Commissioner of Health in a memorandum dated October 22, 1985 that "closure of bathhouses will contribute little if anything to the control of AIDS." (For a vigorous medical opinion to the contrary from a specialist in this field see letter of Stephen S. Calazza, M.D., dated Jan. 24, 1985.) Defendants particularly assail the regulation's inclusion of fellatio as a high risk sexual activity and argue that enforced use of prophylactic sheaths would be a more appropriate regulatory response. They go further and argue that facilities such as St. Mark's, which attempts to educate its patrons with written materials, signed pledges, and posted notices as to the advisability of safe sexual practices, provide a positive force in combating AIDS, and a valuable communication link between public health authorities and the homosexual community. While these arguments and proposals may have varying degrees of merit, they overlook a fundamental principle of applicable law: "It is not for the courts to determine which scientific view is correct in ruling upon whether the police power has been properly exercised. The judicial function is exhausted with the discovery that the relation between means and end is not wholly vain and fanciful, an illusory pretense'" . . . . Justification for plaintiffs' application here more than meets that test.

For the foregoing reasons plaintiffs' application for a [sic] preliminary injunctive relief is granted. . . .

* * *

## Wendy Parmet, *AIDS and Quarantine:*
## *The Revival of an Archaic Doctrine*
### 14 HOFSTRA L. REV. 53, 55–71 (1985)

* * *

Quarantine is one of the oldest forms of public health regulation. The word derives from the Italian *quarantenaria* or the Latin *quadraginta*, which means forty days and refers to the forty day detention placed on ships from plague-ridden ports during the late Middle Ages and early Renaissance. . . . The roots of this form of quarantine have been traced as far back as the Book of Leviticus, which prescribes the ostracism of lepers. Following that Biblical precept, lepers were isolated by official edict throughout medieval Europe.

When the plague struck Europe in the fourteenth century, European cities relied on their experience isolating lepers and denied entrance to persons coming from areas afflicted with the plague. Victims of the plague were isolated in their houses for the duration of the illness, as were all who had come into contact with them. Since the plague is usually spread by fleas and rats, the effectiveness of such measures is questionable. However, lacking a scientific understanding of the disease and its transmission, quarantine was one of the few actions that a community could take. Moreover, it set the precedent for a form of public health regulation that was potentially more effective when later applied to other diseases, such as smallpox, that were easily spread by casual contact between individuals.

In England, an early seventeenth century statute required the isolation of plague victims. According to Blackstone, the violation of this statute was a felony, and the matter was of the "highest importance." In colonial America, quarantine was enforced by both local and colonial governments. The earliest reported local quarantine order in America was in 1622 to combat smallpox in East Hampton, Long Island. Historians have found records of maritime quarantines in Boston as far back as 1647. In 1678, individuals with smallpox in Salem, Massachusetts were isolated by local order.

By the time the federal Constitution was drafted in 1787, quarantine had become a well-established form of public health regulation. Although the Constitution does not mention quarantine, article 1, section 10, acknowledges that states may promulgate and enforce inspection laws. This provision has long been thought to give states the power to keep out articles of commerce that are thought to be infectious. In *Gibbons v. Ogden* [22 U.S. (9 Wheat.) 1 (1824)], Chief Justice Marshall noted in *dicta* that a state had the power to quarantine "to provide for the health of its citizens." Quarantine was thus considered a proper exercise of the states' police power.

In 1796, the federal government enacted the first federal quarantine law in response to a yellow fever epidemic. [Act of May 27, 1796, ch. 31, 1 Stat. 474 (repealed 1799)] That law gave the President the power to assist states in enforcing their own quarantine laws. In 1799, the Act was repealed and replaced with one establishing the first federal inspection system for maritime quarantines. [Act of Feb. 25, 1799, ch. 12, 1 Stat. 619] Thereafter, throughout the nineteenth century, the federal government undertook an increasingly prominent role in implementing maritime quarantines.

It was the states, however, usually acting through localities, that enacted and enforced the quarantine regulations that required the isolation of individuals afflicted with, or exposed to, contagious disease. Cases discussing such state and local quarantines thus set the early precedent as to the government's power to deprive individuals of their liberty in order to protect the public health. Modern commentators have relied upon these cases in discussions of the powers of the state to quarantine people with AIDS. Yet, for the most part, these cases do not reflect the dramatic changes that have occurred in public law and science in the last fifty years. As a result, they must be understood in the context of their times, and their principles should not be applied today without modifications made in light of recent changes in law and science. . . .

## II.  THE LAW OF QUARANTINE

By the mid-to-late nineteenth century, many states had statutes enabling officials to isolate and detain individuals infected with or exposed to contagious diseases. The Massachusetts public health statute of 1797 was typical. Section 1 stated its purpose: "[T]he better preventing the spread of infection . . . ." [Act of June 22, 1797, ch. 16, GEN. LAWS OF MASS. (1822)] The statute gave the selectmen of a town power to:

> take care and make effectual provision in the best way they can, for the preservation of the inhabitants, by removing such sick or infected person or persons, and placing him or them in a separate house or houses, and by providing nurses, attendance, and other assistance and necessaries for them. . . .

Despite the broad authority given to state health officials under the nineteenth century quarantine statutes, prior to the second decade of this century there was little discussion about the constitutionality of the state's power to quarantine individuals. Courts and scholars debated the constitutionality of other state actions taken, but they rarely expressed doubts about the validity of quarantine regulations. At that time, the courts presumed that state actions taken within the police power, which was seen as the sovereign power of the state to protect the peace, health and morals of the public, were constitutional. Since quarantine was clearly designed to protect the public from disease, it was easily assumed to be a proper exercise of the police power.

The tacit acceptance of such broad state power over individuals may be understandable when it is remembered that at that time infectious disease was an ever-present threat. It is not surprising that quarantine was seen as emanating from the "higher ground of public welfare" when epidemics were common, and no one was immune from their terror.

The terror of epidemics and the historical roots of quarantine distinguished it as the example of a legitimate use of the police power. The fact that quarantine regulations were universally held to be both constitutional and beneficent, however, does not mean that the courts totally abrogated all review. To the contrary, courts always conducted a limited review. From the middle of the nineteenth century to approximately the time of World War I, the courts were presented with many quarantine cases. Most of these "classic" cases concerned quarantines imposed for acute infectious diseases such as smallpox, yellow fever, and typhus. In such cases, the courts usually upheld the validity of the quarantine statutes or regulations. Nevertheless, they often questioned the actions of particular government officials. Public health officials received their quarantine authority under specific statutes and regulations, and in order for their actions to be valid they had to follow those enactments.

The validity of a detention, however, was rarely contested. Instead, the issue of official authorization usually arose in an action for damages to property caused by a quarantine.

. . . .

Courts sometimes upheld quarantine orders even when the individuals could not be proven contagious, stating that health officials need not wait until a carrier has made someone ill. And yet, some courts set limits, however weak, on the discretion of health officers. These limits appear in the case of *Kirk v. Wyman*. In *Kirk*, the health officers determined that Miss Kirk, a former missionary, had contagious leprosy and ordered her either to leave the city or be quarantined in a pesthouse which had previously been used only to incarcerate blacks with smallpox. [83 S.C. 372, 65 S.E. 387 (1909)] The court noted that state quarantine statutes were not violative of constitutional rights because:

> [n]either the right to liberty nor the right of property extends to the use of liberty or property to the injury of others. The maxim *Sic utere tuo ut alienum non laedas* applies to the person as well as to the property of the citizen. The individual has no more right of the freedom of spreading disease by carrying contagion on his person, than he has to produce disease by maintaining his property in a noisome condition.

Nevertheless, in a discussion of the constitutional principles governing state and municipal health regulation, the court stated that health officials cannot be given arbitrary power. According to the court, health officials must ensure that "the means used and the extent of the interference were reasonably necessary for the accomplishment of the purpose to be attained." Reviewing the facts under that standard, the court concluded that the board had acted improperly in ordering that Miss Kirk be sent to a pesthouse since she had been safely quarantined in her home and had not made any attempt to violate the quarantine . . .

Although the court in *Kirk* granted broad deference to the health officials, it interceded, perhaps in part because of its sympathy for Miss Kirk, and ordered the officials to adopt a less restrictive alternative by isolating Miss Kirk in a cottage to be built for her outside the city. As the twentieth century progressed, courts became even more willing to scrutinize the decisions of health officers. Ironically, this heightened form of judicial review came as health officials increasingly used their quarantine power against prostitutes and venereal disease.

* * *

Around the time of World War I, health officials began to use quarantine powers against prostitutes on the presumption that they had venereal disease. . . . Until then, quarantine had been used primarily against infectious diseases to which the entire community felt vulnerable . . . [and] was enforced by health officials. But when the power to quarantine was turned against prostitutes, as part of the effort to control venereal disease, a great stigma attached to being quarantined. In addition, it became a complement to police work, a way of holding prostitutes longer than many criminal sentences would allow.

This new association between quarantine and the criminal law led to more petitions for *habeas corpus* and, ultimately, forced courts to recognize that quarantine was not always in the best interest of the individual. The need for judicial review of the facts supporting quarantine, as well as the authority under which it was implemented, became clear. The courts continued to affirm the broad power of health officials to quarantine, but began to demand that health officials base their actions on some reasonable suspicion that the individual was infected.

. . . .

The application of quarantine to prostitutes illustrates how quarantine can be used to harass, isolate and exclude socially disfavored groups.

. . . .

The courts have seldom explicitly addressed the discriminatory potential of quarantine. At the turn of the century, however, at least one federal court did so. In *Wong Wai v. Williamson* [103 F. 1 (C.C.N.D. Cal. 1900)], the court invalidated a quarantine ordinance under the equal protection clause of the fourteenth amendment. The plaintiff was a Chinese resident of San Francisco who challenged a city ordinance that required all Chinese residents of the city to be innoculated against bubonic plague prior to leaving the city. The innoculation, which could cause death, was justified by the city on the grounds that there was plague in the city and Asians as a race were highly susceptible to the disease. The court, however, noted that the regulation discriminated against Asians and could not be justified since the evidence did not support the city's claims. Moreover, the ordinance could not accomplish its stated purpose because the inoculation was only effective if given prior to exposure. The inoculation, in this case, was only administered to Chinese or Asian individuals leaving the city and, therefore, could not possibly stop the spread of disease. The court struck down the regulation, reminding the city that even the police power is subordinate to the Constitution.

. . . .

\* \* \*

# History of Quarantine
(taken from) A History of Quarantine
www.pbs.org/wgbh/nova/typhoid/quarantine.html
(last visited January 2007)

\* \* \*

583    The Council of Lyons restricts lepers from freely associating with healthy persons.

600s    China detains plague-stricken arrivals in Chinese ports.

1179    Third Lateran Council decrees separation from society.

1200    Europe has some 19,000 leprosaria, or houses for leper patients.

1300s  A number of European and Asian countries begin enforcing quarantines of infected regions by encircling them with armed guards.

1348    Venice establishes the world's first institutionalized system of quarantine, giving a council of three the power to detain ships, cargoes, and individuals in the Venetian lagoon for up to 40 days. The act comes in the midst of the Black Death, a plague epidemic that eventually takes the lives of 14 to 15 million people across Europe.

1403    Venice establishes the world's first known maritime quarantine station on an island in the Venetian lagoon.

1629    Sanitary legislation drawn up in Venice requires health officers to visit houses during plague epidemics and isolate those infected in pest-houses situated away from populated areas.

1663    With plague ravaging parts of continental Europe, the English monarchy issues royal decrees calling for the establishment of permanent quarantines.

1700s  All major towns and cities along the eastern seaboard of the United States have now passed quarantine laws.

1701    A Massachusetts statute stipulates that all individuals suffering from plague, smallpox, and other contagious diseases must be isolated in separate houses.

1712    A plague epidemic around the Baltic Sea leads England to pass the Quarantine Act. During a mandatory 40-day quarantine for arriving ships, goods cannot be removed and serious breaches of the act can result in the death penalty.

1738    With smallpox and yellow fever threatening to strike New York, the City Council sets up a quarantine anchorage off Bedloe's Island (home of the Statue of Liberty today).

1832    After about 30,000 people in Britain alone die in a cholera epidemic in 1831-1832, New York mandates in June 1832 that no ship can approach within 300 yards of any dock if its captain suspects or knows the ship has cholera aboard

1850-   Following horrific epidemics of plague and cholera that spread through
1851    Europe from Egypt and Turkey towards the middle of the 19th century, the first international sanitary conference is held in Paris, with an eye to making quarantine an international cooperative effort. . . .

1863    New York State's new Quarantine Act calls for a quarantine office run by a health officer who has the power to detain any ship entering the port of New York for as long as he deems necessary.

1879    Amid concern about yellow fever, the U.S. Congress establishes the National Board of Health, in part to assume responsibility for quarantine in cases where states' actions had proven ineffective.

1890s   As the era of bacteriology arrives, with major diseases like typhoid and cholera determined to arise from germs, the length and nature of quarantine evolves, now often based on the life cycles of specific microbes.

1892    When an Asiatic cholera epidemic reaches the U.S. in the fall, President Benjamin Harrison has his surgeon general issue an order holding that "no vessel from any foreign port carrying immigrants shall be admitted to enter any port of the United States until such vessel shall have undergone quarantine detention of twenty days. . . .

1893    The U.S. Congress passes the National Quarantine Act. The act creates a national system of quarantine while still permitting state-run quarantines. . . .

1894    Epidemics of plague in China, Hong Kong, and Taiwan, as well as in India two years later, fly in the face of arguments promulgated by most European scientists of the day that the widespread scourges that ransacked Europe in the middle ages are history.

1900    [A] Chinese [lumberyard] proprietor dies of bubonic plague in the Chinese quarter of San Francisco. Authorities immediately rope off the 15-block neighborhood, quarantining roughly 25,000 Chinese.

1902    The Pan American Sanitary Bureau is established. It is the first of a series of international health organizations formed in the 20th century.

1903    In an attempt to isolate tuberculosis patients, the New York City Department of Health opens a quarantine facility at Riverside Hospital on North Brother Island, an islet in the East River. Mary Mallon, aka

"Typhoid Mary," begins what becomes a total of 26 years of quarantine here in 1907. . . .

1916   When an epidemic of polio strikes New York residents, authorities begin forcibly separating children from their parents and placing them in quarantine.

1917-  During World War I, American authorities incarcerate more than
1919   30,000 prostitutes in an effort to curb the spread of venereal disease.

1944   The Public Health Service Act is codified, clearly establishing the quarantine authority of the federal government, which has controlled all U.S. quarantine stations since 1921.

1945   Baltimore adopts an ordinance giving health authorities the power to isolate at the city's hospitals those patients with syphilis or gonorrhea who refuse penicillin treatment

1949   To help stem the spread of tuberculosis, Seattle creates a locked ward for TB sufferers who deny treatment.

1967   The U.S. Department of Health, Education, and Welfare transfers responsibility for quarantine to what is now the Centers for Disease Control and Prevention (CDC).

1986   Treating the first cases of HIV/AIDS in the country as a public health emergency, Cuba begins compulsory, indefinite quarantine for citizens testing positive for HIV.

1990s  To help control multi-drug-resistant tuberculosis, New York City detains more than 200 people who refuse voluntary treatment, confining most of them to the secure ward of a hospital for about six months.

2003   An outbreak of severe acute respiratory syndrome, or SARS, in Asia and Canada occurs in the spring. Officials credit the use of both isolation (for those sick with SARS) and quarantine (for those exposed to the sick) with forestalling an even more severe epidemic. In April, President George W. Bush adds SARS to the list of quarantinable diseases.

## NOTES AND QUESTIONS

**1.** *St. Marks Baths* is an example of public health regulating places rather than people. Although there were many calls at the beginning of the HIV/AIDS epidemic to respond with mandatory screening followed by quarantine, this strategy was only employed in Cuba. Why wasn't quarantine applied in the U.S. (and in other countries) for HIV/AIDS? Is this an example of so-called "AIDS exceptionalism" or a reflection of the disease process itself?

There are, of course, many reasons for not using quarantine with HIV/AIDS, and you should be able to list them. Nonetheless, the Cuban strategy has its defenders, and HIV/AIDS has grown to be an uncontrolled pandemic. The U.S. did, however, use quarantine on Guantanamo in 1992 and 1993 to confine Haitian immigrants who were HIV positive. This confinement facility was effectively shut down by Judge Sterling Johnson as being a violation of consti-tutional, statutory and regulatory rights. *Haitian Centers Council v. Sale*, 817 F. Supp. 336 (1993). *See* George J. Annas, *Detention of HIV-Positive Haitians at Guantanamo: Human Rights and Medical Care*, 329 NEW ENG. J. MED. 589 (1993); and Ron Bayer, *Controlling AIDS in Cuba: The Logic of Quarantine*, 320 NEW ENG. J. MED. 1022 (1989). A related early program was an attempt to screen all international travelers, as well as immigrants, for HIV. *See* Larry Gostin et al., *Screening Immigrants and International Travelers for the Human Immunodeficiency Virus*, 322 NEW ENG. J. MED. 1743 (1990). Current strategies rely as much or more on treatment than prevention, although they work synergistically. See, *e.g.*, materials in Chapter Eight.

**2.** HIV/AIDS and TB have been called co-diseases, since when HIV attacks a person's immune system it permits latent TB to become active, and fatal without treatment. There is also current concern that new strains of drug-resistant TB, termed XDR for "extremely drug resistant" may be developing. This new form of TB is resistant to both the first and second line of anti-TB drugs, including isoniazid, rifampin, ethambutol, streptomycin, kanamycin, and ciprofloxacin. At the Toronto AIDS conference in 2006 an early report from South Africa described a new MDR TB strain that had killed 52 of 53 patients in a rural hospital. Lawrence K. Altman, *Doctors Warn of Powerful and Resistant Tuberculosis Strain*, NEW YORK TIMES, August 18, 2006 at A4. Although it might seem like quarantine was a reasonable response, in fact the individuals with this form of TB are so sick they are unable to leave the hos-pital, and isolation is both reasonable and unlikely to be rejected by the patient.

**3.** Compare the use of the word "quarantine" in Professor Parmet's article with the definitions presented at the beginning of this chapter. It seems likely that Professor Parmet is using the word in a manner that, at times, is closer to our understanding of the term "compulsory isolation."

**4.** As the Parmet article relates, in *Wong Wai* (1900) a federal court rebuked the city of San Francisco for discriminatory treatment of Chinese people in its efforts to control bubonic plague. Soon thereafter, the city authorized its board of health to adopt quarantines that the board might adjudge "necessary to pre-vent the spreading of contagious or infectious diseases." Finding that nine deaths from plague had occurred in a particular 12-block area of the city that housed between 10–15,000 people, the board of health promptly ordered that area quarantined. Jew Ho, a grocer living there, filed another suit in federal court, alleging, *inter alia*, that within the quarantine area the authorities failed to segregate infected persons and households from those unafflicted, thereby increasing risks to the latter; that the area itself was unreasonably large, thereby increasing rather than reducing the likelihood that any disease would spread (both within and beyond the quarantine limits); and that some areas within the quarantine area had actually been plague-free for some time. *Jew Ho v. Williamson*, 103 F.10 (C.C.N.D. Cal. 1900).

The same federal judge who decided *Wong Wai* determined that the quaran-tine was in fact drawn and applied as Jew Ho alleged, and ruled that it was unconstitutional on two grounds. First, it was "not a reasonable regulation to accomplish the purposes sought," but rather was "unreasonable, unjust, and oppressive, and therefore contrary to the laws limiting . . . [state and local] police powers. . . ." To understand the court's reasoning here, recall first (from *Jacobson,* decided several years later but on principles well-established by 1900) that legislation, or government action undertaken pursuant thereto, requires at least a "rational fit" between ends and means.

Recall, too, that this level of judicial review is not very demanding; courts applying it usually *defer* to, and do not aggressively re-scrutinize, the judgments already made about such matters by legislatures and boards of health. Finally, be aware that the court found no fault with either the authorities' "declared purpose" of controlling the spread of bubonic plague (the "ends") or with the proper use of quarantine under state police powers (one of the generally-permissible "means"). Yet — even under this familiar, apparently-minimal "rationality" scrutiny — the court found *this* quarantine's enforcement utterly indefensible. Can you determine why? Do you agree?

The second basis for the court's decision to strike down enforcement of the quarantine was that it violated equal protection because it discriminated against the Chinese. Jew Ho had alleged, and the court found, that despite its benign and neutral wording, the quarantine was enforced *only* against Chinese persons and not those of other races. Indeed it appears that San Francisco did not contest this claim, and defended its discriminatory application of the quarantine on the ground "that the Chinese may communicate the disease from one to the other." (This may roughly translate to: "Plague is not a problem as long as it remains in Chinatown"). In an understatement of vast proportion, the court said simply that this "is not [a] sufficient" basis for sustaining the law: the "purpose to enforce [the law] 'with an evil eye and an unequal hand'" was a classic, straightforward violation of equal protection.

Do you think the court's decision on the first ground was at all influenced by its findings and conclusions as to the second?

## D.  CASE STUDY: SARS

### CDC, FACT SHEET: BASIC INFORMATION ABOUT SARS
(Jan. 2004)
www.cdc.gov/ncidod/sars/pdf/factsheet
(last visited August 2006)

* * *

Severe acute respiratory syndrome (SARS) is a viral respiratory illness caused by a coronavirus, called SARS-associated coronavirus (SARS-CoV). SARS was first reported in Asia in February 2003. Over the next few months, the illness spread to more than two dozen countries in North America, South America, Europe, and Asia before the SARS global outbreak of 2003 was contained.

According to the World Health Organization (WHO), a total of 8098 people worldwide became sick with SARS during the 2003 outbreak. Of these, 774 died. In the United States, only eight people had laboratory evidence of SARS-

CoV infection. All of these people had traveled to other parts of the world with SARS. SARS did not spread more widely in the community in the United States.

In general, SARS begins with a high fever (temperature greater than 100.4°F.) Other symptoms may include headache, an overall feeling of discomfort and body aches. Some people also have mild respiratory symptoms at the outset. About 10 percent to 20 percent of patients have diarrhea. After 2 to 7 days, SARS patients may develop a dry cough. Most patients develop pneumonia.

The main way that SARS seems to spread is by close person-to-person contact. The virus that causes SARS is thought to be transmitted most readily by respiratory droplets (droplet spread) produced when an infected person coughs or sneezes. Droplet spread can happen when droplets from the cough or sneeze of an infected person are propelled a short distance (generally up to 3 feet) through the air and deposited on the mucous membranes of the mouth, nose or eyes of persons who are nearby. The virus also can spread when a person touches a surface or object contaminated with infectious droplets and then touches his or her mouth, nose or eye(s). In addition, it is possible that the SARS virus might spread more broadly through the air (airborne spread) or by other ways that are not now known.

In the context of SARS, close contact means having cared for or lived with someone with SARS or having direct contact with respiratory secretions or body fluids of a patient with SARS. Examples of close contact include kissing or hugging, sharing eating or drinking utensils, talking to someone within three feet, and touching someone directly. Close contact does not include activities like walking by a person or briefly sitting across a waiting room or office.

CDC worked closely with WHO and other partners in a global effort to address the SARS outbreak of 2003. For its part, CDC took the following actions:

— Activated its Emergency Operations Center to provide round-the-clock coordination and response.

— Committed more than 800 medical experts and support staff to work on the SARS response.

— Deployed medical officers, epidemiologists, and other specialists to assist with on-site investigations around the world.

— Provided assistance to state and local health departments in investigating possible cases of SARS in the United States.

— Conducted extensive laboratory testing of clinical specimens from SARS patients to identify the cause of the disease.

— Initiated a system for distributing health alert notices to travelers who may have been exposed to cases of SARS.

MARK A. ROTHSTEIN ET AL., QUARANTINE AND ISOLATION:
LESSONS LEARNED FROM SARS, A REPORT TO THE
CENTERS FOR DISEASE CONTROL AND PREVENTION
44–59, 23–26 (2003)
*available at* www.louisville.edu/bioethics/
cdc-collaborating-center/SARS.pdf
(last visited January 2007)

\* \* \*

Canada was among the countries hardest hit by SARS. Only the People's Republic of China, Hong Kong, and Taiwan had more probable SARS cases. Toronto was the Canadian city most affected [by] the outbreak. The first (index) SARS case in Toronto was a 78-year-old woman, Mrs. K, who returned home to Toronto on February 23, 2003 from a trip to Hong Kong to visit relatives. Mrs. K, who was never hospitalized, died on March 5 after the onset of an illness later determined to be SARS. Her son, Mr. T, became ill on February 27, was admitted to Scarborough Hospital (Grace Division) on March 7, and died on March 13. Transmission of SARS traceable to Mrs. K is thought to have included 224 other persons in Toronto alone. In all of Canada, there were 438 SARS cases, including 251 probable (1 active) and 187 suspect (0 active) cases. All of the probable cases were reported in two provinces, Ontario, which includes Toronto, and British Columbia. Suspect cases were reported in four other provinces (Alberta, New Brunswick, Prince Edward Island, and Saskatchewan).

. . . .

. . . Opinions differ about the capability of the Canadian government to respond to SARS or other SARS-like outbreaks. As one commentator stated, "I have a concern about whether or not in the long run our public health-care system will be able to meet the demands placed by new illnesses like SARS. . . . [N]o one is directly accountable or responsible for public health." Concerns like this may be related, in part, to the decentralized nature of Canadian public health governance, with authority formally delegated to a multitude of federal, provincial, and local entities.

[The authors then describe the political and legal structure of Canada. See pp. 44–53 of the original document.]

On June 12, 2003, SARS was added to the Quarantine Act's schedule of infectious and contagious diseases, together with an established incubation period, thereby bringing SARS cases within the ambit of federal public health authority. [T]he Act provides the Minister of Health with a multitude of powers related to the control of infectious disease. One important means of exercising public health authority in the wake of the SARS outbreak was to develop, coordinate, and provide specific guidance for both public and private entities, including public health workers and health professionals, in identifying and managing SARS cases and related health matters within their jurisdictions. At the federal level, the Department of Health has developed a large number of guidance documents intended to assist both public and private entities to respond to specific SARS-related health matters. These include the following: definition of persons under SARS investigation; definition of a SARS case; interim guidelines for public health authorities in the management of probable and suspect SARS cases; definitions of geo-linked persons for hospital surveillance for SARS; public health protocol for persons meeting the "geo-linked person" definition; recommended laboratory testing for probable SARS cases and SARS contact cases; advisory for laboratory biosafety; guidelines for health care providers in the identification, diagnosis, and treatment of adults with SARS; guidelines for the use of respirators (masks) among health care workers; and recommendations and guidelines for public health officials for managing probable or suspect SARS cases among air travelers.

. . .

In contrast to other provincial and local governments — with the exception of British Columbia and to a lesser extent Alberta — only Ontario and the municipality of Toronto have had to invoke their public health authority in a significant and large-scale manner to respond to the SARS outbreak within their jurisdictions. . . .

On March 25, 2003, in the face of a rising number of SARS cases in the Toronto area, the Ontario government took the critical step of designating SARS as a reportable, communicable, and virulent disease under the province's Health Protection and Promotion Act, which authorized public health authorities to issue orders to detain and isolate persons for purposes of preventing SARS transmission. Eventually, about 30,000 persons in Toronto were quarantined. That number is similar to the number of persons who were quarantined due to the SARS outbreak in Beijing, China, but for the latter the number of probable SARS cases (2500) was ten times larger than Toronto's (about 250).

The fast use of isolation in Toronto occurred early in the SARS outbreak, when the physician treating the index case's son, Mr. T, had Mr. T placed in hospital isolation for suspected tuberculosis (at no time before Mr. T's death was his SARS established) and requested that other family members isolate themselves at home as they, too, might be at risk for tuberculosis infection. Unfortunately, these control measures occurred too late to contain the spread of SARS in Toronto. Mr. T, who had entered Scarborough Hospital through the emergency department, was left in the emergency department for 18–20 hours despite a physician's hospital admission order, and only later admitted to the hospital's Intensive Care Unit (ICU). When he was finally examined by a physician, a tuberculosis isolation order was issued and Toronto Public Health was notified as a routine matter of a possible tuberculosis case. During Mr. T's long wait in the Scarborough Hospital emergency department for admission to the ICU and his short time in the ICU before tuberculosis was suspected, other patients and staff were exposed to SARS. At the time there was no indication that these individuals were at risk of contracting or spreading any communicable disease, let alone SARS.

When tuberculosis was ruled out and public health officials and physicians began to understand the implications of Mr. T's case, steps were taken to remove other members of Mrs. K's family, some of whom were reporting illness, to negative pressure isolation rooms in other area hospitals. These steps undoubtedly limited the spread of SARS. Combining the information from the WHO's international health alert for atypical pneumonia with reports of the

Scarborough Hospital cases, both Toronto Public Health and provincial public health authorities activated their emergency response plans. A "Code Orange" (which required all area hospitals to go into emergency mode) was issued, under which area hospitals were required to suspend non-essential services, limit visitors, issue protective equipment for staff, and establish special isolation units for "potential SARS patients." Asymptomatic contacts of SARS patients were not isolated within health facilities, but were asked to adhere to a 10-day home quarantine.

The risk of acquiring SARS was greatest for persons (staff, patients, and visitors) within rather than outside of health care facilities, including doctors' offices; health care workers accounted for over 40% of all SARS patients in Toronto. Tragically, the early SARS patients who were seen in health care facilities were simply not identified in time to implement more rigorous infection control procedures. Moreover, it is not clear that health care workers were always provided with uniform or consistent advice or guidelines regarding the quarantine or isolation of persons with or suspected of having SARS, that adequate protective equipment was provided to health care workers within these hospital or clinic settings, or that health care administrators or workers were diligent about adhering to infection control precautions or procedures. Concerns about a lack of uniform guidance for quarantine were expressed by an *ad hoc* Scientific Advisory Committee of volunteer experts, which found that "different public health units seemed to have different thresholds for the use of quarantine."

Directives issued by Ontario health authorities instructed hospitals to isolate all patients with fever and respiratory symptoms in the hospital or in the hospital emergency department until SARS had been ruled out. Most hospitals took special precautions for inpatients with respiratory symptoms suggestive of infectious diseases. In Phase I of the Toronto SARS outbreak (March 13–25, 2003), over 20 Toronto area hospitals admitted and cared for SARS patients. No single facility was designated as a "SARS hospital," because both provincial and Toronto area officials feared that such a step would overwhelm the facility so designated. For this reason, capacity for SARS clinical management, including isolation of SARS patients and adequate infection control measures, was built into multiple facilities throughout the Greater Toronto area. Two hospitals (Sunnybrook and Woman's) in the Greater Toronto area appeared to carry the largest volume of SARS patients during Phase I. Unfortunately, many of these two hospitals' physicians with relevant expertise or experience in SARS clinical management were themselves ill or in quarantine. Despite the hospitals' requests for staff support, other Toronto area hospitals were either unable or unwilling to provide assistance. Needed support was obtained only after provincial authorities retained a private placement agency to help with recruitment of health care workers.

In Phase II of the Toronto SARS outbreak (May 23–June 30, 2003), four hospitals (later termed the SARS Alliance) were designated as SARS facilities. The "Code Orange" described above for Toronto area hospitals was later extended to all Ontario hospitals, meaning they, too, were required to suspend non-essential services, limit visitors, create isolation units for SARS patients, and issue protective equipment (gowns, masks, and goggles) for exposed staff.

Some concern was expressed over whether the Code Orange was justified or overly broad.

No persons in transit into or out of Canada were actually quarantined or isolated, although clearly the federal government has the authority to take such measures in appropriate cases. In 2002, Health Canada transferred its airport quarantine responsibilities to the Canada Customs and Revenue Agency, but at the time of the SARS outbreak, neither Health Canada nor the Customs and Revenue Agency appeared prepared to discharge their quarantine responsibilities under the federal Quarantine Act Regulations, which soon after the SARS outbreak in Canada had been amended to include SARS. For ships, particularly cruise ships, Health Canada's protocol for handling SARS cases was not released until mid-June, after the SARS outbreak had begun to fade.

SARS screening for airline passengers took place at Canadian airports, but this screening relied primarily upon information cards that were distributed to and completed by both incoming and outbound passengers. In-person screening questions and secondary assessments were conducted only as needed. Thermal scanners were used in a pilot project at the Toronto and Vancouver (British Columbia) airports. As of August 27, 2003, 6.5 million screening transactions had taken place at Canadian airports, with about 9100 passengers referred for further SARS assessment by screening nurses or quarantine officers. None of the passengers who underwent further assessment was found to meet the criteria for a probable or suspect SARS case. The pilot thermal scanner screened 2.4 million passengers, with 832 referred for further assessments, and none met the criteria for a probable or suspect SARS case.

In Toronto, home and workplace quarantines were often imposed for what were definitive "contact" cases, meaning cases in which persons were known to have been in close physical proximity to a probable SARS case with inadequate or no protection from possible exposure. Contact cases included family and household members of SARS patients, hospital visitors and other non-SARS patients within hospitals who may have been exposed to SARS patients, health care staff who provided treatment to SARS patients without adequate protective equipment, and persons at workplaces who may have been exposed to co-workers with SARS. Provided they were timely identified and contacted, these persons were urged to remain at home for a 10-day period, with monitoring, usually by telephone, by a local public health worker.

It should be noted that once the provincial emergency was declared by the Ontario Prime Minister's office, provincial authorities assumed the lead for delivery of all main SARS messages to the public. However, this public information function was often delegated by provincial authorities to the Toronto municipal government. One concern among some commentators was that there were too many "talking heads," including government officials, whose opinions on the SARS outbreak appeared to diverge. According to these critics, there often appeared to be no coherent official or governmental communications strategy aimed at "dispelling the sense of deepening crisis" posed by the SARS outbreak. Interestingly, one of the most apt characterizations of the capacity of the federal and provincial governments to work collectively in their response to the SARS outbreak was provided by the Canadian federal government: "Only weak mechanisms exist in public health for collaborative decision making or systematic data sharing across governments. Furthermore, governments have not adequately sorted out their roles and responsibilities during a national health crisis. The SARS outbreak has highlighted many areas where inter jurisdictional collaboration is suboptimal; so far from being seamless, the public health system showed a number of serious gaps."

Given the acknowledged deficiencies in cross jurisdictional coordination in the response to the SARS outbreak, it is quite likely that the coordination with the international community and the U.S. with respect to the SARS outbreak could likewise be considered suboptimal. As the report further noted, it "is unlikely that most other provinces [aside from Ontario] are in a better position, and the federal capacity to support one or more provinces facing simultaneous health crises is limited.

The federal, provincial, and local governments used a variety of means to convey up-to-date information regarding the SARS outbreak to the public, as well as to health professionals. Features of the public health education and communication measures taken by the government generally and by public health authorities specifically included regular updates to their own websites. Additionally, Toronto Public Health established a SARS Hotline. Hotline staff, primarily public health nurses, provided callers with health information and counseling and case and contact identification, and the recognition and follow-up of emerging issues in SARS-affected institutions and communities. At the height of the outbreak the Hotline had 46 staff on the day shift and 34 staff on the evening shift, including individuals with special language skills. The Hotline received over 300,000 calls between March 15 and June 24, 2003, with a peak of 47,567 calls in a single day.

. . .

Both federal (the Quarantine Act) and provincial laws (*e.g.*, Ontario's Health Protection and Promotion Act, British Columbia's Health Act) regarding quarantine and/or isolation authorize — and may even require — law enforcement agencies to assist public health authorities to effect the quarantine and/or isolation of persons subject to quarantine orders. During the SARS outbreak in Toronto, law enforcement personnel were used to enforce the quarantine of patients with SARS at area hospitals, serve orders as needed, and conduct "spot checks" on persons who were quarantined. On at least one occasion, law enforcement personnel were also used to investigate and try to apprehend and charge a person who broke quarantine and subsequently infected a co-worker, but the person died from the illness. Almost all persons who were asked to submit to quarantine did so voluntarily. In only 27 cases was a written order mandating quarantine issued under Ontario's Health Protection and Promotion Act.

Certain actions taken by the federal and provincial governments may have had the effect of increasing public acceptance of SARS-control measures. For example, the federal government has amended its employment insurance regulations under the Employment Insurance Act to remove the waiting period for sickness benefits for certain persons placed under SARS quarantine, as well as to remove the requirement that certain persons under SARS quarantine obtain a medical certificate as a condition of receiving sickness benefits.

The federal government also provided special employment insurance coverage for health care workers who were unable to work because of SARS and who were not otherwise eligible for benefits under the government's Employment Insurance Act, as well as tax and mortgage payment relief to persons who were facing difficulties making tax or mortgage payments because of SARS. The Ontario government enacted the SARS Assistance and Recovery Strategy Act, which provides certain qualified persons with unpaid leave in the event the person is unable to work due to a SARS-related event, such as being under individual medical investigation or having to provide care for or assistance to a person due to a SARS-related matter.

The use of quarantine and isolation measures in Toronto cannot be characterized as a uniform, coordinated (and perhaps optimal) response to the SARS outbreak, which is not surprising given the highly decentralized way in which public health functions in Canada are organized. The recently released federal Canadian government report mentioned earlier, *Learning from SARS: Renewal of Public Health Canada*, appears to confirm this, stating, "[t]he SARS experience illustrated that Canada is not adequately prepared to deal with a true pandemic." The report suggests comprehensive, large scale reorganization of public health systems within Canada, including the prospect of establishing a national, federal public health agency with the requisite authority to respond to disease outbreaks and emergencies similar to SARS, and with appropriate linkages to other government departments and agencies engaged in public health activities. However, concerning public health activities at the local level, it is argued by officials of Toronto Public Health that at least with respect to Toronto, the "isolation of people who were symptomatic with SARS (i.e., "cases") served to protect the public from infection by separating those who were ill from those who were well." The same might be said of the quarantine of persons who were not symptomatic with SARS but who may have been at increased risk of acquiring or transmitting SARS.

* * *

[In other countries affected by] the SARS outbreak, different types of quarantine and isolation measures were used by public health authorities to control SARS transmission. Isolation was used for persons who posed the greatest risk of transmission, persons who met the criteria used by public health officials for probable SARS cases. Almost all probable SARS cases were isolated in health facilities, generally inpatient acute care hospitals, in which these individuals were actually diagnosed. Often, persons in quarantine, such as persons who met the criteria used by public health officials as suspect SARS cases (*e.g.*, persons who may have been in recent contact with a probable SARS case and are experiencing fever and a cough or breathing difficulty), were subsequently placed in isolation when their symptoms met the criteria for probable SARS cases. Unfortunately, many SARS cases were only diagnosed upon investigation of death or autopsy.

In contrast to isolation, quarantine methods varied greatly, often simply because a particular quarantine method appeared to be the most intuitive and timely response in light of how little was known about the actual risk of transmission. For example, the quarantine of definitive "contact" cases or persons who were known to have been in close physical proximity and who had inadequate or no protection from possible exposure to a probable SARS case or setting, such as household or family members, was perhaps the most intuitive, and in retrospect, rational measure, given what became known about the likely route of transmission (i.e., droplets). This was often referred to as home quarantine or "home isolation," in which the contact cases were urged to remain at home for a 10-day period, with follow-up, usually by telephone, by a local public health worker.

The quarantine of contact cases was also used for health care workers (*e.g.*, emergency medical services or ambulance personnel), under circumstances in which health care workers may have had "either an exposure to a SARS patient or a setting where SARS has been transmitted" while lacking adequate protection from such exposure. These quarantines were called "work quarantines." Health care workers could continue to work in the health facility where they were exposed as long as they remained well. Persons who were subject to work quarantine were required to follow home quarantine rules during the time they were not at work. Persons who were not health care workers but who may have been exposed within a health care facility were also subject to quarantine. . . . Similar quarantines were imposed on other worksites where persons who, although not in the position of providing health care services, were nonetheless known to have been in proximity to and had inadequate or no protection from possible exposure to a probable SARS case. Persons were required to remain in quarantine for the 10-day period, and in some cases, their workplaces were closed for business.

In situations where persons' proximity or possible exposure to probable or suspect SARS cases was less certain, less coercive measures were used. These quarantine methods included "snow days," the closure of schools, child care facilities, or other buildings or locations at which large numbers of people usually gathered (*e.g.*, markets, public services, homeless shelters), and the cancellation or postponement of public events. At the other extreme, highly restrictive measures were used in China, including the cordoning off of certain neighborhoods and villages and restrictions on travel, including the closure of public transit.

While legal authority may have existed or was thought to exist for these quarantine methods, the use of so many different quarantine measures, often without apparent regard to the particularized risk for which control was sought, may have served to undermine public credibility. It is clear that a more considered, careful, and evidence-based approach to quarantine and isolation is needed.

Regardless of the wisdom of quarantine and isolation in particular circumstances, these measures are only part of the public health response to an epidemic. Typically the ordering of quarantine for SARS triggered a whole system of public health measures. Contact tracing was an essential part of the strategy, and this required a staff of trained epidemiologists, public health nurses, and other professionals. Quarantine orders had to be served, and public health officers and law enforcement personnel were used in the countries we studied. Some individuals did not want to stay at home during quarantine because they were afraid of infecting family members. In Singapore, individuals under quarantine had a choice of staying at home or at a designated center (a resort taken over by the government). Taiwan used a public housing center that had not yet opened, military facilities, and a home for the elderly as quarantine facilities. In Hong Kong, "holiday camps" were used for homeless people and those who did not want home confinement. On the other hand, some people did not want to leave their homes because there would be nobody to care for their pets. Every country developed a system for providing meals and other social services.

The vast majority of people under quarantine in all of the countries obeyed requests to stay at home without requiring a court order. Some individuals, however, attempted to escape their confinement, and a variety of means were needed to ensure compliance. For example, in Singapore, three telephone calls were made per day to the home of each individual in quarantine to confirm that the individual was there. People who were known to work at night were called at night. Electronic cameras were used to verify that people were at home, and people in quarantine were required to take their temperature on camera. Anyone initially violating quarantine had an electronic tag put on his or her leg (there were 26 cases). In all of the countries, police officers were charged with locating and confining individuals who violated quarantine.

. . .

Isolation is relatively straightforward scientifically, politically, and socially. It seems to make sense to confine individuals who are ill with a communicable disease and to limit their contacts. Neither the affected individuals nor potential contacts of the person are likely to object to such measures. Similarly, it will not be complicated to decide whom to isolate, where to do so, or for how long. Quarantine, however, is very complicated, and it raises a series of difficult questions of public health, public health law, and public policy.

At the outset, it should be clear that the purpose of quarantine is not to stop immediately all transmission of infection. Not only is this likely to be nearly impossible, but the severity of the measures needed would be extremely unpopular and therefore the necessary level of compliance would be difficult to achieve. The purpose of quarantine is to reduce the incidence of new cases. . . .

The contours of quarantine will vary depending on a variety of factors, including the mode of transmission (*e.g.*, close contact, airborne), the likelihood of transmission per contact event, the length of communicability, and the recovery rate. In the case of SARS, as a new infection, quarantine policy needed to be designed and implemented in the absence of definitive scientific information about the infection rate or the course of the illness.

Although scientific considerations will inform the policy decisions surrounding quarantine, they should not necessarily dictate the results. For example, as the definition of "close contact" is broadened, more people will be quarantined. As the criteria for quarantine are broadened, the absolute number of infected (pre-symptomatic) people in quarantine will increase, but the percentage of infected people in quarantine will decline. This is analogous to a screening test with a high degree of sensitivity and a low degree of specificity generating numerous false positives.

Putting large numbers of people in quarantine may be politically unpopular. It also strains the resources of health care, public health, social service, and law enforcement agencies and may seriously damage the local and national economy. The length of the quarantine period, both on an individual and jurisdictional basis, also is more than a narrow issue of infection control. As the time for quarantine is increased, the rate of compliance will decline. Furthermore, a long period of quarantine may lead to substantial morbidity and mortality from the inability to provide health care services for other conditions.

There seems to be general public support for quarantine if it is applied fairly and reasonably. A complicating factor, however, is that it is often impossible to tell when the need for quarantine will end. Thus, in Toronto, the second wave of quarantine was the most difficult for a variety of psychological and social reasons.

A lack of alternatives made the use of quarantine and isolation an important element of controlling SARS in Canada, China, Hong Kong, Singapore, Taiwan, and Vietnam. These jurisdictions had a high rate of compliance with quarantine and isolation. It is not clear whether the United States would have the same compliance rate in a comparable epidemic. Many of the Asian countries are well known for their communitarian culture, and Canada is also known for its commitment to social solidarity as evidenced by its health care system. By contrast, the United States is a heterogeneous society with a strong tradition of individualism and skepticism about government.

* * *

## George J. Annas, *The Statue of Security: Post-9/11 Epidemics*
### 38 J. HEALTH L. 319, 331–42 (2005)

* * *

The SARS epidemic was our first, and so far only, post-9/11 contagious disease epidemic, but it also returned us to late 19th century Ellis Island days in that its cause and mode of transmission were initially unknown, there is no diagnostic test for it, there is no vaccine, and there is no effective treatment. But SARS also appeared in a society equipped with instant global communication that made management of people through information much more important than management of people through police actions. With the internet information now spreads like a virus, but much faster.

It is probably still too early to reach firm conclusions about which containment methods were or were not the most effective in containing the disease. Nonetheless, since the epidemic has ended in all 30 countries in which suspected SARS cases were reported, and only a few countries used quarantine (detained individuals who showed no symptoms), it seems reasonable to conclude that quarantining "contacts" or even "close contacts" was unnecessarily harmful to those affected. It is not only liberty that is at stake in deciding about quarantine, but the effectiveness of public health itself in the 21st century. This is because to be effective in preventing disease spread from either a new epidemic or a bioterrorist attack, public health officials must also prevent the spread of fear and panic. Maintenance of public trust is essential to achieve this.

When any new contagious disease appears, public health officials must answer three related questions: should contacts be quarantined?, what test should be used to determine who qualifies as a "contact"?, and should quarantine be voluntary or mandatory? China has been rightly criticized for failing to promptly alert the international community to the existence of a possibly new and contagious virus. Had information about the initial outbreak been properly shared, SARS might never have spread beyond China. Nonetheless when, with the active intervention of the World Health Organization, the epidemic was publicly recognized, China reacted vigorously, even harshly, especially in Beijing and Hong Kong. Mass quarantines were initiated involving two universities, four hospitals, seven construction sites, and other facilities, like apartment complexes. Sixty percent of the approximately 30,000 people quarantined in mainland China were detained at centralized facilites, the remainder were permitted to stay at home. Those quarantined were "close contacts," defined as someone who has shared meals, utensils, place of residence, a hospital room, or a transportation vehicle with a probable SARS patient, or visited a SARS patient or been in contact with the secretions of a SARS patient anytime after 14 days before the SARS patient developed symptoms.

Based on the evidence available, it seems reasonable to conclude that these mass quarantines in China had little or no effect on the epidemic. Moreover, the imposition of quarantine led to panic that could have spread the disease if identification of contacts was necessary to contain SARS. When a rumor spread that Bejing itself might be placed under martial law, *China News Service* reported that 245,000 migrant workers from impoverished Henan province fled the city to return home. Even in Hong Kong's Amory Gardens, the site of the initial cluster of SARS cases in Hong Kong, when officials came to relocate residents to a quarantine facility they found no one at home in more than half of the complex's 264 apartments. People were able to evade the police even though the police were working closely with public health officials.

Canada had the only major outbreak of SARS outside of Asia, and it was limited to the Toronto area. Canada had about 440 probable or suspect SARS cases, resulting in 40 deaths, but many more lives were directly affected. Approximately 30,000 people were quarantined, although unlike China, almost all Canadians who were quarantined were confined to their own homes — and staying home, or "sheltering in place" seems to have become the new standard for isolating and protecting individuals in public health emergencies, at least in democracies.

Canadian officials were generally level-headed in their advice to the public, but seem to have overreacted on two occasions. In mid-April, 2003, before Easter, Ontario health officials published full-page newspaper ads asking anyone who had even one symptom of SARS (severe headache, severe fatigue, muscle aches and pains, fever of 38 Celsius or higher, dry cough and shortness of breath) to stay home for a few days. Ontario's health minister said, "This is a time when the needs of a community outweigh those of a single person." Again, in June, during the second wave of infections in Ontario, the health minister, responding to reports that some people were not completing their 10 day home quarantines, said "I don't know how people will like this, but we can chain them to a bed if that's what it takes." While the request may have arguably been reasonable, the threat was not. At a June 2003 WHO meeting on SARS, Health Canada's senior director general, Paul Gully, noted that intra-hospital transmission was the "most important amplifier of SARS infections" and wondered aloud about the utility of the widespread home quarantines during the Canadian epidemic. His reasoning was that very few of those quarantined wound up exhibiting symptoms of SARS.

There were few cases of SARS in the U.S. and no deaths. The Centers for Disease Control and Prevention (CDC) worked with the World Health Organization and other countries to identify the SARS virus, and issued guidelines and recommendations in press conferences and on its website. Perhaps the most important recommendations involved travel. In this cate-gory the CDC issued both travel alerts (which consist of a notification of an outbreak of a specific disease in a geographic area and suggests ways to reduce the risk of infection and what to do if you become ill), and travel advisories (which include the same information, but further recommend against nonessential travel because the risk of disease transmission is considered too high). No attempt was ever made to prohibit Americans from traveling any-where, although the federal government probably has the authority to do this for international travel (*e.g.*, through passport limitations) should the risk of disease become extreme. Nor do there seem to have been any attempts in the U.S. by public health officials to quarantine asymptomatic contacts of SARS patients.

The CDC also issued reasonable guidance to businesses with employees returning from areas affected with SARS, recommending that while in areas with SARS those "with fever or respiratory symptoms should not travel and should seek medical attention" and upon return asymptomatic travelers "should be vigilant for fever and respiratory symptoms over the 10 days after departure." Most important, the CDC noted that "those persons need not limit their activities and should not be excluded from work, meetings, or other pub-lic areas, unless fever or respiratory symptoms develop." In bold letters on its guidelines it underlined the point: "At this time, CDC is not recommending quarantine of persons returning from areas with SARS." The president did, nonetheless, add SARS to the outdated federal list of "quarantinable commu-nicable diseases" on April 4, 2003, and customs and immigration officials were given the authority to detain those entering the U.S. who were suspected of having SARS. This authority was not exercised.

Of course, the public can overreact on its own, and in some cases clearly did — as restaurants in Chinatowns in New York and Boston were virtually empty for a time. The worst offenders were not the uninformed public, how-ever, but academic institutions, some of which forbade their faculty and stu-dents to travel to areas that had SARS cases, or required them to spend ten days after they returned in self-imposed quarantine and obtain a physician's certificate that they did not have SARS before returning to campus. Academic institutions with similar policies included both Harvard and Boston

University, even though the Boston Public Health Commission had reasonably advised on April 9, 2003:

> At this point there is no evidence to suggest that a person without symptoms may infect others with SARS. In the absence of fever or respiratory symptoms, anyone who has traveled to high-risk areas or has been exposed to SARS patients may continue normal activities — isolation or quarantine is not recommended. Persons should not be excluded from school or work.

Anita Barry, director of communicable disease control at the Boston Public Health Commission had warned only four days earlier: "The biggest challenge for now with SARS is fear and rumor and panic." As a general matter, local public health officials acted very responsibly, even under extreme pressure. Although there were no quarantines in the U.S., there were cases in which isolation of symptomatic individuals was advised or mandated by local public health departments. In New York, 27 people were advised by the city health department to stay home for a period of ten days after their SARS fever had returned to normal. In addition, two individuals in New York City and one in Dallas were ordered to be isolated in hospitals because it was suspected they had SARS. The first of these was a young student on a tour around the world. He sought medical care in a New York City hospital and was diagnosed as a suspect case. He would have been quarantined at home, but had none, so he was ordered by the Department to remain in the hospital for ten days after his fever abated, and an unarmed security guard was posted at his door to enforce the order. He was offered an attorney to advise him about fighting the order, but refused. Ten days after the resolution of his fever he left town and has not been heard of since. The second case involved a person who was voluntarily in the hospital, but who became restless and wanted to leave before the ten days was up. He was ordered to stay, and put under guard as well.

The third case, from Dallas, also sought care in a hospital and was diagnosed as a suspect case. He gave a false address. The Dallas County Department of Health and Human Services sought and obtained a court order requiring him to remain in the hospital for ten days. At the hearing all in attendance (including the judge) "were provided with protective gear to wear to avoid any possible exposure to the disease while in the presence of the patient." This alone made it virtually certain that the judge would find the patient a potential danger to the public and order continued isolation, which he did.

In the midst of the SARS epidemic, New York City did, however, change its health code to permit the city's health commissioner to order the quarantine of individuals who "may" endanger the public health because of smallpox, pneumonic plague, or other severe communicable disease. In addition, a contact may also be quarantined: someone who "has been or may have been" in "close, prolonged, or repeated association with a case or carrier." This change in the code from permitting the quarantine of people who actually pose a danger to the public health and who have actually been in close contact with infected individuals, to those who "may" pose a danger and those who "may" have been in close contact with them is breathtaking in its invitation to arbitrariness. Given this, it is disturbing that not one person showed up to testify at the April 28, 2003 public hearing on this change. In the case of SARS, for example, which the revised rules specifically reference in a section on "post-publication changes," the new regulation would have permitted the department to quarantine New York's entire Chinatown area since all residents there "may" have been in contact with someone who "may" have SARS. No one (thankfully) seems to have even suggested such a rerun of the totally arbitrary San Francisco Chinatown quarantine, allegedly for plague. Nonetheless, it is worth noting that even 19th century U.S. courts, while granting extremely broad powers to public health agencies, condemned the arbitrary use of quarantine, even for smallpox, requiring public health officials to show "facts which warranted isolation."

SARS may return, but the CDC is to be commended for providing the U.S. with a credible and open official (the CDC director, Julie Gerberding, herself) who informed Americans about what they could voluntarily do to avoid contracting or spreading the disease. Nationally, encouragement of sensible voluntary responses became policy, and no state invoked any emergency powers, including quarantine, in response to SARS. As a general rule, sick people seek treatment and accept isolation to obtain it — people do not want to infect others, especially their family members, and will voluntarily follow reasonable public health advice to avoid spreading disease. SARS, like the threat of a bird flu pandemic, emphasizes that effective public health today must rely on actions taken at the national and international level, and that public health should be seen primarily as a global issue. Virtually every country in the world had to take some action to limit the exposure of its people to the disease.

SARS was a major public health challenge; but it is no less a medical challenge. At the beginning of the 21st century, sick people seek medical care. Individuals believed to be infected with the disease were (and continue to be) cared for one-by-one by physicians and nurses in hospitals. In fact, one of the salient aspects of the SARS epidemic is that many (in some countries, most) infections were actually acquired in hospitals, and many of those infected, and some who died, were physicians and nurses who cared for the patients. The dedication of the physicians and nurses who treated SARS patients was exemplary. Neither public health nor medicine alone could have effectively dealt with SARS. The old distinctions between medicine and public health are blurring, and perhaps the most important message is that public health and medicine must work together to be effective. Of course, SARS is not HIV/AIDS, which is not smallpox, which is not plague or tuberculosis or bioterrorism. Each infectious disease is different, and epidemiology provides the key to any effective public health and medical response to a new disease. The rapid exchange of information, made possible by the internet and an interconnected group of laboratories around the world (set up primarily for influenza identification and tracking), were critical to combating fear with knowledge. Information really does travel faster than even a new virus, and managing information is the most important task of modern public health officials. People around the world, provided with truthful, reasonable information by public health officials who are interested in both their health and human rights will follow their advice.

Isolating sick people seems to have been critical to containing SARS, but better infection-control techniques in hospitals, and adherence to them, are equally necessary. Quarantining contacts, where it was attempted, seems to have been both ineffective (in that many, if not most, contacts eluded quarantine) and useless (in that almost none of those quarantined developed SARS). Mass quarantine is a relic of the past that seems to have outlived its usefulness. Attempts at mass quarantine, as evidenced by the experience in China, are now likely to create more harm than they prevent. They do this both by imposing unnecessary restrictions on liberty on those quarantined, and by encouraging potentially infected people to flee from public health officials.

\* \* \*

## NOTES AND QUESTIONS

**1.** As with tuberculosis, SARS is clearly a serious disease, although, thus far, a major outbreak of SARS has been avoided. But consider some of the characteristics of SARS that make it and diseases like it particularly troubling: Much like TB, people infected with SARS may not know they have it, at least initially. Thus people can be exposed and infected, but asymptomatic for up to 10 days, during which time they can travel and potentially expose many other people. Even when symptoms start, they are indistinguishable from many, more common, and less lethal viral infections such as influenza (although as discussed in the Pandemic Influenza Preparedness and Response Plan, an outbreak of influenza can be a public health problem of epidemic proportions as well; *see* Note 5, *infra*). Yet, once these symptoms start, even a casual contact with a person infected with SARS can lead to an infection.

One of the most troubling aspects of the SARS outbreaks in 2003 was the number of health care workers who contracted SARS while caring for hospitalized patients who had not been diagnosed with SARS. To make matters worse, there was no apparent cure or treatment for people with SARS; the disease merely ran its course and was often fatal.

For additional information on SARS, see www.cdc/gov/ncidod/sars/ (last visited February 2005); for more information on SARS from an international perspective, see www.who.int/csr/sars/en/ (last visited February 2005).

**2.** The effects of the SARS epidemic on the United States were limited — more of a warning of what might happen in the future than a first encounter with a full-blown epidemic. Nonetheless, some efforts were made to control the initial and future spread of the disease. As reported by Rothstein:

> The CDC's Global Migration and Quarantine Division has coordinated efforts to prevent and control the spread of infectious diseases with other federal agencies, state and local health departments, the travel industry, and other organizations. The Division has eight permanent quarantine stations at major points of entry staffed by 30 permanent quarantine inspectors. During the SARS outbreak staffing and presence were augmented to 23 quarantine stations (15 new ports of entry) and 150 additional staff in order to provide information to

travelers arriving from SARS-affected countries via airplanes, ships or land; distributing health alerts to travelers with information regarding symptoms of SARS and what to do if they should develop SARS-like symptoms; examining travelers aboard airplanes and ships who have been reported as being ill with SARS-like symptoms; providing updates to other government agencies; and working with the CDC SARS investigation team and local and state health departments. SARS-specific yellow health alert cards were distributed to over 2.7 million arriving passengers disembarking from over 11,000 flights and 62 ships over a three-month period.

. . . .

**3.** Even if there is not another outbreak of SARS, there are many other new and "nasty" infectious diseases that could create a similar pandemic scenario: West Nile virus, Hantavirus, Ebola virus, Nipah virus, Hendra virus, just to name a few that have recently drawn some attention. Are there really more such diseases today and are these contemporary threats any different from those that humans have faced throughout history? In May of 2003, the IOM convened a panel of experts to address that question. Their answers were not comforting and, in general, affirmed the popular impression that there is a surge in new diseases. To explain that apparent trend they pointed to 13 factors that encourage the development of new diseases:

— microbial adaptation

— human susceptibility to infection

— climate and weather changes

— changing ecosystems

— changes in human demographics and behavior

— increased economic development and land use

— international travel and commerce

— spread of technology and industry

— breakdown of public health measures

— poverty and social injustice

— war and famine

— lack of political will

— bioterrorism

Obviously, not all of these factors are references to new phenomena. But the panel made particular reference to the modern trend towards the manipulation of the natural environment, the increasing number of large, crowded urban areas, and the increased level of travel and international commerce. They also noted that many of the new diseases have lived for some time in animals, and have spread to humans more frequently as more people move into habitats that were previously used predominantly by other animals.

For the full report, see IOM, MICROBIAL THREATS TO HEALTH: EMERGENCE, DETECTION, AND RESPONSE (2003) available to read at www.nap.edu/books. 030908864X/html (last visited February 2005).

**4.** In general terms, the states have the primary legal responsibility for responding to outbreaks of infectious diseases; but given the inter-jurisdictional and international nature of diseases like SARS or the avian flu, obviously the federal government has co-equal and, in some cases, preemptive authority.

Title 42 U.S.C. § 264 authorizes the Secretary of the DHHS to make and enforce regulations necessary to prevent the introduction, transmission, and spread of communicable diseases from foreign countries into the United States, and from one state to another. Section 264 specifically authorizes the federal government to use isolation and quarantine measures to achieve its purposes; however, it appears to limit the authority to use quarantine and isolation to specific communicable diseases that have been identified by executive orders from the President. The President added SARS to the list by Executive Order 13295, issued April 3, 2003; he added "flu viruses that are causing, or have the potential to cause, a pandemic" to the list by Executive Order 13375 issued April 1, 2005. Thus both diseases now fall within federal regulatory jurisdiction. It is worth noting that the list still includes yellow fever (transmitted by mosquitoes) and cholera (transmitted through ingestion of bacteria in water or food), added long ago and never deleted, which do not really belong there.

For regulations further detailing the federal powers with regard to inter-state communicable diseases under § 264, see the materials and notes on influenza, in Section E, *infra*, discussing the regulations adopted under this statute (42 C.F.R. § 70 *et seq.*) For similar regulations with regard to foreign communicable diseases, see 42 C.F.R. § 71 *et seq.*

In June 2002, President Bush signed the Public Health Security and Bioterrorism Preparedness and Response Act of 2002. Among the provisions of that legislation was a clarification of the federal authority to extend isolation and quarantine measures not only to people who are infectious but also to people who have been exposed to a communicable disease and may potentially become infectious; the legislation also had provisions that clarified procedures for expediting the executive orders under § 264.

Prior to the SARS outbreak, the list of federal diseases subject to federal quarantine authority under § 264 had not been updated since 1983 and was limited to cholera, diphtheria, tuberculosis, plague, small pox, yellow fever, and viral hemorrhagic fevers. Following the outbreak, SARS was added to the list as noted above. This essentially gave CDC and other federal health officials the authority to isolate or quarantine anyone who was considered infectious or who had been exposed to anyone who was considered infectious. This authority was, however, never exercised during the SARS outbreak.

For a broader discussion of the interrelation of federal and state authority in these situations, see James J. Misrahi, Joseph A. Foster, Frederic E. Shaw & Martin S. Cetron, *HHS/CDC Legal Response to SARS Outbreak,*

EMERGING INFECTIOUS DISEASES, Volume 10, No. 2 (February 2004) *available at* www.cdc.gov/ncidod/EID/ (last visited August 2006). For additional discussion of the authority of state and federal agencies, see Chapter Eight, *infra*.

**5.** For current and proposed *federal* rules on interstate quarantine, promulgated by the CDC, see Section E, *infra*.

## E.   CASE STUDY: INFLUENZA

In the following excerpt, Historian John Barry describes the experience of Paul Lewis, a Navy physician-scientist in Philadelphia asked to diagnose sailors taken ill with what turned out to be influenza (often called "Spanish Flu") in September 1918.

### JOHN M. BARRY, THE GREAT INFLUENZA: THE EPIC STORY OF THE DEADLIEST PLAGUE IN HISTORY
### 2–5 (2004)

\* \* \*

. . . The blood that covered so many of them did not come from wounds, at least not from steel or explosives that had torn away limbs. Most of the blood had come from nosebleeds. A few sailors had coughed the blood up. Others had bled from their ears. Some coughed so hard that autopsies would later show they had torn apart abdominal muscles and rib cartilage. And many of the men writhed in agony or delirium; nearly all those able to communicate complained of headache, as if someone were hammering a wedge into their skulls just behind the eyes, and body aches so intense they felt like bones breaking. A few were vomiting. Finally the skin of some of the sailors had turned unusual colors; some showed just a tinge of blue around their lips or fingertips, but a few looked so dark one could not tell easily if they were Caucasian or Negro. . . .

. . . [W]hatever was attacking these sailors was not only spreading, it was spreading explosively.

And it was spreading despite a well-planned, concerted effort to contain it. This same disease had erupted ten days earlier at a navy facility in Boston. . . .

. . . .

Philadelphia navy authorities had taken [Milton] Rosenau's warnings seriously, especially since a detachment of sailors had just arrived from Boston, and they had made preparations to isolate any ill sailors should an outbreak occur. They had been confident that isolation would control it.

Yet four days after the Boston detachment arrived, nineteen sailors in Philadelphia were hospitalized with what looked like the same disease. Despite their immediate isolation and that of everyone with whom they had had contract, eighty-seven sailors were hospitalized the next day. They and their contacts were again isolated. But two days later, six hundred men were hospitalized with this strange disease. The hospital ran out of empty beds, and hospital staff began falling ill. . . . Meanwhile, [navy] personnel from Boston, and now Philadelphia, had been and were being sent throughout the country as well.

. . . .

. . . In 1918 an influenza virus emerged — probably in the United States — that would spread around the world. . . . Before that world-wide pandemic faded away in 1920, it would kill more people than any other outbreak of disease in human history. Plague in the 1300's killed a far larger proportion of the population — more than one-quarter of Europe — but in raw numbers influenza killed more than plague then, more than AIDS today.

The lowest estimate of the pandemic's worldwide death toll is twenty-one million, in a world with a population less than one-third today's. That estimate comes from a contemporary study of the disease and newspapers have often cited it since, but it is almost certainly wrong. Epidemiologists today estimate that influenza likely caused at least fifty million deaths worldwide, and possibly as many as one hundred million.

. . . Normally influenza chiefly kills the elderly and infants, but in the 1918 pandemic roughly half of those who died were young men and women in the prime of their life, in their twenties and thirties. . . .

. . . .

. . . Although the influenza pandemic stretched over two years, perhaps two-thirds of the deaths occurred in a period of twenty-four weeks, and more than half of those deaths occurred in even less time, from mid-September to early December 1918. Influenza killed more people in a year than the Black Death of the Middle Ages killed in a century; it killed more people in twenty-four weeks than AIDS has killed in twenty-four years.

. . . .

Yet the story of the 1918 influenza virus is not simply one of havoc, death, and desolation, of a society fighting a war against nature superimposed on a war against another human society.

. . . .

For the influenza pandemic that erupted in 1918 was the first great collision between nature and modern science. It was the first great collision between a natural force and a society that included individuals who refused either to submit to that force or to simply call upon divine intervention to save themselves from it, individuals who instead were determined to confront this force directly, with a developing technology and with their minds.

\* \* \*

## DEPARTMENT OF HEALTH AND HUMAN SERVICES, HHS
### PANDEMIC INFLUENZA PLAN
17–21, 32 (November 2005)
*available at* www.hhs.gov/pandemicflu/plan/pdf/
HHSPandemicInfluenzaPlan.pdf
(last visited January 2007)

\* \* \*

Emergence of a human influenza virus with pandemic potential presents a formidable response challenge. If such a strain emerged in one or a few isolated communities abroad or within the U.S. and was detected quickly, containment of the outbreak(s), though very difficult, might be feasible, thereby preventing or significantly retarding the spread of disease to other communities. Containment attempts would require stringent infection-control measures such as bans on large public gatherings, isolation of symptomatic individuals, prophylaxis of the entire community with antiviral drugs, and various forms of movement restrictions  possibly even including a quarantine.

The resources required for such vigorous containment would almost certainly exceed those available in the affected communities. Thus, if a containment attempt is to have a chance of succeeding, the response must employ the assets of multiple partners in a well coordinated way. For isolated outbreaks outside the U.S., this means effective multinational cooperation in executing containment protocols designed and exercised well in advance. For isolated outbreaks within the U.S., this would require effective integration of the response assets of local, state, and federal governments and those of the private sector.

The National Response Plan (NRP), based on the principles of incident management, provides an appropriate conceptual and operational framework for a multi-party response to an outbreak of a potential influenza pandemic in one or a few U.S. communities. In particular, the NRP is designed to engage the response assets of multiple public and private partners and bring them to bear in a coordinated way at one or a few incident sites.

If efforts to contain isolated outbreaks within the U.S. were unsuccessful, and influenza spread quickly to affect many more communities either simultaneously or in quick succession — the hallmark of a pandemic — response assets at all levels of government and the private sector would be taxed severely. Communities would need to direct all their influenza response assets to their own needs and would have little to spare for the needs of others. Moreover, as the number of affected communities grows, their collective need would spread the response assets of states and the federal government ever thinner. In the extreme, until a vaccine against the pandemic virus would become available in sufficient quantity to have a significant impact on protecting public health, thousands of communities could be countering influenza simultaneously with little or no assistance from adjacent communities, the state, or the federal government. Preparedness planning for pandemic influenza response must take this prospect into account.

## Planning Assumptions

Pandemic preparedness planning is based on assumptions regarding the evolution and impacts of a pandemic. Defining the potential magnitude of a pandemic is difficult because of the large differences in severity for the three 20th century pandemics. While the 1918 pandemic resulted in an estimated 500,000 deaths in the U.S., the 1968 pandemic caused an estimated 34,000 U.S. deaths. This difference is largely related to the severity of infections and the virulence of the influenza viruses that caused the pandemics. The 20th century pandemics have also shared similar characteristics. In each pandemic, about 30% of the U.S. population developed illness, with about half seeking medical care. Children have tended to have the highest rates of illness, though not of severe disease and death. Geographical spread in each pandemic was rapid and virtually all communities experienced outbreaks.

Pandemic planning is based on the following assumptions about pandemic disease:

- Susceptibility to the pandemic influenza subtype will be universal.

- The clinical disease attack rate will be 30% in the overall population. Illness rates will be highest among school-aged children (about 40%) and decline with age. Among working adults, an average of 20% will become ill during a community outbreak.

- Of those who become ill with influenza, 50% will seek outpatient medical care.

- The number of hospitalizations and deaths will depend on the virulence of the pandemic virus. Estimates differ about 10-fold between more and less severe scenarios. Because the virulence of the influenza virus that causes the next pandemic cannot be predicted, two scenarios are presented based on extrapolation of past pandemic experience (Table 1).

- Risk groups for severe and fatal infections cannot be predicted with certainty. During annual fall and winter influenza season, infants and the elderly, persons with chronic illnesses, and pregnant women are usually at higher risk of complications from influenza infections. In contrast, in the 1918 pandemic, most deaths occurred among young, previously healthy adults.

- The typical incubation period (the time between acquiring the infection until becoming ill) for influenza averages 2 days. We assume this would be the same for a novel strain that is transmitted between people by respiratory secretions.

- Persons who become ill may shed virus and can transmit infection for one-half to one day before the onset of illness. Viral shedding and the risk for transmission will be greatest during the first two days of illness. Children will shed the greatest amount of virus and, therefore, are likely to pose the greatest risk for transmission.

**Table 1. Number of Episodes of Illness, Healthcare Utilization, and Deaths Associated with Moderate and Severe Pandemic Influenza Scenarios**

| Characteristic | Moderate (1958/68-like) | Severe (1918-like) |
|---|---|---|
| Illness | 90 million (30%) | 90 million (30%) |
| Outpatient Medical care | 45 million (50%) | 45 million (50%) |
| Hospitalization | 865,000 | 9,900,000 |
| ICU care | 128,750 | 1,485,000 |
| Mechanical ventilation | 64,875 | 742,500 |
| Deaths | 209,000 | 1,983,000 |

- On average, about two secondary infections will occur as a result of transmission from someone who is ill. Some estimates from past pandemics have been higher, with up to about three secondary infections per primary case.

- In an affected community, a pandemic outbreak will last about six to eight weeks. At least two pandemic disease waves are likely. Following the pandemic, the new viral subtype is likely to continue circulating and to contribute to seasonal influenza.

- The seasonality of a pandemic cannot be predicted with certainty. The largest waves in the U.S. during 20th century pandemics occurred in the fall and winter. Experience from the 1957 pandemic may be instructive in that the first U.S. cases occurred in June, but no community outbreaks occurred until August, and the first wave of illness peaked in October.

## Doctrine for a Pandemic Influenza Response

HHS will be guided by the following principles in initiating and directing its response activities:

1. In advance of an influenza pandemic, HHS will work with federal, state, and local government partners and the private sector to coordinate pandemic influenza preparedness activities and to achieve interoperable response capabilities.

2. In advance of an influenza pandemic, HHS will encourage all Americans to be active partners in preparing their states, local communities, workplaces, and homes for pandemic influenza and will emphasize that a pandemic will require Americans to make difficult choices. An informed and responsive public is essential to minimizing the health effects of a pandemic and the resulting consequences to society.

3. In advance of an influenza pandemic, HHS, in concert with federal partners, will work with the pharmaceutical industry to develop domestic vaccine production capacity sufficient to provide vaccine for the entire U.S. population as soon as possible after the onset of a

pandemic and, during the pre-pandemic period, to produce up to 20 million courses of vaccine against each circulating influenza virus with pandemic potential and to expand seasonal influenza domestic vaccine production to cover all Americans for whom vaccine is recommended through normal commercial transactions.

4.  In advance of an influenza pandemic, HHS, in concert with federal partners and in collaborations with the States, will procure sufficient quantities of antiviral drugs to treat 25% of the U.S. population and, in so doing, stimulate development of expanded domestic production capacity sufficient to accommodate subsequent needs through normal commercial transactions. HHS will stockpile antiviral medications in the Strategic National Stockpile, and states will create and maintain local stockpiles.

5.  Sustained human-to-human transmission anywhere in the world will be the triggering event to initiate a pandemic response by the United States. Because we live in a global community, a human outbreak anywhere means risk everywhere.

6.  The U.S. will attempt to prevent an influenza pandemic or delay its emergence by striving to arrest isolated outbreaks of a novel influenza wherever circumstances suggest that such an attempt might be successful, acting in concert with WHO and other nations as appropriate. At the core of this strategy will be basic public health measures to reduce person-to-person transmission.

7.  At the onset of an influenza pandemic, HHS, in concert with federal partners, will work with the pharmaceutical industry to procure vaccine directed against the pandemic strain and to distribute vaccine to state and local public health departments for pre-determined priority groups based on pre-approved state plans.

8.  At the onset of an influenza pandemic, HHS, in collaboration with the states, will begin to distribute and deliver antiviral drugs from public stockpiles to healthcare facilities and others with direct patient care responsibility for administration to pre-determined priority groups.

. . .

## HHS Actions for Pandemic Influenza Preparedness and Response

HHS will follow the WHO published guidance for national pandemic planning, which defines pandemic activities in six phases. WHO Phases 1 and 2 are the Interpandemic Period, which includes phases where no new influenza virus subtypes have been detected in humans.

The Pandemic Alert Period includes a phase when human infection with a novel influenza strain has been identified, but no evidence has been found of transmission between people or, at most, rare instances of spread to a close contact (WHO Phase 3), and includes phases where person-to-person transmission is occurring in clusters with limited human-to-human transmission (WHO Phases 4 and 5). WHO Phase 6 is the Pandemic Period, in which there is increased and sustained transmission in the general population. . . .

Each pandemic phase is associated with a range of preparedness and response activities directed by the Secretary of Health and Human Services, after consultation with international authorities and others, as necessary. Given that an influenza pandemic may not unfold in a completely predictable way, decision-makers must regularly reassess their strategies and actions and make adjustments as necessary. . . .

* * *

# NOTES AND QUESTIONS

**1.** Outbreaks of influenza can present a major public health problem even if they do not appear as "pandemics." In the United States, cases of "the flu" generally start appearing in late fall and continue through the winter. During a typical year, more than 36,000 Americans will die and over 100,000 will be hospitalized. The risk is particularly high for people over the age of 65, people with chronic heart or lung diseases, people with metabolic diseases, people with impaired immune systems, and children under the age of two. Vaccination is the major public health strategy for limiting the incidence and spread of influenza.

**2.** Influenza viruses are grouped into three types: A, B, and C. Humans can be infected with all three types, but type A is the most common and causes more severe illness. Influenza A viruses are further divided into subtypes or strains on the basis of the number of their protein components, hemagglutinin (H) and neuraminidase (N). The 1918 epidemic was caused by influenza A (H1N1). Less severe pandemics occurred in 1957 and 1968 (influenza A (H3N2)). The influenza virus constantly changes the structure of its H and N proteins, because it lacks a "proofreading" mechanism that can repair mutations in replicating its genetic material. This change is called "antigenic drift," and is responsible for annual variations in the influenza that appears in winter seasons around the world. Influenza vaccines must take antigenic drift into account, so vaccine producers try to predict what subtype of influenza is likely to appear each year. Most annual changes are relatively minor, so that vaccines remain relatively effective against any unexpected variation. However, every 10 to 40 years, the virus mutates so dramatically that the human immune system does not recognize it and existing vaccines offer little protection. Such a virus can cause a pandemic — an epidemic that spreads to several countries. This happened with the influenza pandemic in 1918, which claimed more lives than both World Wars, the Korean War, and the Vietnam War combined. Sarah F. Fujimura, *The Purple Death: The Great Flu of 1918*, 8 PERSPECTIVES IN HEALTH MAG., 28, 30 (2003), *available at* www.paho.org/English/DD/PIN/Number18_article5.htm.

We have had one notorious experience with governmental planning for influenza — the so-called "swine flu" epidemic of 1976. Swine flu was expected to be especially serious, and the federal government took the lead in educating the public and attempting (unsuccessfully) to vaccinate the entire population of the country, along with other preventive steps. The flu that year turned out to be nothing particularly hazardous, resulting in a loss of credibility for public health and some presumably-unnecessary morbidity and mortality arising from the widespread vaccination that was in fact achieved (more than 10 million people in 2.5 months). For the authoritative account — which is thorough, fascinating, and illuminating — see RICHARD E. NEUSTADT & HARVEY V. FINEBERG, THE EPIDEMIC THAT NEVER WAS: POLICY-MAKING & THE SWINE FLU AFFAIR (1983).

**3.** As described by the material in this section, the possibility that a new strain of the influenza will emerge creates the threat of a pandemic in the United States, one that could cause many times more deaths, straining both public and private resources, and raising the possibility that more draconian measures might be required to limit the spread of influenza through the population. The "bird" flu (officially identified as H5N1 avian flu virus) represents a prime example, one which has garnered considerable attention over the past couple of years.

In March 2006, Secretary of Health and Human Services Michael O. Leavitt issued a report specifically addressing pandemic planning for avian flu. Leavitt's report described the nature of the virus, the risks of its causing pandemic disease, and some of the potential consequences, suggesting that an outbreak of "bird flu" could potentially cause hundreds of thousands of deaths, jeopardize the economy, and disrupt virtually all activities that involve human-to-human contact. The report identified and described five critical national planning priorities: monitoring disease spread to report rapid response; developing vaccines and vaccine production capacity; stockpiling antiviral medications and other countermeasures; coordinating federal, state, and local preparation; and enhancing outreach and communications planning. For more on the "bird flu" see www.who.int/csr/disease/avianinfluenza_influenza/ (last visited August 2006); www.cdc.gov/flu/avian/ (last visited August 2006).

Are we ready for such an event? The PANDEMIC INFLUENZA PLAN and Secretary Leavitt's report outline the possible scenarios that we may face and the manner in which the federal, state, and local government will respond. For updates and additional references, see www.PandemicFlu.gov/ (last visited May 2006).

There appears to be no shortage of reports and plans, especially at the national level. *See* HOMELAND SECURITY COUNCIL, NATIONAL STRATEGY FOR PANDEMIC INFLUENZA: IMPLEMENTATION PLAN (May 2006) found at www.white house.gov/homeland/nspi_implementation (last visited May 2006). There is also a broader NATIONAL RESPONSE PLAN (NRP) adopted in 2005. For further details, see also discussion of that agency and other matters relating to homeland security in Section E *infra*. Increasingly, the states are also preparing similar plans. *See, e.g.,* www.azdhs.gov/pandemicflu/index.htm (Arizona plan).

**4.** Mostly we have plans and checklists rather than resources to deal with a potential flu pandemic. But we are nonetheless better off than when President Bush first discussed his reaction to a flu pandemic in the fall of 2005. He suggested that Congress should consider empowering the military to be the "first responders" in any national disaster. Later, the president suggested that the U.S. should confront the risk of a bird flu pandemic by giving him the power to use the U.S. military to quarantine "part[s] of the country" experiencing an "outbreak." Bush said he got the idea by reading John Barry's excellent account of the 1918 Spanish flu pandemic, THE GREAT INFLUENZA, which opened this section. Although quarantine was only used successfully in that pandemic once, on the island of American Samoa, Barry in his afterword suggests (sensibly) that we need a national plan to deal with a future influenza pandemic. Barry has also said that his other suggestions were only ones that he hoped public health officials and ethicists would consider — but they do read like policy recommendations to some, and apparently including the president. He wrote, for example, "if there is any chance to limit the geographical spread of the disease, officials must have in place the legal power to take extreme quarantine measures." And this recommendation comes shortly after his praise for countries that "moved rapidly and ruthlessly to quarantine and isolate anyone with or exposed to" SARS. In response to the Bush "plan" George Annas wrote an op/ed in the *Boston Globe*:

> Planning makes sense. But planning for "brutal" or "extreme" quarantine of large numbers of people or of areas of the United States makes no sense, and actually creates many more problems than it could possibly solve. First, historically mass quarantines of healthy people who may have been exposed to a pathogen have never worked to control a pandemic, and have almost always done more harm than good because they usually involve vicious discrimination against classes of people who are seen as "diseased" and dangerous. Second, the notion that ruthless quarantine was responsible for preventing a SARS pandemic is a public health myth.

* * *

> Sick people should be treated, but we don't need the military to force treatment. Even in extremes like the anthrax attacks, people seek out and demand treatment. Sending soldiers to quarantine large numbers of people is most likely to create panic, and cause people to flee (and spread disease), as it did in China where a rumor during the SARS epidemic that Beijing would be quarantined led to 250,000 people fleeing the city that night. Not only can't we evacuate Houston [during Hurricane Rita], we cannot realistically quarantine its citizens. The real public health challenge will be shortages of health care personnel, hospital beds, and medicine. Plans to militarize quarantine miss the point in a pandemic. The enemy is not sick or exposed Americans — it is the virus itself. And effective action against any flu virus demands its early identification, and the quick development, manufacture, and distribution of a vaccine and treatment modalities.

> In 1918 the Spanish flu was spread around the U.S. primarily by soldiers, and it seems to have incubated primarily on military bases. It is a misreading of history that a lesson from 1918 is to militarize mass quarantine to contain the flu. And neither medicine nor public health are what they were in 1918; having public health rely on mass quarantine today is like having our military rely on trench warfare in Iraq. What has

not changed in the past century, however, is the fact that national flu policy will be determined by national politics. In World War I, as Barry recounts, this policy demanded that there be no public criticism of the federal government. That policy was a disaster, and did prevent many potentially effective public health actions. Today's presidential substitution of a military quarantine solution for credible public health planning will also be counterproductive and ineffective in the event of a real pandemic, leaving all U.S. citizens sick with the flu to wonder, like the citizens of New Orleans told to go to the Convention Center and the Superdome for help, why the federal government has abandoned them.

George J. Annas, Op/Ed, BOSTON GLOBE, Oct. 8, 2005, at A15.

**5.** One practical problem for lawyers attempting to assess what can and cannot be done in response to an outbreak of SARS, influenza, or some other fast-spreading communicable disease, is sorting out the authority of their state and the federal government in these matters. For an interesting effort by the CDC to coordinate the various state and federal laws in what they call a "legal roadmap," see CDC, ROADMAP TO U.S. STATE LEGAL AUTHORITIES: SEPARATION AND DETENTION OF PERSONS FOR PURPOSES OF CONTROLLING THE SPREAD OF COMMUNICABLE DISEASES, *available at* www.phppo.cdc.gov/od/phlp/ roadmap (last visited February 2005). *See also* discussion of "legal preparedness" in notes to Section E, *infra*.

**6.** If anything close to the type of pandemic suggested in these materials actually occurs, then virtually every individual and institutional actor — both within and without government — is likely to be affected. For one interesting and demonstrative example of how to prepare for a flu or other pandemic event, see FLORIDA STATE COURTS, STRATEGY FOR PANDEMIC INFLUENZA: KEEPING THE COURTS OPEN IN A PANDEMIC (March 2006).

**7.** What would most Americans do if confronted with a governmental effort to isolate or quarantine a large number of people? Even if there is constitutional authority to do so, and that authority has been properly delegated to a state or federal agency, will isolation or quarantine really work in a society that is often distrustful of "big government" and rather individualistic in its behavior? For one view, see Mark A. Rothstein, *Are Traditional Public Health Strategies Consistent With Contemporary American Values?*, 77 TEMPLE L. REV. 175 (2004).

For some anecdotal indications of what Americans might do, see the descriptions of the various 18th and 19th century epidemics in Chapter One. Consider also the *Jew Ho* case in Section C, Note 4, *supra*.

What would you do?

**8.** In addition to this chapter's exploration of infectious diseases capable of causing public health disasters, we have had recent experience with other threats to public health, including West Nile virus, Eastern equine encephalopathy, and tularemia. Sometimes, rare but frightening conditions also cause considerable public unease, as in the case of bovine spongiform encephalopathy (BSE), popularly known as "mad cow disease," a disease that is largely confined to cattle but, some believe, could be spread to humans who consume infected meat. For background, see Litjen Tan, et al., *Risk of Transmission of Bovine Spongiform Encephalopathy to Humans in the United States: Report of the Council on Scientific Affairs, American Medical*

*Association,* 281 JAMA 2330 (1999); *see also Ranchers Cattleman Action Legal Fund United Stockgrowers of America v. Department of Agriculture,* 2005 LEXIS 17360 (9th Cir. 2005) (overturning an injunction that had attempted to stop the issuance of an agency rule allowing the re-introduction of Canadian beef into the United States after "mad cow disease" had been found in some Canadian livestock). For further exploration of how public risk perception can shape social responses to disease, see Chapter Six, *infra.*

### Federal Rules on Interstate Quarantine

In connection with federal planning for control of "bird flu" and other contagious diseases that fall within federal jurisdiction (explained in Note 4 of the SARS readings, sec. D, *supra*), the CDC is undertaking proposed revisions to its rules on interstate quarantine. Among other things, the rules would require airlines to submit detailed passenger lists to the CDC (rather than to the Federal Aviation Administration), to identify anyone with a communicable disease.

Two documents follow: first, parts of the existing CDC rules on interstate quarantine; and next, the CDC's proposed revisions to those rules (announced in November 2005 and, at this time, still pending and under consideration). In reviewing both documents, consider the changes that would be made to the existing rules, and their purpose, impact, and justification.

---

### 42 C.F.R. Part 70 (2004) Interstate Quarantine

#### § 70.1 General definitions.

As used in this part:

(a) Communicable diseases means illnesses due to infectious agents or their toxic products, which may be transmitted from a reservoir to a susceptible host either directly as from an infected person or animal or indirectly through the agency of an intermediate plant or animal host, vector, or the inanimate environment.

(b) Communicable period means the period or periods during which the etiologic agent may be transferred directly or indirectly from the body of the infected person or animal to the body of another.

(c) Conveyance means any land or air carrier, or any vessel as defined in paragraph (h) of this section.

(d) Incubation period means the period between the implanting of disease organisms in a susceptible person and the appearance of clinical manifestation of the disease.

[subsections 70.1(e)-(h) omitted]

#### § 70.2 Measures in the event of inadequate local control.

Whenever the Director of the Centers for Disease Control and Prevention determines that the measures taken by health authorities of any State or possession (including political subdivisions thereof) are insufficient to prevent the spread of any of the communicable diseases from such State or possession to any other State or possession, he/she may take such measures to prevent such spread of the diseases as he/she deems reasonably necessary, including inspection, fumigation, disinfection, sanitation, pest extermination, and destruction of animals or articles believed to be sources of infection.

### § 70.3 All communicable diseases.

A person who has a communicable disease in the communicable period shall not travel from one State or possession to another without a permit from the health officer of the State, possession, or locality of destination, if such permit is required under the law applicable to the place of destination. Stopovers other than those necessary for transportation connections shall be considered as places of destination.

### § 70.4 Report of disease.

The master of any vessel or person in charge of any conveyance engaged in interstate traffic, on which a case or suspected case of a communicable disease develops shall, as soon as practicable, notify the local health authority at the next port of call, station, or stop, and shall take such measures to prevent the spread of the disease as the local health authority directs.

### § 70.5 Certain communicable diseases; special requirements.

The following provisions are applicable with respect to any person who is in the communicable period of cholera, plague, smallpox, typhus or yellow fever, or who, having been exposed to any such disease, is in the incubation period thereof:

(a) Requirements relating to travelers.

(1) No such person shall travel from one State or possession to another, or on a conveyance engaged in interstate traffic, without a written permit of the Surgeon General or his/her authorized representative.

(2) Application for a permit may be made directly to the Surgeon General or to his/her representative authorized to issue permits.

(3) Upon receipt of an application, the Surgeon General or his/her authorized representative shall, taking into consideration the risk of introduction, transmission, or spread of the disease from one State or possession to another, reject it, or issue a permit that may be conditioned upon compliance with such precautionary measures as he/she shall prescribe.

(4) A person to whom a permit has been issued shall retain it in his/her possession throughout the course of his/her authorized travel and comply with all conditions prescribed therein, including presentation of the permit to the operators of conveyances as required by its terms.

[subsection 70.5(b) omitted]

### § 70.6 Apprehension and detention of persons with specific diseases.

Regulations prescribed in this part authorize the detention, isolation, quarantine, or conditional release of individuals, for the purpose of preventing the introduction, transmission, and spread of the communicable diseases listed in an Executive Order setting out a list of quarantinable communicable diseases, as provided under section 361(b) of the Public

Health Service Act. Executive Order 13295, of April 4, 2003, contains the current revised list of quarantinable communicable diseases, and may be obtained at www.cdc.gov, or at www.archives.gov/federal-register. If this Order is amended, DHHS will enforce that amended order immediately and update this reference.

# Centers For Disease Control, Proposed Quarantine Regulations, Notice of Proposed Rulemaking
70 Fed. Reg. 71892 (Nov. 30, 2005)

## Sec. 70–.1 Scope and definitions.

*Provisional quarantine* means the detention on an involuntary basis of a person or group of persons reasonably believed to be in the qualifying stage of a quarantinable disease until a quarantine order has been issued or until the Director [of the CDC] determines that provisional quarantine is no longer warranted.

*Qualifying stage* means (i) A communicable stage of the disease; or (ii) A pre-communicable stage, if the disease would be likely to cause a public health emergency if transmitted to other persons.

*Quarantine* means the holding on a voluntary or involuntary basis, including the isolation, of a person or group of persons in such place and for such period of time as the Director deems necessary or desirable to prevent the spread of infection or illness.

*Quarantinable diseases* means any of the communicable diseases listed in an Executive Order . . .

. . .

## Sec. 70.13 Screenings to detect ill persons.

The Director may, at airports or other locations, conduct screenings of persons or groups of persons to detect the presence of ill persons. Such screenings may be conducted through visual inspection, electronic temperature monitors, or other means determined appropriate by the Director to detect the presence of ill persons.

## Sec. 70.14 Provisional quarantine.

(a) The Director may provisionally quarantine a person or group of persons who the Director reasonably believes to be in the qualifying stage of a quarantinable disease and: (1) moving or about to move from one state to another state; or (2) a probable source of infection to persons who will be moving from a state to another state.

(b) Provisional quarantine shall commence upon: (1) the service of a written provisional quarantine order; (2) a verbal provisional quarantine order; or (3) actual movement restrictions placed on the person or group of persons.

(c) Provisional quarantine shall end three business days after provisional quarantine commences . . .

(e) A persons or group of persons subject to provisional quarantine may be offered medical treatment, prophylaxis or vaccination, as the Director deems necessary to prevent the introduction, transmission or spread of the disease; such persons may refuse such medical treatment, prophylaxis, or vaccination, but remain subject to provisional quarantine.

### Sec. 70.16 Quarantine.

(a) The Director may issue a quarantine order whenever the Director reasonably believes that:

(1) a person or group of persons are in the qualifying stage of a quarantinable disease . . . and either (2) moving or about to move from a state to another state; or (3) a probable source of infection to persons who will be moving from a state to another state.

\* \* \*

# NOTES AND QUESTIONS

**1.** As a matter of nomenclature, note that the CDC's use of the word "quarantine" appears in some places to connote what we would consider to be involuntary isolation. (Compare the definitions from the sidebar at the beginning of this chapter).

**2.** The CDC's proposed rule-changes, which have not been promulgated as of September 2006, drew almost unanimous objection. The following comments on the proposed changes were submitted by the New England Coalition for Law and Public Health:

> The CDC's legal analysis that accompanied the publication of the proposed regulations (legal analysis) acknowledges that "freedom from physical restraint is a 'liberty' interest protected by the Due Process Clause . . ." 70 Fed. Reg. at 71895. Oddly, however, it cites as authority for that statement the case of the civil commitment of a convicted child sex molester, *Kansas v. Hendricks*, 521 U.S. 346 (1997). Moreover, it describes the case as noting that "while freedom from physical restraint is at the core of the liberty protected by the Due Process Clause, that liberty is not absolute." 70 Fed. Reg. at 71895. *Kansas v. Hendricks* stands not for the meaningless proposition that liberty is not absolute, but for the critical principle that both grounds for civil commitment must be proved in order to justify civil commitment — even in the case of a convicted sex offender who has served his prison sentence. Indeed, in *Hendricks*, the Supreme Court said, "A finding of dangerousness, standing alone, is ordinarily not sufficient ground upon which to justify indefinite involuntary commitment. We have sustained civil commitment statutes when they have coupled proof of dangerousness with the proof of some additional factor, such as 'mental illness' or 'mental abnormality.'" 521 U.S. at 358. This additional factor is intended to limit commitment to "those who suffer from volitional impairment rendering them dangerous beyond their control." *Id*. The Court again emphasized the necessity of a showing that a person lacks control over

dangerous behavior in *Kansas v. Crane*, 534 U.S. 407, 411 (2002) ("there must be proof of serious difficulty in controlling behavior").

These cases and their progeny make clear that, by itself, neither illness nor dangerousness is a constitutionally adequate basis for involuntary detention. Both must be present in ways that create the risk of harm to others. Therefore, no statute or regulation can meet constitutional standards of due process unless it requires evidence of both the presence of a serious contagious disease and the probability that the person will actually infect others if not involuntarily confined.

The proposed regulations do not meet these standards. . . .

    . . .

One of the most notable inventions of the proposed regulations is the institution of a puzzling new procedure called "provisional quarantine," which is actually just involuntary detention — without probable cause or a warrant or a hearing — for up to 3 business days. Proposed 42 C.F.R. §§70.15 and 71.18. The purpose of such detention appears to be to allow the CDC time to figure out whether there is probable cause or even reasonable suspicion that a person actually has a contagious disease that will be transmitted to others and could therefore justifiably be subjected to quarantine under the statute or Constitution. Thus, the provisional quarantine provisions appear to be simply a way to avoid meeting any constitutional standards whatsoever prior to involuntarily detaining people.

This conclusion is supported by the text of the legal explanation which states:

> A provisional quarantine order is likely to be premised on the need to investigate based on reasonable suspicion of exposure or infection, whereas a quarantine order is more likely to be premised on a medical determination that the individual actually has one of the quarantinable diseases. Thus, during this initial three business day period, there may be very little for a hearing officer to review in terms of factual and scientific evidence of exposure or infection. Three business days may be necessary to collect medical samples, transport such samples to laboratories, and conduct diagnostic testing, all of which would help inform the Director's determination that the individual is infected with a quarantinable disease and that further quarantine is necessary. In addition, because provisional quarantine may last no more than three business days, allowing for a full hearing, with witnesses, almost guarantees that no decision on the provisional quarantine will actually be reached until after the provisional period has ended, thus making such a hearing virtually meaningless in terms of granting release from the provisional quarantine. 70 Fed. Reg. at 71896.

CDC's arguments for failing to provide any oversight for up to *3 business days* is unconvincing and constitutionally troubling. Proposed 42 C.F.R. §§70.15(c) and 71.16(c). When there is a weekend or holiday, the provisional quarantine provisions could permit unreviewable detention for up to 6 days. The use of business days is itself puzzling in this context, since it suggests that the CDC does not work on weekends or holidays, even during a threatened epidemic. If a disease is so dangerous that it is arguably necessary to detain someone without evidence that he has the disease, why would public health officials and laboratories be unavailable to work over the weekend?. . . .

New England Coalition for Law and Public Health, Comments on Interstate and Foreign Quarantine Regulations Proposed by the Centers for Disease Control and Prevention, 42 C.F.R Parts 70 and 71, Feb. 3, 2006, *available at* www.cdc.gov/ncidod/dq/npgm/viewcomments_feb.htm

Comments on the proposed revisions submitted by the Center for Biosecurity of University of Pittsburgh on January 28, 2006 included the following:

The proposed revisions . . . are in many instances inconsistent with available scientific understanding of the nature of person-to-person disease transmission. This is particularly the case with pandemic influenza. The basic premise of the proposed revision, that the identification and quarantine of airline passengers showing symptoms of influenza infection will significantly diminish the spread of pandemic flu, is highly questionable and unsupported by data . . .

Specific issues:

. . .

6) **Monitoring only interstate flights for patients who need to be quarantined does not make sense.** To prevent spread of infection between states, why would the CDC single out air travel? Why do the proposed rules not apply to interstate train or bus travel? If preventing ill patients from crossing state lines is so fundamentally important to protecting public health, why only apply this principle to air travel? Since this would be impossible, why single out air travel?

. . .

8) **The rule proposes that arriving persons can be ordered to a medical examination and then placed into provisional quarantine. This element of the proposed rules is highly concerning on a number of levels.** This places unwarranted authority in a single individual ("the quarantine officer") whose medical training is not clearly articulated in the rule. Who will provide medical attention/care and legal resources for these quarantined individuals? Do these individuals have to get their own counsel at their own cost? The details of the administrative hearing which may follow a three day provisional quarantine period are unclear. Who is the "hearing officer"? Is it a judge? A doctor? What are the rights of the detained/quarantined individual?

Jennifer B. Nuzzo, SM, Donald A. Henderson, MD, MPH, Tara O'Toole, MD, MPH, Thomas V. Inglesby, MD, *Comments from the Center for Biosecurity of University of Pittsburgh Medical Center on Proposed Revisions to 42 CFR 70 and 71 (Quarantine Rules)*, www.cdc.gov/ncidod/dq/nprm/viewcomments_jan.htm (last visited January 28, 2006).

**3.** There are practical problems with this proposal as well, especially the small number of quarantine stations that actually exist to do the screening at airports and other ports of entry. The CDC recognizes this, and has advocated an increase in the number of so-called quarantine "stations" in the United States. However, even if the number were increased, they do not offer a feasible means of preventing contagious disease in the United States. As the Institute of Medicine recently reported, "Unlike their namesakes, today's quarantine stations are not stations *per se*, but rather small groups of individuals located at major U.S. airports." INSTITUTE OF MEDICINE, COMMITTEE ON MEASURES TO ENHANCE THE EFFECTIVENESS OF THE CDC QUARANTINE STATION EXPANSION PLAN FOR U.S. PORTS OF ENTRY, QUARANTINE STATIONS AT PORTS OF ENTRY PROTECTING THE PUBLIC'S HEALTH 1 (Sivitz, LB, Stratton K & Benjamin, GC, eds., 2005). The IOM describes these stations as follows:

> Unlike physical areas that travelers pass through, the term "station" in this report refers to a group of one to eight individuals located at an airport, land crossing, or seaport who perform activities designed to help mitigate the risk that a microbial and other threats of public health significance may enter the United States or affect travelers in this country. As noted above, all of the established stations (as of May 2005) are located at airports. Although the staff have offices and one or more patient isolation rooms, most interactions between quarantine station staff and travelers or crew take place in public areas of the terminals.

*Id.* at 20.

As of May 2005, there were a total of 8 "stations" in the country. By the month of November, the number rapidly increased to 18, according to the CDC's website. The proposed rules would authorize the CDC to establish hospitals and stations. However, it is impossible to believe that the CDC would be able to create a presence at every one of the 474 points of international travel into the United States. The current 18 "stations" cover only 3.8% of U.S. ports of entry. At best, the CDC hopes to ultimately have 25 stations, which would represent 5% of all ports of entry.

**4.** A year after Katrina, and the confusion about authority to call on the U.S. military to respond not only to emergencies such as floods, but also to public health emergencies such as a pandemic flu, the President signed the John Warner National Defense Authorization Act of 2007 on October 17, 2006. Included in the Act (H.R. 5122) is the following amendment to Section 333 of Title 10 (U.S.C.):

(a)  USE OF ARMED FORCES IN MAJOR PUBLIC EMERGENCIES—

    (1)  The President may employ the armed forces, including the National Guard in Federal service, to—

        (A)  restore public order and enforce the laws of the United States when, as a result of natural disaster, epidemic, or other serious public health emergency, terrorist attack, or incident, or other condition in any State or possession of the United States, the President determines that—

(i) domestic violence has occurred to such an extent that the constituted authorities of the State or possession are incapable of maintaining public order; and

(ii) such violence results in a condition described in paragraph (2); or

(B) suppress, in a State, any insurrection, domestic violence, unlawful combination, or conspiracy results in a condition described in paragraph (2).

(2) A condition described in the paragraph is a condition that—

(A) so hinders the execution of the laws of a State or possession, as applicable, and of the United States within that State or possession, that any part or class of its people is deprived of a right, privilege, immunity, or protection named in the Constitution and secured by law, and the constituted authorities of the State or possession are unable, fail, or refuse to protect that right, privilege, or immunity, or to give that protection; or

(B) opposes or obstructs the execution of the laws of the United States or impedes the course of justice under those laws.

(3) In any situation covered by paragraph (1)(B), the State shall be considered to have denied the equal protection of the laws secured by the Constitution.

This legislation passed Congress with virtually no debate and no public attention or comment. Nonetheless, Senator Edward Kennedy did applaud Senator Warner for the law on the floor of the Senate, saying that the authority of the President to use the military inside the U.S. needed to be clarified: "Late August last year, New Orleans and gulf coast residents saw the devastation nature can sow. We are now in another hurricane season. Communicable disease like SARS and avian flu are still real risks. No one needs reminding that bin Laden and al-Qaeda are still are still out there. We need to clarify the applicability of this law to modern problems." Cong. Rec., Sept. 29, 2006, S108060. Do you agree? Are we better off or worse off with this law? How are terrorism, natural disaster, insurrections, and epidemics alike? How are they different?

## F.  EMERGENCY PREPAREDNESS FOR BIOTERRORISM AND EPIDEMICS

This final section explores mass public health emergencies created by contagious disease, whether through an act of bioterror or a widespread, naturally-occuring epidemic. The focus of subsection 1 is on overall public health planning for such emergencies; as such, it concentrates, inevitably, primarily on actions that may be taken by the administrative arms of government at the federal, state and local levels. Subsection 2 focuses more explicitly on "legal planning" — consideration of the adequacy of current legal tools for effectively responding to such events, and exploration of changes in law that may enhance that response. Of course, the distinction between these two subtopics is imperfect, since much of what government can and will do is controlled by the powers and constraints of existing law. Nonetheless, the distinctive focus of subsection 2 on what might be called "public health law reform" seems warranted as we contemplate these unwelcome threats.

## 1.  Planning for Public Health Emergencies: Policy and Administrative Aspects

### Thomas V. Inglesby et al., *A Plague on Your City: Observations from TOPOFF*
32 CLINICAL INFECTIOUS DISEASE 436, 437–38 (2001)

\* \* \*

The U.S. Congress, in an effort "to assess the nation's crisis and consequence management capacity under extraordinarily stressful conditions," directed the Department of Justice to conduct an exercise that would engage key personnel in the management of mock chemical, biological or cyber-terrorist attacks.

TOPOFF was a $3 million drill that tested the readiness of top government officials to respond to terrorist attacks directed at multiple geographic locations. It was the largest exercise of its kind to date. The exercise, which took place in May 2000 in three cities in the United States, simulated a chemical weapons event in Portsmouth, N.H., a radiological event in the greater Washington, D.C. area, and a bioweapons event in Denver, Colo. The bioterrorism component of the exercise centered on the release of an aerosol of *Yersinia pestis*, the bacteria that causes plague. Denver was selected in part because it had received domestic preparedness training and equipment. . . .

This article seeks to identify the medical and public health observations and lessons discovered in the biological weapons component (i.e., the Denver component) of the TOPOFF exercise. . . .

. . . .

Officials were involved in the event as participants, controllers, or observers. Participants were the actual players of the exercise and, in general, operated within the parameters of their usual roles and authorities. Controllers maintained the structure of the exercise, which helped guide the unfolding scenario. Observers were generally agency heads who had policy responsibilities relevant to the events of the exercise. A number of health agencies (including the county health agency, the state health agency, the Centers for Disease Control and Prevention [CDC], The Office of Emergency Preparedness, and elements of the Public Health Service, as well as three hospitals in the Denver area [Swedish Medical Center, Medical Center of Aurora and Denver Health Medical Center]) participated in the exercise. Many persons from these institutions worked around the clock for days in attempts to cope with the unfolding medical and public health crisis depicted in the exercise.

TOPOFF was intended to be "player driven" which meant that the participants' decisions and the subsequent consequences were to be the primary drivers in the shaping of the exercise. . . .

The scope and complexity of the exercise were such that many of the events that occurred in the exercise could only be "notional" (i.e., they could not be acted out and, thus, occurred on paper only). Examples of notional events that occurred in the exercise included situations in which "thousands of panicked persons . . . [were] flooding into emergency departments" and "one million persons . . . [were] advised to stay in their homes." All media communication during the exercise was transmitted through the "Virtual News Network" (VNN). VNN was the virtual news agency that was used in the exercise to interview the exercise participants, to hold press conferences, and to disseminate information (notionally) to the public. No actual news agencies were involved in the exercise, nor was any of the news that was reported on VNN actually disseminated to the public.

. . . [TOPOFF was intended to be conducted without advance knowledge on the part of participants, a goal that was not not fully realized]. However, a number of participants, including participants from the three hospitals, did not have advance knowledge of when the exercise was to begin or what weapons agent was to be used; they knew only that a bioterrorism exercise would take place sometime in May.

. . .

The exercise began on May 20, 2000, and ended on May 23.

## OVERVIEW OF THE EXERCISE

*May 17.* An aerosol of plague (*Y. pestis*) bacilli is released covertly at the Denver Performing Arts Center.

*May 20 (day 1 of exercise).* The Colorado Department of Public Health and Environment receives information that increasing numbers of persons began to seek medical attention at Denver area hospitals for cough and fever during the evening of May 19 . . . By early in the afternoon of May 20, 500 persons with these symptoms have received medical care; 25 of the 500 have died. The Department of Public Health and Environment notifies the CDC of the increased volume of sick patients. Plague is confirmed first by the state laboratory and subsequently, in a patient specimen, by the CDC lab at Ft. Collins, CO. . . .

A public health emergency is declared by the state health officer. The state health officer places an official request for support from the Department of Health and Human Services' Office of Emergency Preparedness. The governor's Emergency Epidemic Response Committee . . . assembles to respond to the unfolding crisis. Thirty-one CDC staff are sent to Denver. The CDC is notified by the Denver police and the Federal Bureau of Investigation (FBI) that a dead man has been found with terrorist literature and paraphernalia in his possession; his cause of death is unknown. Hospitals and clinics in the Denver area, which just a day ago were dealing with what appeared to be an unusual increase in influenza cases, are recalling staffs, implementing emergency plans, and seeking assistance in the determination of treatment protocols and protective measures. By late afternoon, hospital staff are beginning to call in sick, and antibiotics and ventilators are becoming more scarce. Some hospital staff have donned protective respiratory equipment.

The governor issues an executive order that restricts travel (including travel by bus, rail, and air) into or out of 14 Denver metropolitan counties; he also commandeers all antibiotics that can be used to prevent or treat plague. During a VNN press conference, at which a number of agencies are represented, the Denver police is informed that an outbreak of the plague has occurred in the city after a terrorist attack, and it is told of the governor's executive order. The public is also told to seek treatment at a medical facility if they are feeling ill or if they have been in contact with a known or suspected case of plague. Those who are healthy are directed to stay in their homes and to avoid public gatherings. The public is told that the disease can spread from person to person only "if you are within six feet of someone who is infected and coughing," and they are told that dust masks effectively prevent the spread of disease. . . . It is announced that the governor is working with the President of the United States to resolve the crisis and that federal resources are being brought in to support the state agencies. By the end of the day, 783 cases of pneumonic plague have occurred; 123 persons have died.

*May 21 (day 2 of exercise).* VNN reports that a "national crash effort" is under way that aims to move large quantities of antibiotics to the region as the CDC brings in its "national stockpile," but the quantity of available antibiotics is uncertain. The report explains that early administration of antibiotics is effective in the treatment of plague, but that antibiotic treatment must be started within 24 hours of the development of symptoms. A few hours later, a VNN story reports that hospitals are running out of antibiotics.

A "push-pack" from the National Pharmaceutical Stockpile (NPS) arrives in Denver, but there are great difficulties in moving antibiotics from the stockpile delivery point to the persons who need it for treatment and prophylaxis. Out-of-state cases begin to be reported. The CDC notifies bordering states of the epidemic. Cases are reported in England and Japan. Both Japan and the World Health Organization (WHO) request technical assistance from the CDC.

A number of hospitals in Denver are full to capacity, and by the end of the day, they are unable to see or to admit new patients. Thirteen hundred ventilators from the NPS are to be flown to Colorado. The number of bodies in hospital morgues is reported to have reached critical levels. By 5:00 p.m. mountain time, the CDC has performed an epidemiological investigation on 41 cases. The U.S. Surgeon General flies to Colorado to facilitate communications issues. Many states are now requesting components of the NPS from the CDC. By the end of the day, 1871 plague cases have occurred in persons throughout the United States, London, and Tokyo. Of these, 389 persons have died.

*May 22 (day 3 of exercise).* Hospitals are understaffed and have insufficient antibiotics, ventilators, and beds to meet demand. They cannot manage the influx of sick patients into the hospitals. Medical care is "beginning to shut down" in Denver. A total of 151 patient charts have been reviewed by state and federal health officials who are pursuing the epidemiological investigation. There are difficulties getting antibiotics from the NPS to the facilities that need them. Details of a distribution plan are still not formalized.

Officials from the Department of Public Health and Environment and the CDC have determined that secondary spread of disease appears to be occurring. The population in Denver is encouraged to wear face masks. The CDC advises that Colorado state borders be cordoned off to limit further spread of plague throughout the United States and other countries. Colorado officials express concern about their ability to get food and supplies into the state. The governor's executive order is extended to prohibit travel into or out of the state of Colorado. By noon, there are reports of 3060 U.S. and international patients with pneumonic plague, 795 of whom have died.

*May 23 (day 4 of exercise)*. There are conflicting reports regarding the number of sick persons and dead persons. Some reports show an estimated 3700 cases of pneumonic plague with 950 deaths. Others are reporting more than 4000 cases and more than 2000 deaths. . . .

   . . .

# NOTES AND QUESTIONS

**1.** Inglesby describes a number of what he terms "lessons" from the exercise. Generally he notes that issues of "leadership, the role of authorities, and the processes of decision-making" were all "highly problematic," and that political considerations often received more attention from "experts" than they might have received from elected officials. He continues:

> Some participants attributed these difficulties to the decision-making processes of public health agencies. One observer commented about how "in public health, more decision-making is through democratic processes and consensus building, but for some decisions, this cannot work." . . . Another observer remarked, "the time frame that public health is accustomed to dealing with is not what is needed for bioterrorism. . . . Some from the CDC, state and local health agencies tried to look at this as a standard epidemiological investigation. In absolutely no way would this [scenario allow] a normal epidemiological investigation." . . .

> The flow of information was another major concern of the participants. . . . It is also unlikely that health departments would have had the resources to acquire and analyze data rapidly enough to know the rate of secondary transmission or to pinpoint the outbreak's origin as quickly as was portrayed in the exercise. Without rapid access to this information and other data, decision-makers would have been even more ill-positioned to make important decisions, such as how and when to distribute antibiotics, make recommendations for containment measures, or communicate public education messages.

>    . . .

> The large numbers of ill persons seeking medical care was one of the most serious challenges identified by the exercise, according to one senior health department official. Even at the outset of the epidemic, hospitals were quickly seeing far more cases than they could handle. Notional patient visits to the emergency department at one hospital were double

and then triple the normal volumes. Within the short timeframe of the exercise, they quickly escalated to ten times the usual caseload.

*Id.* at 439–41. With specific regard to quarantine and isolation of individuals, Inglesby noted:

> Perhaps the issues that provoked the greater concerns and uncertainties with regard to TOPOFF were the series of containment measures that were undertaken to control the spread of the epidemic. . . .

> Early in the crisis, antibiotic prophylaxis and isolation of individual patients in hospitals were the primary epidemic containment measures. Less than one full day into the exercise, the epidemic was rapidly spreading — long before health authorities had sufficient time to characterize the common source of the outbreak, the rate of secondary transmission, the response to antibiotics, or the results of other containment measures. The unfolding situation precipitated a series of increasingly stringent containment measures. By the end of the first day, the Emergency Epidemic Response Committee issued a travel advisory that restricted travel in 16 Denver metropolitan counties. However, as one person noted, "the public was not [heeding] the voluntary travel advisory." Some people, in fact, were reported to have been racing out of the state. As part of the travel advisory, persons were advised to stay home unless they were close contacts of persons with diagnosed plague or were feeling sick; in the case of the latter, they were directed to seek medical care. As one observer noted, "They told one million people to stay in their homes. How would we have enforced this?" When asked what would be possible if the situation actually required it, the police and National Guard admitted to the Emergency Epidemic Response Committee that they would be unable to keep people at home. Another participant commented that, by the end of the exercise, "people had been asked to stay in their homes for 72 hours. . . . How were they supposed to get food or medicine?"

> . . . .

> When health officials were informed (by inject) on May 22 (5 days after the release of plague) that there were now more than 3000 persons with pneumonic plague, "it was not clear who they [the victims] were, where they lived, where they were exposed, how many of them were secondary cases.". . .

> The governor's Emergency Epidemic Response Committee, in consultation with the CDC, discussed issuing an executive order that would close the Colorado state borders and the Denver International Airport. Not all committee members agreed that the borders should or could be closed . . .

> Comments offered by one senior health participant summarized the implications and lessons of disease containment:

>> Many previous bioterrorism exercises dealt with non-contagious diseases. It is just beginning to dawn on us how dramatically different this was as the exercise ended. It terminated arbitrarily and

many issues were left unresolved. It is not clear what would have happened if it had gone on. . . . Competition between cities for the NPS has already broken out. It had all of the [characteristics] of an epidemic out of control.

*Id.* at 441–42.

**2.** For additional descriptions of the TOPOFF exercise and the lessons that may have been learned, see Thomas V. Inglesby, *Observations from the TOPOFF Exercise*, 116 PUB. HEALTH REP. 64 (Supp. 2 2001); Richard E. Hoffman & Jane E. Norton, *Lessons Learned From a Full-Scale Bioterrorism Exercise*, 6 EMERGING INFECTIOUS DISEASES 652 (2000).

Since the first TOPOFF, there have been several other simulated exercises, testing the ability of federal, state, and local public health agencies to respond collectively to a disaster — often demonstrating some of the same organizational and management problems encountered in the Colorado exercise. For one example, see Joint Center for Lessons Learned, *Smallpox Strikes Puerto Rico in Bioterrorism Exercise*, J. HOMELAND SECURITY (August 9, 2004) (*available at* www.homelandsecurity.org/journal/articles (last visited April 2005); *see also* a simulated smallpox attack on Oklahoma City, described at www.homelandsecurity.org/darkwinter (last visited April 2005).

According to that homeland security website, the Oklahoma exercise demonstrated five "learning points": biological weapons could threaten vital national security interests; current organizational structures are not well suited to managing a biological attack; there is no surge capacity in our health system; dealing with the media is critical; and should a contagious bioweapon pathogen be used, containing the spread of disease will present significant ethical, political, cultural, operational, and legal challenges.

TOPOFF 2 was held in May of 2003: a simulated release of the plague in Chicago. As of the Spring of 2005, plans were in place for "TOPOFF 3," a simulation of a smallpox outbreak in New Jersey and a chemical attack in Connecticut. *See* www.dhs.gov/dhs.public/ (last visited April 2006).

**3.** The Department of Homeland Security seems especially fond of running exercises like TOPOFF and involving the public health community in them. The primary rationale for such exercises is to "educate, train, or develop interorganizational and interjurisdictional relationships." As a committee of the Institute of Medicine has put it: ". . . having partnerships is preferable to working in isolation. Furthermore, some level of organization and coordination is essential to help avoid chaos; rehearsing processes may lead to smoother functioning of complex response systems, and in the event of an emergency, for example, a smallpox attack, having personnel that possess certain knowledge and skills (*e.g.*, smallpox diagnosis, vaccination, and search and containment) is better than having personnel that did not receive such education and training."

Nonetheless, the Committee concluded that although the assumptions underlying the utility of such exercises are reasonable, "The overall effectiveness of exercises as a preparedness strategy has not been well demonstrated, and research is needed to determine, for example, whether exercises could be considered predictors of successful response, what type of exercise would have the greatest positive influence on preparedness, what exercises are most cost-effective, and the best way to assess opportunity costs posed by conducting exercises." COMMITTEE ON SMALLPOX VACCINATION PROGRAM IMPLEMENTATION, INSTITUTE OF MEDICINE, THE SMALLPOX VACCINATION PROGRAM: PUBLIC HEALTH IN AN AGE OF TERRORISM 308-309 (2005).

## Joseph Barbera et al., *Large-Scale Quarantine Following Biological Terrorism in the United States*
### 286 JAMA 2711 (2001)

\* \* \*

Throughout history, medical and public health personnel have contended with epidemics. . . . Historically, quarantine was a recognized public health tool used to manage some infectious disease outbreaks, from the plague epidemic in the 13th century to the influenza epidemics of the 20th century. During the past century in the United States, professional medical and public health familiarity with the practice of quarantine has faded. . . . Despite this lack of modern operational experience local, state, or federal incident managers commonly propose or have called for quarantine in the early or advanced stages of bioterrorism exercises. . . . A striking example of the inclination to resort to quarantine was demonstrated during a recent federally sponsored national terrorism exercise, TOPOFF 2000. . . .

Given the rising concerns about the threat of bioterrorism and the concomitant renewed consideration of quarantine as a possible public health response to epidemics, it is important that the implications of quarantine in the modern context be carefully analyzed.

## QUARANTINE v. ISOLATION

. . . In the historical context, quarantine was defined as detention and enforced segregation of persons suspected to be carrying a contagious disease. Travelers or voyagers were sometimes subjected to quarantine before they were permitted to enter a country or town and mix with the inhabitants. . . .

Unfortunately, during modern bioterrorism response exercises, this term has been used broadly and confusingly to include a variety of public health disease containment measures, including travel limitations, restrictions on public gatherings, and isolation of sick individuals to prevent the spread of disease. The authors believe that it is most appropriate to use quarantine to refer to compulsory physical separation, including restriction of movement, of populations or groups of healthy people who have been potentially exposed to a contagious disease, or to efforts to segregate these persons within specified geographic areas. . . . We use the term isolation to denote the separation and confinement of individuals known or suspected . . . to be infected with a contagious disease to prevent them from transmitting disease to others. . . .

## LEGISLATIVE FRAMEWORK FOR DISEASE CONTAINMENT

[The article then discusses the distribution of responsibilities between local and state government and the general inadequacy of local and state legislation concerning quarantine.]

The federal government has the authority to enact quarantine when presented with the risk of transmission of infectious disease across state lines. . . . [T]he CDC is the federal agency authorized to manage federal quarantine actions. The implementation apparatus for such an order could involve other agencies. . . . The federal government may also assert supremacy in managing specific intrastate incidents if so requested by that state's authorities or if it is believed that local efforts are inadequate. . . .

For travelers seeking to enter the United States, the CDC has the authority to enact quarantine. . . . While rarely used, detention of arriving individuals, including U.S. citizens, is authorized to prevent the entry of specified communicable disease into the United States.

Currently, federal law authorizes cooperative efforts between the federal government and the state relating to planning, training, and prevention of disease epidemics and other health emergencies. Despite this, lines of authority between federal and state/local jurisdictions have not been sufficiently tested to ensure that all essential parties have clear understanding of the boundaries and interface between these potentially conflicting authorities. In a large-scale or rapidly evolving natural or deliberate biological incident, confusion and conflict in this public health authority may result. . . .

. . . .

## KEY CONSIDERATIONS IN QUARANTINE DECISIONS

In most infectious disease outbreak scenarios, there are alternatives to large-scale quarantine that may be more medically defensible, more likely to effectively contain the spread of the disease, less challenging to implement, and less likely to generate unintended adverse consequences. Decisions to invoke quarantine, therefore, should be made only after careful consideration of 3 major questions. . . .

### 1. Do Public Health and Medical Analyses Warrant the Imposition of Large-Scale Quarantine?

Decision makers must consider whether large-scale quarantine implementation at the time of discovery of a disease outbreak has a reasonable scientific chance of substantially diminishing the spread of disease. There is no valid public health or scientific justification for any type of quarantine in the setting of disease outbreaks with low or no person-to-person transmission, such as anthrax. Despite this, quarantine has been invoked in anthrax bioterrorism hoaxes in recent years. Among the many diseases that are termed contagious, only a limited number could pose a serious risk of widespread person-to-person transmission. Of these contagious diseases with potential for widespread person-to-person transmission, only a limited number confer sufficient risk of serious illness or death to justify consideration of sequestration of large groups or geographic areas. In addition to the agent characteristics, available treatment and prophylaxis options also create the context for the decision process. Public health responses must be accurately tailored to meet the specific risks and resource needs imposed by individual agents.

There are imaginable contexts in which a large-scale smallpox outbreak would generate a reasonable consideration for quarantine. But even in the setting of a bioterrorist attack with smallpox, the long incubation period almost ensures that some persons who were infected in the attack will have traveled great distances from the site of exposure before the disease is recognized or quarantine could be implemented. . . .

## 2. Are the Implementation and Maintenance of Large-Scale Quarantine Feasible?

Is there a plausible way to determine who should be quarantined? Are there practically available criteria for defining and identifying a group or a geographic area that is at higher risk of transmitting a dangerous disease? As noted, depending on the disease-specific incubation period and due to the mobility of modern society, it is probable that a population exposed to a biological weapon will have dispersed well beyond any easily definable geographic boundaries before the infection becomes manifest and any disease containment measures can be initiated. Even within a specific locale, it will be initially impossible to clearly define persons who have been exposed and, therefore, at risk of spreading the disease. A quarantine of a neighborhood would potentially miss exposed individuals, but a large-scale quarantine of a municipality could include many with no significant risk of disease. Currently proposed or functional health surveillance systems have not yet demonstrated adequate proficiency in rapid disease distribution analysis.

Are resources available to enforce the confinement? The human and material resources that would be required to enforce the confinement of large groups or persons, perhaps against their will, would likely be substantial, even in a modest-sized quarantine action. The behavioral reaction of law enforcement or military personnel charged with enforcing quarantine should also be considered. It is possible that fear of personal exposure or public reaction to enforcement actions may compromise police willingness to enforce compliance.

Can the quarantined group be confined for the duration during which they could transmit the disease? Quarantine will not be over quickly. The period during which confined persons could develop disease might be days or weeks, depending on the specific infectious agent. Development of illness among detainees could prolong the confinement of those remaining healthy. Resources and political resolve must be sufficient to sustain a quarantine of at least days, and probably weeks. Furthermore, the multiple needs of detainees must be addressed in a systematic and competent fashion. . . .

## 3. Do the Potential Benefits of Large-Scale Quarantine Outweigh the Possible Adverse Consequences?

. . . .

What are the health risks to those quarantined? . . . [T]here are U.S. historical examples in which persons with clear evidence of infection with a contagious disease have been quarantined together with persons with no evidence of infection. It is now beyond dispute that such measures would be unethical today, but a recent event illustrates that this ethical principle might still be disregarded or misunderstood [citing an incident in which an airplane full of passengers was isolated because one passenger had suspicious symptoms].

What are the consequences if the public declines to obey quarantine orders? It is not clear how those quarantined would react to being subjected to compulsory confinement. Civilian noncompliance with these public health efforts could compromise the action and even become violent. Historical quarantine incidents have generated organized civil disobedience and wholesale disregard for authority. . . . Some might lose confidence in government authorities and stop complying with other advised public health actions (*e.g.*, vaccination, antibiotic treatment) as well. The possibility also exists for development of civilian vigilantism to enforce quarantine. . . . The rules of engagement that police are expected to follow in enforcing quarantine must be explicitly determined and communicated in advance. Protection of police personnel and their families against infection would be essential to police cooperation.

What are the consequences of restricting commerce and transportation to and from the quarantined area? Halting commercial transactions and the movement of goods to and from quarantined areas will have significant economic effects that may be profound and long term and reach well beyond the quarantined area. Much modern business practice relies on just-in-time supply chains. Shortages of food, fuel, medicines and medical supplies, essential personnel, and social services (sanitation) should be anticipated and provisions must be in place to deal with such issues. Post-quarantine stigmatization of the geographic location and of the population quarantined should be anticipated.

## CONCLUSIONS AND RECOMMENDATIONS

. . .

The essential first step in developing any disease containment strategy is to determine if the disease is communicable. If not, then no consideration of quarantine should be pursued. If the disease of concern is contagious, then the specific mechanism of disease transmission must drive the disease containment strategy (*e.g.*, spread by cough at close distances or possibly over long range, as has occurred in smallpox outbreaks; or spread through person-to-person contact, as in Ebola outbreaks). Some progress in delineating disease containment strategies for bioterrorism-induced outbreaks has already occurred in the form of consensus public health and medical recommendations, though more diseases must be addressed and public health actions examined. Political leaders in particular need to understand that a single strategy for limiting the spread of all contagious diseases is not appropriate and will not work. The political consequences of public health actions such as large-scale quarantine must also be carefully examined and understood. Modern U.S. disaster response has consistently focused on assistance to those directly affected; in the case of bioterrorism, response will focus on both those potentially and actually infected. With implementation of quarantine, the perception may be that those potentially and actually infected have instead been secondarily harmed by response actions.

In an outbreak of a contagious disease, disease containment may be more effectively achieved using methods that do not attempt to contain large groups of people. As noted, persons with clinical or laboratory evidence demonstrating infection with a contagious disease should be isolated, separate from those who do not have clinical or laboratory evidence of that disease. Depending on the illness, this isolation may be primarily respiratory, body fluid, or skin contact isolation rather than full physical separation from all healthy people.

Additionally, population-based public health intervention strategies should also be considered. Depending on the context, rapid vaccination or treatment programs, widespread use of disposable masks (with instructions), short-term voluntary home curfew, restrictions on assembly of groups (*e.g.*, schools, entertainment sites) or closure of mass transportation (buses, airliners, trains, and subway systems) are disease containment steps that may have more scientific credibility and may be more likely to result in diminished disease spread, more practically achievable, and associated with less adverse consequences. For clarity, these alternative disease control measures should not be termed quarantine or quarantine actions.

. . .

During large-scale contagious disease outbreaks, decision makers would be critically dependent on the availability of timely, accurate information about what is happening and what interventions are desirable and feasible. Emergency management and public health officials will need real-time case data and the analytic capacity to determine the epidemiological parameters of the outbreak to make the most appropriate disease containment decisions. Clinicians will seek information about the natural history and clinical management of the illness and ongoing analyses of the efficacy of treatment strategies. Rapid communication between the medical and public health communities may be especially important and in most locales is currently not conveyed by electronic means or though routine, well-exercised channels.

. . .

Positive incentives may help to persuade the public to take actions that promote disease containment. The ready provision of adequate medical expertise, appropriate vaccines or antibiotics, or distribution of disposable face masks to the public in specific circumstances are examples of incentives that may positively influence population behavior to promote disease containment. Allowing family members to voluntarily place themselves at some defined, calculated risk of infection to care for their sick loved ones might encourage participation in a community's overall disease containment strategy. . . .

. . .

The development of strategies for communicating with the public throughout a disease outbreak is of paramount importance. . . . Once public credibility is lost, it will be difficult or impossible to recover. A well-informed public that perceives health officials as knowledgeable and reliable is more likely to volunteer to comply with actions recommended to diminish the spread of the disease. Effective information dissemination would work to suppress rumors and anxiety and enlist community support.

It is clear that public health strategies for the control of potential epidemics need to be carefully reevaluated. This process should ensure that civil rights and liberties are kept at the forefront of all discussions. . . . Further delineation of the authority to impose quarantine is required, and the political and psychological implications must be addressed. Given the complex multidisciplinary nature of the problem, further analysis of possible disease containment strategies would ideally include experts from the fields of medicine, public health, emergency management, law, ethics, and public communication. . . .

*  *  *

## NOTES AND QUESTIONS

**1.** The threat of a fast-spreading infectious disease, whether introduced by terrorists or by Mother Nature, presents unique problems that will be measured not only in terms of the immediate impact — widespread illness and death — but in terms of long-term social and economic consequences. A fast-spreading disease would quickly exhaust local first-aid and medical resources, and, possibly, even the food and water supply. People would stop reporting to work (and some of those people would have first-response and medical responsibilities). The state and the federal governments may act to support local efforts, but even their resources may be at best only able to contain the spread of the disease. Scenarios involving hundreds or even thousands of casualties are imaginable.

What would happen then? The result might be a loss of confidence in the ability of the government to govern, possibly even a loss of respect for the rule of law. Most Americans have ambivalent feelings about "big government" intervention, but most Americans also have lived their lives in a world in which they could confidently assume that their government, big or otherwise, could maintain order and resolve virtually any widespread problem. For them, an unchecked epidemic disease would be a unique and potentially unsettling experience.

**2.** As several of the articles excerpted in this chapter argue, Americans need to increase their level of preparation for what appears to be the inevitable: either a naturally created, fast-moving outbreak of an infectious disease, or the release by terrorists of some comparable biological threat. Indeed, "preparedness" seems to be the new buzz word of public health policymaking. But what exactly do we have to do to be *prepared*? Part of the answer may simply be to educate ourselves and overcome the "it can't happen here" complacency that many Americans seem to exhibit, or at least exhibited until the fall of 2001. Other suggestions are more concrete:

— more and more coordinated laboratories to identify diseases and biological agents better and quicker;

— more and better trained staff for state and local health departments;

— better (and more sophisticated) communication among local, state, and federal agencies, between government agencies and private health care providers, and between private providers — even those who normally compete for the same health care business and don't like to talk freely to each other;

— better communication between public health agencies and the mass media;

— better education of private health care workers as to what to do (*e.g.,* identify and report signs of contagious diseases) and what *not* to do (*e.g.,* prescribe antibiotics to patients who are worried about future terrorist attacks).

There has been only some improvement in public health preparedness since 9/11, mostly in the areas of communications, response plans and staff training. National Association of County and City Health Officers, *The Impact of Federal Funding on Local Bioterrorism Preparedness,* RESEARCH BRIEF, Issue 5, No.9 (April 2004). For a more recent assessment of bioterrorism preparedness and public health agencies, see http://healthyamericans.org/state/bioterror/ (last visited August 2006).

All of the "preparedness" recommendations, of course, apply to the public health system generally and not just to that portion of the public health infrastructure that is designed to respond to bioterrorism or the outbreak of an epidemic disease. All of these recommendations also sound like good ideas. But how do we make these things happen? Just dedicate more money to these sorts of activities? Increase federal oversight of state and local public health agencies? Create independent private organizations to assess our preparedness and any future progress? Do we need a "super-agency" or a "bioterrorist czar"?

More basically, why haven't these problems been fixed already? After all, none of these recommendations is anything more than common sense. Who has failed: our leaders, our policymakers, or all of us who select and support them?

**3.** The Stafford Disaster Assistance and Emergency Relief Act provides for federal assistance to the states in the cases of natural emergencies and disasters, as in the case of floods or hurricanes. *See* 42 U.S.C. § 5121 *et seq.* Note, however, that Stafford Act assistance is not available in the case of biological or disease-related disasters or emergencies.

Apart from the Stafford Act authority, several federal agencies have statutory authority to act in public health and related emergencies, including the Department of Health and Human Services, the Department of Defense and the Department of the Interior, all generally coordinated through the Department of Homeland Security created in 2002.

As described in the notes to Section D *supra*, there are several documents outlining the responsibilities of these federal agencies in the event of a pandemic outbreak or other large, fast-moving biological event. The plan excerpted in Section D is only one example. The NATIONAL RESPONSE PLAN (NRP) adopted by the Bush Administration in 2005 attempts to specify which agencies will have what responsibilities, how decisions within and across agencies will be made, and the factors that will determine how and when federal resources will be allocated in a wide range of emergencies. For its full text, see www/dhs.gov/dhs/public/ (last visited April 2006); see also the NATIONAL INCIDENT MANAGEMENT SYSTEM (NIMS) describing the structural arrangements among the various agencies that may respond to these types of emergencies.

While these "master plans" and, especially, the NRP, represent a great deal of work and decision making, what exactly are they? Are they enforceable? Do they carry any legal significance or are they merely a kind of public pronouncement? Is any agency or any person really bound to act in accordance with these plans? One possible suggestion is that they are more of a process than a set of rules: They may provide the vehicle through which various state and federal officials and their staffs interact and, on a provisional basis, create a decision making framework in the expectation that they will be able to communicate better and more effectively when the next disaster arrives.

For a good discussion of the need for such administrative arrangements (and the problems that they are attempting to mitigate), see the evaluation of the response to Hurricane Katrina at www.whitehouse.gov/reports/katrina-lessons-learned (last visited August 2006).

**4.** An event with consequences like those of a "bioterrorist attack" need not, of course, come from sources outside of the United States or, for that matter, necessarily be an intentional attack. The release of a fast-spreading infectious disease could be accidental or due to the careless practices of otherwise legitimate researchers. For one discussion of the likelihood of such an event, see NATIONAL RESEARCH COUNCIL, NATIONAL ACADEMIES, BIOTECHNOLOGY RESEARCH IN AN AGE OF TERRORISM 17–29 (2004) (available online at http://newton.nap.edu/catalog/10827.html (last visited August 2006).

## 2. Planning for Public Health Emergencies: Legal Aspects

### CENTER FOR LAW AND PUBLIC HEALTH, MODEL STATE EMERGENCY HEALTH POWERS ACT
#### (2001)

[Note that the authors of the Act, led by Professor Larry Gostin, have published three major versions of this Act, the first dated October 23, 2001, the second dated December 21, 2001, and the third prepared as a "Model State Public Health Act" as part of their TurningPoint exercise, dated September, 2003; the portions reprinted here are from the December 21, 2001 version]

\* \* \*

**ARTICLE I. TITLE, FINDINGS, PURPOSES, AND DEFINITIONS**

. . .

Section 103. **Purposes.** . . .

(a) To require the development of a comprehensive plan to provide for a coordinated, appropriate response in the event of a public health emergency . . .

. . . .

## Section 104. **Definitions.**

. . . .

(m) A "**public health emergency**" is an occurrence of imminent threat of an illness or health condition that:

(1) is believed to be caused by any of the following:

    (i)   bioterrorism;

    (ii)  the appearance of a novel or previously controlled or eradicated infectious agent or biological toxin;

    (iii) [*a natural disaster*;]

    (iv) [*a chemical attack or accidental release*; *or*]

    (v) [*a nuclear attack or accident*]; and

(2) poses a high probability of any of the following harms:

    (i)   a large number of deaths in the affected population;

    (ii)  a large number of serious or long-term disabilities in the affected population; or

    (iii) widespread exposure to an infectious or toxic agent that poses significant risk of substantial future harm to a large number of people in the affected population.

\* \* \*

## ARTICLE II. PLANNING FOR A PUBLIC HEALTH EMERGENCY

## Section 201. **Public Health Emergency Planning Commission.**

The Governor shall appoint a Public Health Emergency Planning Commission ("the Commission"), consisting of the State directors, or their designees, of agencies the Governor deems relevant to public health emergency preparedness, a representative group of state legislators, members of the judiciary, and any other persons chosen by the Governor. The Governor shall also designate the chair of the Commission.

. . . .

## Section 202. **Public Health Emergency Plan**

(a) The Commission shall, within six months of its appointment, deliver to the Governor a plan for responding to a public health emergency, that includes provisions or guidelines on the following: (1) Notifying and communicating with the population during a state of public health emergency in compliance with this Act; (2) Central coordination of resources, manpower, and services, including coordination of responses by State, local, tribal, and federal agencies; (3) The location, procurement, storage, transportation, maintenance, and distribution of essential materials, including but not limited to medical supplies, drugs, vaccines, food, shelter, clothing and beds; (4) Compliance with the reporting requirements in Section 301; (5) The continued, effective operation of the judicial system including, if deemed necessary, the identification and training of personnel to serve as emergency judges regarding matters of isolation and quarantine as described in this Act; (6) The method of evacuating populations, and housing and feeding the evacuated populations; (7) The identification and training of health care providers to diagnose and treat persons with infectious diseases; (8) The vaccination of persons, in compliance with the provisions of this Act; (9) The treatment of persons who have been exposed to or who are infected with diseases or health conditions that may be the cause of a public health emergency; (10) The safe disposal of infectious wastes and human remains in compliance with the provisions of this Act; (11) The safe and effective control of persons isolated, quarantined, vaccinated, tested, or treated during a state of public health emergency; (12) Tracking the source and outcomes of infected persons; (13) Ensuring that each city and county within the State identifies the following:

> (i) sites where persons can be isolated or quarantined in compliance with the conditions and principles for isolation or quarantine of this Act; (ii) sites where medical supplies, food, and other essentials can be distributed to the population; (iii) sites where public health and emergency workers can be housed and fed; and (iv) routes and means of transportation of people and materials. . . .

> . . . .

## ARTICLE III. MEASURES TO DETECT AND TRACK PUBLIC HEALTH EMERGENCIES

## Section 301. **Reporting.**

. . . A health care provider, coroner, or medical examiner shall report all cases of persons who harbor any illness or health condition that may be potential causes of a public health emergency. Reportable illnesses and health conditions include, but are not limited to, the diseases caused by the biological agents listed in 42 C.F.R. § 72, app. A (2000) and any illnesses or health conditions identified by the public health authority. . . . In addition to the foregoing requirements for health care providers, a pharmacist shall report any unusual or increased prescription rates, unusual types of prescriptions, or unusual trends in pharmacy visits that may be potential causes of a public health emergency . . .

> . . . .

## Section 303. **Information sharing.**

. . . Whenever the public safety authority or other state or local government agency learns of a case of a reportable illness or health condition, an unusual cluster, or a suspicious event that may be the cause of a public health emergency, it shall immediately notify the public health authority.

  . . .

## ARTICLE IV. DECLARING A STATE OF PUBLIC HEALTH EMERGENCY

### Section 401. **Declaration.**

A state of public health emergency may be declared by the Governor upon the occurrence of a "public health emergency". . . . Prior to such a declaration, the Governor shall consult with the public health authority and may consult with any additional public health or other experts as needed. The Governor may act to declare a public health emergency without consulting with the public health authority or other experts when the situation calls for prompt and timely action.

### Section 402. **Content and Declaration.**

A state of public health emergency shall be declared by an executive order that specifies: (a) the nature of the public health emergency, (b) the political subdivision(s) or geographic area(s) subject to the declaration, (c) the conditions that have brought about the public health emergency, (d) the duration of the state of the public health emergency, if less than thirty (30) days, and (e) the primary public health authority responding to the emergency.

### Section 403. **Effect of Declaration.**

The declaration of a state of public health emergency shall activate the disaster response and recovery aspects of the State, local, and inter-jurisdictional disaster emergency plans in the affected political subdivision(s) or geographic area(s) . . .

  . . .

. . . The public health authority shall have primary jurisdiction, responsibility, and authority for: (1) Planning and executing public health emergency assessment, mitigation, preparedness response, and recovery for the State; (2) Coordinating public health emergency response between State and local authorities; (3) Collaborating with relevant federal government authorities, elected officials of other states, private organizations or companies; (4) Coordinating recovery operations and mitigation initiatives subsequent to public health emergencies; and (5) Organizing public information activities regarding public health emergency response operations.

After the declaration of a state of public health emergency, special identification for all public health personnel working during the emergency shall be issued as soon as possible. The identification shall indicate the authority of the bearer to exercise public health functions and emergency powers during the state of public health emergency. Public health personnel shall wear the identification in plain view.

. . . .

## Section 404. Enforcement.

During a state of public health emergency, the public health authority may request assistance in enforcing orders pursuant to this Act from the public safety authority. The public safety authority may request assistance from the organized militia in enforcing the orders of the public health authority.

. . . .

. . .

## ARTICLE V. SPECIAL POWERS DURING A STATE OF PUBLIC HEALTH EMERGENCY: MANAGEMENT OF PROPERTY

## Section 501. Emergency measures concerning facilities and materials.

The public health authority may exercise, for such period as the state of public health emergency exists, the following powers over facilities or materials: (a) To close, direct and compel the evacuation of, or to decontaminate or cause to be decontaminated any facility of which there is reasonable cause to believe that it may endanger the public health. (b) To decontaminate or cause to be decontaminated, or destroy any material of which there is reasonable cause to believe that it may endanger the public health.

. . . .

## Section 502. Access to and control of facilities and property — generally.

The public health authority may exercise, for such period as the state of public health emergency exists, the following powers concering facilities, materials, roads, or public areas: (a) To procure, by condemnation or otherwise, construct, lease, transport, store, maintain, renovate, or distribute materials and facilities as may be reasonable and necessary to respond to the public health emergency, with the right to take immediate possession thereof. Such materials and facilities include, but are not limited to, communication devices, carriers, real estate, fuels, food, and clothing. (b) To require a health care facility to provide services or the use of its facility if such services or use are reasonable and necessary to respond to the public health emergency as a condition of licensure, authorization or the ability to continue doing business in the state as a health care facility. The use of the health care facility may include transferring the management and supervision of the health care facility to the public health authority for a limited or unlimited period of time, but shall not exceed the termination of the declaration of a state of public health emergency. (c) To inspect, control, restrict, and regulate by rationing and using quotas, prohibitions on shipments, allocation, or other means, the use, sale, dispensing, distribution, or transportation of food, fuel, clothing and other commodities, as may be reasonable and necessary to respond to the public health emergency. . . .

. . . .

## Section 505. **Control of health care supplies.**

. . . .

During a state of public health emergency, the public health authority may procure, store, or distribute any anti-toxins, serums, vaccines, immunizing agents, antibiotics, and other pharmaceutical agents or medical supplies located within the State as may be reasonable and necessary to respond to the public health emergency, with the right to take immediate possession thereof. . . .

. . . .

## ARTICLE VI. SPECIAL POWERS DURING A STATE OF PUBLIC HEALTH EMERGENCY: PROTECTION OF PERSONS

## Section 601. **Protection of persons.**

During a state of public health emergency, the public health authority shall use every available means to prevent the transmission of infectious disease and to ensure that all cases of contagious disease are subject to proper control and treatment.

. . . .

## Section 602. **Medical examination and testing.**

During a state of public health emergency the public health authority may perform physical examinations and/or tests as necessary for the diagnosis or treatment of individuals. (a) Medical examinations or tests may be performed by any qualified person authorized to do so by the public health authority. (b) Medical examinations or tests must not be such as are reasonably likely to lead to serious harm to the affected individual. (c) The public health authority may isolate or quarantine, pursuant to Section 604, any person whose refusal of medical examination or testing results in uncertainty regarding whether he or she has been exposed to or is infected with a contagious or possibly contagious disease or otherwise poses a danger to public health.

. . . .

## Section 603. **Vaccination and treatment.**

During a state of public health emergency the public health authority may exercise the following emergency powers over persons as necessary to address the public health emergency: (a) To vaccinate persons as protection against infectious disease and to prevent the spread of contagious or possibly contagious disease. Vaccination may be performed by any qualified person authorized to do so by the public health authority. A vaccine to be administered must not be such as is reasonably likely to lead to serious harm to the affected individual. To prevent the spread of contagious or possibly contagious disease the public health authority may isolate or quarantine, pursuant to Section 604, persons who are unable or unwilling for reasons of health, religion, or conscience to undergo vaccination pursuant to this Section. (b) To treat persons exposed to or infected with disease. Treatment may be administered by any qualified person authorized to do so by the public health authority. Treatment must not be such as is reasonably likely to lead to serious harm to the affected individual. To prevent the spread of contagious or possibly contagious disease the public health authority may isolate or quarantine, pursuant to Section 604, persons who are unable or unwilling for reasons of health, religion, or conscience to undergo treatment pursuant to this Section.

. . . .

## Section 604. **Isolation and quarantine.**

(a) During the public health emergency, the public health authority may isolate or quarantine an individual or groups of individuals. This includes individuals or groups who have not been vaccinated, treated, tested, or examined pursuant to Sections 602 and 603. The public health authority may also establish and maintain places of isolation and quarantine, and set rules and make orders. Failure to obey these rules, orders, or provisions shall constitute a misdemeanor. (b) The public health authority shall adhere to the following conditions and principles when isolating or quarantining individuals or groups of individuals:

(1) Isolation and quarantine must be by the least restrictive means necessary to prevent the spread of a contagious or possibly contagious disease to others and may include, but are not limited to, confinement to private homes or other private and public premises.

(2) Isolated individuals must be confined separately from quarantined individuals.

(3) The health status of isolated and quarantined individuals must be monitored regularly to determine if they require isolation or quarantine.

(4) If a quarantined individual subsequently becomes infected or is reasonably believed to have become infected with a contagious or possibly contagious disease he or she must promptly be removed to isolation.

(5) Isolated and quarantined individuals must be immediately released when they pose no substantial risk of transmitting a contagious or possibly contagious disease to others.

(6) The needs of persons isolated and quarantined shall be addressed in a systematic and competent fashion, including, but not limited to, providing adequate food, clothing, shelter, means of communication with those in isolation or quarantine and outside these settings, medication, and competent medical care.

(7) Premises used for isolation and quarantine shall be maintained in a safe and hygienic manner and be designed to minimize the likelihood of further transmission of infection or other harms to persons isolated and quarantined.

(8) To the extent possible, cultural and religious beliefs should be considered in addressing the needs of individuals, and establishing and maintaining isolation and quarantine premises.

Persons subject to isolation or quarantine shall obey the public health authority's rules and orders; and shall not go beyond the isolation or quarantine premises. Failure to obey these provisions shall constitute a misdemeanor. . . .

## Section 605. **Procedures for isolation and quarantine.**

. . . .

(a) The public health authority may temporarily isolate or quarantine an individual or groups of individuals through a written directive if delay in imposing the isolation or quarantine would significantly jeopardize the public health authority's ability to prevent or limit the transmission of a contagious or possibly contagious disease to othe rs. The written directive shall specify the following: (i) the identity of the individual(s) or groups of individuals subject to isolation or quarantine; (ii) the premises subject to isolation or quarantine; (iii) the date and time at which isolation or quarantine commences; (iv) the suspected contagious disease if known. . . . A copy of the written directive shall be given to the individual to be isolated or quarantined or, if the order applies to a group of individuals and it is impractical to provide individual copies, it may be posted in a conspicuous place in the isolation or quarantine premises. Within ten (10) days after issuing the written directive, the public health authority shall file a petition pursuant to Section 605(b) for a court order authorizing the continued isolation or quarantine of the isolated or quarantined individual or groups of individuals.

(b) The public health authority may make a written petition to the trial court for an order authorizing the isolation or quarantine of an individual or groups of individuals. A petition shall specify the following: (i) the identity of the individual(s) or groups of individuals subject to isolation or quarantine; (ii) the premises subject to isolation or quarantine; (iii) the date and time at which isolation or quarantine commences; (iv) the suspected contagious disease if known; (v) a statement of compliance with the conditions and principles for isolation and quarantine of Section 604(b); and (vi) a statement of the basis upon which isolation or quarantine is justified in compliance with this Article. . . . Notice to the individuals or groups of individuals identified in the petition shall be accomplished within twenty-four (24) hours in accordance with the rules of civil procedure. A hearing must be held on any petition filed pursuant to this subsection within five (5) days of filing of the petition. In extraordinary circumstances and for good cause shown the public health authority may apply to continue the hearing date on a petition filed pursuant to this Section for up to ten (10) days, which continuance the court may grant in its discretion giving due regard to the rights of the affected individuals, the protection of the public's health, the severity of the emergency and the availability of necessary witnesses and evidence. The court shall grant the petition if, by a preponderance of the evidence, isolation or quarantine is shown to be reasonably necessary to prevent or limit the transmission of a contagious or possibly contagious disease to others. An order authorizing isolation or quarantine may do so for a period not to exceed thirty (30) days. The order shall (a) identify the isolated or quarantined individuals or groups of individuals by name or shared or similar characteristics or circumstances; (b) specify factual findings warranting isolation or quarantine pursuant to this Act; (c) include any conditions necessary to ensure that isolation or quarantine is carried out within the stated purposes and restrictions of this Act; and (d) be served on affected individuals or groups of individuals in accordance with the rules of civil procedure. . . .

An individual or group of individuals isolated or quarantined pursuant to this Act may apply to the trial court for an order to show cause why the individual or group of individuals should not be released. The court shall rule on the application to show cause within forty-eight (48) hours of its filing. If the court grants the application, the court shall schedule a hearing on the order to show cause within twenty-four (24) hours from issuance of the order to show cause. The issuance of an order to show cause shall not stay or enjoin an isolation or quarantine order. An individual or groups of individuals isolated or quarantined pursuant to this Act may request a hearing in the trial court for remedies regarding breaches to the conditions of isolation or quarantine. . . .

In any proceedings brought for relief under this subsection, in extraordinary circumstances and for good cause shown, the public health authority may move the court to extend the time for a hearing, which extension the court in its discretion may grant giving due regard to the rights of the affected individuals, the protection of the public's health, the severity of the emergency and the availability of necessary witnesses and evidence.

A record of the proceedings pursuant to this Section shall be made and retained. In the event that, given a state of public health emergency, parties can not personally appear before the court, proceedings may be conducted by their authorized representatives and be held via any means that allows all parties to fully participate.

The court shall appoint counsel at state expense to represent individuals or groups of individuals who are or who are about to be isolated or quarantined pursuant to the provisions of this Act and who are not otherwise represented by counsel. . . .

In any proceedings brought pursuant to this Section, to promote the fair and efficient operation of justice and having given due regard to the rights of the affected individuals, the protection of the public's health, the severity of the emergency and the availability of necessary witnesses and evidence, the court may order the consolidation of individual claims into group or claims [sic] where: (i) the number of individuals involved or to be affected is so large as to render individual participation impractical; (ii) there are questions of law or fact common to the individual claims or rights to be determined; (iii) the group claims or rights to be determined are typical of the affected individuals' claims or rights; and (iv) the entire group will be adequately represented in the consolidation.

. . . .

## Section 608. **Licensing and appointment of health personnel.**

The public health authority may exercise, for such period as the state of public health emergency exists, the following emergency powers regarding licensing and appointment of health personnel: (a) To require in-state health care providers to assist in the performance of vaccination, treatment, examination, or testing of any individual as a condition of licensure, authorization, or the ability to continue to function as a health care provider in this State. (b) To appoint and prescribe the duties of such out-of-state emergency health care providers as may be reasonable and necessary to respond to the public health emergency. . . . Any out-of-state emergency health care provider appointed pursuant to this Section shall not be held liable for any civil damages as a result of medical care or treatment related to the response to the public health emergency unless such damages result from providing, or failing to provide, medical care or treatment under circumstances demonstrating a reckless disregard for the consequences so as to affect the life or health of the patient. . . .

. . . .

## ARTICLE VIII. MISCELLANEOUS

. . . .

## Section 804. **Liability.**

Neither the State, its political subdivisions, nor, except in cases of gross negligence or willful misconduct, the Governor, the public health authority, or any other State or local official referenced in this Act, is liable for the death of or any injury to persons, or damage to property, as a result of complying with or attempting to comply with this Act or any rule or regulations promulgated pursuant to this Act during a state of public health emergency.

. . . .

During a state of public health emergency, any private person, firm or corporation and employees and agents of such person, firm or corporation in the performance of a contract with, and under the direction of, the State or its political subdivisions under the provisions of this Act shall not be civilly liable for causing the death of, or injury to, any person or damage to any property except in the event of gross negligence or willful misconduct.

. . . .

\* \* \*

## Kenneth R. Wing, *Policy Choices and Model Acts: Preparing for the Next Public Health Emergency*
13 HEALTH MATRIX 71 (2003)

\* \* \*

Let me start with some unkind comments about "model acts" and their drafters. Circulating a "model act" is the most cumbersome and ineffective way I can think of to inform the general public or state policymakers concerning important policy choices. If in fact the Center's experts or the CDC or anyone else has a clear vision of what needs to be done by the various states to prepare for the next public health emergency, they should say so — as clearly and specifically as possible — and provide the rest of us with a descriptive explanation of that vision and some insightful defense of the necessity and feasibility of achieving it. . . . If and when a state wants to adopt the Center's recommmendations, surely someone will have to convert those policy choices into statutory terms. That's what statute drafting is all about: It's a technical and instrumental job, but it's one that ought to follow — not precede — the more fundamental task of deciding what that statute ought to say. For that matter, even if a state decides to do any or all of what the Center has proposed, just how to draft appropriate legislation to implement that choice will depend greatly upon the pre-existing legal structure of that particular state, something that varies from jurisdiction to jurisdiction. A one-size-fits-all "model act" would be of marginal value even for this purpose. More importantly, a "model act" is of virtually no value in doing what really needs to be done now: informing our state policymakers of the choices they should consider and the merits of the alternatives that face them.

But even to the extent that I can figure out what is proposed by the "model act" or how such measures might work . . . I'm not impressed with either the authors' ideas or their craftsmanship. As I decode the December [2001] draft, there are three major elements of the "model act": First, the "model act" would create what the authors' call an emergency planning commission. Second, the act would require the reporting of various indicia of infectious diseases and other public health risks by health care providers; and it would create a "public health authority" empowered to investigate these reports and other potential causes of a public health emergency. Third, the "model act" would specify those circumstances under which the governor may declare a public health emergency and it would create a series of extraordinary powers concerning the public use of private property and the confinement of individuals during such an emergency. . . .

The emergency planning commission is described by Article II of the "model act" as a commission of legislators, judges, local public health officials, and other "interested persons" appointed by the governor who are empowered to write a "public health emergency plan," essentially a description of how the federal, state, and local governments will react and share authority in a public health emergency. It is hard to evaluate or critique this proposal without knowing more specifically what its authors have in mind. . . . If the objective of Article II is that the state should empanel — as states so often do — still another study commission or advisory body, it seems unnecessary to include this commission in an already cumbersome legislative package. I would argue that it is also inappropriate: Study commissions are hardly an efficient or expeditious vehicle for making important and difficult decisions. The December draft has a nonexclusive list of 15 categories of issues that the commission is required to address within a six month-time frame. Why create a study commission for this particular set of choices, leaving these choices to be reconsidered within the state legislature once the commission has completed its study? Why *now,* when common sense and recent events would dictate that speed is of the political essence?

On the other hand, if Article II of the "model act" is proposing a regulatory agency or that any of the commission's decisions would be binding, it is indeed an extraordinary proposal: Create a new governmental agency with members drawn from the various branches of government and include both local officials and "other interested persons." Give that body policymaking authority with minimal statutory limits on its scope. That's heady stuff. I can speculate that this agency would do lots of things — both good and bad — but again I return to essentially the same questions: What does the Center think this agency can and will do and why do they think it will do so better than the normal lawmaking apparatus of the states? It's nice to be original — but why? Why this sort of commission and to what end? . . .

I also know that if a state were to create the type of commission suggested by the "model act" and give it binding regulatory authority, there would be serious constitutional objections to such legislation. The principles of separation of powers impose limits on the legislature's ability (a) to delegate legislative-type decisions to independent agencies, and (b) to give any authority to a governmental body made up of members of a mix of judicial, legislative, and executive actors. For that matter, no state law can authorize a commission to exercise binding authority over what the federal government can do, which is among the things that the "model act" empowers the commission to address. . . .

Article III requires that health care providers (and coroners and medical examiners) report "all cases of persons who harbor any illness or health condition that may be potential causes of a public health emergency" to a [designated] state agency within 24 hours." Pharmacists are similarly required to report any unusual or increased use of prescription drugs that may indicate a public health emergency. (Veterinarians, live stock owners, and others have similar obligations with regard to animal diseases.) The information requirements are extensive: providers are required to report the name, address, medical condition, location, and essentially any other information that is considered relevant to the "potential cause of a public health emergency."

The public health authority (described in Article I of the "model act" as some designated state or local agency) is charged with the authority to investigate these reports, track individuals, and, if I am reading the "model act" correctly, "ensure that they are subject to proper control measures. . . ."

I have no doubt that all states need to collect and analyze data on infectious diseases and other public health risks quickly and effectively. I also have no doubt that the states should structure and empower some agency to respond to identified public health risks. Indeed, all states do so in one way or another. My questions concerning the reporting requirements, the public health authority, and the broad investigational powers that would be created under the "model act," however, are not unlike those outlined above: Why should a state create such an extensive system of reporting and in this particular manner? Anyone familiar with the experience of tracking AIDS and HIV exposure knows that mandatory disclosure of individual-identifying data can be counterproductive (not to mention politically volatile). . . . The extent of the power of the public authority to investigate these reports is not clear from the "model act" but, as written, it is virtually without limit. As such, it is notable — and somewhat ironic — that there are no provisions for the protection of confidentiality or privacy written into the statute although, in a later article of the "model act," the authors have had the foresight to immunize public officials from liability for exceeding their powers.

More to the point, is there any evidence — from the events of September 11, 2001, or otherwise — that suggests such laws should be in place? Are state or local agencies even equipped to handle this volume of information? What would be the impact on the behavior of people seeking medical attention? Again, interesting ideas are interesting ideas, but a proposed solution to a problem — let alone a "model act" — has to be tied to some assessment of the problem and its underlying causes. Why enact this type of legislation at this time? Many states have enacted comparable regulatory requirements but in much more limited circumstances — reporting of gun shot wounds for instance — and under much more carefully prescribed limits on the government's investigational response. Even those programs are controversial. State and local public health agencies have long struggled to maintain a user-friendly public image and a posture that emphasizes their public health — not their public safety character. The public health authority created by the "model act" would permanently obliterate that distinction. . . .

Article IV of the "model act" authorizes the governor to declare a "state of public health emergency." It specifies the power of the state legislature to terminate the state of emergency after sixty days (premised on certain legislative findings). In Articles V and VI the extraordinary powers that can be exercised by the state during a declared public health emergency are described. . . . But even apart from the concerns I have with the extent of the emergency powers envisioned by the authors of the "model act," I have a more basic constitutional concern with Article IV.

Under the constitutional structure in most states, the governor, as the chief executive, has inherent powers to act in an emergency, apart from any gubernatorial powers that may be created by the state's statutes. The exact limits on the governor's emergency powers are not clear, as, by their nature, they are infrequently exercised and litigated.

. . . .

. . . [T]he "model act" — by defining what can be done by whom and under what circumstances — would necessarily limit the authority of the governor to act in any ways other than those set out in that legislation. If I were in the governor's office, or even just concerned about the integrity of that office, I would be opposed to such a proscriptive effort — especially one in an area of such immediate concern. Among other concerns, would I want the scope of my authority in a public health emergency to be limited to that which is the end-product of a legislative debate? Politics being politics, isn't it just as likely that that legislation will be influenced by people who want to tie the governor's hands — possibly for reasons wholly unrelated to public health emergencies? More to the point, the next public health emergency may involve nuclear exposure or some result of Mother Nature's, not some bioterrorist's, wrath. A statute drawn in anticipation of the most recent public health emergency may actually inhibit the discretion of the governor to act in another unanticipated fashion. The fact that what happens next may be what no one has anticipated is, after all, undeniably part of our post-September 11, 2001, world.

. . . .

I would rather accept the *status quo*: The governor is empowered to act in an emergency in whatever way she thinks appropriate. The courts can adjudicate the legitimacy of those actions on a case-by-case basis. The legislatures can enact, *post hoc*, remedial legislation. With most problems in most times, that is, admittedly, not a recipe for good public policymaking. For emergencies of the sort we are considering here, it is the proper and more workable order of action. And that's not just my own idea of good policy, it's the way the state and federal constitutions read or, to be more accurate, it is what has been read into our constitutional structure in order to make it workable. . . .

As noted earlier, the powers outlined in Articles V and VI of the "model act" have drawn the most public attention and controversy . . .

The provisions of Articles V and VI only outline the powers that the "model act" would allow the state during a declared emergency. In statutory interpretation, as in so many other things in life, the devil may be found in the details as often as in the broad outlines of an enactment. Words like "reasonable and necessary" and "preponderance of the evidence" carry a lot of legal baggage. The details of how and when isolation orders would be issued might create a program so constrained that it becomes a rare event, even in emergencies. Again, if the authors of the "model act" really want the states to consider authorizing public officials to do what the language of the "model act" suggests, we would be all better served with a textual description of what is proposed and, most importantly, some justification for creating what, even in its broad outlines, appears to be a public health version of martial law.

I could go through these subsections line-by-line, or spend hours (or pages) raising questions about the "temporary" isolation of groups of people without notice or requiring medical providers to participate in mass testing programs as a condition of their licensure or any one of a number of other specific provisions. But my basic question would in all cases have the same common element: Why? What is it that we have learned about the public health risks that we face that would counsel creating this elaborate and draconian apparatus? What is it that we cannot do now, under existing statutory enactments or through the implied powers of the governor, that we need to empower some public authority to do through such sweeping legislation? Why, for that matter, recommend that state legislatures even consider such legislation — given the media circus that would likely surround such deliberations? There are lots of theories of liberty and reasoned justifications for its denial. Under most, individual and economic liberty is assumed the *status quo* and its denial is selectively justified and done so in a particularized fashion. Why do we need all of what is outlined in the "model act"?

I can think of circumstances under which some individuals may have to be isolated or quarantined involuntarily. There might even be extraordinary circumstances under which isolation or quarantine should be mandated on the basis of a "group" — although again I find myself wondering exactly what the authors meant by such terminology in Articles V and VI. I also can imagine events that would necessitate some massive marshalling of medical resources, both public and private. But why create the regulatory apparatus for doing so in advance? Why do so in such plenary and heavy-handed terms? Is there any reality-based evidence that American providers need to be regulated in such a fashion during an emergency? Why not improve education and communication and funding such that providers can and will do what the "model act" would simply require under penalty of criminal sanctions? Again I reflect on what we learned in the Fall of 2001 about the behavior in a public health emergency of government officials, medical care providers, businesses and property owners, and thousands of ordinary Americans. Not then nor now do I find myself wishing that the Model State Emergency Health Powers Act had been in effect. There are some things I do wish had been in existence and will be in the next comparable scenario: more funding for state and local health departments, new procedures for communicating across jurisdictions and from public health to public safety agencies, better training for emergency medical personnel, and so on. I find little to suggest that what we need is the ability to quickly suspend civil rights and to empower public health officials to command and control all public and private resources. If my state is ever faced with a public health emergency, I would prefer that we respond to it on a case-by-case basis and in the *ad hoc* way anticipated under our constitutional system.

Surely what we need in the state of Washington and in many other states is a discussion of how to prepare for the next public health emergency. I strongly suspect that that discussion will focus quickly on staffing, infrastructure, and other resource and organizational problems. We also should discuss the adequacy of our state's legal structure. Among other things, we should immediately figure out the parameters of the governor's emergency powers under our state's constitutional structure. . . . It is possible that we may decide that given our constitutional structure and existing statutory framework remedial legislation should be adopted. But it's also possible that nothing more can or should be added to our legal structure. We may find instead that what we need is more resources and more expertise and better coordination of both. Not incidentally, to the extent that we do decide to empower a public health authority to do some of the more draconian things outlined in the "model act," both as a political and constitutional matter, we should be doubly sure that the resources and expertise are available to do those things accurately and effectively.

It is entirely possible that the most basic assumption underlying the "model act" is flawed. If in fact there is a need for some remedial legislation of the type outlined in the "model act," or, for that matter, any other, it may need to be federal legislation, not state legislation. Anthrax doesn't respect state borders or jurisdictional niceties. Whatever public health emergency we experience in Washington is likely to be a problem for Oregon and Idaho and, for that matter, Canada as well. Think about the number of Washingtonians that get on and off airplanes, trains, or Interstate 5 each day. In both practical *and* constitutional terms, public health emergencies that reach across state borders can only be resolved at the federal level. That may not be what conservative politicians like to hear, but interstate problems, including interstate public health emergencies are the province of congressional, not state authority; for that matter, interstate activities are one area in which the states *cannot* act even in the absence of federal action. As I have said so often above, I have a hard time deciphering what the authors of the "model act" envision we need, but it seems rather odd to me that they have chosen to implement that vision through a model *state* law. At the very least, it would seem the federal/state issue deserves some prefatory attention in their proposal, particularly as it is quite possible that at least portions of their vision could only be enacted as a matter of *federal* law.

\* \* \*

## Lawrence O. Gostin, *When Terrorism Threatens Health: How Far Are Limitations on Personal and Economic Liberties Justified?*
### 55 FLA. L. REV. 1105, 1159–69 (2003)

\* \* \*

. . . The relative low cost, ease of transport, and difficulty of detection makes bioweapons attractive to those intending to inflict harm and widespread fear on civil society. The fact that several countries have developed such weapons and fringe groups have used them (with minor success), is further evidence that bioweapons are technically feasible and that some people desire the capability. Biological agents already have been used within the United States, and there are strong indicators that the public health infrastructure is currently unprepared to cope with a large-scale attack. These risks require society to contemplate measures designed to avert an attack or minimize the impact should an attack occur.

The question faced is not whether the government should have liberty-limiting authority designed to cope with an attack, but what powers the state should have under what circumstances. American society prizes liberty and freedom, openness and tolerance; these values are part of the national identity and seem sometimes to rise to the level of inviolable tenets. These values, important in their own right, need to be balanced against equally valid values of population health and safety.

The task for society is to grant government power in a way that clearly separates the warranted from the unwarranted. That task is difficult enough even though most clear thinkers agree in principle about the legitimacy of state action in these contexts. What is still more difficult is setting justifiable boundaries for state action to address moderate risk situations where government cannot be sure of the precise parameters of the threat society faces. How can the law help assure that citizens' lives are secure, while preserving their values?

The answer to this question first requires a careful balance between individual and collective interests. The law must seriously consider authentic . . . claims to human dignity and tolerance of [diversity and individual choice]. At the same time, legal scholars should recognize that individual choices are shaped by the social context in which people live. The law also must take account of bona fide group interests, including a community's claim to a certain level of health, safety, and security. The law's objective, then, should be to take both private (personal freedom) and public (the social dimensions of human existence) interests seriously, recognizing that neither is dispensable.

The problem with constructing legal standards and procedures for state action is that any formulation necessarily expresses a preference for one set of interests over another, even if government seeks to respect both. Setting the legal standard too high effectively thwarts legitimate collective interests because, in practice, government action is chilled if not blocked. Setting the standard too low results in the opposite error of excessive deference to state action. The law cannot calibrate precisely enough to split the difference exactly.

. . . [T]here is no reason, *a priori*, for choosing one set of values over the other. In particular, I do not concede that liberalism should be the default preference. Rights, in other words, do not invariably trump common good. Thus, if government can point to a moderate risk and propose interventions that are reasonably well targeted and not unduly burdensome, the law should permit a sphere of state action. By doing so, each person bears a small burden (equitably distributed), but as members of a community all gain in the social exchange.

My refusal to cede to the primacy of individualism is animated by my concern for public safety in a health emergency. It is important that the government has the authority to act quickly should a bioterrorist attack occur. Quick action will be required on the part of both federal and local governments to minimize the impact of the attack and to protect the population. The federal government will need to move supplies from the National Pharmaceutical Stockpile in ways that distribute resources fairly and quickly enough to help those affected. Similarly, plans designed to mobilize experts from the CDC must provide for a prompt response, and the federal government must be prepared to provide support for state and local governments that may be overwhelmed by the sudden drastic increase in public health needs.

State and local governments must have the ability to act quickly as well. If a contagious disease agent is used, compulsory powers, like quarantine, will be effective only if they are used during the early stages of the outbreak. Otherwise, those who were initially infected will spread the disease to their contacts, and those contacts to their own contacts, until the geographical area affected is too vast to make quarantine plausible and effective. Laws and regulations that provide for compulsory powers in a fair and expeditious manner must be in place in order to avoid delays that would render the quarantine moot. In addition, state and local governments must have surveillance mechanisms in place for early detection. Timely identification of a health threat will facilitate distribution of needed resources (*e.g.*, medical personnel, medicine, and hospital equipment) in an equitable and expedient way. While careful consideration of policy choices and extensive deliberation are hallmarks of democracy, this reflection must take place now, so that when the government is called upon to act, it is able to do so in time to be useful.

. . . .

A successful framework would allow the government to act quickly in response to an emergency, but not allow individual liberties to be reduced to an unacceptable level. The best way to work toward this balance is to make use of traditionally successful mechanisms, like the democratic process, checks and balances, clear criteria for decision making, and judicial procedures designed to control the abuse of power by governmental agencies. In addition, the framework could adopt the modern concept of "shielding" — the governmental duty to engage the community in voluntary measures of self-protection as a "less restrictive alternative" to compulsion. . . .

. . . .

Public health policy is riddled with contradictions. Agency officials seek power without constraint. Since they are "experts," they resist substantive or procedural fetters on their decisions. Public health officials often distrust the lay public or their elected representatives, believing they do not understand the sciences of public health and are ill-suited to make sound judgments about infectious disease. The liberal public, on the other hand, prefers strict limits on agency action. They, in turn, often do not trust "experts" to provide objective information and respect individual rights.

The resolution of these differences should take place in the policy making branch of government. Legislators, although not experts, have a fiduciary duty to the public, which should include assuring the public's health and safety. At the same time, the legislature is accountable to the electorate and should avoid undue restrictions on individual freedoms. Legislatures obviously cannot make detailed choices in response to an emergency but, as suggested below, should put in place clear criteria and procedures for agency action.

. . . .

The legislature also should specify clear criteria for the exercise of public health powers. Objective standards have at least two positive effects. First, the political branch of government specifies in advance of a threat the conditions under which it will countenance the use of compulsion. The legislature, as discussed above, can deliberate about the appropriate conditions for coercion and remains politically accountable. Second, the use of clear criteria has a constraining effect on public health agencies. Deciding ahead of time what elements must be present for the executive branch to intervene offers some protection against policy based on suspect motives or irrational public fear. By circumscribing the conditions under which agencies can exercise power, it is possible to permit effective action while reigning in governmental excesses.

Most existing infectious disease statutes afford agencies broad discretion without setting clear standards for the exercise of power. This approach affords public health officials broad authority and makes it difficult to hold them accountable. Although health officials may prefer wide statutory mandates that grant them flexibility, they are not well served by such legislative inattention to standards. If agencies need to exercise strong power, they are more likely to gain political and public acceptance if they can point to a clear legislative standard supporting their decisions.

. . . .

Clear standards for agency action can limit discretion, helping ensure that power is exercised only where needed. Yet, there is still a need for procedural safeguards. Procedural due process has an instrumental and normative value in the context of a public health emergency. Primarily, due process helps ensure that compulsory powers are correctly applied. By affording individuals the right to a fair hearing, there is increased certainty that the individual actually is infectious, poses a risk to others, and cannot or will not comply with public health advice.

. . . .

Some scholars advocate government engagement with the community to promote measures of self-protection — a modern concept known as "shielding." Shielding operates on a macro-level, known as "community-shielding," and on a micro-level, labeled "self-shielding." . . .

Shielding often is seen as an alternative to compulsory measures. Scholars particularly urge its use as a non-coercive model of mass civil confinement: "a form of insulation wherein individuals and groups employ a self-imposed isolation, or quarantine, within their natural surrounding for a temporary period of time." Under this reasoning, government, far in advance of an actual attack, should "prepare the public to stay in place voluntarily, to resist the impulse to flee to family and friends outside the initial danger zone."

The shielding concept could usefully be placed within the legal framework for bioterrorism preparedness by requiring government to supplement (although not supplant) compulsory powers with voluntary approaches. As a form of least drastic means, the law would require public health authorities to provide mechanisms for keeping the public informed about the health emergency, its effects, and the ways in which the public can minimize the impact of the event on themselves and their communities. Preparing a means of effective communication is important in gaining the public's trust and avoiding panic. In addition, it allows the state to use the resources of the community effectively.

Public cooperation is important to the success of counter-bioterrorism interventions. If resources, like medicines, vaccines, or other supplies, need to be distributed, the public will need to follow public health advice and approach distribution points in a rational state of mind to prevent chaos. Similarly, if quarantine or isolation is mandated, the cooperation of the public is crucial to its success. A panicked public will require a much greater force of peacekeepers — police or the National Guard, for instance — to maintain order. Building the public's trust through communicating correct and timely information is crucial to successful management of any emergency.

. . . .

* * *

## Oregon Revised Statutes §§ 401.654, 401.657
### (Selected Provisions Related to Health Services in a Public Health Emergency)

### § 401.654. Registry of emergency health care providers established

(1) The Department of Human Services may establish a registry of emergency health care providers who are available to provide health care services during an emergency or crisis. The department may require training related to the provision of health care services in an emergency or crisis as a condition of registration.

(2) The department shall issue identification cards to health care providers included in the registry established under this section that:

(a) Identify the health care provider;

(b) Indicate that the health care provider is registered as an Oregon emergency health care provider;

(c) Identify the license or certification held by the health care provider;

(d) Identify the health care provider's usual area of practice if that information is available and the department determines that it is appropriate to provide that information.

(3) The department by rule shall establish a form for identification cards issued under subsection (2) of this section.

(4) The department shall support and provide assistance to the Office of Emergency Management in emergencies or crises involving the public health or requiring emergency medical response.

. . . .

### § 401.657 Emergency health care center, designation

(1) The Department of Human Services may designate all or part of a health care facility or other location as an emergency health care center. Upon the Governor declaring a state of emergency under § 401.055 or proclaiming a state of impending public health crisis after determining that a threat to the public health is imminent and likely to be widespread, life-threatening and of a scope that requires immediate medical action to protect the public health, emergency health care centers may be used for:

(a) Evaluation and referral of individuals affected by the emergency . . . .

(b) Provision of health care services; and

(c) Preparation of patients for transportation.

(2) The department may enter into cooperative agreements with local public health authorities that allow local public health authorities to designate emergency health care centers under this section.

(3) An emergency health care center designated under this section must have an emergency operations plan and a credentialing plan that governs the use of emergency health care providers registered under § 401.654 and other

health care providers who volunteer to perform health care services at the center under § 401.651 to § 401.670. The emergency operations plan and credentialing plan must comply with rules governing those plans adopted by the department.

\* \* \*

# Selected Provisions of The Federal Volunteer Protection Act
## 42 U.S.C. §§ 14503, 14504

### § 14503. Limitation on liability for volunteers

(a) Liability protection for volunteers. Except as provided in subsections (b) and (d) of this section, no volunteer of a nonprofit organization or governmental entity shall be liable for harm caused by an act or omission of the volunteer on behalf of the organization or entity if —

(1) the volunteer was acting within the scope of the volunteer's responsibilities in the nonprofit organization or governmental entity at the time of the act or omission;

(2) if appropriate or required, the volunteer was properly licensed, certified, or authorized by the appropriate authorities for the activities or practice in the State in which the harm occurred, where the activities were or practice was undertaken within the scope of the volunteer's responsibilities in the nonprofit organization or governmental entity;

(3) the harm was not caused by willful or criminal misconduct, gross negligence, reckless misconduct, or a conscious, flagrant indifference to the rights or safety of the individual harmed by the volunteer; and

(4) the harm was not caused by the volunteer operating a motor vehicle, vessel, aircraft, or other vehicle for which the State requires the operator or the owner of the vehicle, craft, or vessel to—

(A) possess an operator's license; or

(B) maintain insurance.

(b) Concerning responsibility of volunteers to organizations and entities. Nothing in this section shall be construed to affect any civil action brought by any nonprofit organization or any governmental entity against any volunteer of such organization or entity.

(c) No effect on liability of organization or entity. Nothing in this section shall be construed to affect the liability of any nonprofit organization or governmental entity with respect to harm caused to any person.

(d) Exceptions to volunteer liability protection. If the laws of a State limit volunteer liability subject to one or more of the following conditions, such conditions shall not be construed as inconsistent with this section:

(1) A State law that requires a nonprofit organization or governmental entity to adhere to risk management procedures, including mandatory training of volunteers.

(2) A State law that makes the organization or entity liable for the acts or omissions of its volunteers to the same extent as an employer is liable for the acts or omissions of its employees.

(3) A State law that makes a limitation of liability inapplicable if the civil action was brought by an officer of a State or local government pursuant to State or local law.

(4) A State law that makes a limitation of liability applicable only if the non-profit organization or governmental entity provides a financially secure source of recovery for individuals who suffer harm as a result of actions taken by a volunteer on behalf of the organization or entity. A financially secure source of recovery may be an insurance policy within specified limits, comparable coverage from a risk pooling mechanism, equivalent assets, or alternative arrangements that satisfy the State that the organization or entity will be able to pay for losses up to a specified amount. Separate standards for different types of liability exposure may be specified.

(e) Limitation on punitive damages based on actions of volunteers. . . . Punitive damages may not be awarded against a volunteer in an action brought for harm based on the action of a volunteer acting within the scope of the volunteer's responsibilities to a nonprofit organization or governmental entity unless the claimant establishes by clear and convincing evidence that the harm was proximately caused by an action of such volunteer which constitutes willful or criminal misconduct, or a conscious, flagrant indifference to the rights or safety of the individual harmed. [This provision] does not create a cause of action for punitive damages and does not preempt or supersede any Federal or State law to the extent that such law would further limit the award of punitive damages.

(f) Exceptions to limitations on liability. . . . The limitations on the liability of a volunteer under this chapter shall not apply to any misconduct that —

(A) constitutes a crime of violence . . . or act of international terrorism . . . for which the defendant has been convicted in any court;

(B) constitutes a hate crime. . . .

(C) involves a sexual offense, as defined by applicable State law, for which the defendant has been convicted in any court;

(D) involves misconduct for which the defendant has been found to have violated a Federal or State civil rights law; or

(E) where the defendant was under the influence (as determined pursuant to applicable State law) of intoxicating alcohol or any drug at the time of the misconduct.

## § 14504. Liability for noneconomic loss

(a) General rule. In any civil action against a volunteer, based on an action of a volunteer acting within the scope of the volunteer's responsibilities to a nonprofit organization or governmental entity, the liability of the volunteer for noneconomic loss shall be determined in accordance with subsection (b) of this section.

(b) Amount of liability

(1) In general. Each defendant who is a volunteer, shall be liable only for the amount of noneconomic loss allocated to that defendant in direct proportion to the percentage of responsibility of that defendant (determined in accordance with paragraph (2)) for the harm to the claimant with respect to which that defendant is liable. The court shall render a separate judgment against each defendant in an amount determined pursuant to the preceding sentence.

(2) Percentage of responsibility. For purposes of determining the amount of noneconomic loss allocated to a defendant who is a volunteer under this section, the trier of fact shall determine the percentage of responsibility of that defendant for the claimant's harm.

\* \* \*

# NOTES AND QUESTIONS

**1.** If and when federal agencies respond to a local or state public health problem, there are a myriad of legal problems involved in sorting out who can do what and under which circumstances. Americans need to be prepared, but American lawyers need to enhance their level of *legal preparedness* as well.

First of all, state and local public health laws need to be understood, coordinated, and, where necessary, revised in preparation for the next terrorist attack or epidemic outbreak. Many local and state public health laws were devised in other contexts and other eras. Moreover, laws allowing for quarantine or isolation are likely to be out-of-date and in need of revision.

What other laws need to be examined and revised? More broadly, what else should lawyers be doing to prepare themselves?

One group of thoughtful commentators, representing diverse professions within public health, has attempted to specify the elements of the public health system's legal preparedness that will need to be improved in order for the legal community to respond effectively to a bioterrorist or epidemic event:

The first step in fleshing out the concept of public health legal preparedness is to unpack its four core elements. . . .

Laws or legal authorities clearly are the beginning point for public health legal preparedness, just as epidemiology is for outbreak investigation. Laws are the authoritative utterances of public bodies and come in many stripes, among them statutes, ordinances, and judicial rulings as well as the policies of such public bodies as school boards, mosquito control districts, transportation commissions, and land use planning bodies.

At the operational level, public health laws also include such "implementation tools" as executive orders, administrative rules and regulations, memoranda of understanding (*e.g.*, between health departments and private hospitals for surge capacity or between health departments and law enforcement agencies for joint investigation of suspected terrorism), and mutual aid agreements among localities, states, or nations.

Laws, however, are neither self-creating nor self-enforcing. Thus the second core element is the competencies of the people who serve as the agents of public health legal preparedness. In the public sector these include elected officials, public health professionals, their legal counsel, government agency administrators, judges, law enforcement officials, and others. In the private sector are included medical practitioners, hospital and health plan administrators, community organizations, a wide range of service and advocacy organizations, and their legal counsel. Also important are the researchers, educators, and other scholars who develop the science base for public health legal preparedness and who educate practitioners in public health law. . . .

The third core element is information for these agents' use in shaping and applying public health laws. Examples include repositories of public health laws, updates on new enactments and judicial rulings, reports on innovations and public health law "best practices," and public health law practice guidelines. A surprising finding is how rare such information resources are. With some exceptions, there appear to be few, if any, published manuals on public health emergency law for government and hospital attorneys, "bench books" for judges to brief themselves on evidentiary standards for public health search warrants and quarantine orders, or databases of extant state and municipal public health emergency statutes and regulations.

The fourth core element is coordination of legal authorities across the multiple sectors that bear on public health practice and policy and across the vertical dimension of local-state-federal-international jurisdictions. Coordination is critical precisely because the public health system is richly multidisciplinary, multi-sectoral, and cross-jurisdictional.

Anthony Moulton, Richard N. Gottfried, Richard A. Goodman, Anne M. Murphy & Raymond D. Rawson, *What is Public Health Legal Preparedness?* 31 J.L. MED. & ETHICS 672, 674 (2003).

**2.** The interplay of federal and state authority may be particularly problematic. Any use of federal authority will have to be implemented under some specific federal statute (and not just be based on the existence of some connection to interstate commerce, as the Barbera article in section F[1] seems to imply) and may only be triggered, in some cases, by specific presidential declaration. Nor does the invitation of a state, by itself, legitimatize federal action. At least at the agency level, all federal action must derive from some federal statutory foundation.

We have already encountered one example of this, in connection with the CDC's statutory authority to prevent diseases from entering the country and to regulate transmission across state lines, including the power to impose quarantine. See Section E, *supra*, discussing 42 U.S.C. § 264 and its implementing regulations (both existing and proposed). Note that 42 C.F.R. § 70.2 provides for federal intervention when a state or local government's efforts to stop the spread of an infectious disease are inadequate; presumably this would provide some basis for federal action, even without the invitation or consent of a state. In addition, 42 U.S.C. § 243 authorizes CDC to act in concert with state or local public health authorities in matters relating to infectious diseases where the CDC is *requested* to do so.

Even where there is statutory authority for the CDC to act in matters relating to bioterrorism or in a naturally-occurring epidemic, there still may be legal problems associated with federal intervention. The legality of the use of military resources is a particularly problematic (and politically volatile) problem that lawyers should be prepared to address — and, as with all other decisions made in these circumstances — address very quickly. The Posse Comitatus Act, 18 U.S.C. § 1385, is a general prohibition on the use of military forces to enforce domestic criminal laws. Among other things, this would prevent the use of the army or other Department of Defense personnel in the enforcement of state or local isolation or quarantine laws, even if other federal personnel, such as those from the CDC, are involved in the implementation of those activities. The President does have the constitutional authority to authorize the use of military force — essentially declaring martial law. The Insurrection Act, 10 U.S.C. §§ 331–334, also allows the President to authorize the use of military personnel in emergencies. There is also limited authority under 10 U.S.C. § 382 for the Secretary of defense to extend assistance to the Department of Justice in some bioterroist emergencies. Otherwise, federal military personnel may have to limit their roles to "support" of other federal agencies and avoid engaging in what could be considered a violation of the Posse Comitatus Act.

Establishing the statutory basis for federal action, of course, is only one step in establishing the legal framework within which federal, state, and local public health agencies can act in concert. A myriad of other legal questions will have to be answered. (For just one example, see 42 U.S.C. § 233, limiting liability for health workers who participate in certain specified smallpox countermeasures.) Moreover, as illustrated in the TOPOFF exercise, some of the most difficult legal decisions will have to be made as part of the rapid implementation of the activities that these statutes and regulations authorize. Simply deciding who can decide certain legal questions will be difficult.

**3.** The full (and most recent) version of the Model State Emergency Health Powers Act can be found at the Center's website, www.publichealth law.net (last visited April 2006). The model act has drawn a considerable amount of commentary, much of it critical, but it has sparked a healthy debate and led to the consideration and, in some cases, enactment of legislation in a number of states. For a defense of the model act, see James G. Hodge, Jr., *Bioterrorism Law and Policy: Critical Choices for Public Health*, 30 J.L. Med. & Ethics 254 (2002).

George Annas has been a particularly vocal critic of the act and its underlying philosophy. As he stated in an article written in the same symposium as the Wing article:

> Of course, state public health, police, fire, and emergency planners should be clear about their authority, and to the extent the model act encourages states to review their emergency laws this is constructive. On the other hand, many of the provisions of this model act, especially those giving authority of public health officials over physicians and hospitals, and authority to quarantine without meaningful standards, seem to be based on the assumption that neither physicians nor the

public are likely to cooperate with public health officials in the after-math of a bioterrorist attack, and that panic is likely. . . .

[There are] three major objections to the initial version of the model act. First, it is far too broad, applying as it does not just to a smallpox attack, but to non-emergency conditions as diverse as our annual flu epidemic and the HIV epidemic. Second, although it may make sense to put public health officials in charge of responding to a smallpox attack, it may not make sense to put them in charge of responding to every type of a bioterrorism event. . . .

The third objection to the act is that there is no evidence from either 9/11 or the anthrax attacks that physicians, nurses, or members of the public panic, are reluctant to cooperate in responding to a bioterrorism attack, or are reluctant to take drugs or vaccines recommended by public health officials. . . .

There is no chance that every, or even many, states will adopt the suggested act as written, so if uniformity is seen as necessary or desir-able, only a federal statute can provide it. Obviously, it is also much more important what states like New York and California (large states that are likely bioterror targets) do than what states like Montana, Wyoming or Arkansas do. So far, only a few states, like Delaware, Oklahoma, and South Carolina, have adopted the suggested act whole-sale. More typically states have ignored it, or like California, have con-sidered it and rejected it outright. Other states, like Minnesota, have modified their quarantine laws, but have updated them to be consis-tent with contemporary medical ethics and constitutional rights, rather than making them more arbitrary.

George J. Annas, *Blinded by Terrorism: Public Health and Liberty in the 21st Century*, 13 HEALTH MATRIX 33, 50–52, 60 (2003). For development of some of these same critiques, see George J. Annas, *Bioterrorism, Public Health, and Civil Liberties*, 346 NEW ENG. J. MED. 1337–1342 (2002). See also his response to Gostin's Florida Law Review article, *Puppy Love, Bioterrorism, Civil Rights, and Public Health*, 55 FLA. L. REV. 1171 (2003).

**4.** With specific regard to Florida's version of the "Model Act", which was based on the October 23, 2001 version, Annas has written:

There has been an epidemic of new state laws addressing public health powers in the event of a bioterrorist attack or epidemic since 9/11. Florida's is by far the most extreme. Perhaps because it was the site of the first anthrax letter attack, Florida was fertile grounds for all sorts of so-called antiterrorist legislation. Within a year of September 11, the Florida legislature passed, and Governor Jeb Bush signed, 21 bills related to terrorism. One of these 21 bills (2002–269) was based at least in part on the CDC-sponsored model, adopting the scheme of declaring a public health emergency to trigger additional government powers, and vesting this power in the state's "health officer." The state officer's emergency powers are in four categories: (1) the shipment of drugs in the state, (2) the provision of bulk drugs by pharmacists, (3) the temporary licensing of certain health care practitioners, and

(4) power over individuals. There are major problems will all of the provisions (especially the extraordinarily broad definition of "public health emergency" which, for example, would include the annual flu epidemics and HIV disease), but section 4, on the power over individuals, is so out of step with anything else in the rest of the country, and so inconsistent with basic human rights and constitutional law, that it warrants scrutiny. The operative section gives the State Health Officer the following power over individuals in a public health emergency:

4. Ordering an individual to be examined, tested, vaccinated, treated, or quarantined for communicable diseases that have significant morbidity or mortality and present a severe danger to public health. Individuals who are unable or unwilling to be examined, tested, vaccinated, or treated for reasons of health, religion, or conscience may be subjected to quarantine.

a. Examination, testing, vaccination, or treatment may be performed by any qualified person authorized by the State Health Officer.

b. If the individual poses a danger to the public health, the State Health Officer may subject the individual to quarantine. If there is no practical method to quarantine the individual, the State Health Officer may use any means necessary to treat the individual.

Any order of the State Health Officer given to effectuate this paragraph shall be immediately enforceable by a law enforcement officer . . .

This section of the Florida law can be usefully contrasted to a Minnesota law on the same subject, which rather than trading off civil liberties for security, takes a human rights and health approach. Specifically, the Minnesota law provides: "individuals have a fundamental right to refuse medical treatment, testing, physical or mental examination, vaccination, participation in experimental procedures and protocols, collection of specimens and preventative programs" even in a public health emergency.

All four parts of this provision are extreme, and each shows how public health can drastically overreact to a perceived threat in ways that are counterproductive to public health and devastating to human rights. The first part, relating the "ordering an individual to be examined . . ." makes no public health sense at all, because there is no characteristic of the individual that gives rise to any suspicion or reason to believe that the individual either has the disease in question or has been exposed to the disease. Instead, the mere presence of a disease in Florida that the state health officer designates as creating a "public health emergency" authorizes anyone designated as "qualified" by the state health officer to order anyone to be "examined, tested, vaccinated, treated or quarantined." Mere refusal results in quarantine, without *any* evidence even of exposure to disease, let alone that the person is a threat to others. This is not public health, but authorization for a public health police state. This police-suspect model is the core mistake of the entire approach: Americans (Floridians) are not the enemy in a bioterrorist attack, and to prearrange a response that has the police seek out, confine, and forceably inject innocent Floridians is makes no scientific or public health sense. The enemy is the bioterrorist — although neither current law nor this Florida statute would permit police to do the things to a suspected bioterrorist it authorizes police to do to innocent Floridians. This law not only misses the target, it shoots in the wrong direction altogether.

But the third part, 4(b), is the most extreme and offensive and it is difficult to believe that anyone in the legislature actually read it. The first sentence makes perfect sense, and summarizes the law in virtually every state: "If the individual poses a danger to the public health, the State Health Officer may subject the individual to quarantine," at least so long as the phrase "provided this is the least restrictive alternative available" is understood. But the second sentence has no legal pedigree at all (at least outside of totalitarian states): "If there is no practical method to quarantine the individual, the State Health Officer may use any means to vaccinate or treat the individual." This could be labeled the "torture exception." If the risk is big enough to society, we can torture bioterrorists (and their victims!). But governments cannot engage in torture (or slavery or murder) under any circumstances under applicable international human rights treaties, even where the very survival of their country is at risk. Article 7 of the International Covenant on Civil and Political Rights is unambiguous: "No one shall be subjected to torture or to cruel, inhuman or degrading treatment or punishment. In particular, no one shall be subjected without his free consent to medical or scientific experimentation." And article 7 is one of the articles from which no derogation is permitted, even "in time of a public emergency which threatens the life of the nation." Because this section authorizes the violation of international law prohibition on torture, it is shocking to see it as part of a public health law.

For almost all potential bioterrorist agents there is neither a vaccine nor an effective treatment; and even for garden variety new epidemics that could qualify as public health emergencies under the statute, like SARS, no approved treatment exists. So, what can this provision possibly mean? That the state health officer can compel the use of potentially dangerous experimental drugs? But this is a fundamental violation not only of international law, but also of basic U.S. constitutional law, and U.S. federal drug law. No state law can, of course, overturn any, let alone all, of these higher laws. Even assuming that there is an approved vaccine that could also serve as a treatment if delivered to an exposed person quickly (the smallpox vaccine seems to have been what whoever drafted this language was likely thinking about), what justification can there be for forcing the vaccination "by any means"? The state gives only one, "if there is no practical method to quarantine the individual." But the entire statute is based on the premise that state public health officials know how to respond to a public health emergency, and should have the power to quarantine if needed.

This provision undercuts the assumption that state public health officials have done any planning at all, and instead assumes that the state will not be able to even provide quarantine facilities where needed — although it can also be read more cynically, to say the state need not provide quarantine for vaccination refusers but can simply force vaccination on everyone. Either way, there is no constitutional or human rights justification for forced treatment. Americans have a constitutional right to refuse any medical treatment, even lifesaving treatment. It is also a fundamental principle of medical ethics that patients have the right to informed choice, and the right to refuse any medical intervention. An emergency may justify very short periods of confinement of individuals who public health officials believe pose a risk to others, but nothing justifies this type of "treatment."

Perhaps the only good news about the Florida statute is that even in the wake of 9/11 and the drumbeat of the threat of a possible smallpox attack, no other state has passed anything like it. The Florida legislature, and its governor, should be ashamed.

George J. Annas, *Puppy Love: Bioterrorism, Civil Rights, and Public Health*, 55 FLA. L. REV. 1171, 1182–90 (2003).

**5.** There are many dimensions to the term "preparedness" when describing the potential ability of local, state, and federal governments to respond to public health emergencies. Perhaps the most fundamental is structuring the legal authority of each level of government to allow the various governmental agencies to perform the tasks that such emergencies will require.

One problem has to do with amassing the individual and institutional providers in sufficient numbers and in appropriate locations — and in timely fashion — to respond to public health needs. Obviously the existing distribution of hospitals, physicians, and other health care providers, both within and without the public sector, does not anticipate the immediate needs for emergency care, mass vaccination or treatment, or long-term confinement of thousands or even millions of people. Individual providers, supplies, even equipment will have to be mobilized and moved quickly, often across jurisdictional lines. Our experience on September 11, 2001, and in other emergencies has demonstrated that many individual providers will volunteer to support such efforts, even at great personal sacrifice, but even the logistics of moving and organizing volunteers can be problematic.

The problems encountered by physicians and other health care providers who attempt to volunteer their services during various public health disasters are particularly troublesome. After Hurricane Katrina, for example, there were numerous reports of groups of providers who are denied access to disaster areas because local officials could not determine whether they were legally authorized to provider services in that jurisdiction. Other reports documented incidents of government officials attempting to *prevent* volunteers from entering disaster areas for fear that they could not coordinate their efforts.

The Oregon statute excerpted above is an attempt by one state to mitigate the impact of some of these problems, particularly the likelihood that any amassing of emergency services will likely be encumbered by the various state licensing, credentialing, and other regulatory laws that, during more normal times, are intended to insure that the services available are of sufficient quality, but that in an emergency could frustrate the efforts of public agencies and the willingness of private providers to respond to the needs of the moment. Lost in the details of this legislation is the essential objective: to allow the state public health authorities to authorize individual and institutional providers to provide services that may otherwise be beyond the scope of state and local regulatory limits.

Note how much of the impact of the legislation is limited to circumstances where the governor has declared a specific emergency. Note also that the details of this statute are largely left to be completed by various local and state agencies, and by various providers. Does this make sense — or does it just pass along the real decision making to other already over-burdened actors?

Is this statute enough? What other provisions might a state want to add to such legislation? What are the risks of doing so?

**6.** One aspect of the preparedness problem has focused on civil liability. Again, both individual and institutional providers may be willing to participate in the response to an emergency or a disaster, but they may fear that providing emergency services under such conditions may run the risk of civil liability for negligence. This is particularly true for providers who may be licensed in one jurisdiction but called to provide services in another.

Many states have already enacted "Good Samaritan" laws to insulate from negligence-liability, but not usually from gross negligence-liability, providers (and, in some cases, others) who give first aid and other services in emergencies, although most of these statutes anticipated scenarios more akin to roadside emergencies. Other states have broader liability-limiting laws and some have enacted laws after September 11, 2001, anticipating their application in larger public health emergencies or disasters. Both state and federal law also provide some immunity from lawsuits for providers who are acting as governmental agents. Nonetheless, the potential for civil liability is still perceived as a problem, although for injured citizens, the bigger problem is negligent responders.

The federal statute excerpted above was one effort to mitigate the potential threat of liability for those who volunteer to work for a government or non-profit agency. Note, of course, that it is not complete immunity, it is limited; and that the various qualifications of the statute would make it inapplicable to many volunteers. Is this sufficient? Should this be expanded? Conversely, does it go too far? Can you imagine scenarios where liability would be appropriate, but barred by this statute? If most negligence-based liability relies on some assessment of whether the defendant acted unreasonably, is it really likely that a court would regard a volunteer as violating the appropriate standard of conduct?

**7.** There is a federal program that avoids both the problem of inter-jurisdictional credentialing and mitigates the threat of malpractice liability for providers and other volunteers who cross jurisdictions. The federal government's National Disaster Medical System (NDMS) is the country's most comprehensive, organized system for providing medical care in the wake of natural or manmade disasters. *See* www.oep-ndms.dhhs.gov/ (last visited August 2006). NDMS, formerly part of the Department of Health and Human Services (DHHS) and now part of the Department of Homeland Security (DHS), consists of pre-organized, existing teams of volunteer physicians and other medical professionals who train together regularly for disaster response and are subject to being called by the Department at any time to handle mass casualties and other national medical emergencies. The medical teams operated in New York City after the 9/11 attacks, for example. (NDMS also includes teams in nursing, pharmacy and veterinary medicine.) Medical team members work as temporary federal employees during deployment; their licensure and certification is recognized by all states, and they are covered by the Federal Tort Claims Act in the event of any claim of malpractice.

After NDMS was transferred to DHS, DHHS initiated a new program for volunteers, although without the advantages provided by federal employee status mentioned above. The Public Health Security and Bioterrorism Preparedness Act of 2002 contained provisions directing the DHHS to create a program called Emergency System for Advanced Registration of Volunteer Health Professional (ESAR-VHP). The federal agency provides funding for states to develop volunteer registration systems, but does not control their activities or volunteers. *See* www.hrsa.gov/esarvhp/ (last visited August 2006). Perhaps for this reason, the act encourages states to enact legislation such as the Oregon statute excerpted *supra*, provides guidelines for state programs, and provides federal funds for related activities. *See, e.g.,* Department of Health and Human Services, *Emergency System for Advance Registration of Volunteer Health Professionals (ESAR-VHP): Legal and Regulatory Issues* (draft May 2006) (includes a list of various state public health emergency laws).

**8.** Another potential problem involves the constitutional limits on joint, multi-state efforts to plan for public health emergencies and disasters. Under the commerce clause, only Congress can regulate interstate commerce, and while there are some "grey areas" within which an individual state can act in the absence of federal action, one constitutional limit is clear: Only with congressional approval can two or more states join together in some sort of cooperative effort. Such an activity is interstate commerce almost by definition. In response, Congress enacted a federal law authorizing the Emergency Management Assistance Compact, Pub. L. No. 104–321. Among other things, this allows qualifying states to share identity-sensitive information, make arrangement for accepting out-of-state licensed professionals, and clarifying the applicability of civil liability laws. For the most part, however, the terms of the compact only apply to agents of the state, not private volunteers (in the absence of additional state legislation). For additional information on EMAC, see www.emacweb.org/ (last visited August 2006).

# Chapter 4

# PUBLIC HEALTH SURVEILLANCE AND MEDICAL INFORMATION PRIVACY

## A. INTRODUCTION

Sound public health policy depends importantly on accurately identifying health risks and effective methods of decreasing or eliminating those risks. What is causing young men and women in a coastal city to fall ill with vomiting and dizziness — a bacterium in the water, a virus spread by sneezing, a chemical in the workplace, a saboteur or terrorist plot? How can it be eliminated? Can a viral or chemical agent be removed from the water supply or industrial process? If not, can it be reduced to a tolerable level? This chapter examines the public health programs that gather the information to answer such questions.

Section B provides background on the history and evolution of what is today called public health surveillance, beginning with case reports of contagious diseases at a time when medicine had no way to control epidemics, to current and proposed programs to collect information about people and their chronic diseases, DNA, and personal behaviors in data banks that could be electronically linked and accessed for use by physicians, public health policy makers, commercial marketing companies, and researchers. The explosion of information and the technology that makes it easy to use can create tensions between government's legitimate need for good information about the health risks and public policy protecting personal privacy, and this section briefly reviews the sources of law governing information privacy. Section C presents major relevant U.S. Supreme Court decisions analyzing constitutional protection for information privacy. The remainder of the chapter examines surveillance programs that illustrate how information can be used for public health activities ranging from controlling epidemics to conducting research and policy analysis. This review begins with contagious diseases in Section D, focusing on HIV case reporting, which became controversial in part because it highlighted the role of case reporting in identifying people who can be subjected to compulsory isolation, discussed in Chapter Three. Section E considers whether and when surveillance programs are conducting research with identifiable data that would require individual consent, and whether the Health Insurance Portability and Accountability Act (HIPAA) Privacy Rule clarifies or muddies the decision. The boundaries of the government's power to compel information disclosure are further explored in Section F, concerning cancer, chronic diseases, and environmental surveillance programs, and Section G, concerning genetic information, newborn screening, and DNA banking. Throughout the chapter, the recurring questions are: What kind of information does government need to protect public health? When can government demand

your personal health information without your consent or even your knowledge?[1]

Three themes are threaded though the materials in this chapter. First, the value of good information for public health policy sometimes competes for primacy with the values of personal autonomy and privacy. Reasonable people weigh the two differently, often depending upon whether they are the observers or the observed. Second, the way in which courts balance the two depends importantly on the procedural posture of the cases they decide. For example, different statutes may authorize the ongoing collection of data or require a subpoena for specific documents. Personal health information is subject to a fragmented array of laws governing information privacy, often with ambiguous or unsettled applications and exceptions. The choice of law (or laws) turns not only on what information is collected, but who collects it, from whom, how it collected, how it is used, whether it is kept secure and confidential, and whether and how it is further disclosed to third parties and for what purpose.

Finally, the explosion of data relevant to public health is challenging traditional conceptions of the types of information that should not be obtained without individual consent and information that should be shared without consent for the good of all, as well as what counts as a public health justification for such data collection. The apex of disease surveillance may have been the decades between 1955 and 1985, when public health officials were most true to Alexander Langmuir's admonition that surveillance should be "information for action" and largely focused on communicable diseases. Courts have generally deferred to public health assessments that personal health information is necessary for "public health purposes" or "disease control." Today, courts and public health practitioners may mean quite different things by those terms. With public health attention turned to "epidemics" of cancer, diabetes and obesity, the meaning of "disease control" as a justification for surveillance may undergo reexamination.

## B.  OVERVIEW OF PUBLIC HEALTH SURVEILLANCE

### Ruth L. Berkelman et al., *Public Health Surveillance,* *in* 2 OXFORD TEXTBOOK OF PUBLIC HEALTH
759, 759-60 (Roger Detels et al., eds., 4th ed. 2002)

* * *

Public health surveillance is the epidemiological foundation for modern public health.

. . . .

---

[1] This chapter does not cover law enforcement demands for information for purposes of criminal prosecutions. *See* Chapter Six for related materials on drug testing.

## Definition

In 1963, Langmuir defined disease surveillance as 'the continued watchfulness over the distribution and trends of incidence through the systematic collection, consolidation, and evaluation of morbidity and mortality reports and other relevant data' together with timely dissemination to those who 'need to know'. In 1968, the 21st World Health Assembly described surveillance as the systematic collection and use of epidemiological information for the planning, implementation, and assessment of disease control; in short, surveillance implied 'information for action.'

. . . Thus, health information systems (for example, registration of births and deaths, routine abstraction of hospital records, health surveys in a population) that are general and not linked to specific prevention and control programmes do not, by themselves, constitute surveillance. However, data collected from ongoing health information systems may be useful for surveillance purposes when systematically analysed and applied on a timely basis.

## History

. . . Possibly, the first public health action that can be attributed to surveillance occurred in the 1300s when public health authorities in a port near the Republic of Venice prevented passengers from coming ashore during the time of epidemic bubonic plague in Europe. The first Bill of Mortality was issued in London in 1532 as a consequence of fear of a plague epidemic. . . .

William Farr is recognized as the founder of the modern concept of surveillance. As Superintendent of the Statistical Department of the General Registrar's Office in Great Britain from 1839 to 1879, he collected, analysed, and interpreted vital statistics and disseminated the information in weekly, quarterly, and annual reports. . . . [and] took the responsibility of seeing that action was taken on the basis of his analyses.

In the nineteenth century, . . . Edwin Chadwick . . . investigated the relationship between environmental conditions and disease. . . . Louis Rene Villerme . . . analysed the relation between poverty and mortality in Paris. In the United States, Lemuel Shattuck also published data that related deaths, infant and maternal mortality, and infectious diseases to living conditions. He further recommended standardized nomenclature for cause of disease and death, and the collection of health data that included sex, age, locality, and other demographic factors. The first international list of causes of death was developed in 1893.

Increasingly, elements of surveillance were applied to aid in detecting epidemics and in preventing and controlling infectious diseases. In 1899 the United Kingdom began compulsory notification of selected infectious diseases. National morbidity data collection on plague, smallpox, and yellow fever was initiated in 1878 in the United States and by 1925 all states were reporting weekly to the United States Public Health Service on the occurrence of selected diseases. In the public health context, the term surveillance was increasingly applied to programmes of reporting selected infectious diseases in a population, with less emphasis on its application to quarantine of individuals.

Similar reporting activities were occurring in Europe at about the same time. . . . However, many of the morbidity and mortality reporting systems . . . were still largely developed for long-term archival functions.

[Surveillance became important to public health activities in the 1950s.] In 1955 acute poliomyelitis among recipients of the poliomyelitis vaccine in the United States threatened national vaccination programmes that had just begun. [Ed.: This refers to the Cutter incident.]. . . . [The CDC and state health departments] developed an intensive national surveillance systems [to report polio cases]. The surveillance data assisted epidemiologists in demonstrating that the problem was limited to a single manufacturer of the vaccine and allowed the vaccination programme to continue. . . . During the worldwide malaria control programme, surveillance was used to determine areas of continued transmission and to focus spraying efforts, as well as to document those areas without malaria. With the subsequent decline in malaria control efforts, surveillance data have documented the re-emergence of malaria in many areas of the world. . . .

Surveillance was also the foundation for the successful global campaign to eradicate smallpox. When the campaign began in 1967, efforts were focused on achieving a high vaccination level in countries with endemic smallpox; however, it was soon evident that the programme based on surveillance to target vaccination in limited areas would be more efficient. Smallpox reporting sources, usually medical facilities, were contacted on a routine basis. . . .

[Perhaps the greatest surveillance success story was that of HIV/AIDS.] Even before . . . HIV was identified, surveillance data contributed to identifying modes of transmission, population groups at risk for infection, and, equally important, population groups not at risk for infection. These data have been instrumental in directing public health resources to programmes, preventing further spread of HIV, and averting widespread public hysteria.

The need for a strong infrastructure for surveillance systems is currently being re-emphasized not only as countries face the emergence and re-emergence of infectious diseases but also as a result of the increasing threat of biological terrorism.

The potential usefulness of surveillance as a public health tool to address problems beyond infectious disease was emphasized in 1968 when the 21st World Health Assembly recommended the application of surveillance principles to a wider scope of problems, including cancer, atherosclerosis, and social problems such as drug addiction. Many of the principles of surveillance traditionally applied to acute infectious diseases have also been applied to chronic diseases and conditions, although some differences in surveillance techniques have been observed. . . .

In addition to the increased scope of health problems under surveillance, the methods of surveillance have expanded from general disease notification systems to include survey techniques, sentinel health-provider systems, and other approaches to data collection. . . .

The assimilation of computers into the workplace has made possible more efficient data collection as well as more rapid and sophisticated analyses. In the United States, all state health departments are linked to the CDC by computer for the routine collection and dissemination of selected data on notifiable conditions. . . .

The explosive development of technology will include the development of high-capacity storage devices, expansion of the capabilities of the internet, use of local- and wide-area networks for entry of surveillance data at multiple computers simultaneously, and development of new programming tools, video and computer integration, and voice and pen input. . . .

\* \* \*

# NOTES AND QUESTIONS

1. The chapter by public health scholars Berkelman, et al., uses the phrase "public health surveillance" in lieu of more traditional terms like "case reporting" or "disease surveillance." In the middle to late twentieth century, the term disease surveillance replaced "case reporting" in order to encompass newer and more sophisticated methods of data collection, including research studies like sample surveys, seroprevalence surveys, and capture-recapture studies. The more recent and even more generic "public health surveillance" expands the definition beyond disease to encompass all matters of interest to public health. This definition captures the positive, protective role of public health. Since September 11, 2001, at least one public health scholar has used the term "health intelligence" to describe collecting and linking multiple sources of data about health and health risks.

2. Statutory requirements for reporting certain diseases were first adopted in European countries in the late 1800s. Rhode Island required tavern owners to report customers with smallpox, yellow fever and cholera to local officials as early as 1741, but Michigan adopted the first American compulsory reporting law in 1893. All states now have "case reporting" laws requiring physicians (and often hospitals, laboratories and other health entities with relevant knowledge) to report to the state or local health department cases of "notifiable," "communicable," or "dangerous" diseases — contagious infections that could be easily (and involuntarily) transmitted to others through the air, like tuberculosis, by touching the same objects, like smallpox, or by drinking the same water, like cholera. Most states also include sexually transmitted infections (STIs), such as syphilis and gonorrhea, as well as diseases that are new or not yet understood but which appear to be communicable, like SARS. Diseases like the common cold or influenza are not included, because they do not cause severe illness (in most cases; but see the discussion of influenza in Chapter Three). Reports were first made by sending a post card to the health department; more detailed forms followed. (An example can be seen in Section D, *infra*.) Beyond diseases, all states require reports of injuries like bullet wounds or injuries from firearms, knives, or other sharp instruments,

primarily for the purpose of criminal investigations. Cases of child abuse and, more recently in most states, elder abuse must be reported to the social services or health department to permit an investigation into whether the person needs protection. Cases requiring urgent intervention are reported by telephone. Electronic transmission is developing, but spotty. The basic structure of case reporting systems today differs little from the original design. In addition, births, deaths, marriages, divorces, and fetal deaths must be reported for compiling vital statistics.

3. Mandatory reporting laws can be a source of controversy. The rapid increase in data collection of all types and the expansion of public health into areas traditionally reserved to physicians on the one hand and biomedical researchers on the other have begun to test both the state's power to compel the production of information and the law's protection of individual autonomy and control of one's personal information. Instead of privacy being what Justice Brandeis called the "right most valued by civilized men," *Olmstead v. United States*, 277 U.S. 438, 478 (1928) (dissenting), it may become the right most challenged by technology and curiosity. Many in the public health community and their representatives have begun to argue that identifiable information about individuals should be more freely available to government agencies without the person's knowledge or consent. Critics of this view do not dispute the value of information, but rather the need for so much identifiable information. They argue that both government agencies and commercial industry always offer a plausibly good reason for obtaining identifiable information without consent, so that such purposes offer no principled protection for privacy.

The threshold legal question in surveillance is whether the state can compel information to be reported without the consent of the person the information is about (*e.g.*, a patient) or the person holding the information (*e.g.*, a physician). The answer is, of course, it depends.

Specifically, it depends upon whether the information is personally identifiable and also upon one or more of the following factors:

- What use will be made of the information, immediately and in the future, and by whom

- Whether subsequent uses will be made with or without consent

- Whether the information will be linked or combined with information from other sources that makes identification possible

- Whether the information will be disclosed to third parties and whether they will subsequently disclose it to fourth and fifth parties

- Whether the information will be kept secure and inaccessible to anyone not authorized to view it, and kept or destroyed after use

- Whether there is an enforceable duty to keep the information secure and confidential on the part of all parties who receive or view it

4. Shortly before the first mandatory reporting law was enacted, Warren and Brandeis published their classic exposition of "the right to privacy," the amorphous collection of rights and duties protecting individual control over

one's person and reputation. Samuel D. Warren & Louis D. Brandeis, *The Right to Privacy*, 4 HARV. L. REV. 193, 196 (1890). Since that time, the scope and bounds of individual autonomy to control personal information have been developed and debated, but not fully delineated. In *Katz* v. *United States*, 389 U.S. 347, 350, n. 5 (1967), the United States Supreme Court noted, "Virtually every governmental action interferes with personal privacy to some degree. The question in each case is whether that interference violates a command of the United States Constitution." Protections against government intrusions into different personal and private matters can be found in the Fourth Amendment's protection against unreasonable searches and seizures; the First Amendment's protection of freedom of association; and the Fifth Amendment's protection of liberty. The U.S. Supreme Court has distinguished the line of constitutional cases protecting information privacy or "the individual interest in avoiding disclosure of personal matters," (*see Whalen v. Roe, infra*) from the cases protecting personal autonomy in personal decision making concerning family, marriage, procreation, and raising children, but the lines blur when sensitive information is at issue. (*See* Chapter Two.) Federal courts of appeal have also recognized that the Fourteenth Amendment protects a person's privacy interest in personal information, especially medical information.

**5.** Beyond constitutional protection, federal statutes and regulations provide some specific protections for personal information that vary with whether the entity seeking the information is public or private, the type of information sought, and how it is to be used. (*See* Box.) There is no single comprehensive federal (or state) privacy law governing all personal information or even all medical information in all hands, resulting in a patchwork with both gaps and some overlap. The major federal effort at protecting privacy resulted in the Privacy Act of 1974. Congressional hearings on the bill offer a useful history of privacy concerns. *Privacy: The Collection, Use and Computerization of Personal Data (Part 2): Joint Senate Hearings before the Ad Hoc Subcomm. on Privacy and Information Systems of the Comm. on Government Operations and Subcomm. on Constitutional Rights of the Comm. on the Judiciary*, 93rd Cong. 2240, 2246 (1974). The Act created the Privacy Protection Study Commission, whose final 1977 report remains perhaps the most complete analysis of general privacy issues in print. PRIVACY PROTECTION STUDY COMMISSION, PERSONAL PRIVACY IN AN INFORMATION SOCIETY (1977). Still, most agencies are subject to their own statutory rules. For example, the Public Health Service Act prohibits information obtained by the National Center for Health Statistics from being used for any other purpose without consent and from being published in identifiable form without consent. 42 U.S.C. § 242m. More recently, the Department of Health and Human Services issued its HIPAA Privacy Rule, discussed in Section E below, to provide more consistency in the protection of medical records, but the Rule applies only to specifically covered entities and allows state laws that are more protective of privacy to govern where they apply. Despite recent publicity surrounding revelations of federal surveillance of domestic telephone calls and international banking activity, the substantive law has changed little in the past quarter century. *See* Joy Pritts et al., *The State of Health Privacy: An Uneven Terrain*, (Institute for Health Care Research and Policy, 1999).

---

Federal Laws Regulating the Privacy of Health Information

- Privacy Act of 1974

- Computer Matching and Privacy Protection Act

- Electronic Communications Privacy Act (1986)

- Family Educational Rights and Privacy Act

- Freedom of Information Act

- Gramm-Leach-Bliley Act

- Food, Drug and Cosmetic Act

- The Children's Online Privacy Protection Act (1998)

- U.S. Safe Harbor Privacy Principles (Developed to comply with European Union Directive on Data Protection)

- Health Research Extension Act (1985), Public Health Service Act § 491, and Federal Policy for the Protection of Human Subjects ("Common Rule"), 42 C.F.R. Part 46.

- Substance Abuse Confidentiality Requirements, Public Health Service Act §543 (substance abuse and chemical dependency treatment information) and 42 C.F.R. Part 2

- Fair and Accurate Credit Transactions Act (amending the Fair Credit Reporting Act)

- Health Insurance Portability and Accountability Act, Health Information Security and Privacy Regulations, 42 C.F.R. Parts 160 and 164.

---

**6.** Privacy protections can also be found in state constitutional, statutory, and common law. State common law typically recognizes a cause of action for breach of confidentiality against a physician who reveals a patient's medical information without the patient's consent (out of court). Different causes of action for invasion of privacy are available against those who obtain private information to which they are not otherwise entitled without the person's consent. The reasons for protecting medical information were cogently summarized in *Alberts v. Devine,* 395 Mass. 59, 66 (1985):

We continue to recognize a patient's valid interest in preserving the confidentiality of medical facts communicated to a physician or discovered by the physician through examination. "The benefits which inure to the relationship of physician-patient from the denial to a physician of any right to promiscuously disclose such information are self-evident. On the other hand, it is impossible to conceive of any countervailing benefits which would arise by according a physician the right to gossip about a patient's health." "To foster the best interest of the patient and to insure a climate most favorable to a complete recovery, men of medicine have urged that patients be totally frank in their discussions with their physicians. To encourage the desired candor, men of law have formulated a strong policy of confidentiality to assure patients that only they themselves may unlock the doctor's silence in regard to those private disclosures. The result which these joint efforts of the two professions have produced . . . has been urged or forecast in *una voce* by commentators in the field of medical jurisprudence." [Internal citations omitted.]

State statutes cover a wide range of specific circumstances. Medical licensure laws or regulations may treat breach of confidentiality as unprofessional conduct subject to disciplinary action. Licensure laws governing other health professionals and health care facilities contain comparable requirements for patient confidentiality and medical recordkeeping. Rules of evidence specify certain permitted disclosures and grant testimonial privileges. Laws governing research specify privacy protections, while other disease-specific laws strictly limit the disclosure of information about specific diseases, like HIV test results or substance abuse treatment. State public records laws often contain exceptions to public disclosure for medical and other confidential information. Both statutory and common law also specify circumstances in which a person may be compelled to reveal personal medical information, such as in a lawsuit in which the person's medical condition is at issue. For a recent example, see *John B. v. Bridget B.*, 137 P.3d 153 (Cal. 2006). Mandatory reporting statutes are the best known exceptions to allowing individuals to decide who can obtain their private health information.

Resources on laws affecting privacy are available from the Georgetown Privacy Project at www.healthprivacy.org (last visited August 2006) (updated compilations and commentary on privacy laws at the state and federal levels), and the Electronic Privacy Information Center, a privacy advocacy organization at www.epic.org (last visited August 2006) (laws and news concerning all types of privacy issues, including medical privacy).

**7.** The National Center for Health Statistics (NCHS) in the CDC is a good source of vital statistics concerning births, deaths, disease and injury for the country. *See* www.cdc.gov/nchs (last visited August 2006). The NCHS funds several types of state data collection programs and conducts research studies to describe numbers and rates of disease and disability (morbidity) and death (mortality) in the population as a whole and among subgroups defined by such characteristics as age, sex, race, and residence. Such data can be essential to determine whether a public health problem exists, its magnitude, and whom it most affects. Among the most basic information resources are data on the leading causes of death. Causes of death are categorized according to the INTERNATIONAL STATISTICAL CLASSIFICATION OF DISEASES, INJURIES AND DEATHS, published by the World Health Organization. Historically, deaths were classified as attributable to one cause. Since 1955, the NCHS has been able to tabulate contributing causes of death. The following table presents the most recent data on causes of death in the United States. How would the ranking of causes of death influence public health policy?

| Cause of Death | Total Number of Deaths |
| --- | --- |
| All causes | 2,398,365 |
| 1. Heart disease | 654,092 |
| 2. Malignant neoplasms (cancers) | 550,270 |

|  |  |
|---|---|
| 3.  Cerebrovascular diseases (stroke, etc.) | 150,147 |
| 4.  Chronic lower respiratory disease | 123,884 |
| 5.  Accidents (unintentional injuries) | 108,694 |
| 6.  Diabetes mellitus | 72,815 |
| 7.  Alzheimer's disease | 65,829 |
| 8.  Influenza and pneumonia | 61,472 |
| 9.  Nephritis, nephrotic syndrome and nephrosis | 42,762 |
| 10.  Septicemia | 33,464 |
| 11.  Suicide | 31,647 |
| 12.  Chronic liver disease | 26,549 |
| 13.  Essential (primary) hypertension and hypertensive renal disease | 22,953 |
| 14.  Parkinson's disease | 18,018 |
| 15.  Pneumonitis due to solids and liquids | 16,959 |

Arialdi M. Miniño et al., *Deaths: Preliminary Data for 2004*, NAT. VITAL STAT. REP., June 28, 2006, at 1,4.

\* \* \*

## C.  COMPULSORY REPORTING OF MEDICAL INFORMATION

### WHALEN v. ROE
### 429 U.S. 589 (1977)

Stevens, Justice.

\* \* \*

The constitutional question presented is whether the State of New York may record, in a centralized computer file, the names and addresses of all persons who have obtained, pursuant to a doctor's prescription, certain drugs for which there is both a lawful and an unlawful market.

The District Court enjoined enforcement of the portions of the New York State Controlled Substances Act of 1972 which require such recording on the ground that they violate appellees' constitutionally protected rights of privacy. We noted probable jurisdiction of the appeal by the Commissioner of Health, and now reverse.

Many drugs have both legitimate and illegitimate uses. In response to a concern that such drugs were being diverted into unlawful channels, in 1970 the New York Legislature created a special commission to evaluate the State's drug control laws. The commission found the existing laws deficient in several respects. There was no effective way to prevent the use of stolen or revised prescriptions, to prevent unscrupulous pharmacists from repeatedly refilling prescriptions, to prevent users from obtaining prescriptions from more than one doctor, or to prevent doctors from overprescribing, either by authorizing an excessive amount in one prescription or by giving one patient multiple prescriptions. In drafting new legislation to correct such defects, the commission consulted with enforcement officials in California and Illinois where central reporting systems were being used effectively.

The new New York statute classified potentially harmful drugs in five schedules. Drugs, such as heroin, which are highly abused and have no recognized medical use, are in Schedule I; they cannot be prescribed. Schedules II through V include drugs which have a progressively lower potential for abuse but also have a recognized medical use. Our concern is limited to Schedule II, which includes the most dangerous of the legitimate drugs.[2]

With an exception for emergencies, the Act requires that all prescriptions for Schedule II drugs be prepared by the physician in triplicate on an official form. The completed form identifies the prescribing physician; the dispensing pharmacy; the drug and dosage; and the name, address, and age of the patient. One copy of the form is retained by the physician, the second by the pharmacist, and the third is forwarded to the New York State Department of Health in Albany. A prescription made on an official form may not exceed a 30-day supply, and may not be refilled.

The District Court found that about 100,000 Schedule II prescription forms are delivered to a receiving room at the Department of Health in Albany each month. They are sorted, coded, and logged and then taken to another room where the data on the forms is recorded on magnetic tapes for processing by a computer. Thereafter, the forms are returned to the receiving room to be retained in a vault for a five-year period and then destroyed as required by the statute. The receiving room is surrounded by a locked wire fence and protected by an alarm system. The computer tapes containing the prescription data are kept in a locked cabinet. When the tapes are used, the computer is run "off-line," which means that no terminal outside of the computer room can read or record any information. Public disclosure of the identity of patients is expressly prohibited by the statute and by a Department of Health regulation. Willful violation of these prohibitions is a crime punishable by up to one year in prison and a $2,000 fine. At the time of trial there were 17 Department of Health employees with access to the files; in addition, there were 24 investigators with authority to investigate cases of overdispensing which might be identified by the computer. Twenty months after the effective date of the Act, the computerized data had only been used in two investigations involving alleged overuse by specific patients.

A few days before the Act became effective, this litigation was commenced by a group of patients regularly receiving prescriptions for Schedule II drugs, [and] by doctors who prescribe such drugs. . . . Appellees offered evidence tend-

---

[2] These include opium and opium derivatives, cocaine, methadone, amphetamines, and methaqualone. Pub. Health Law § 3306. These drugs have accepted uses in the amelioration of pain and in the treatment of epilepsy, narcolepsy, hyperkinesia, schizo-affective disorders, and migraine headaches.

ing to prove that persons in need of treatment with Schedule II drugs will from time to time decline such treatment because of their fear that the misuse of the computerized data will cause them to be stigmatized as "drug addicts."

The District Court held that "the doctor-patient relationship is one of the zones of privacy accorded constitutional protection" and that the patient-identification provisions of the Act invaded this zone with "a needlessly broad sweep," and enjoined enforcement of the provisions of the Act which deal with the reporting of patients' names and addresses.

## I

The District Court found that the State had been unable to demonstrate the necessity for the patient-identification requirement on the basis of its experience during the first 20 months of administration of the new statute. There was a time when that alone would have provided a basis for invalidating the statute. *Lochner* v. *New York,* 198 U.S. 45. . . . The holding in *Lochner* has been implicitly rejected many times. State legislation which has some effect on individual liberty or privacy may not be held unconstitutional simply because a court finds it unnecessary, in whole or in part. For we have frequently recognized that individual States have broad latitude in experimenting with possible solutions to problems of vital local concern.

The New York statute challenged in this case represents a considered attempt to deal with such a problem. It is manifestly the product of an orderly and rational legislative decision. It was recommended by a specially appointed commission which held extensive hearings on the proposed legislation, and drew on experience with similar programs in other States. There surely was nothing unreasonable in the assumption that the patient-identification requirement might aid in the enforcement of laws designed to minimize the misuse of dangerous drugs. For the requirement could reasonably be expected to have a deterrent effect on potential violators as well as to aid in the detection or investigation of specific instances of apparent abuse. At the very least, it would seem clear that the State's vital interest in controlling the distribution of dangerous drugs would support a decision to experiment with new techniques for control. For if an experiment fails — if in this case experience teaches that the patient-identification requirement results in the foolish expenditure of funds to acquire a mountain of useless information — the legislative process remains available to terminate the unwise experiment. It follows that the legislature's enactment of the patient-identification requirement was a reasonable exercise of New York's broad police powers. The District Court's finding that the necessity for the requirement had not been proved is not, therefore, a sufficient reason for holding the statutory requirement unconstitutional.

## II

Appellees contend that the statute invades a constitutionally protected "zone of privacy." The cases sometimes characterized as protecting "privacy" have in fact involved at least two different kinds of interests. One is the individual interest in avoiding disclosure of personal matters, and another is the interest in independence in making certain kinds of important decisions. Appellees argue that both of these interests are impaired by this statute. The mere existence in readily available form of the information about patients' use of Schedule II drugs creates a genuine concern that the information will become publicly known and that it will adversely affect their reputations. This concern makes some patients reluctant to use, and some doctors reluctant to prescribe, such drugs even when their use is medically indicated. It follows, they argue, that the making of decisions about matters vital to the care of their health is inevitably affected by the statute. Thus, the statute threatens to impair both their interest in the nondisclosure of private information and also their interest in making important decisions independently.

We are persuaded, however, that the New York program does not, on its face, pose a sufficiently grievous threat to either interest to establish a constitutional violation.

Public disclosure of patient information can come about in three ways. Health Department employees may violate the statute by failing, either deliberately or negligently, to maintain proper security. A patient or a doctor may be accused of a violation and the stored data may be offered in evidence in a judicial proceeding. Or, thirdly, a doctor, a pharmacist, or the patient may voluntarily reveal information on a prescription form.

The third possibility existed under the prior law and is entirely unrelated to the existence of the computerized data bank. Neither of the other two possibilities provides a proper ground for attacking the statute as invalid on its face. There is no support in the record, or in the experience of the two States that New York has emulated, for an assumption that the security provisions of the statute will be administered improperly. And the remote possibility that judicial supervision of the evidentiary use of particular items of stored information will provide inadequate protection against unwarranted disclosures is surely not a sufficient reason for invalidating the entire patient-identification program.

Even without public disclosure, it is, of course, true that private information must be disclosed to the authorized employees of the New York Department of Health. Such disclosures, however, are not significantly different from those that were required under the prior law. Nor are they meaningfully distinguishable from a host of other unpleasant invasions of privacy that are associated with many facets of health care. Unquestionably, some individuals' concern for their own privacy may lead them to avoid or to postpone needed medical attention. Nevertheless, disclosures of private medical information to doctors, to hospital personnel, to insurance companies, and to public health agencies are often an essential part of modern medical practice even when the disclosure may reflect unfavorably on the character of the patient. Requiring such disclosures to representatives of the State having responsibility for the health of the community, does not automatically amount to an impermissible invasion of privacy.

Appellees also argue, however, that even if unwarranted disclosures do not actually occur, the knowledge that the information is readily available in a computerized file creates a genuine concern that causes some persons to decline needed medication. The record supports the conclusion that some use of Schedule II drugs has been discouraged by that concern; it also is clear, however, that about 100,000 prescriptions for such drugs were being filled each month prior to the entry of the District Court's injunction. Clearly, therefore, the statute did not deprive the public of access to the drugs.

Nor can it be said that any individual has been deprived of the right to decide independently, with the advice of his physician, to acquire and to use needed medication. Although the State no doubt could prohibit entirely the use of particular Schedule II drugs, it has not done so. This case is therefore unlike those in which the Court held that a total prohibition of certain conduct was an impermissible deprivation of liberty. Nor does the State require access to these drugs to be conditioned on the consent of any state official or other third party. Within dosage limits which appellees do not challenge, the decision to prescribe, or to use, is left entirely to the physician and the patient.

We hold that neither the immediate nor the threatened impact of the patient-identification requirements in the New York State Controlled Substances Act of 1972 on either the reputation or the independence of patients for whom Schedule II drugs are medically indicated is sufficient to constitute an invasion of any right or liberty protected by the Fourteenth Amendment.

. . . .

## IV

A final word about issues we have not decided. We are not unaware of the threat to privacy implicit in the accumulation of vast amounts of personal information in computerized data banks or other massive government files. The collection of taxes, the distribution of welfare and social security benefits, the supervision of public health, the direction of our Armed Forces, and the enforcement of the criminal laws all require the orderly preservation of great quantities of information, much of which is personal in character and potentially embarrassing or harmful if disclosed. The right to collect and use such data for public purposes is typically accompanied by a concomitant statutory or regulatory duty to avoid unwarranted disclosures. Recognizing that in some circumstances that duty arguably has its roots in the Constitution, nevertheless New York's statutory scheme, and its implementing administrative procedures, evidence a proper concern with, and protection of, the individual's interest in privacy. We therefore need not, and do not, decide any question which might be presented by the unwarranted disclosure of accumulated private data — whether intentional or unintentional — or by a system that did not contain comparable security provisions. We simply hold that this record does not establish an invasion of any right or liberty protected by the Fourteenth Amendment.

\* \* \*

## PLANNED PARENTHOOD v. DANFORTH
### 428 U.S. 52, 80-81 (1976)

[The Court struck down provisions of a Missouri statute requiring pregnant women to obtain their husband's consent to an abortion and requiring minors to obtain parental consent to an abortion. The Court upheld the recordkeeping requirement, as follows:]

Blackmun, Justice.

\* \* \*

Recordkeeping. Sections 10 and 11 of the Act impose recordkeeping require-ments for health facilities and physicians concerned with abortions irrespec-tive of the pregnancy stage. Under § 10, each such facility and physician is to be supplied with forms "the purpose and function of which shall be the preser-vation of maternal health and life by adding to the sum of medical knowledge through the compilation of relevant maternal health and life data and to mon-itor all abortions performed to assure that they are done only under and in accordance with the provisions of the law." The statute states that the infor-mation on the forms "shall be confidential and shall be used only for statisti-cal purposes." The "records, however, may be inspected and health data acquired by local, state, or national public health officers." Under § 11 the records are to be kept for seven years in the permanent files of the health facility where the abortion was performed.

\* \* \*

[T]here are important and perhaps conflicting interests affected by record-keeping requirements. On the one hand, maintenance of records indeed may be helpful in developing information pertinent to the preservation of maternal health. On the other hand, as we stated in Roe, during the first stage of preg-nancy the State may impose no restrictions or regulations governing the med-ical judgment of the pregnant woman's attending physician with respect to the termination of her pregnancy. . . .

Recordkeeping and reporting requirements that are reasonably directed to the preservation of maternal health and that properly respect a patient's con-fidentiality and privacy are permissible. As to the first stage [of pregnancy], one may argue forcefully, as the appellants do, that the State should not be able to impose any recordkeeping requirements that significantly differ from those imposed with respect to other, and comparable, medical or surgical pro-cedures. We conclude, however, that the provisions of §§ 10 and 11, while per-haps approaching impermissible limits, are not constitutionally offensive in themselves. Recordkeeping of this kind, if not abused or overdone, can be use-ful to the State's interest in protecting the health of its female citizens, and may be a resource that is relevant to decisions involving medical experience and judgment. The added requirements for confidentiality, with the sole exception for public health officers, and for retention for seven years, a period not unreasonable in length, assist and persuade us in our determination of the constitutional limits. As so regarded, we see no legally significant impact or consequence on the abortion decision or on the physician-patient relation-ship. We naturally assume, furthermore, that these recordkeeping and record-maintaining provisions will be interpreted and enforced by Missouri's Division of Health in the light of our decision with respect to the Act's other provisions, and that, of course, they will not be utilized in such a way as to accomplish, through the sheer burden of recordkeeping detail, what we have held to be an otherwise unconstitutional restriction. . . .

\* \* \*

# THORNBURGH v. AMERICAN COLLEGE OF OBSTETRICIANS AND GYNECOLOGISTS
### 476 U.S. 747, 765–68 (1986)

[The Court struck down the provisions of a Pennsylvania statute requiring (1) delivering specified information to a woman seeking an abortion; (2) reports on abortions that would be available to the public; (3) a particular standard of care when aborting a viable fetus; and (4) a second physician to be present during an abortion, without an express medical-emergency exception. This excerpt from the majority opinion deals with reporting requirements.]

Blackmun, Justice.

\* \* \*

Section 3214(a) (8), part of the general reporting section, incorporates § 3211(a). Section 3211(a) requires the physician to report the basis for his determination "that a child is not viable." It applies only after the first trimester. The report required by §§ 3214(a) and (h) is detailed and must include, among other things, identification of the performing and referring physicians and of the facility or agency; information as to the woman's political subdivision and State of residence, age, race, marital status, and number of prior pregnancies; the date of her last menstrual period and the probable gestational age; the basis for any judgment that a medical emergency existed; the basis for any determination of nonviability; and the method of payment for the abortion. The report is to be signed by the attending physician.

. . . .

Despite the fact that § 3214(e) (2) provides that such reports "shall not be deemed public records," within the meaning of the Commonwealth's "Right-to-Know Law," each report "shall be made available for public inspection and copying within 15 days of receipt in a form which will not lead to the disclosure of the identity of any person filing a report." Similarly, the report of complications, required by § 3214(h), "shall be open to public inspection and copying." A willful failure to file a report required under § 3214 is "unprofessional conduct" and the noncomplying physician's license "shall be subject to suspension or revocation."

The scope of the information required and its availability to the public belie any assertions by the Commonwealth that it is advancing any legitimate interest. In *Planned Parenthood of Central Missouri v. Danforth*, we recognized that recordkeeping and reporting provisions "that are reasonably directed to the preservation of maternal health and that properly respect a patient's confidentiality and privacy are permissible." But the reports required under the Act before us today go well beyond the health-related interests that served to justify the Missouri reports under consideration in *Danforth*. Pennsylvania would require, as Missouri did not, information as to method of payment, as to the woman's personal history, and as to the bases for medical judgments. The Missouri reports were to be used "only for statistical purposes." They were to be maintained in confidence, with the sole exception of public health officers. . . . "The decisive factor was that the State met its burden of demonstrating that these regulations furthered important health-related state concerns."

The required Pennsylvania reports, on the other hand, while claimed not to be "public," are available nonetheless to the public for copying. Moreover, there is no limitation on the use to which the Commonwealth or the public copiers may put them. The elements that proved persuasive for the ruling in *Danforth* are absent here. The decision to terminate a pregnancy is an intensely private one that must be protected in a way that assures anonymity. JUSTICE STEVENS, in his opinion concurring in the judgment in *Bellotti* v. *Baird*, 443 U.S. 622, 655 (1979), aptly observed:

> It is inherent in the right to make the abortion decision that the right may be exercised without public scrutiny and in defiance of the contrary opinion of the sovereign or other third parties."

> A woman and her physician will necessarily be more reluctant to choose an abortion if there exists a possibility that her decision and her identity will become known publicly. Although the statute does not specifically require the reporting of the woman's name, the amount of information about her and the circumstances under which she had an abortion are so detailed that identification is likely. Identification is the obvious purpose of these extreme reporting requirements. The "impermissible limits" that *Danforth* mentioned and that Missouri approached have been exceeded here.

We note, as we reach this conclusion, that the Court consistently has refused to allow government to chill the exercise of constitutional rights by requiring disclosure of protected, but sometimes unpopular, activities. Pennsylvania's reporting requirements raise the specter of public exposure and harassment of women who choose to exercise their personal, intensely private, right, with their physician, to end a pregnancy. Thus, they pose an unacceptable danger of deterring the exercise of that right, and must be invalidated.

* * *

# PLANNED PARENTHOOD v. CASEY
## 505 U.S. 833, 900-901 (1992)

[The Court upheld provisions of a Pennsylvania statute, including a 24-hour period between consent and performance of abortions, but struck down a requirement that women notify their husbands and, in the following excerpt, upheld part of a reporting requirement.]

O'Connor, Kennedy and Souter, Justices.

* * *

Under the recordkeeping and reporting requirements of the statute, every facility which performs abortions is required to file a report stating its name and address as well as the name and address of any related entity, such as a controlling or subsidiary organization. In the case of state-funded institutions, the information becomes public.

For each abortion performed, a report must be filed identifying: the physician (and the second physician where required); the facility; the referring physician or agency; the woman's age; the number of prior pregnancies and prior abortions she has had; gestational age; the type of abortion procedure; the date of the abortion; whether there were any pre-existing medical conditions which would complicate pregnancy; medical complications with the abortion; where applicable, the basis for the determination that the abortion was medically necessary; the weight of the aborted fetus; and whether the woman was married, and if so, whether notice was provided or the basis for the failure to give notice. Every abortion facility must also file quarterly reports showing the number of abortions performed broken down by trimester. In all events, the identity of each woman who has had an abortion remains confidential.

In *Danforth*, we held that recordkeeping and reporting provisions "that are reasonably directed to the preservation of maternal health and that properly respect a patient's confidentiality and privacy are permissible." . . . The collection of information with respect to actual patients is a vital element of medical research, and so it cannot be said that the requirements serve no purpose other than to make abortions more difficult. Nor do we find that the requirements impose a substantial obstacle to a woman's choice. At most they might increase the cost of some abortions by a slight amount. While at some point increased cost could become a substantial obstacle, there is no such showing on the record before us.

Subsection (12) of the reporting provision requires the reporting of, among other things, a married woman's "reason for failure to provide notice" to her husband. This provision in effect requires women, as a condition of obtaining an abortion, to provide the Commonwealth with the precise information we have already recognized that many women have pressing reasons not to reveal. Like the spousal notice requirement itself, this provision places an undue burden on a woman's choice, and must be invalidated for that reason.

* * *

## NOTES AND QUESTIONS

1. *Whalen v. Roe* has been cited most often for the general principle that the due process clause of the constitution protects the "individual['s] interest in avoiding disclosure of personal matters." It has also been cited by commentators for the broad proposition that the state is free to require the reporting of personal medical information without patient consent for almost any reason that might be considered helpful to public health or safety. Does the case support these expansive readings of its holding? The statement that information privacy is protected by the constitution merely describes first principles without suggesting the scope or limits of that protection. Determining what kind of information deserves what kind of protection in what circumstances remains open for development. In contrast, the statement that information may be mandated when it might prove useful to government is more conclusory (always a dangerous approach in interpreting Court decisions) and leaves less room for the nuance necessary in the many different types of cases that involve information disclosure.

The reporting requirement in *Whalen* was initiated and upheld as a means of identifying criminal offenders: patients who attempted to obtain controlled substances and physicians who prescribed them without a medical reason. Can this rationale wholly apply in cases involving the reporting of medical information having no relationship with criminal activity? Might the state have made the prescription or possession of the same drugs for *any* reason a criminal offense? *See Boruki v. Ryan*, 827 F.2d 836, 841 n. 7 (1st Cir. 1987) ("Additional factors apparently underlying the Court's ruling were that the State could have proscribed use of the drugs entirely, and that the decision of whether to use the drugs, within certain prescription limits, was left entirely to the physician and patient."). In *Whalen*, the law at issue was part of the Controlled Substances Act, which criminalized the non-medical prescription or possession of controlled substances, but the data were collected and held by the health department, not law enforcement. How would health agencies become involved in the investigation or prosecution of a criminal offense? (*See* the discussion in Chapter Three concerning the relationship between public health and law enforcement in detaining and isolating people with communicable diseases.) Compare the Supreme Court's approach to the reporting of drug prescriptions in *Whalen* to the reporting of pregnant women who used illegal drugs in *Ferguson v. City of Charleston* in Chapter Six ("Because law enforcement involvement always serves some broader social purpose or objective, under respondents' view, virtually any nonconsensual suspicionless search could be immunized under the special needs doctrine by defining the search solely in terms of its ultimate, rather than immediate, purpose. Such an approach is inconsistent with the Fourth Amendment.").

**2.** The *Whalen* Court did not require the state to demonstrate that the reporting law was actually *necessary* to deter or investigate drug crimes, as plaintiffs requested. Instead, the Court appeared confident that the state would repeal the law if it proved to be ineffective or a waste of time or money. Was the Court's confidence well-founded? Not all mandatory reporting laws, or any laws for that matter, are the result of "an orderly and rational legislative decision." Moreover, legislatures rarely bother to repeal unnecessary or even wasteful programs unless there is a major scandal, public outcry or budget crunch. Individuals who object to such programs may find it easier to avoid getting care where they will be reported than to lobby the legislature for repeal. In addition, once the program is in place, a new constituency of groups that benefit from the program is likely to develop. In the case of reporting laws, agencies and private organizations that use the data collected pursuant to reporting laws tend to favor continued reporting, even if their own goals differ from that which justified the program in the first place. For example, substance abuse agencies that have nothing to do with criminal drug diversion may use the data to estimate the number of drug users or trends in the use of specific drugs, or to predict the cost of future treatment programs. Thus, the program may enjoy considerable support in some quarters even if it is not meeting its original goals. There is nothing inherently wrong with retaining a program that no longer serves its original purpose, as long as it now serves a purpose that, by itself, would justify creating the program in the first place. Whether a particular mandatory reporting program meets this test can be a close question.

**3.** Justice Brennan, concurring in *Whalen*, was concerned with the potential for widespread dissemination of personal information that computers might permit:

> What is more troubling about this scheme, however, is the central computer storage of the data thus collected. Obviously, as the State argues, collection and storage of data by the State that is in itself legitimate is not rendered unconstitutional simply because new technology makes the State's operations more efficient. However, as the example of the Fourth Amendment shows, the Constitution puts limits not only on the type of information the State may gather, but also on the means it may use to gather it. The central storage and easy accessibility of computerized data vastly increase the potential for abuse of that information, and I am not prepared to say that future developments will not demonstrate the necessity of some curb on such technology. . . . In this case, as the Court's opinion makes clear, the State's carefully designed program includes numerous safeguards intended to forestall the danger of indiscriminate disclosure. Given this serious and, so far as the record shows, successful effort to prevent abuse and limit access to the personal information at issue, I cannot say that the statute's provisions for computer storage, on their face, amount to a deprivation of constitutionally protected privacy interests, any more than the more traditional reporting provisions.

429 U.S. at 606-07.

Should *Whalen* be interpreted to mean that the state may require personally identifiable information to be reported for any plausible reason as long as the information is kept secure? What kinds of information would be susceptible to mandatory reporting using that reasoning? Assurance of enforceable protection of confidentiality appears to be a necessary requirement *in addition* to those of demonstrating that the disclosure is a reasonable means of achieving a legitimate state interest and does not offend reasonable expectations of privacy. The few courts that have addressed the question whether the state violates individual privacy by requiring the reporting of personally identifiable information have emphasized that authorizing legislation contains specific requirements that the personal information be kept confidential, in a secure location, and not be disclosed further, with penalties for any violation of these requirements. *See ACT-UP Triangle v. Comm'n for Health Servs. of North Carolina*, 345 N.C. 699, 483 S.E.2d 388 (N.C. 1997) (upholding an AIDS reporting law that enforced the confidentiality of medical records with criminal and civil penalties); *Treants Enters. v. Onslow County*, 83 N.C. App. 345, 350, 358 S.E.2d 365, 374 (1986), *aff'd*, 320 N.C. 776, 360 S.E.2d 783 (1987) (finding that a county licensing ordinance which required companionship services to keep permanent records of their patrons and "grants authority to any law enforcement officer to inspect the records" violated the state and federal constitutions).

In *Whalen*, the Court focused on the possibility of information being disclosed to the public at large. However, that was not the only or even necessarily the primary concern of the plaintiffs. They considered the initial report to the health department itself to be a harmful disclosure. Later cases sometimes conflate these two distinct disclosures. However, more recent cases indicate that the initial disclosure to the health department is the threshold concern; the possibility of disclosure to the public remains part of the "secondary" issue of protecting confidentiality, which appears to mean that a person's identifiable information should not be disclosed to third parties, either deliberately or negligently. *See, e.g., Tucson Woman's Clinic v. Eden*, 371 F3d 1173, 1193 (9th Cir. 2004) ("Even if a law adequately protects against *public* disclosure of a patient's private information, it may still violate informational privacy if an unbounded number of government employees have access to the information.")

**4.** The *Danforth, Thornburgh,* and *Casey* cases represent the rest of the Supreme Court's body of decisions concerning mandatory reporting laws. In each of these cases, the Court accepted the value of collecting health information, but with the caveat that it was "reasonably directed to the preservation of maternal health." *Danforth*, 428 U.S. at 80. As in *Whalen*, however, it did not analyze whether reporting was necessary for this purpose. The law offered no benefit to those reported, but permitted the collection of data that might be used in research to identify health risks or better procedures in the future. Instead, the decisions appear to turn on whether the law "respects a patient's confidentiality and privacy." *Id.* Here, the key concern was whether a woman could be identified from the information reported. In *Thornburgh*, the Court examined the possibility of identification even where the law did not require names to be reported. In *Casey*, it upheld a later Pennsylvania law that did not require reporting the woman's name, even though the information required was somewhat detailed. The Court recognized that state mandatory reporting laws could chill the exercise of constitutionally protected rights when they require the reporting of protected activities, and struck down the requirement to report a woman's reason for not notifying her husband of the abortion. The Court's attention to the types of information at issue and the potential for identification suggest an increasing sophistication with the benefits and risks of data collection.

These decisions suggest that when disclosure of information threatens the exercise of important rights of personal autonomy, more careful scrutiny of the state's purpose is warranted. Lower courts have used this reasoning to apply heightened scrutiny where sexual or health information is at issue. *See Sheets v. Salt Lake County*, 45 F.3d 1383, 1387 (10th Cir. 1995) (disclosure of sexual or health information may violate a person's right to information privacy unless the disclosure serves a compelling state interest in the least intrusive manner); *Walls v. Petersburg*, 895 F.2d 188, 192 (4th Cir. 1990) ("The more intimate or personal the information, the more justified is the expectation that it will not be subject to public scrutiny."); *Fraternal Order of Police v. City of Philadelphia*, 812 F.2d 105, 110 (3d Cir. 1987) ("Most circuits appear to apply an 'intermediate standard of review' for the majority of confidentiality violations, . . . with a compelling interest analysis reserved for 'severe intrusions' on confidentiality."). *See John B. v. Superior Court*, 38 Cal. 4th 1177, 137 P.3d 153, 45 Cal. Rptr. 3d 316 (2006) (addressing discovery requests for medical records of HIV infection, the court found that where a plaintiff seeks "discovery from a defendant concerning sexual matters protected by the constitutional right of privacy, the intrusion upon sexual privacy may only be done on the basis of practical necessity and the compelled disclosure [must] be narrowly drawn to assure maximum protection of the constitutional interests at stake" (internal quotes omitted)); There remains some uncertainty about whether more careful scrutiny is required because the type of information itself at issue is especially sensitive or important, or because disclosure of that information would affect the exercise of an important aspect of personal liberty. Further, courts use different levels of scrutiny for somewhat similar types of information, suggesting that there is room for future debate on analytic approaches.

It is worth pondering why the Supreme Court has only reviewed mandatory reporting laws involving drug crimes and abortion, not contagious diseases, injuries, or other conditions. Drug crimes and abortion appear in a significant number of all cases the Court agreed to decide. They also represent major public health concerns. Might there be other reasons? Perhaps few people are aware of disease reporting laws. Perhaps most people are happy to have their information used. How likely is it that patients who disagree might object to a mandatory reporting law?

**5.** Several different lines of cases consider the power of state agencies to subpoena medical records. *See Schachter v. Whalen*, 581 F.2d 35 (2d Cir. 1978) (finding a state medical licensure board could subpoena patient medical records for purposes of investigating a physician's professional conduct in treating patients with laetrile or MA-7); and *U.S. v. Westinghouse, infra.* Also distinct is the authority of law enforcement agencies to obtain medical records when the records may provide evidence that the patient or physician committed a crime. For interesting recent examples, *see Rush Limbaugh v. Florida*, 2004 Fla. App. LEXIS 14653 (Ct. App. Fla. 2004); *New York City Health & Hosp. Corp. v. Morgenthau (In re Grand Jury Investigation)*, 98 N.Y.2d 525; 779 N.E.2d 173; 749 N.Y.S.2d 462 (2002).

\* \* \*

# NORTHWESTERN MEMORIAL HOSPITAL v. ASHCROFT
## 362 F.3d 923 (7th Cir. 2004)

Posner, Judge.

\* \* \*

The government appeals from an order by the district court quashing a subpoena commanding Northwestern Memorial Hospital in Chicago to produce the medical records of certain patients on whom Dr. Cassing Hammond had performed late-term abortions at the hospital using the controversial method known variously as "D & X" (dilation and extraction) and "intact D & E" (dilation and evacuation). . . .

The subpoenaed records, apparently some 45 in number, are sought for use in the forthcoming trial in the Southern District of New York of a suit challenging the constitutionality of the Partial-Birth Abortion Ban Act of 2003. Dr. Hammond is one of the plaintiffs in that suit and will also be testifying as an expert witness. The district court held that the production of the records is barred by regulations issued under the Health Insurance Portability and Accountability Act of 1996 (HIPAA), and let us begin there.

[The court concludes that the HIPAA Privacy Rule, discussed in Section E of this Chapter, does not bar production of the records, even though it does not supersede state laws that are more protective of privacy and Illinois law prohibits the disclosure of even redacted medical records in judicial proceedings.]

All that [HIPAA] should be understood to do, therefore, is to create a procedure for obtaining authority to use medical records in litigation. Whether the records are actually admissible in evidence will depend among other things on whether they are privileged. And the evidentiary privileges that are applicable to federal-question suits are given not by state law but by federal law, *Fed. R. Evid. 501*, which does not recognize a physician-patient (or hospital-patient) privilege. Rule 501 in terms makes federal common law the source of any privileges in federal-question suits unless an Act of Congress provides otherwise. We do not think HIPAA is rightly understood as an Act of Congress that creates a privilege.

The purely procedural character of the HIPAA standard for disclosure of medical information in judicial or administrative proceedings is indicated by the procedure for disclosure in response to a subpoena or other process; the notice to the patient must contain "sufficient information about the litigation or proceeding in which the protected health information is requested to permit the individual to raise an objection to the court." The objection in court would often be based on a privilege — the source of which would be found elsewhere than in the regulations themselves.

. . . .

. . . Northwestern Memorial Hospital concedes that there is no federal common law physician-patient privilege. It is not for us — especially in so summary a proceeding as this litigation to quash the government's subpoena — to create one. . . .

The district court did not reach a further ground urged by Northwestern Memorial Hospital for quashing the government's subpoena, which is simply that the burden of compliance with it would exceed the benefit of production of the material sought by it. *Fed. R. Civ. P. 45(c) (3) (A) (iv)*. However, . . . the judge made findings that are highly germane to — indeed arguably dispositive of — the Rule 45(c) issue. He pointed out that the "government seeks these records on the *possibility* that it may find something therein which would affect the testimony of Dr. Hammond adversely, that is, for its potential value in impeaching his credibility as a witness. What the government ignores in its argument is how little, if any, probative value lies within these patient records." He contrasted the dearth of probative value "with the potential loss of privacy that would ensue were these medical records used in a case in which the patient was not a party" and concluded that "the balance of harms resulting from disclosure severely outweighs the loss to the government through non-disclosure."

These findings were solidly based. The hospital had urged both the lack of probative value of the records and the loss of privacy by the patients. The government had responded in generalities, arguing that redaction would eliminate any privacy concern and that since Dr. Hammond had "made assertions of fact about his experience and his patients that plaintiffs are using to support their claim that, without a health exception, the Act is unconstitutional," the government should be permitted to test those assertions; but the government had not indicated what assertions these were or how the records might bear on them. . . .

At the oral argument we pressed the government's lawyer repeatedly and hard for indications of what he hoped to learn from the hospital records, and drew a blank. . . . The lawyer did suggest that if Hammond testified that patients with leukemia are better off with the D & X procedure than with the conventional D & E procedure but the medical records indicate that not all abortion patients with leukemia undergo D & X abortions, this would both impeach Hammond and suggest that D & X is not the only medically safe abortion procedure available to pregnant women afflicted with leukemia. But such information would be unlikely to be found in *Hammond's* records, given his strongly expressed preference for using the D & X method in the case of patients in fragile health. The information would be much more likely to be found in the records of physicians who perform D & E rather than D & X abortions on such women. Those records, however, the government didn't seek.

[The Court here explains that, the district judge's findings in effect "weighed the competing hardships" of complying with the subpoena. Because of an impending trial of this case, the Court decided remand was not necessary and would weigh the hardships itself.]

Like the district judge, we think the balance weighs in favor of quashing the subpoena. The government does not deny that the hospital is an appropriate representative of the privacy interests of its patients. But it argues that since it is seeking only a limited number of records and they would be produced to it minus the information that would enable the identity of the patient to be determined, there is no hardship to either the hospital or the patients of compliance. The argument is unrealistic and incomplete. What is true is that the *administrative* hardship of compliance would be modest. But it is not the only or the main hardship. The natural sensitivity that people feel about the disclosure of their medical records — the sensitivity that lies behind HIPAA — is amplified when the records are of a procedure that Congress has now declared to be a crime. Even if all the women whose records the government seeks know what "redacted" means, they are bound to be skeptical that redaction will conceal their identity from the world. . . . These women . . . doubtless . . . are also aware that hostility to abortion has at times erupted into violence, including criminal obstruction of entry into abortion clinics, the fire-bombing of clinics, and the assassination of physicians who perform abortions.

Some of these women will be afraid that when their redacted records are made a part of the trial record in New York, persons of their acquaintance, or skillful "Googlers," sifting the information contained in the medical records concerning each patient's medical and sex history, will put two and two together, "out" the 45 women, and thereby expose them to threats, humiliation, and obloquy. "[W]hether the patients' identities would remain confidential by the exclusion of their names and identifying numbers is questionable at best. The patients' admit and discharge summaries arguably contain histories of the patients' prior and present medical conditions, information that in the cumulative can make the possibility of recognition very high.". . .

Even if there were no possibility that a patient's identity might be learned from a redacted medical record, there would be an invasion of privacy. Imagine if nude pictures of a woman, uploaded to the Internet without her consent though without identifying her by name, were downloaded in a foreign country by people who will never meet her. She would still feel that her privacy had been invaded. The revelation of the intimate details contained in the record of a late-term abortion may inflict a similar wound.

If Northwestern Memorial Hospital cannot shield its abortion patients' records from disclosure in judicial proceedings, moreover, the hospital will lose the confidence of its patients, and persons with sensitive medical conditions may be inclined to turn elsewhere for medical treatment. . . .

The government has had repeated opportunities to articulate a use for the records that it seeks, and it has failed to do so. What it would like to prove at the trial in New York, to refute Dr. Hammond, is that D & E is always an adequate alternative, from the standpoint of a pregnant woman's health, to the D & X procedure. But the government has failed to explain how the record of a D & X abortion would show this. . . .

None of the records is going to state that Dr. Hammond said that he performed a D & X although he believed that a D & E would be just as good. We thought the government might be hoping to find in the records evidence that Hammond had lied when he said he had performed a D & X on a woman who had leukemia or a woman who had breast cancer, but at argument the government disclaimed any such suggestion. We're still at a loss to understand what it hopes to gain from such discovery. (We begged the government's lawyer to be concrete.) Of course, not having seen the records, the government labors under a disadvantage, although it has surely seen other medical records. And of course, pretrial discovery is a fishing expedition and one can't know what one has caught until one fishes. But *Fed. R. Civ. P. 45(c)* allows the fish to object, and when they do so the fisherman has to come up with more than the government has been able to do in this case despite the excellence of its lawyers.

. . . .

Were the government sincerely interested in whether D & X abortions are ever medically indicated, one would have expected it to seek from Northwestern Memorial Hospital statistics summarizing the hospital's experience with late-term abortions. Suppose the patients who undergo D & X abortions are identical in all material respects (age, health, number of weeks pregnant, and so on) to those who undergo procedures not forbidden by the Partial-Birth Abortion Ban Act. That would be potent evidence that the D & X procedure does not have a compelling health rationale. No such evidence has been sought. . . . A variant of the suggested approach would be to obtain a random sample of late-term abortion records from various sources and then determine, through good statistical analysis, whether the patient characteristics that lead Dr. Hammond to perform a D & X lead other physicians to perform a conventional D & E instead, and whether there are differences in the health consequences for these two groups of women. If there are no differences, the government might have a good defense of the Act.

Gathering records from Hammond's patients alone will not be useful; but if the government has *other* records (say, from VA hospitals) already in its files, then records of Hammond's procedures might enable a useful comparison. The government hasn't suggested doing anything like that either. Its motives in seeking individuals' medical records remain thoroughly obscure.

The fact that quashing the subpoena comports with Illinois' medical-records privilege is a final factor in favor of the district order's action. [C]omity "impels federal courts to recognize state privileges where this can be accomplished at no substantial cost to federal substantive and procedural policy." Patients, physicians, and hospitals in Illinois rely on Illinois' strong policy of privacy of medical records. They cannot rely completely, for they are not entitled to count on the state privilege's being applied in federal court. But in a case such as this in which, so far as we can determine, applying the privilege would not interfere significantly with federal proceedings, comity has required us not to apply the Illinois privilege, but to consider with special care the arguments for quashing the subpoena on the basis of relative hardship under *Fed. R. Civ. P. 45(c)*.

\* \* \*

## AID FOR WOMEN v. FOULSTON
### 427 F. Supp. 1093 (D. Kan. 2006)

Marten, Judge.

\* \* \*

Plaintiffs seek to prevent enforcement of Kansas Attorney General Phill Kline's application of the state mandatory reporting statute, through an Attorney General's Opinion [the "Kline Opinion"], to consensual underage sexual activity. [The action was brought pursuant to 42 U.S.C. § 1983 seeking declaratory and injunctive relief by licensed professionals.] Specifically . . . this case turns on whether Kan. Stat. Ann. § 38–1522, commonly referred to as the "Kansas reporting statute," requires reporting of all consensual underage sexual activity as sexual abuse.

. . . [N]either side objects to the reporting of: 1) incest; 2) sexual abuse of a child by an adult; and 3) sexual activities involving a child under the age of twelve. Therefore, the only issue presented is whether consensual underage sexual activity must be reported under the Kansas reporting statute. After extensive review of the record, this court holds that the Kansas reporting statute: 1) does not make all underage sexual activity inherently injurious; and 2) requires that the reporter have reason to suspect both injury and that the injury resulted from illegal sexual activity, as defined by Kansas law, before reporting is required. In addition, to require reporting in accordance with Attorney General Kline's opinion would violate a minor's limited right of informational privacy. Thus, this court permanently enjoins enforcement of Kan. Stat. Ann. § 38–1522 in any manner inconsistent with this decision, which includes the Kline Opinion.

. . . .

As part and parcel of [the state's interest in protecting children], Kansas requires reporting to the state government whenever certain persons have "reason to suspect that a child has been injured as a result of . . . sexual abuse." The mandatory reporting requirement extends to various medical and health care providers, school officials, law enforcement, child care service providers, social workers, counselors, and emergency response personnel. . . . "Willful and knowing failure to make a report" is a misdemeanor criminal offense. . . . [S]exual activity of minors younger than sixteen is illegal, regardless of whether the activity is voluntary or the sexual activity involves an agemate. The only exception to this criminal ban is in the case of consensual sexual contact between a person under sixteen and that person's spouse. Kansas has long allowed twelve-year-old females and fourteen-year-old males to marry with parental or judicial consent, although the Kansas legislature is now considering raising these ages.

. . . .

[The state Department of Social and Rehabilitative Services] has a longstanding policy of screening out consensual underage sexual activity. [Earlier Attorney Generals' opinions required reporters to determine whether sexual activity caused harm.] . . . [O]n June 18, 2003, Kansas Attorney General Phill Kline issued an opinion seeking to significantly change the standard for reporting. His opinion, in part, states:

> Kansas law clearly provides that those who fall under the scope of the reporting requirement must report any reasonable suspicion that a child has been injured as a result of sexual abuse, which would be any time a child under the age of 16 has become pregnant. As a matter of law such child has been the victim of rape or one of the other sexual abuse crimes and such crimes are inherently injurious.

In reaching this conclusion, the Attorney General looked beyond the statute's language and beyond the law of the State of Kansas. His opinion that the minor's pregnancy is "inherently injurious" eliminated the reporter's discretion to determine whether the minor had been "injured." Further, as the Attorney General's opinion acknowledges, such "inherent injury" reaches beyond a minor's pregnancy:

> We are aware that although this opinion is limited to the question posed, the consequences of the conclusion reach further. Other situations that might trigger a mandated reporter's obligation, because sexual activity of a minor becomes known, include a teenage girl or boy who seeks medical attention for a sexually transmitted disease, a teenage girl who seeks medical attention for a pregnancy, or a teenage girl seeking birth control who discloses she has already been sexually active.

Thus, if all illegal sexual activity of a minor is considered sexual abuse and is per se injurious, then pursuant to the Kline Opinion, a mandatory reporter must automatically report any indication that a minor is sexually active.

. . . .

[The reporting statute] recognizes that a mandatory reporter must identify two things: 1) there is reason to suspect that the child has been injured; and 2) the injury resulted from sexual abuse. . . . [T]he legislature has defined "sexual abuse" in Article 35, Chapter 21 of the Kansas Statutes. However, it has not defined "injury."

. . . .

The legislature included a very specific phrase in the statute: "reason to suspect that a child has been injured as a result of . . . sexual abuse. . . ." This phrase vests a degree of discretion in the reporter not only to determine suspected sexual abuse, but also resulting injury. The legislature acknowledged that not all illegal sexual activity involving a minor necessarily results in "injury;" thus, not all unlawful sexual activity warrants reporting. . . .

Therefore, the court finds that the legislature's inclusion of the phrase "reason to suspect that a child has been injured" requires reporters to determine if there is a reason to suspect injury resulting from sexual abuse. "Injury" and "sexual abuse" are distinct concepts under the statute. Any attempt to conflate the meaning of these terms is contrary to a plain reading of this statute.

. . . .

The narrow constitutional issue before this court is whether minor patients have a right to informational privacy concerning consensual sexual activity with an age-mate where there is no evidence of force, coercion, or power differential. Plaintiffs argue that . . . confidentiality is a cornerstone of treating adolescents and that automatic reporting of all illegal, but non-injurious, sexual activity will deter their minor patients' access to health care. Defendants argue that the state interest in reporting of sexual abuse trumps a minor's privacy interests.

An individual's right to informational privacy may be implicated when the government compels disclosure of that individual's personal sexual or health-related information to the government and/or to other third parties. Compelled disclosure may violate an individual's right to informational privacy unless the disclosure serves a compelling state interest in the least intrusive manner. To determine whether information is of such a personal nature that it demands constitutional protection, the court considers: "1) if the party asserting the right has a legitimate expectation of privacy; 2) if disclosure serves a compelling state interest; and 3) if disclosure can be made in the least intrusive manner." A "legitimate expectation of privacy," is based "at least in part, upon the intimate or otherwise personal nature of the material." . . .

Plaintiffs provided credible evidence of irreparable harm at trial. First, the Kline Opinion places plaintiffs on notice that they may be prosecuted for not reporting illegal sexual activity of minors. . . .

Second, considering the Kline Opinion, plaintiffs do not have fair notice of what is reportable under the statute. . . .

. . . .

Third, based upon the testimony and other evidence, serious questions arise as to whether minors will continue to seek timely medical care and psychological services if all illegal sexual activity is automatically reported. . . .

Since medical and psychological care providers have an obligation to disclose the scope of confidentiality at the onset of treatment, underage minors will be aware of the limits of confidentiality and the potential for state notification of underage sexual activity. . . .

. . . Mandatory reporting of all sexual activity to a state agency can be more frightening given the potential for criminal liability. If minors are told that there may be an investigation, they may be more inhibited in seeking care. Further, minors who otherwise would seek medical care with their parents' involvement may be deterred by the potential to involve their parents in a criminal investigation.

Automatic mandatory reporting of illegal sexual activity involving a minor will change the nature of the relationship between a health care provider and the minor patient to some degree. Based on studies that evaluated the effects of parental notification, there will be a significant decrease in minors seeking care and treatment related to sexual activity. In the context of a reporting statute, the effects may be greater since a state agency will be notified of the alleged "sexual abuse." According to several witnesses, in the long-term, forgoing or delaying medical care leads to risks to minors including the worsening of existing medical conditions and the spreading of undiagnosed diseases. The Wisconsin study indicates that at a minimum, young persons report that they will engage in riskier behavior if confidential care is not available. The cumulative, credible medical evidence presented at trial indicates that minors face irreparable harm in the face of a reporting statute that requires automatic disclosure of all illegal sexual activity.

Finally, . . . SRS Director Sandra Hazlett stated that the Kline Opinion would increase the number of intake reports, increasing the workload without a corresponding increase in funding. Besides overwhelming state agencies, reporting all sexual activity as sexual abuse tends to trivialize actual sexual abuse.

. . . .

The state has a strong interest in protecting minors and promoting public health. But this interest is at its ebb in the present action, where the Attorney General's Opinion goes beyond the scope of the reporting statute, potentially criminalizing the decisions health care providers make in utmost good faith, and solely with the physical and emotional health of their patients in mind. The Attorney General's over-expansive interpretation of the reporting statute not only fails to serve the public interest, it actually serves to undermine it by causing minors to avoid seeking medical services and potentially overburdening SRS.

. . . .

[Permanent injunction granted.]

* * *

# NOTES AND QUESTIONS

**1.** As part of the defense of constitutional challenges to the Partial Birth Abortion Ban Act, 18 U.S.C. § 1531, the U.S. Attorney General sought medical records about abortion from hospitals and physicians in several cities, including Chicago, San Francisco, and New York. Resistance to the government's subpoenas met with slightly different court decisions. In *Planned Parenthood Federation of America, Inc. v. Ashcroft*, 2004 U.S. Dist. LEXIS 3383 (N.D. Cal. 2004), Judge Phyllis J. Hamilton did not consider the HIPAA Privacy Rule, but, like the 7th Circuit later, found the government's request to be "irrelevant, unduly burdensome" and that the patients' right to privacy outweighed the government's interest in disclosure, and quashed the subpoena. The federal district court for the Southern District of New York had ordered New York-Presbyterian Hospital to comply with the Justice Department's subpoena on the ground that the records were relevant to the litigation. *National Abortion Federation v. Ashcroft*, 2004 U.S. Dist. LEXIS 4530 (S.D.N.Y. 2004). That decision was appealed to the Court of Appeals for the Second Circuit, which remanded the case, indicating some doubt as to the government need for the records. (The U.S. Supreme Court granted certiorari to review the constitutionality of the Act itself; its decision is expected in 2007. See discussion in Chapter Two.) The Attorney General's Office ultimately abandoned its attempt to obtain medical records, including those in New York, without irrevocably renouncing future subpoenas.

The Attorney General used civil litigation and subpoenas to obtain evidence that could support Congress's finding that so-called partial birth abortions are never medically necessary. Why would the Attorney General want only records of D & X abortions? The *Northwestern Memorial Hospital* decision suggests more useful data to determine medical need for specific abortion procedures. Where might such data be found? State laws requiring reports of abortions may not include the type of procedure performed or complications. Should such information also be reported? (See the discussion of the HIPAA Privacy Rule's exception for "public health" in Section E of this Chapter.)

*Northwestern Memorial Hospital* focuses on the justification for compliance with a subpoena in a civil lawsuit: "The only issue for us is whether, given that there is a potential psychological cost to the hospital's patients, and a potential cost in lost goodwill to the hospital itself, from the involuntary production of the medical records even as redacted, the cost is offset by the probative value of the records. . . ." 362 F.3d at 930. Compare this type of balancing with that used in *Whalen v. Roe*. To what degree must the legislature demonstrate the state's need for information to defend the constitutionality of a compulsory reporting law? What difference might there be between the need for information to pursue a lawsuit and the need for information to develop public policy?

**2.** *Northwestern Memorial Hospital* presents a more sophisticated analysis of the kinds of information that might identify individuals than had earlier U.S. Supreme Court decisions. Judge Posner is quite sensitive to how medical information might be disseminated and how patients might react, even to data that does not include names. Compare his conclusions with those of the U.S. Supreme Court in *Casey*, *supra*. For an analysis and demonstration of ways in individuals can be identified from a few bits of data in apparently "de-identified" data, see Latanya Sweeney, *Maintaining Patient Confidentiality When Sharing Medical Data Requires a Symbiotic Relationship Between Technology and Policy* (MIT Artificial Intelligence Lab. Working Paper No. AIWP-WP344b, 1997). Judge Manion, dissenting in part in *Northwestern Memorial Hospital*, dismissed the fear of disclosure emphasized by Judge Posner in the following language: "In fact, there is no reason to believe that the women themselves have any idea that their records are among the few sought by the government in this case. But even if they knew, no one else ever would, because all of the information that could reasonably be used to identify them will be redacted, and none of the information — not even the redacted non-identifying information — will ever be made public, much less paraded in court or placed on the Internet. . . ." Judge Manion may be correct that the women would not know that their records were sought or submitted. Is this a reason to permit or prohibit their discovery? In this case, the government obtained a protective order for the records it subpoenaed. Protective orders can be and are granted in cases in which the information meets the requirements for discovery or submission in evidence and also warrants protection against disclosure outside the litigation.

**3.** *Foulston* presents an unusual use of a state reporting law. Critics claimed that the state attorney general was using the law as a pretext to investigate medical records to identify minors who had abortions. Regardless of the motives for the "Klein opinion," there may be other reasons for the state or a state agency to seek information from surveillance programs in the future. Can you think of some? The opinion notes that sexually transmitted diseases might be evidence of criminal sexual acts. Could data collected pursuant to STI reporting laws be a source of evidence for a criminal investigation? What if the district attorney simply wanted to see who might be engaging in criminal sexual conduct?

The opinion in *Foulston* details considerable expert testimony that the reporting law, enacted in 1982, if applied to all sexual activity in minors, would discourage adolescents from seeking necessary medical care. Are adolescents different from adults in this respect? The court also noted that reporting laws can create a conflict of interest for physicians, because they have an obligation to maintain patient confidentiality and also to violate that confidentiality when required by law. It added, "Because many licensed professionals play a dual role as both mandatory reporters and care providers, the confidentiality between licensed professionals and patients should be breached only sparingly. . . . [C]onfidentiality is the "cornerstone" of the doctor-patient relationship." Perhaps for this reason, physicians testified at trial that "they personally do not report all cases of underage sexual activity. . . ." The court found that "there is no indication that under-reporting is or has been a problem under the Kansas statute," and that the local district attorney had never prosecuted anyone for not reporting abuse in her 17 years in office. Does this failure to report indicate that physicians are using appropriate discretion, adhering to their duty to act in the best interests of their patients, committing a criminal offense, or acting as conscientious objectors?

* * *

## D.  CONTAGIOUS DISEASE SURVEILLANCE

### Background

At the end of the nineteenth century, tuberculosis (TB) was the leading cause of death in the United States. To control the disease, Dr. Hermann M. Biggs wanted information on where the disease was concentrated and made the then controversial recommendation that physicians in New York City report cases of TB to the city health department. *See generally*, C-E.A. WINSLOW, THE LIFE OF HERMANN M. BIGGS: PHYSICIAN AND STATESMAN OF THE PUBLIC HEALTH (1929). Biggs was then Director of the Bacteriological Laboratory of the Department of Health and encouraged public education about how to avoid TB transmission. In 1897, the city adopted a compulsory reporting ordinance, but bills to rescind it were introduced in each of the next two years, in part because of physician opposition to reporting. To encourage voluntary cooperation among resistant physicians, Biggs offered a carrot — free (often overnight) laboratory analysis of sputum specimens to confirm or deny the presence of TB. Physicians gained useful diagnostic information for their patients, and Dr. Biggs got his surveillance data. Patterns of TB cases provided evidence that tuberculosis was a communicable disease, which some physicians had doubted. Physicians began to appreciate the medical value of collecting data on a population of patients and became willing to report their charity patients. *Id.* Nonetheless, physicians objected to reporting their private patients, believing that it would violate physician-patient confidentiality or stigmatize their paid medical practice. In these early years, fewer than half of the cases of active TB were reported to the health department.

Today, physicians generally accept and support case reporting of certain diseases for certain purposes. At the same time, physicians often have little incentive to spend uncompensated time completing reporting forms. Thus, state legislation requires physicians to report cases of "notifiable" diseases to the state or local health department. Some states specify the diseases in the statute, while others authorize the health commissioner to designate diseases for reporting by regulation or rule. Most statutes limit notifiable diseases to those that qualify as contagious and easily transmissible to others. The terminology used depends on when the laws were enacted, with many using terms common in the early twentieth century, like "communicable" or simply "dangerous." The subgroup of sexually transmitted infections (STIs), called venereal diseases in the past, like syphilis, gonorrhea, and canchroid, caused particular concern in the periods surrounding World War I and II. ( *See* the discussion of the history of quarantine in Chapter Three.) An example of a reporting law is shown in Figure 1, *infra*.

The number of diseases required to be reported has grown substantially. The CDC and the Council of State and Territorial Epidemiologists (CSTE), a professional membership association of epidemiologists employed primarily by state and local departments of health and originally initiated by the CDC, annually recommend diseases for reporting. The CDC manages the National Notifiable Disease Surveillance System (NNDSS), which collects reports of cases of notifiable diseases that are voluntarily submitted to CDC by the states. *See* CDC, NATIONAL NOTIFIABLE DISEASE SURVEILLANCE SYSTEM, www.cdc.gov/epo/dphsi/nndsshis.htm (last visited Aug. 2006). (The proposed federal Biopreparedness Act of 2005 would create a mandatory national reporting system with the same name.) By 1999, CSTE and CDC recommended reporting 52 diseases and four medical conditions. Sandra Roush et al., *Mandatory Reporting of Diseases and Conditions by Health Care Professionals and Laboratories*, 282 JAMA 164, 166 (1999). As Table I shows, the diseases recommended for reporting are no longer limited to those that pose an imminent threat of contagion or even person to person transmission. CSTE/CDC recommendations are highly influential. States, however, have no obligation to accept them and sometimes do not. For example, in 1995 and 1996, CSTE/CDC recommended adding elevated blood lead levels, silicosis, and tobacco use. While some states require the reporting of elevated blood lead levels in children, because lead can cause growth and mental deficits in children less than 6 years of age, no state has required the reporting of tobacco use — yet.

The uses of disease reports have also changed. States that require reporting rarely subject people to compulsory isolation; although partner notification is still used to let others know they may be at risk. Instead, health regulations typically recommend approaches tailored to the specific disease, the mode of transmitting any infection, and the availability of medical treatment. *See, e.g.*, Reportable Diseases, 105 MASS. CODE REGS. § 300.200. For example, the recommendations for food handlers with Amebiasis or Giardiasis are restrictions from work until diarrhea has resolved and they have one negative stool sample, while people with cutaneous anthrax are told not to touch other people until their lesions are healed or they are free of anthrax bacilli. People with Hepatitis B are barred from donating blood or organs and counseled on how to avoid transmission to others. There are no restrictions for reported cases of diseases like arbovirus infection, botulism, encephalitis, or Hansen's disease (leprosy). As noted in the *Axelrod* case, *infra*, interventions can be tailored to the specific risk presented: "the Sanitary Code in general presents a situation where flexibility and that adaptation of the legislative policy to infinitely variable conditions constitute the essence of the program."

## FIGURE 1

*Surveillance and Control of Diseases Dangerous to the Public Health and Access to Medical Records*, 105 MASS. CODE REGS. 300.190-300.191

*300.190: Surveillance and Control of Diseases Dangerous to the Public Health*

The Department and local boards of health are authorized to conduct surveillance activities necessary for the investigation, monitoring, control and prevention of diseases dangerous to the public health. Such activities shall include, but need not be limited to:

(A) Systematic collection and evaluation of morbidity and mortality reports.

(B) Investigation into the existence of diseases dangerous to the public health in order to determine the causes and extent of such diseases and to formulate prevention and control measures.

(C) Identification of cases and contacts.

(D) Counseling and interviewing individuals as appropriate to assist in positive identification of exposed individuals and to develop information relating to the source and spread of illness.

(E) Monitoring the medical condition of individuals diagnosed with or exposed to diseases dangerous to the public health.

(F) Collection and/or preparation of data concerning the availability and use of vaccines, immune globulins, insecticides and other substances used in disease prevention and control.

(G) Collection and/or preparation of data regarding immunity levels in segments of the population and other relevant epidemiological data.

(H) Ensuring that diseases dangerous to the public health are subject to the requirements of 105 CMR 300.200 and other proper control measures.

*300.191: Access to Medical Records and Other Information*

The Department or local boards of health are authorized to obtain, upon request, from health care providers and other persons subject to the provisions of 105 CMR 300.000 *et seq.*, medical records and other information that the Department or the local board of health deems necessary to carry out its responsibilities to investigate, monitor, prevent and control diseases dangerous to the public health.

**Table I.**

CDC, *Nationally Notifiable Infectious Diseases — United States 2006*
www.cdc.gov/epo/dphsi/phs/infdis2006.htm

| | |
|---|---|
| AIDS | Meningococcal disease |
| Anthrax | Mumps |
| Arboviral diseases (*e.g.*, Eastern equine encephalitis; West Nile virus disease) | Pertussis |
| | Plague |
| Western equine encephalitis virus disease | Poliomyelitis, paralytic |
| | Psittacosis |
| Botulism | Q Fever |
| Brucellosis | Rabies |
| Chancroid | Rocky Mountain spotted fever |
| *Chlamydia trachomatis*, genital infections | Rubella |
| | Rubella, congenital syndrome |
| Cholera | Salmonellosis |
| Coccidioidomycosis | (SARS-CoV) disease |
| Cryptosporidiosis | Shiga toxin-producing Escherichia coli |
| Cyclosporiasis | |
| Diphtheria | Shigellosis |
| Ehrlichiosis | Smallpox |
| Giardiasis | Streptococcal disease, invasive, Group A |
| Gonorrhea | |
| *Haemophilus influenzae*, invasive disease | Streptococcal toxic-shock syndrome |
| | Streptococcus pneumoniae |
| Hansen disease (leprosy) | Syphilis |
| Hantavirus pulmonary syndrome | Syphilis, congenital |
| Hemolytic uremic syndrome, post-diarrheal | Tetanus |
| Hepatitis, viral, acute (A, B, C) | Toxic-shock syndrome |
| Hepatitis, viral, chronic (B, C) | (other than Streptococcal) |
| HIV infection | Trichinellosis (Trichinosis) |
| Influenza-associated pediatric mortality | Tuberculosis |
| | Tularemia |
| Legionellosis | Typhoid fever |
| Listeriosis | Vancomycin |
| Lyme disease | Varicella (morbidity) |
| Malaria | Varicella (deaths only) |
| Measles | Yellow fever |

Note: Several diseases are divided into different manifestations, *e.g.*, adult/pediatric; animal/human; and viral variants.

# NEW YORK STATE SOCIETY OF SURGEONS v. AXELROD

## 77 N.Y.2d 677, 572 N.E.2d 605, 569 N.Y.S.2d 922 (1991)

Simons, Judge.

\* \* \*

Petitioners are four medical organizations whose membership consists of New York State physicians. Respondents are the Commissioner of Health and the New York State Public Health Council. In February of 1988, petitioners sent a letter to the Commissioner of Health requesting that infection with the human immunodeficiency virus (HIV infection) be added to the lists of communicable and sexually transmissible diseases pursuant to Public Health Law § 225(5) (h) and § 2311.[3] The Commissioner denied the request on the ground that designation would be contrary to the health of the public because it would discourage cooperation of affected individuals and would lead to the loss of confidentiality for those infected with the disease. Petitioners then commenced this . . . proceeding contending that the statutes imposed a duty on respondents to add HIV infection to the lists or, alternatively, if designation was a matter of discretion, that respondents' refusal to list HIV infection was arbitrary and capricious.

The Commissioner of Health is appointed by the Governor with the consent of the Senate and is charged with the responsibility of taking "cognizance of the interests of health and life of the people of the state, and of all matters pertaining thereto" (Public Health Law § 204[1]; § 206[1][a]). . . . The Public Health Council . . . appointed by the Governor . . . establishes health and health-related regulations, known as the Sanitary Code of the State of New York, subject to approval by the Commissioner (Public Health Law § 225[4]). The list of communicable diseases is promulgated by the Council with the approval of the Commissioner pursuant to Public Health Law § 225(4) and (5)(h). The list of sexually transmissible diseases is promulgated by the Commissioner pursuant to Public Health Law § 2311. Both are set forth in the Sanitary Code.

HIV infection is a communicable disease. It is transmitted by sexual contact, intravenous drug use or transfusions of infected blood. It can also spread from an infected mother to her infant during pregnancy or at the time of birth. Studies show no evidence that the infection is transmitted by casual contact. Individuals with HIV infection may or may not develop signs of infection and the disease can lead to AIDS. AIDS is a disease which damages the individual's immune system: those who develop it are vulnerable to unusual infections and cancers that do not generally pose a threat to anyone whose immune system is intact. At the present time there is no known cure for AIDS and the percentage of HIV infected individuals who will develop it is not known.

Petitioners contend first that the provisions of section 225(5) (h) and section 2311 require respondents to list HIV infection as a communicable and sexually transmissible disease. We do not construe those sections as imposing a

---

[3] Petitioners originally requested that respondents designate AIDS as a communicable and a sexually transmitted disease. They subsequently expanded the request to include any status of HIV seropositivity (see, Public Health Law § 2780 [definitions]).

flat, unvarying duty on respondents to designate as such every communicable or sexually transmissible disease in the Sanitary Code.

Section 225(5) (h) of the Public Health Law provides that "[the] sanitary code may . . . designate the communicable diseases which are dangerous to the public health." Petitioners noting that HIV infection is both "communicable" and "dangerous to the public health," contend that the statute requires respondents to list it. The Legislature's use of the permissive word "may," however, supports the conclusion that designation is left to the discretion of respondents. Indeed, we find no language in Public Health Law § 225(5) (h) that arguably could be construed as mandating that they list all communicable diseases.

Our construction of the statute is confirmed by the language found in section 225(4) and (5) (a) of the Public Health Law. Section 225(4) authorizes the Council, with the approval of the Commissioner, to "establish, and from time to time, amend and repeal sanitary regulations, to be known as the sanitary code of the state of New York." Subdivision (5) of the same section provides that the Sanitary Code "may," "deal with any matters affecting the security of life or health or the preservation and improvement of public health in the state of New York". . . . [I]n *Chiropractic Assn. v Hilleboe* [we] stated that "the Sanitary Code in general presents a situation where flexibility and the adaptation of the legislative policy to infinitely variable conditions constitute the essence of the program." That observation is pertinent to respondents' powers to amend and adapt the Sanitary Code in order to deal with changing public health concerns regarding HIV infections.

The Commissioner of Health is vested with similar discretion under section 2311 of the Public Health Law. That section provides that the Commissioner shall promulgate a list of sexually transmissible diseases, "such as gonorrhea and syphilis." In determining the diseases to be included in such list, the Commissioner "shall consider those conditions principally transmitted by sexual contact and the impact of particular diseases on individual morbidity and the health of newborns."

Petitioners assert that because HIV infection is principally transmitted by sexual contact and has an impact on individual morbidity and the health of the newborns, respondents must include it on the list of sexually transmissible diseases. However, the statute does not require that every sexually transmitted disease be listed. It identifies the type of diseases to be covered, "such as gonorrhea and syphilis," and directs the Commissioner to "consider" conditions transmitted by sexual contact. Under the terms of the statute, the Commissioner has the discretion to "determin[e] the diseases to be included in such list." The discretionary nature of the power conferred is confirmed by the legislative history of the statute. As originally proposed, section 2311 could have been read as requiring that all sexually transmitted diseases be listed. Governor Carey vetoed it for that reason. . . .

There are valid reasons for giving the Commissioner discretion in these matters. Placement of any disease on the communicable or sexually transmitted disease lists triggers statutory provisions relating to isolation and quarantine, reporting, mandatory testing, and contact tracing — provisions which, for public health reasons, may not be appropriate in dealing with every type of communicable or sexually transmissible disease. The Commissioner has determined, for example, that no public health purpose is served by placing influenza, a communicable disease, and chlamydia, a sexually transmissible disease, on the lists. Whether HIV infection should be listed or not involves a similar determination by respondents after considering the circumstances attendant to the disease.

Petitioners urge alternatively that if respondents have discretion in these matters, their determination in this case is arbitrary and capricious because they failed to consider the pervasive and serious effect of the disease on the public as a whole and petitioners in particular. They argue that the reporting, mandatory testing and contact tracing requirements contained in the communicable and sexually transmissible disease statutes are crucial in controlling the spread of HIV infection and necessary to allow them to determine whether patients are infected with the disease so that they can take appropriate precautions during treatment.

Our review is limited to whether respondents' determination is rationally based, i.e., whether it is unreasonable, arbitrary or capricious. We cannot substitute our judgment for that of qualified experts in the field of public health unless their judgment is "without justification." We conclude that in this case the evidence in the record provides a rational basis for respondents' determination.

Respondents have declined to add HIV infection to the lists because the provisions triggered by that designation — isolation and quarantine, reporting, mandatory testing and contact tracing — are, in their opinion, ineffective and impractical in dealing with it.

Petitioners acknowledge that isolation and quarantine would not be appropriate for HIV infection because there is no evidence that it is spread by casual contact. Their argument is directed to the provisions of the statute requiring reporting, testing and contact tracing. Under existing requirements, New York State and New York City health officials already have access to reported cases of HIV infection, including most confirmatory test results. Thus, the inquiry narrows to whether respondents' determination to forego contact tracing and mandatory testing of those infected with HIV is rational. In support of their decision, respondents note that, as a practical matter, mandatory testing and contact tracing will not lead to control and prevention because many persons infected with HIV are not tested until their symptoms become apparent and symptoms may not develop for many years. In the interim, between infection and the appearance of symptoms, an individual may have multiple needle sharing, sexual contacts or both. These factors would make contact tracing, without the voluntary cooperation of the infected individuals, an almost impossible task. Moreover, HIV antibodies may take months to develop and infected individuals who have not yet developed antibodies may be capable of carrying and transmitting the disease. Thus, while contact tracing has historically been a useful public health tool in stemming epidemics of readily discoverable communicable diseases which have a short incubation period, that is not the nature of HIV infections.

In addition to these practical limitations, respondents argue that mandatory testing and contact tracing would prevent individuals with HIV infection from cooperating with public health officials. This is so because of the fatal and incurable nature of HIV infection and the segment of the population which has in the past been most affected by that disease. Respondents note that most people affected have strong reasons to avoid disclosing that they have AIDS or HIV infection and confidentiality is critical to them. Intravenous drug users, who make up an ever increasing percentage of new AIDS cases, are engaged in behavior which is illegal and there is little reason to believe they will cooperate with health authorities in identifying their needle sharing contacts. Similar disincentives exist for homosexuals and others at risk of HIV infection because disclosure can result in discrimination in housing, employment and health care. Respondents contend that counseling and active voluntary cooperation are essential to alter private sexual and drug abuse practices which spread HIV infection and they maintain that infected individuals will come forward for counseling and testing only if they are assured that testing will not be coerced and that their test results will remain confidential.

Respondents' approach is in accord with the State policy underlying article 27-F of the Public Health Law, a statute enacted to promote voluntary testing for HIV infection. As the Governor emphasized in approving the act, "by enacting this bill, New York rejects coercive measures. As experience in other states has shown, mandatory testing of broad population groups is neither effective nor desirable."

The relief petitioners seek is inconsistent with that legislation. In article 27-F, the Legislature has mandated that written informed consent must be obtained from an individual prior to the performance of any HIV-related test. By contrast, informed consent is not required to test for communicable or sexually transmissible diseases generally. Moreover, article 27-F sets strict limits on contact tracing. For example, it permits physicians to warn an identified contact if they believe the contact is in danger, but precludes the physician from revealing the subject's identity. Any individual who does not want a physician to notify contacts can obtain anonymous testing pursuant to section 2781 of the Public Health Law. No such limitations exist on contact tracing once a disease is listed as communicable. Finally, article 27-F provides a mechanism for assuring anonymity and confidentiality of test results). No comparable protections are provided to an individual once the disease has been listed as communicable or sexually transmissible.

Finally, respondents' approach to the problem is supported by leading health authorities. The United States Centers for Disease Control has adopted guidelines for dealing with HIV infection which include voluntary testing, counseling and confidentiality of personal information. Similarly, the Institute of Medicine, National Academy of Sciences, has concluded that mandatory testing and contact tracing are inappropriate, at this stage, to deal with the spread of HIV infection. We conclude, therefore, that respondents' determination that designating HIV infection as a communicable or sexually transmissible disease would be detrimental to the public health is rational.

Accordingly, the order of the Appellate Division [holding that designation was discretionary with respondents and that their decision was reasonable] should be affirmed, with costs.

* * *

Figure 2

Physician's Name: _____
(Last, First, M.I.)

Hospital/Facility: _____

Phone No.: ( ) _____

Person
Completing Form: _____

Medical
Record No.: _____

Phone No.: ( ) _____

- *Patient identifier information is not transmitted to CDC!* -

## VIII. CLINICAL STATUS

| CLINICAL RECORD REVIEWED: | Yes [1] No [0] | ENTER DATE PATIENT WAS DIAGNOSED AS: | Asymptomatic (Including acute retroviral syndrome and persistent generalized lymphadenopathy): | Mo. Yr. ☐☐ | Symptomatic (not AIDS): | Mo. Yr. ☐☐ |

| AIDS INDICATOR DISEASES | INITIAL DIAGNOSIS Def. Pres. | INITIAL DATE Mo. Yr. | AIDS INDICATOR DISEASES | INITIAL DIAGNOSIS Def. Pres. | INITIAL DATE Mo. Yr. |
|---|---|---|---|---|---|
| Candidiasis, bronchi, trachea, or lungs | [1] NA | ☐☐☐ | Lymphoma, Burkitt's (or equivalent term) | [1] NA | ☐☐☐ |
| Candidiasis, esophageal | [1] [2] | ☐☐☐ | Lymphoma, immunoblastic (or equivalent term) | [1] NA | ☐☐☐ |
| Carcinoma, invasive cervical | [1] NA | ☐☐☐ | Lymphoma, primary in brain | [1] NA | ☐☐☐ |
| Coccidioidomycosis, disseminated or extrapulmonary | [1] NA | ☐☐☐ | Mycobacterium avium complex or M.kansasii, disseminated or extrapulmonary | [1] [2] | ☐☐☐ |
| Cryptococcosis, extrapulmonary | [1] NA | ☐☐☐ | M. Tuberculosis, pulmonary* | [1] [2] | ☐☐☐ |
| Cryptosporidiosis, chronic intestinal (>1 mo. Duration) | [1] NA | ☐☐☐ | M. Tuberculosis, disseminated or extrapulmonary* | [1] [2] | ☐☐☐ |
| Cytomegalovirus disease (other than liver, spleen, or nodes) | [1] NA | ☐☐☐ | Mycobacterium, of other species or unidentified species, disseminated for extrapulmonary | [2] | ☐☐☐ |
| Cytomegalovirus retinitis (with loss of vision) | [1] [2] | ☐☐☐ | Pneumocystis carinii pneumonia | [1] [2] | ☐☐☐ |
| HIV encephalopathy | [1] NA | ☐☐☐ | Pneumonia, recurrent, in 12 mo. period | [1] [2] | ☐☐☐ |
| Herpes simplex chronic ulcer(s) (>1 mo. duration); or bronchitis, pneumonitis or esophagitis | [1] NA | ☐☐☐ | Progressive multifocal leukoencephalopathy | [1] NA | ☐☐☐ |
| Histoplasmosis, disseminated or extrapulmonary | [1] NA | ☐☐☐ | Salmonella septicemia, recurrent | [1] NA | ☐☐☐ |
| Isosporiasis, chronic intestinal (>1 mo. duration) | [1] NA | ☐☐☐ | Toxoplasmosis of brain | [1] [2] | ☐☐☐ |
| Kaposi's sarcoma | [1] [2] | ☐☐☐ | Wasting syndrome due to HIV | [1] NA | ☐☐☐ |

Def. = definitive diagnosis　　Pres. = presumptive diagnosis　　　　* RVCT CASE NO.: ☐☐☐☐☐☐☐

● If HIV tests were not positive or were not done, does this patient have an immunodeficiency that would disqualify him/her from the AIDS case definition?　[1] Yes　[0] No　[9] Unknown

## IX. TREATMENT/SERVICES REFERRALS

Has this patient been informed of his/her HIV infection?　[1] Yes　[0] No　[9] Unk.

This patient's partners will be notified about their HIV exposure and counseled by:
[1] Health department　[2] Physician/provider　[3] Patient　[9] Unknown

| This patient received or is receiving | Yes No Unk. |
|---|---|
| ● Anti-retroviral therapy for HIV treatment | [1] [0] [9] |
| ● PCP prophylaxis | [1] [0] [9] |

This patient has been enrolled at:
| Clinical Trial | Clinic |
|---|---|
| [1] NIH-sponsored | [1] NRSA-sponsored |
| [2] Other | [2] Other |
| [3] None | [3] None |
| [4] Unknown | [4] Unknown |

This patient is receiving or has been referred for:
|  | Yes No NA Unk. |
|---|---|
| ● HIV related medical services | [1] [0] – [9] |
| ● Substance abuse treatment services | [1] [0] [8] [9] |

This patient's medical treatment is primarily reimbursed by:
| [1] Medicaid | [2] Private insurance/HMO |
|---|---|
| [3] No coverage | [4] Other Public Funding |
| [7] Clinical trial/government program | [9] Unknown |

**FOR WOMEN:**
● This patient is receiving or has been referred for gynecological or obstetrical services　[1] Yes　[0] No　[9] Unknown
● Is this patient currently pregnant?　[1] Yes　[0] No　[9] Unknown
● Has this patient delivered live-born infants?　[1] Yes (if delivered after 1977, provide birth information below for the most recent birth)　[0] No　[9] Unknown

| CHILD'S DATE OF BIRTH: Mo. Day Yr. | Hospital of Birth: _____ | Child's Soundex | Child's State Patient No. |
|---|---|---|---|
|  | City: _____ State: _____ | ☐☐☐☐ | ☐☐☐☐☐ |

Would you like the health department to provide (circle Yes or No or A,B,C, and D below)
(A) Post-test counseling: Yes or No (B) Referral for social work/support services: Yes or No
(C) Partner notification: Yes No or (D) Info. about TDH HIV Drug Assistance Program: Yes or No
!!! IMPORTANT NOTICE !!!
IF "YES" TO ANY OF THE ABOVE, PLEASE INFORM YOUR PATIENT THAT HE/SHE WILL BE
CONFIDENTIALLY CONTACTED BY A HEALTH DEPARTMENT REPRESENTATIVE

**Figure 2 (*Continued*)**

# NOTES AND QUESTIONS

**1.** The *Axelrod* opinion illustrates the discretion typically allowed to state health officials to determine whether cases of disease should be reported to the state by law. The petitioners in *Axelrod* were physicians who wanted to know whether their patients were HIV positive. What might have influenced physicians to advocate for making HIV infection a reportable disease? At the time the *Axelrod* case was decided, many physicians were worried about becoming infected with HIV as a result of treating HIV positive patients. In 1990, Dr. David Acer, a dentist in Florida, was found to be the most likely source of HIV infection in five of his patients, including Kimberly Bergalis, although the precise mechanism of transmission has never been determined. CDC, *Update: Transmission of HIV Infection during an Invasive Dental Procedure — Florida*, MORBIDITY & MORTALITY WKLY. REP., Jan. 18, 1991, at 21. Senator Jesse Helms advocated a $10,000 fine and a 10-year prison sentence for HIV positive physicians who practiced medicine. Some physicians began to advocate for testing physicians for HIV, perhaps in order to justify testing their patients; the risk of transmission from patient to physician was at least verifiable, while the risk of transmission from physician to patient remained unknown and probably infinitesimal. In 1991, the American Medical Association issued a statement that "Physicians who are HIV positive have an ethical obligation not to engage in any professional activity which has an identifiable risk of transmission of that infection to the patient." AM. MED. ASS'N, STATEMENT ON HIV-INFECTED PHYSICIANS (Jan. 17, 1991). For a description of the general controversy and an argument that physicians have no duty to disclose their HIV status because it does not affect their ability to practice medicine, but should refrain from engaging in any medical procedure that they cannot perform safely and competently for any reason, see Leonard H. Glantz, Wendy K. Mariner & George J. Annas, *Risky Business: Setting Public Health Policy for HIV Infected Health Care Professionals*, 70 THE MILBANK Q. 43 (1992).

Judge Simons' opinion in *Axelrod* states that persons with certain reportable diseases could be subjected to isolation and mandatory testing and contact tracing. As discussed in Chapter Three, isolation can be imposed on the basis of clearly defined standards. Is the judge correct that persons can also be tested for a disease without consent?

**2.** In the early twentieth century, courts upheld the state's power to require physicians to report cases of communicable disease to the health department. *See* JAMES A. TOBY, PUBLIC HEALTH LAW 110 (3d ed. 1947). Decided before the development of antibiotics and most vaccines, those cases recognized that little could be done to stop the spread of contagious disease besides separating those who were infected from those who were not. The need for immediate intervention made it important to find people with a serious contagious disease as quickly as possible. Only a few reported decisions since the 1960s involve disease reporting laws, primarily HIV/AIDS reporting. In *Middlebrooks v. State Board of Health*, 710 So. 2d 891 (Ala. 1998), a physician had provided certain statistical data, but refused to provide the names and addresses of his patients with HIV and AIDS as required by Alabama's reporting statute. The court upheld the State Board of Health's power to compel the disclosure in a summary decision without explaining the reasons for its conclusion. The lack of cases on reporting laws and the limited explanations for the decisions that exist could mean that these courts consider reporting laws generally within the state's power to protect public health. Alternatively, it might mean that the courts have not yet been forced to present a clear statement of their reasoning.

**3.** The most immediate use of communicable disease reports still is to investigate the source of a possible epidemic or outbreak of contagious disease and remove the hazard or limit (control) the spread of disease. Indeed, formal case reporting systems may be more valuable in investigating an ongoing outbreak than in discovering it in the first place. *See* Robert A. Weinstein, *Planning for Epidemics — The Lessons of SARS*, 350 NEW ENG. J. MED. 23, 24 (2004) ("The recent high-profile epidemics [*e.g.*, those of SARS, West Nile virus, anthrax, and monkeypox] were all first identified by alert clinicians."). Because outbreaks are now rare, however, outbreak investigations occupy a small proportion of state surveillance program activities. In the case of a serious disease, public health investigators interview the person reported to determine where he or she might have been exposed to a virus, for example. They also typically ask who the patient has had contact with, so that those people can be interviewed to see if they also became infected. Contacts of these persons may also be investigated. This process, known as contact tracing, can continue until the source of the problem is found and, ideally, eliminated. If the disease has an environmental source, such as contaminated water for cholera or food for salmonella, investigators may be able to find the source and remove the danger. If the disease is spread by personal contact, like STIs and TB, public health nurses can advise the patient's contacts to seek medical testing and treatment and, if they are not infected, how to avoid infection. Partner notification traces a reported person's sexual or household contacts in order to let them know that they have been exposed to a contagious disease. Because of its association with sexual activity, partner notification can be a sensitive matter. The more stigma that is attached to the disease being investigated, the more reluctant patients may be to reveal their sexual contacts to a public health investigator. Partner notification programs have mixed results, depending upon the state and the disease in question. *See* Matthew R. Golden et al., *HIV Partner Notification Programs in the United States: A National Survey of Program Coverage and Results*, 31 SEXUALLY TRANSMITTED DISEASES 709 (2004). New York City's health department reported less success in contacting partners than elsewhere: "Of 4312 persons with newly diagnosed HIV infection in 2003, information on these persons' partners was available for less than a fifth and testing results were confirmed for fewer than 200 partners." Thomas R. Frieden et al., *Applying Public Health Principles to the HIV Epidemic*, 353 NEW. ENG. J. MED. 2397 (2005).

**4.** Historically, reports for contagious diseases submitted to state health departments included the patient's name. Reporting systems were originally designed to prevent an epidemic, so health officials often needed to meet the patient. In some cases, it may have been necessary to seek a court order to isolate the person or quarantine a house. Knowledge of personal identity is obviously necessary in such circumstances. When the AIDS epidemic emerged in 1981, states began to require the reporting of symptomatic AIDS cases in the same way sexually transmitted diseases were reported — with the patient's name. Some states simply added AIDS to the list of communicable diseases that were required to be reported. Many, however, adopted separate statutes so that AIDS cases would not automatically be subject to control measures like isolation that applied to other contagious diseases. One reason for this approach was that AIDS was considered incurable and isolation would have to last a lifetime if it were imposed solely because a person had AIDS. This seemed unnecessary and unjust to many, especially the growing number of AIDS advocacy groups. In addition, Supreme Court decisions recognizing more explicit constitutional protection of personal autonomy militated against imposing compulsory measures on people with a disease that was spread, not inadvertently through the air, but by particular behavior, such as unprotected sex and sharing syringes.

After 1985, with the development of reliable diagnostic tests for the HIV virus and antiretroviral therapies and better survival rates for people with HIV infection, some states began to adopt laws requiring the reporting of HIV cases in addition to AIDS cases. HIV/AIDS advocacy organizations objected to including names and other identifiable information. They also believed that names were unnecessary for the purpose of the reports and feared that the identities of individuals would be shared or disclosed to employers, insurers, or others who would discriminate against those reported. (This had not been a major impediment when AIDS reporting laws were first adopted in the early 1980s, probably because most AIDS patients then were too ill to work and insurance coverage was rarely available.) Many people at particular risk for HIV sought testing at centers that did not require their names in order to avoid such problems. There was concern that if names were required, they would not seek testing and might inadvertently infect others if they were in fact HIV positive. Opponents of named HIV reporting pointed to a few cases in which unauthorized people obtained lists of reported names or where old computers were sold to the public with lists of names still on the hard drive. Public health departments, justly proud of their tradition of maintaining confidentiality of individual identities, defended both the need for the information and their ability to keep records confidential. The terminology for reporting systems changed. Reporting systems that require a person's name are now called "confidential reporting," instead of "named" reporting, to indicate that identifiable information is collected but kept confidential within the health department. Systems that do not require or collect names are called "anonymous reporting."

The Institute of Medicine summarized the controversy surrounding the adoption of HIV reporting as follows:

> Public health authorities justified reporting of HIV infection on several grounds. Reporting would alert public health officials to the presence of individuals with a lethal infection; would allow officials to counsel them about what they needed to do to prevent further transmission; would assure the linkage of infected persons with medical and other services [if public health officials referred them to accessible facilities]; and would permit authorities to monitor the incidence and prevalence of infection. In the following years, the CDC continued to press for name-based reporting of HIV cases. . . . Political resistance persisted however, and HIV cases typically became reportable by name only in states that did not have large cosmopolitan communities with effectively organized gay constituencies or high AIDS caseloads. By 1996, although 26 states had adopted HIV case reporting, they represented jurisdictions with only approximately a quarter of total reported AIDS cases.

INSTITUTE OF MEDICINE, MEASURING WHAT MATTERS: ALLOCATION, PLANNING, AND QUALITY ASSESSMENT FOR THE RYAN WHITE CARE ACT 78 (2004) [hereinafter IOM, MEASURING WHAT MATTERS].

*ACT-UP Triangle v. Comm'n for Health Servs. of North Carolina*, 345 N.C. 699, 483 S.E.2d 388 (N.C. 1997), illustrates that resistance. The North Carolina Commission on Health Services adopted a rule to eliminate anonymous HIV testing (which did not record names) at local health departments by September 1994. Advocacy groups and individuals petitioned the Commission to rescind the new rule and to keep offering anonymous testing. Although the court recognized that "arguments can and have been made that the previous program of exempting HIV testing from the reporting requirements is the better policy," it concluded that confidential testing did not violate petitioners' rights to privacy. The court found that the Commission's decision was based on sufficient evidence in the record and was not arbitrary or capricious; it concluded that it did not have authority to override the exercise of agency discretion properly exercised. The Court did not confront the question whether the state could grant such discretion to the agency without infringing on the constitutional rights of its residents.

**5.** In Massachusetts, California, Maryland, and a few other states with large numbers of people with HIV, physicians recorded a code (numbers or letters) instead of the name on the report that went to the heath department. In other states, the physician submitted the name, but the health department replaced it with a code. The most common code in use is the Soundex code. The U.S. National Archives and Records Administration and other organizations use a Soundex code for genealogical and other types of searches and provide instructions on how to construct a Soundex code for names. *See* www. archives.gov/research_room/genealogy/census/soundex.html (last visited Aug. 2006). (The code uses the first letter of a person's surname followed by three numbers assigned to the consonants next appearing in the name. The numbering rules are uniform across agencies and websites: 1 = B, F, P, V; 2 = C, G, J, K, Q, S, X, Z; 3 = D, T; 4 = L; 5 = M, N; 6 = R; 0 = no additional letters in name. For example, the name Washington is coded W252, and Gutierrez is coded G362. The result gives a phonetic result without the vowels or the consonants H, W and Y. Some websites automatically convert a surname to a soundex code with a click of the mouse: *See, e.g.,* www.geocities.com/Heartland/Hills/ 3916/soundex.html (last visited Aug. 2006). Some states add elements like date of birth to the Soundex code to create a unique identifier. In California, until recently, the provider sent the health department the Soundex code, plus the date of birth, gender, and the last 4 digits of the social security number of a patient being reported with HIV infection.

Physicians, hospitals and laboratories send completed case report forms to the state health department, either in paper or electronic form. The health department periodically compiles the case reports and sends them on to the CDC's surveillance unit, after removing the physician's name and replacing the patient's name with a Soundex code and adding a 6-digit date of birth and residence at diagnosis. (An example of a report form to the CDC is shown in Figure 2.) One pilot study of six states found that a major activity of their surveillance programs was compiling reports for submission to the CDC. The Public Health Service Act authorizes CDC to collect, conduct research, and publish information about diseases. Public Health Service Act § 301(a), 42 U.S.C. § 241(a). The CDC has stated that the use of the Soundex code protects the confidentiality of a person's identity "because a person's name cannot be inferred from a phonetic Soundex code." CDC, SOUNDEX — REFERENCE GUIDE 2 (Dec. 1999), *available at* www.cdc.gov/od/hissb/docs/Soundex.pdf (last visited Aug. 2006) ("Soundex data are permitted for transfer to CDC because a person [sic] name cannot be inferred from a phonetic Soundex code. By using Soundex in conjunction with other demographic data such as date of birth and sex, CDC programs are able to identify duplicate name reports while adhering to patient confidentiality and privacy laws.").

Is it possible to convert a Soundex code back into a person's name? Would the additional information contained on the form permit identification? Do the concerns about the possibility of identification discussed in *Thornburgh* and *Northwestern Memorial Hospital, supra,* apply here?

**6.** Providers and health care facilities are typically required to submit a report every time they see a patient with a reportable disease, and laboratories every time they conduct a test for the patient. The same person may be reported several times or by several providers or laboratories (duplicate reports). Like any organization that conducts statistical analyses, the CDC wants to determine which reports refer to the same person so that one person is not counted more than once. Reports with names or the Soundex code enable the CDC to do so. "Deduplication" is also possible even if different states use different codes that do not permit identification of the patient. However, CDC has declined to accept reports from states that use such codes on the ground that it is unable to deduplicate them. *See* IOM, MEASURING WHAT MATTERS, *supra* (recommending that the CDC accept HIV reports from all states, regardless of whether names or codes are used, and develop better methods of deduplication).

**7.** The CDC uses the reports it receives from the states for many different purposes. Perhaps the most common is to compile monthly and annual summaries of the number of people in each state and the country as a whole with a specific disease. Periodic reports are published in the CDC's *Morbidity and Mortality Weekly Review* and summaries are available on the CDC website at www.cdc.gov (last visited August 2006). The agency also reviews the reports to see whether a disease is occurring with unusual frequency in particular locations or among specific populations. More detailed analyses may be conducted to determine, for example, whether patients with specific characteristics — like age, race or sex, drug use, or insurance coverage — have a high or low incidence of disease, receive treatment, or survive for given periods of time. The findings can be used to alert both researchers and clinicians to the types of people who might be at risk for a disease.

**8.** Many state surveillance systems, especially those for AIDS and HIV case reports and cancer case registries (discussed in Section F below), depend significantly on federal funding to operate. AIDS case reporting may the most complete because of such funding. A survey conducted for the Institute of Medicine found that "[d]uring 1999-2002, the majority of funds for AIDS and HIV surveillance programs came from the federal government, and in 32 states it was entirely from the federal government." IOM, MEASURING WHAT MATTERS, *supra,* at 241. On average, in the 41 states surveyed, federal funding accounted for more than 95 percent of state budgets used for HIV and AIDS case reporting. States facing lower revenues may curtail or eliminate surveillance programs. California, which endured significant budget cuts in recent years, reduced state funding for its Birth Defects Monitoring Program, for example. *See* STRATEGIES FOR ESTABLISHING AN ENVIRONMENTAL HEALTH SURVEILLANCE SYSTEM IN CALIFORNIA: REPORT OF THE SB 702 WORKING GROUP (California Policy Research Center, 2004), *available at* www.ucop.edu/cprc (last visited August 2006).

Funding may also come with strings attached. In the case of HIV case reporting programs, federal funding provided the carrot or stick that persuaded states that used codes instead of names to change their laws to require the reporting of HIV cases with the name of the patient, often against the advice of the health department, AIDS treatment programs, and advocacy organizations. The circumstances surrounding that change demonstrate not only the influence of federal funding on state law, but also the increasing use of surveillance data in formulas for allocating federal funds among the states, and are described in IOM, MEASURING WHAT MATTERS, *supra*, at 73–85.

**9.** The best defense against infectious disease is an effective vaccine that prevents illness and the ability to transmit the disease. Concerns about avian influenza were eased slightly in 2005 when initial clinical trials of an investigational vaccine appeared promising. The best known immunizations are those for pediatric diseases. The Healthy People 2010 immunization goal is 80 percent of children 19–35 months of age to be vaccinated with DTP, polio, MMR, Hib, and PCV. In 2004, the US substantially exceeded that goal, with well over ninety percent coverage of all but the last two (more recent) vaccines. As of 2004, the CDC National Immunization Survey (NIS) — a telephone survey of households using random digit dialing — estimated that between 92.6 and 95.9 percent of children received adequate doses of the recommended vaccines (diphtheria, tetanus toxoid and pertussis; poliovirus; haemophilus influenzae type b (Hib); measles-mumps-rubella; and hepatitis B). 87.5 percent received varicella (chickenpox) vaccine. 73.2 percent received pneumococcal conjugate vaccine (PCV). Philip J. Smith et al., *Overview of the Sampling Design and Statistical Methods Used in the National Immunization Survey*, 20 AM. J. PREV. MED. 17 (2001). The response rate was 67.4%. Another objective of Healthy People 2010 is to increase participation by children up to 6 years old in immunization registries to 95%.

All states have immunization registries, which collect information from health care providers about the vaccines received by individual children. CDC, *Immunization Information System Progress — United States, 2003*, MORBIDITY & MORTALITY WKLY. REP., July 29, 2005, at 722. *See generally* CDC, NATIONAL VACCINE ADVISORY COMMITTEE, DEVELOPMENT OF COMMUNITY AND STATE-BASED IMMUNIZATION REGISTRIES: REPORT OF THE NATIONAL VACCINE ADVISORY COMMITTEE (1999), *available at* www.cdc.gov/nip/registry/nvac.htm (last visited Aug. 2006). The CDC administers grants to immunization registries in 50 states. Public Health Service Act § 317b. The data are used to estimate what proportion of the population has been vaccinated against different diseases. Individuals for whom specific vaccinations are not recorded can be contacted and reminded to get immunized. Somewhat more sophisticated registries, called immunization information systems (IIS), also can be used to record adverse events associated with vaccination, maintain a lifetime history of vaccinations, and link with electronic medical records.

Although almost all children in the country have been vaccinated for childhood infectious diseases, fewer than half voluntarily participate in an immunization registry. Forty-four percent of children under six are recorded in immunization information systems. Public medical facilities are twice as likely as private providers to submit vaccination information to registries. CDC, *Immunization System Progress, supra*, at 722.

Should states require reporting to immunization registries? The CDC favors such laws so that children can be followed and urged to get all their vaccinations. In addition, the CDC wants to link immunization registries to electronic medical records to make it easy for physicians to report immunization data for their patients. Some of the CDC funded registries already link information from the registry and medical record systems, such as Medicaid or the special Supplemental Nutrition program of Women, Infants, and Children (WIC).

**10.** State and federal public records and freedom of information laws give the public access to government agency records. Specific statutes have been enacted to permit the agencies to keep some health information confidential, including data collected by some surveillance programs. In the absence of such confidentiality laws, members of the public could claim access to disease reports about individuals that were submitted to the health department. For example, in *Thomas v. Morris*, 286 N.Y. 266, 36 N.E.2d 141 (1941), the New York Court of Appeals approved the plaintiff's subpoena for health department records indicating whether the defendant was a typhoid carrier in an action for damages for the death of plaintiff's decedent after eating food prepared and served by the defendant at a hotel restaurant:

> We decide . . . that no privilege attaches to these records and that the public policy of the State as expressed in the Public Health Law and the State Sanitary Code confers no privilege. Privilege does not exist unless conferred by statute. Here the statutes point the other way and seem to require that such records, in so far as they refer to known or suspected typhoid carriers, be made available in a case like this. The Sanitary Code . . . requires local health officers to keep the State Department of Health informed of the names, ages and addresses of known or suspected typhoid carriers, . . . to inform the carrier and members of his household of the situation and to exercise certain controls over the activities of the carriers, including a prohibition against any handling by the carrier of food which is to be consumed by persons other than members of his own household. Why should the record of compliance by the County Health Officer with these salutary requirements be kept confidential? Hidden in the files of the health office, it serves no public purpose except a bare statistical one. Made available to those with a legitimate ground for inquiry, it is effective to check the spread of the dread disease. . . .

> . . . The information in the Health Commissioner's files concerning the defendant, if there be any such information there, was not acquired by the Health Commissioner "in attending a patient in a professional capacity" nor was the information "necessary to enable him to act in that capacity." Although the information may have come to the commissioner from a physician in private practice, the transmittal

from that physician to the public officer was in obedience to the express command of section 25 of the Public Health Law. [That section does not state that the report shall be kept confidential, while other sections concerning reports of TB and two other diseases do provide for confidentiality.] It seems to follow that similar reports as to other communicable diseases are not so privileged.

The court's language may represent an earlier era, but it reflects the basic premise that information collected by public agencies should be available to the public unless expressly exempted by the legislature. It points to the need for statutory requirements for confidentiality if medical information reported to a disease surveillance program should not be made public. Reports that include patient names or other ways to identify an individual have value to people and businesses, including litigants, who seek information about specific individuals. Databases that lack identifying information remain useful for statistical analyses.

Note the distinction between the confidentiality expected of a physician who receives personal information from a patient and the status of a government agency that receives a report from the physician. The physician may have a common law and in some cases a statutory duty to refrain from revealing the patient's information to others. The health department has no such personal or professional relationship with the patient and no duty to protect the patient's confidentiality absent a statutory mandate. When a health department submits surveillance records to a third party, such as the CDC, to be included in a national data collection system, the third party recipient is even further removed from any duty of confidentiality absent statutory prescriptions. The CDC's obligation to protect the confidentiality of reports it receives from the states is based on the Public Health Service Act and regulations, which do not contain the kind of explicit privilege language that the New York court thought necessary to prevent public disclosure.

# E.  PUBLIC HEALTH SURVEILLANCE AND RESEARCH

## Amy L. Fairchild, *Dealing with Humpty Dumpty: Research, Practice, and the Ethics of Public Health Surveillance*
### 31 J.L. Med. & Ethics 615, 615–20 (2003)

* * *

The last third of the twentieth century witnessed the articulation of the ethics governing human subjects research. The federal research legislation and guidelines passed and promulgated in the 1970s built on the Nuremberg Code of 1947 and the 1964 Declaration of Helsinki. All were based on a common set of principles stressing the absolute need to prioritize the rights of the individual over that of society: there could be no exceptions to voluntary participation and informed consent of competent adults in any research protocol. . . . no one could be conscripted into research projects. . . .

In response to the new federal research protections, epidemiologists and ethicists began to discuss whether the principle of informed consent extended to the use of records, and whether the insistence on individual consent would render epidemiological research virtually impossible. . . .

But the discussion . . . did not extend to public health surveillance . . . [which is] based on a principle fundamentally different from that animating biomedical research ethics; individuals may be compelled to do or not do things to protect the common good.

. . . [I]n the 1991 International Guidelines for Ethical Review of Epidemiological Studies, issued by the Council for International Organizations of Medical Sciences (CIOMS) . . . , a relatively narrow definition of public health surveillance was employed to justify exemptions from the requirement of ethical review: "An exception is justified," the guidelines stated, "when epidemiologists must investigate outbreaks of acute communicable diseases. Then they must proceed without delay to identify and control health risks. They cannot be expected to await the formal approval of an ethical review committee." By focusing on the urgency of some surveillance efforts, though, the committee excluded the vast majority of surveillance, which is routine and ongoing. . . .

Blinded HIV Seroprevalence and the Challenge to Surveillance

In 1993, National Institute of Health's (NIH) Office for the Protection from Research Risks (OPRR) received written complaints regarding two CDC studies: a measles vaccine trial intended to compare two different vaccination schedules that the CDC had contracted out to the Kaiser Foundation Research Institute and its own blinded HIV seroprevalence surveillance of childbearing women. [I]it was the serosurvey that raised questions about the bounds between research and practice within the context of federal human research regulations.

The CDC began to explore the feasibility of tracking the HIV epidemic through blinded testing at sentinel hospitals in 1986. When subject to ethical review in the 1980s, experts deemed such screening unproblematic. It involved samples of blood, not identifiable individuals. The privacy of no one could be violated. Informed consent was hence unnecessary. But what made the studies — based on unconsented testing — ethically acceptable also precluded notification of infected individuals. Since there was little that could be done for people with asymptomatic HIV infection in the late 1980s, there was widespread consensus that the blinded surveys were ethically permissible and served a critical public health need.

. . . .

A 12-member OPRR ad hoc advisory group determined that serosurveillance did not fall within the regulatory definition of human subjects research because it met both of two key criteria: first, it "caused no interaction or intervention with living individuals (i.e., the activity resulted in no collection of information or specimens that would not otherwise be obtained)" and, second, it "utilized no information or specimens that could be linked, directly or indirectly, to identifiable living individuals.". . .

[After investigating, OPRR concluded] that "Discussions with CDC personnel indicated that the distinction between human subjects research and routine, non-research public health practice was poorly understood and inconsistently applied."

. . . But while OPRR raised the prospect of formal IRB review for almost all surveillance activities, they required only that CDC develop a program for educating personnel about the regulatory requirements of human subjects research as well as written guidelines for distinguishing research from practice.

. . . Dixie Snider, the CDC's Associate Director for Science in the Office of the Director, assigned Marjorie Speers, his Deputy Director, the task of addressing the OPRR report. Speers came to the CDC from academia, where all studies are considered research, unaware that surveillance "was such a sacred cow."

Prior to its internal examination of what constituted research, Speers explained, the CDC had traditionally employed a procedure-based approach to determining whether an activity required IRB review: "If they did a blood draw," for example, "they were defining it as research." Scientists at the CDC were profoundly resistant to labeling an activity research, in part because of a concern that such a designation would invoke a lengthy IRB review and require informed consent.

It was precisely these concerns that had so worried epidemiologists and other social science researchers following passage of the Privacy Act and National Research Act in 1974. Regulations requiring the protection of privacy and informed consent, they feared, would effectively put an end to their research efforts. At the CDC, the concerns of epidemiologists were compounded by the way in which health officials tended to see the relationship between surveillance efforts and the central mission of public health. Speers recalled that on numerous occasions CDC scientists — on hearing that she had determined a protocol to be human subjects research requiring IRB review — would tell her, "You are killing people because you are making me go to the IRB." . . . In short, the new application of the research regulations "wreaked havoc" on the way things had been done for a century.

    . . . .

The 1979 Belmont Report [by the National Commission for the Protection of Research Subjects of Biomedical and Behavioral Research] defined practice as "interventions that are designed solely to enhance the well-being of an individual patient or client and that have a reasonable expectation of success." Research, in contrast, "designates an activity designed to test a hypothesis, permit conclusions to be drawn, and thereby to develop or contribute to generalizable knowledge (expressed, for example, in theories, principles, and statements of relationships). . . ." The NIH subsequently used the Belmont Report as the basis for the definition of research in its 1981 regulations governing human subjects research: "research is a systematic investigation, including research development, testing and evaluation, designed to contribute to generalizable knowledge."

    . . . .

Although the National Commission formally rejected the notion of intent [as the factor distinguishing practice from research], the first set of CDC guidelines drafted in 1996 made the case that public health surveillance is differentiated from pure research by intent: public health practice is undertaken with "the primary goal . . . to monitor the health of a given population for the purpose of taking public health action." Whereas "The *intent* of research is to contribute to or generate generalizable knowledge; the *intent* of public health practice is to conduct programs to prevent disease and injury and improve the health of communities." [Emphasis added.]

    . . . OPRR . . . advanced the notion . . . that all surveillance was research. This alarmed the CDC as well as the Council of State and Territorial Epidemiologists (CSTE), which protested the position. According to the CDC, "The implications of calling public health surveillance research are broad and far reaching. There are 2088 health departments and over 100 surveillance systems. If all surveillance activities were research, it might mean each local health department would have to form institutional review boards (IRBs) and secure [special CDC assurances that human subjects were being protected] for each system. Whether the surveillance system is mandated by state law is irrelevant. If the research activity is federally funded, it requires assurance of human subjects protection." To the CDC, this was more than a bureaucratic consideration: if surveillance activities were designated research, the CDC feared that "people with TB could prevent their names from being reported to the health department or refuse to provide information about their contacts."

    . . . .

    The Effort to Distinguish Research from Practice

    . . . .

The CDC, which notably relies on the voluntary reporting of surveillance data by the states, is rarely involved in the use of surveillance for public health interventions like contact tracing. It is thus open to considering many of its activities as directed toward generating "new" knowledge based on the collective experience of the states. . . . [H]owever practical their research might be, it remains research requiring IRB review in the minds of many CDC officials.

States, typically operating under statutes mandating departments of health to collect and act on individual-level disease data for the explicit purpose of controlling disease, tended to view most public health surveillance activities as practice. New York State, for example, described the range of activities it undertook to control a typhoid outbreak in 1989, which included not only case reporting and testing but also one cohort and two case control studies conducted by phone on the sixth day of the outbreak. In the case of the two phone studies, participation was not mandatory, but outbreak investigators were not required to inform individuals about what cooperation was required. . . .

While there was little disagreement between the CDC and the states that activities such as outbreak investigation should not be defined as research, the federal government and the states defined research and practice differently when it came to routine surveillance. These differences were not merely semantic, but carried broad consequences. John Middaugh, Alaska's State Epidemiologist, described an instance in which his state was given legislative authority to conduct birth defects surveillance using federal funds. The funding agency viewed the project as research and demanded a state-level IRB review: "Alaska eventually returned the grant funds because the Attorney General did not want to delegate the decision-making process to an IRB.". . .

In response to the comments from a meeting with CSTE, the CDC, in its June 1999 draft "Guidelines for Defining Public Health Research and Non-Research" sought to describe more specifically the activities that constituted research. These efforts at clarification provoked more pointed objections on the part of state and local health officials. The guidelines stated that "If the primary intent is to prevent or control disease or injury and no research is intended at the present time, the project is non-research. If the primary intent changes to generating generalizable knowledge, then the project becomes research." That is, "if subsequent analysis of identifiable private information is undertaken in order to generate or contribute to generalizable knowledge, the analysis constitutes human subjects research that requires IRB review." Thus, a hallmark of public health practice that was not research was that the "intended benefits of the project are primarily or exclusively for the study participants; data collected are needed to assess and/or improve the health of the participants."

The New York City Department of Health responded that "the very essence" of its mission was "to prevent or control disease and injury." In doing so, the department argued, "we derive knowledge that may protect the particular 'victims' before us. However, it may also be that it is too late to help the particular victims, but that the activity, or the information derived from it, becomes generalizable so as to protect the general population." CSTE concurred, arguing that "we are rarely able to conduct an investigation that provides any medical benefit to those already infected." For example, in the case of food-borne outbreak investigations, the "major benefit has been to others than those we identified and obtained data and specimens from."

New York City gave the example of an outbreak investigation of Hepatitis A among young gay men, which was determined to be associated with sexual practices rather than consumption of contaminated food or water: vaccination "was then directed not to the original victims but to the general population of young men who have sex with men. At what stage of this investigation did the Department shift from its 'primary intent' of preventing disease or injury to 'generating generalizable knowledge?'" The department thus adamantly insisted that "Generalizable knowledge can be derived from public health epidemiological investigations, and such investigations can still be deemed not to be human subjects research where there is sufficient statutory authority to conduct the investigation. . . ." And, indeed, New York State Public Health Law specifically noted that "Human research shall not . . . be construed . . . to include epidemiological investigations." For New York City, because surveillance carried the potential for public health impact, broadly construed, this made it practice rather than research, regardless of any research implications it might also carry: "if an inquiry may result in a public health intervention, such as contact notification, Commissioner's Orders or perhaps even rulemaking, then such should be viewed as an epidemiological investigation" that does not constitute research.

Just as surveillance may not always benefit directly the populations from which it was drawn, health officials also drew a distinction between immediate intent and primary intent. CSTE thus explained that it consistently collected data with an eye not only to the present but also the future: "ongoing analysis" of previously collected data sets was "routinely conducted for most, if not all, of the diseases for which data are collected under state law." By review of previous investigations of trichinosis outbreaks, for example, the state health department in Alaska not only developed an early diagnostic test for the disease but also identified an animal species not previously known to harbor trichinella as well as a new subspecies of the disease-causing organism. "We do not view these activities as research" when conducted by the state, "if conducted by an entity other than the state public health agency, we would define it as research and require an outside research to obtain IRB approval." Thus it was the provenance of the undertaking that determined whether an activity was research or practice. By definition, then, what public health departments did was not research.

Most alarming to state and local officials was the very narrow conception of when surveillance clearly represented pure practice. The CDC described only disease reporting "conducted to monitor the frequency of occurrence and distribution of disease or a health condition in the population" and surveillance regimes "in which no analytic (etiological) analyses can be conducted" as practice. "[L]ongitudinal data collection systems (e.g. follow up surveys and registries)" in which "the scope of the data is broad" and includes "more information than occurrence of a health-related problem," in which "analytic analyses can be conducted," and in which "cases may be identified for subsequent studies" were, according to the CDC guidelines, "likely to be research." The CSTE described this as a contradiction in terms: after all, "by its very nature, mandatory disease reporting is intended to be longitudinal data collection" and "to detect the causal agent to prevent future disease or injury."

But it also represented a catch-22 for states: New York City and some states found the narrow definition of non-research surveillance "very troubling" because it conflicted with their legal mandate to collect data. For example, the New York State Sanitary Code, in creating the AIDS registry, authorized the health commissioner, after receiving an initial case report, to collect all information "as may be required for the epidemiologic analysis and study of Acquired Immune Deficiency Syndrome." Thus, for many public health officials, "If an intervention or action is delegated to the health officer by statute or regulation, such intervention is per se ethical and not human subjects research." CSTE broadly concurred that "What distinguishes the activities as non-research at the state level is that the public health authority undertakes them and the data are collected under the authority of explicit state law."

In the end, the CDC addressed the specific state concerns not by altering its guidelines to meet any of the specific challenges raised by the states, but by holding that "intent is different under the authority of a state/local health department versus a university" and that legal authority or mandate to protect the public health also shaped intent: states acted with such power, the CDC did not. In short, "activities can be viewed differently at federal and state levels."

Conclusion: Putting Humpty Dumpty Together Again?

It is clear that public health surveillance is simultaneously both research and practice, in some instances more heavily favoring one component than another. Key stakeholders, moreover, can draw the boundary differently at different moments or recognize it not at all. In 1998 and 1999, for instance, the CDC commissioned the drafting of a Model Public Health Privacy Act to help ensure that states keep all surveillance data secure without impeding surveillance efforts. Some AIDS advocates challenged not only the model act but also the very legitimacy of public health surveillance. Advocates did not explicitly frame the debate in terms of whether surveillance should be considered research or practice, but they worried about how easy it was for health officials to conduct research with surveillance data under the model law and thus attempted to require informed consent for all surveillance for all diseases in a way that would have brought even state-mandated data collection under strict human subjects regulation. But not all disease advocates agree that informed consent was desirable. In the context of cancer surveillance, breast cancer advocates led the fight against efforts to make inclusion in state tumor registries voluntary.

It may be that there are few practical consequences for individuals if an activity is defined as practice rather than research, for it may well be the case that health officials protect the rights of citizens as vigilantly as IRBs protect the rights of those same people when they are defined as research subjects. But using the intent of surveillance to determine whether it is research or practice is a slight of hand that in the end is conceptually unsatisfying. . . .

Thus, the time has come to articulate the ethical principles for public health practice that both justify and limit data collection and use and to envision a mechanism for oversight. To be sure, ethical guidelines governing public health practice would not eliminate the thorny problem of determining when surveillance should be governed by the ethics of medical research and when it should be governed by the ethics of public health practice. Nor would such an ethics provide a practical mechanism for challenging legal mandates for states to acquire, use, and disclose surveillance data. But it would provide a systematic means for evaluating legal mandates to conduct surveillance: a practice is not made ethical simply because it is mandatory. . . .

\* \* \*

## Health Insurance Portability and Accountability Act (HIPAA): Standards for Privacy of Individually Identifiable Health Information
### 45 C.F.R. §§ 164.508–512

§ 164.508 Uses and disclosures for which an authorization is required.

(a) Standard: authorizations for uses and disclosures. — (1) Authorization required: general rule. Except as otherwise permitted or required by this subchapter, a covered entity may not use or disclose protected health information without an authorization that is valid under this section. When a covered entity obtains or receives a valid authorization for its use or disclosure of protected health information, such use or disclosure must be consistent with such authorization.

. . . .

§ 164.510 Uses and disclosures requiring an opportunity for the individual to agree or to object.

A covered entity may use or disclose protected health information, provided that the individual is informed in advance of the use or disclosure and has the opportunity to agree to or prohibit or restrict the use or disclosure, in accordance with the applicable requirements of this section. The covered entity may orally inform the individual of and obtain the individual's oral agreement or objection to a use or disclosure permitted by this section.

. . . .

§ 164.512 Uses and disclosures for which an authorization or opportunity to agree or object is not required.

A covered entity may use or disclose protected health information without the written authorization of the individual, as described in § 164.508, or the opportunity for the individual to agree or object as described in § 164.510, in the situations covered by this section, subject to the applicable requirements of this section. When the covered entity is required by this section to inform the individual of, or when the individual may agree to, a use or disclosure permitted by this section, the covered entity's information and the individual's agreement may be given orally.

(a) Standard: Uses and disclosures required by law. (1) A covered entity may use or disclose protected health information to the extent that such use or disclosure is required by law and the use or disclosure complies with and is limited to the relevant requirements of such law. (2) A covered entity must meet the requirements described in paragraph (c), (e), or (f) of this section for uses or disclosures required by law.

(b) Standard: uses and disclosures for public health activities. (1) Permitted disclosures. A covered entity may disclose protected health information for the public health activities and purposes described in this paragraph to:

(i) A public health authority that is authorized by law to collect or receive such information for the purpose of preventing or controlling disease, injury, or disability, including, but not limited to, the reporting of disease, injury, vital events such as birth or death, and the conduct of public health surveillance, public health investigations, and public health interventions; or, at the direction of a public health authority, to an official of a foreign government agency that is acting in collaboration with a public health authority;

(ii) A public health authority or other appropriate government authority authorized by law to receive reports of child abuse or neglect;

(iii) A person subject to the jurisdiction of the Food and Drug Administration (FDA) with respect to an FDA-regulated product or activity for which that person has responsibility, for the purpose of activities related to the quality, safety or effectiveness of such FDA-regulated product or activity. Such purposes include:

(A) To collect or report adverse events (or similar activities with respect to food or dietary supplements), product defects or problems (including problems with the use or labeling of a product), or biological product deviations;

(B) To track FDA-regulated products;

(C) To enable product recalls, repairs, or replacement, or lookback (including locating and notifying individuals who have received products that have been recalled, withdrawn, or are the subject of lookback); or

(D) To conduct post marketing surveillance;

(iv) A person who may have been exposed to a communicable disease or may otherwise be at risk of contracting or spreading a disease or condition, if the covered entity or public health authority is authorized by law to notify such person as necessary in the conduct of a public health intervention or investigation; or (v) An employer, about an individual who is a member of the workforce of the employer, if:

(A) The covered entity is a covered health care provider who is a member of the workforce of such employer or who provides health care to the individual at the request of the employer: (1) To conduct an evaluation relating to medical surveillance of the workplace; or

(2) To evaluate whether the individual has a work-related illness or injury;

(B) The protected health information that is disclosed consists of findings concerning a work-related illness or injury or a workplace-related medical surveillance;

(C) The employer needs such findings in order to comply with its obligations, under 29 CFR parts 1904 through 1928, 30 CFR parts 50 through 90, or under state law having a similar purpose, to record such illness or injury or to carry out responsibilities for workplace medical surveillance; and

(D) The covered health care provider provides written notice to the individual that protected health information relating to the medical surveillance of the workplace and work-related illnesses and injuries is disclosed to the employer:

. . . .

> (2) Permitted uses. If the covered entity also is a public health authority, the covered entity is permitted to use protected health information in all cases in which it is permitted to disclose such information for public health activities under paragraph (b) (1) of this section.

. . . .

\* \* \*

# NOTES AND QUESTIONS

**1.** The article by Fairchild describes distinctly different views of what counts as research requiring consent for the use of identifiable data. Attempts to differentiate public health practice from research appear to be based on an analogy to the Belmont Report's distinction between medical practice and medical research. The National Commission distinguished medical practice from medical research in order to identify which ethical principles apply to various endeavors by physicians. THE NATIONAL COMMISSION FOR THE PROTECTION OF HUMAN SUBJECTS OF BIOMEDICAL AND BEHAVIORAL RESEARCH. THE BELMONT REPORT: ETHICAL PRINCIPLES AND GUIDELINES FOR THE PROTECTION OF HUMAN SUBJECTS OF RESEARCH (1979), www.hhs.gov/ohrp/humansubjects/guidance/belmont.htm ("For the most part, the term 'practice' refers to interventions that are *designed* solely to enhance the well-being of an individual patient or client and that have a reasonable expectation of success. The purpose of medical or behavioral practice is to provide diagnosis, preventive treatment or therapy to particular individuals. By contrast, the term 'research' designates an activity designed to test an hypothesis, permit conclusions to be drawn, and thereby to develop or contribute to generalizable knowledge (expressed, for example, in theories, principles, and statements of relationships)." As Fairchild describes, some public health officials resist characterizing some (or all) public health surveillance activities as research, perhaps because that might entail obtaining consent from anyone whose identifiable information is collected. *See, e.g.,* James L. Hodge, Jr. & Lawrence O. Gostin, *Public Health Practice v. Research: A Report for Public Health Practitioners including Cases and Guidance for Making Distinctions* (Atlanta, GA, 2004), www.publichealthlaw.net/Research/Affprojects.htm#CSTE (last visited December 2006) (arguing that public health surveillance is not research, because it is conducted by government, intended to benefit the public, and often authorized by legislation).

Mariner argues that the research-practice distinction is misguided and beside the point:

> The question is whether the state can compel the reporting of personally identifiable information for any particular reason. The answer to that question depends upon the scope and limits of government's

sovereign power and whether any particular exercise of that power infringes on constitutionally protected liberties. The answer does not depend on whether something is research or practice. The fact that an activity might be considered "practice" does not mean that participation can be compelled, any more than the fact that a physician's recommendation is part of medical practice means that patients must obey it. . . . There is little point in debating the differences in practice and research when the central question is the state's power to conduct each specific activity without consent.

The idea that there is some special set of endeavors called public health practice may be an illusion. All government agencies can equally call what they do "practice." Indeed, the kind of public health programs and activities that public health officials call practice are precisely the same in kind, if not in subject matter, as those of almost every other government agency, from the Department of Agriculture to the Securities and Exchange Commission. And most of these agencies also conduct research.

The fact that public health is a government function does not exclude surveillance from constitutional constraints. Law enforcement is also a government function, but that does not authorize the police to obtain information about a person in violation of the Fourth Amendment.

Even more far-reaching is the argument that public health surveillance is not research because it *intended* to promote the public good in much the same way that standard medical care is intended to personally benefit a patient. . . . Even the most conscientious researchers see themselves as working for the benefit of humanity, however far in the future that might be. Virtually all public health programs are intended to benefit the population as a whole, whether by stopping an epidemic or by collecting data that might be analyzed to identify a risk that might be studied in the future to determine whether it might cause disease. Since the ultimate goal of all research — and possibly all government action — is to benefit the population, such a sweeping view of intent would virtually eliminate the rights of research subjects. A more immediate and objective standard is necessary to identify what counts as a research activity [requiring consent]. . . .

Wendy K. Mariner, *Mission Creep: Public Health Surveillance and Medical Privacy*, B.U. L. REV. (forthcoming 2007).

**2.** The Health Insurance Portability and Accountability Act (HIPAA) of 1996, Pub. L. 104-191, 110 Stat. 1936 (1996), authorized the Department of Health and Human Services (DHHS) to issue regulations in the event, as happened, that Congress failed to enact federal legislation to protect the privacy of medical information within three years. HIPAA modified health insurance regulation and encouraged health care providers and health insurers to adopt electronic recordkeeping to simplify and expedite insurance administration. HIPAA provisions are codified in 42 U.S.C. §§ 1320d to 1320d-8; 42 U.S.C. § 242k(k).

HIPAA directs the Secretary of HHS to establish "standards and requirements for the electronic transmission of certain health information," and "uniform national standards for the secure electronic exchange of health information." Congress recognized that public support for electronic record-keeping depended importantly on assurance that personal medical information would be kept secure and confidential. A major public concern was the use of such information for commercial marketing by pharmaceutical, medical device and other health services companies. The rules on security have been less controversial than those on privacy, perhaps because there is little dispute over the need for better mechanisms to protect the security of data. *See* GENERAL ACCOUNTING OFFICE, INFORMATION SECURITY: SERIOUS AND WIDESPREAD WEAKNESSES PERSIST AT FEDERAL AGENCIES, GAO/AIMD-00-295 (2000) (noting evidence that security systems at government agencies may not be what those agencies and the public expect). The security rule also makes clear that patients have a right to see their own medical records. The history of HIPAA Privacy Rule can be found in the Introduction to the original rule, Standards for Privacy of Individually Identifiable Health Information, 65 Fed. Reg. 82462 (Dec. 28, 2000), and to the revised rule, Standards for Privacy of Individually Identifiable Health Information, 67 Fed. Reg. 14776 (Mar. 27, 2002). *See also South Carolina Med. Ass'n v. Thompson*, 327 F.3d 346, 348 n.1 (4th Cir. 2003) (explaining effect of HIPAA administrative simplification provisions). The Final Rule took effect April 14, 2003.

As finally issued, the HIPAA Privacy Rule sets forth general rules for the use or disclosure by "covered entities" of "protected health information" (PHI): "A covered entity may not use or disclose protected health information, except as permitted or required by this subpart or by subpart C of part 160 of this subchapter." 45 C.F.R. § 164.502(a). Much of the remainder of Part 164 contains various exceptions, many subject to specific standards in order to qualify for exception. The Rule defines "protected health information" as "individually identifiable health information." 45 C.F.R. § 160.103. In turn, "individually identifiable health information" is information that is created or received by a health care provider, health plan, employer, or health care clearinghouse ('covered entities'), and relates to the past, present, or future physical or mental health or condition of an individual, the provision of health care to an individual, or the past, present, or future payment for the provision of health care to an individual, which identifies the individual or with respect to which there is a reasonable basis to believe the information can be used to identify the individual." 45 C.F.R. § 160.103. 45 C.F.R. § 164.514 defines what is considered identifiable and lists 18 data elements that must be removed for data to be considered non-identifiable. The best understood exception is for patient care. HIPAA does not require that patients provide express consent or authorization for covered entities to use or disclose their health information "for treatment, payment, or health care operations." This is intended to allow physicians and health care facilities to use patient data for regular care, consultations, filing insurance claims for payment, and internal quality assurance reviews, but has generated some confusion over what is included in these concepts. *See Citizens for Health v. Leavitt*, 428 F.3d 167 (3d Cir. 2005) (rejecting a challenge to the Rule's promulgation on the ground that whatever violation of constitutionally protected privacy might occur, it would be "at the hands of private entities," not the government).

The HIPAA statute provides that any privacy regulation issued pursuant to its authority shall "not supercede a contrary provision of State law, if the provision of State law imposes requirements, standards, or implementation specifications that are more stringent than the requirements, standards, or implementation specifications imposed under the regulation." HIPAA § 264(c) (2); *see also* 45 C.F.R. § 164.203 (no federal preemption of a "provision of State law [that] relates to the privacy of individually identifiable health information and is more stringent than a standard, requirement, or implementation specification adopted under [the Privacy Rule].") *See also* HIPAA § 1178(a) (2) (B) (providing that HIPAA does not preempt state law "subject to section 264(c) (2) of [HIPAA that] relates to the privacy of individually identifiable health information."). *Northwestern Memorial Hospital v. Ashcroft* (excerpted in Section C, *supra*), reviews the relationship of HIPAA to other state and federal laws.

Critics of the HIPAA Privacy Rule argue that it may permit the disclosure of more information without consent than prior law. For example, Minnesota Attorney General Mike Hatch writes: "In those few instances where patient authorization is needed, HIPAA permits the health care provider to refuse treatment to a patient who does not sign an authorization form — the "sign or die" provision. . . . HIPAA effectively neutralizes the patient's ability to restrict access to medical information." Mike Hatch, *HIPAA: Commercial Interests Win Round Two*, 86 MINN. L. REV. 1481, 1485 (2002).

**3.** A state or local health department ordinarily is not bound by the HIPAA Privacy Rule, because it would not meet the definition of a covered entity. However, divisions within a health department that provide or fund health care for people (as in substance abuse clinics or cholesterol screening programs) would be covered entities that must comply with the HIPAA Privacy Rule to protect patient information recorded for such services. In effect, one branch of a health department may function like a clinic or hospital; if so, it must ensure compliance with the Rule before transmitting any data to other units of the health department. The Rule does not protect information handled by parties, such as universities and researchers, that are not covered entities. Covered entities that are authorized to disclose PHI to researchers and other non-covered entities must ensure that recipients of the information preserve its confidentiality. Protection against further disclosure by researchers, therefore, depends upon contractual agreements between the covered entity and the researcher. Can individuals whose information is used or disclosed by third party researchers enforce such a contract?

**4.** Section 164.512(b) of the HIPAA Privacy Rule permits — but does not require — covered entities to disclose PHI for certain public health purposes. How would you construe this public health exception? How is this different from § 164.512(a), which permits covered entities to disclose PHI when "required by law"? The public health purposes mentioned in the text of the section are a more limited subset of public health activities than public health professionals might include within the meaning of surveillance and appear to reflect a layperson's understanding of the circumstances that would justify reporting medical information without consent. Since the Rule took effect, there has been some confusion over what kinds of information hospitals and physicians are *permitted* to disclose to public health agencies and what they may be *required* to disclose. State laws governing state agencies often contain authorizations to collect information to enable the agencies to receive information relevant to their functions. That type of authorization does not automatically include the power to compel information without consent. Whether any blanket authorization to an agency to obtain information includes the additional power to seize it from the party who holds it entails an analysis of the specific statute at issue. A federal example is the Cancer Registry Amendments of 2000 discussed in Section F of this Chapter.

**5.** HIPAA does not affect the law governing research with human subjects, including state statutory and common law and the Common Rule in effect for research funded by or submitted to the Department of Health and Human Services, the Food and Drug Administration, and other federal agencies. *See e.g.*, 45 C.F.R. Part 46 (HHS); 21 C.F.R. Parts 50 and 56 (FDA). Because researchers are not covered entities, HIPAA affects researchers only indirectly — when they seek access to information held by a covered entity. It does not allow researchers to conduct research without subject consent that would not be lawful under laws governing research with human subjects. Nor does it authorize covered entities to give researchers information that would not otherwise be authorized under state or federal law. DHHS considers the creation by a covered entity of a database or repository for research (such as a registry) to be itself a research activity, which must comply with the research requirements. And every time the database is used, the use may be a new research study. Of course, studies may use nonidentifiable information without individual consent (and some may obtain a waiver of consent in certain cases), but those that use identifiable information (and do not qualify for a waiver) would require individual consent to the study. For HIPAA rules governing research by covered entities, see 42 C.F.R. § 164.512(i).

As noted in the article by Fairchild, *supra*, public health surveillance activities may include the creation of registries and data repositories and conducting research studies. When might a surveillance program be considered to be collecting data for public health purposes and when might it be considered to be collecting data for research? Even when public health agencies are entitled to obtain data from covered entities, a separate question arises with respect to the later use of that data. Consider the ways in which health departments and federal agencies could use case reports submitted to a surveillance program or registry. The fact that information was lawfully collected by a public health surveillance program does not necessarily imply that it may be disclosed to researchers without the person's consent. Does release to internal health department researchers count as research or as part of surveillance?

* * *

## F.    ENVIRONMENTAL DISEASES: CANCER & OTHER CHRONIC DISEASES

### Background

Environmental hazards include chemical, biological, and physical agents in the indoor or outdoor environment at home or at work, such as pesticides, dioxins, tobacco smoke, and radiation. Some environmental specialists also include social concerns like biomechanical stressors, such as repetitive motion, and psychological stress, as from sexual harassment in the workplace. Of particular concern are environmental hazards that potentially or actually cause illness in humans. Chronic diseases or genetic conditions that may be caused or aggravated by exposure to something in the environment can be considered environmental diseases. Thus, environmental diseases can include any illness or condition that is not an infectious disease caused by a virus, bacterium or parasite.

Environmental surveillance, or tracking as it often called, can mean obtaining information about one or more of the following: the source of an environmental hazard; human exposure to a hazard; or human health outcomes from exposure to the hazard. In order to determine whether a particular chemical, for example, causes disease in human beings, it would be necessary to find out whether the people who are exposed to that chemical ultimately get a particular disease (that is not attributable to some other source). This may require linking exposure to the chemical to specific health outcomes. More sophisticated studies of environmental diseases seek to determine what is produced, when and where it is released, who is exposed to it, and what happens to them later. Such studies could use anonymous data to correlate exposures with disease in populations with specific characteristics, such as workplace, age or sex. Alternatively, identifiable data can be used to link particular individuals with specific environmental exposures. That data could be obtained from medical records, cancer registries or government agencies like the Social Security Administration, Medicare, or worker compensation systems. The type of data that could be obtained from other sources includes a person's name or unique identifier such as social security number, gender, date of birth, diagnostic code (ICD-9) for disease, date of diagnosis, race/ethnicity, address or latitude/longitude of residence, occupational history, school, and smoking history. An efficient environmental health surveillance system would be linked with some or all of these other registries or records.

\* \* \*

# UNITED STATES v. WESTINGHOUSE ELECTRIC CORP.
## 638 F.2d 570 (3d Cir. 1980)

Sloviter, Judge.

\* \* \*

In this case, we attempt to reconcile the privacy interests of employees in their medical records with the significant public interest in research designed to improve occupational safety and health.

The National Institute for Occupational Safety and Health (NIOSH) was established by the Occupational Safety and Health Act of 1970, 29 U.S.C. §§ 651 et seq. (1976). NIOSH has the authority to "develop and establish recommended occupational safety and health standards," and to conduct research concerning occupational safety and health. In particular, it has the authority to conduct a health hazard evaluation, which entails an investigation to determine following a written request by any employer or authorized representative of employees, specifying with reasonable particularity the grounds on which the request is made, whether any substance normally found in the place of employment has potentially toxic effects in such concentrations as used or found.

On February 22, 1978, NIOSH received a written request for a health hazard evaluation from an officer of the International Union of Electrical Workers, Local 601, an authorized representative of the employees at Westinghouse Electric Corporation's plant in Trafford, Pennsylvania. The Trafford plant manufactures, inter alia, electric insulators by means of an epoxy mold process. The complaint concerned two areas in the Trafford plant, the "bushings aisle" or TC-72, and the "epoxy aisle" or TC-74, and alleged that workers were suffering allergic reactions as a result of exposure to methyl ethyl ketone. The Director of NIOSH initiated an investigation pursuant to his authority under 29 U.S.C. § 669(a) (6).

On April 21, 1978, an industrial hygienist and two physicians employed by NIOSH performed a walk-through inspection. They determined that the conditions which led to the complaint concerning TC-72 had been remedied and no further evaluation of that area was required. However, although methyl ethyl ketone was found not to be a potential health hazard, hexahydrophthalic anhydride, or HHPA, was used in significant quantities in TC-74, and the physicians suspected that it might be causing allergic reactions in some workers. The physicians therefore recommended that environmental and medical testing be done regarding the presence and effect of HHPA in the TC-74 area.

Dr. Thomas Wilcox, a Medical Project Officer in . . . NIOSH, and G. Edward Burroughs, an industrial hygienist, visited the site and requested access to the company's medical records of potentially affected employees in the TC-74 area. A Westinghouse official replied that access would be difficult because the records were considered confidential. [A footnote describes the records at issue as including "the employee's reported medical history," and "reports of physical examinations given to employees at the time they are hired," which "generally includes a chest x-ray, a pulmonary function test, hearing and visual tests, a blood count, an examination by a medical doctor."]

. . . .

Thereafter, the Director of NIOSH issued a subpoena duces tecum to Westinghouse's custodian of records at the Trafford plant, requiring the production of "(medical) records of all employees presently employed in the TC-74 area and the medical records of all employees who formerly worked in the TC-74 area and who now work elsewhere in the plant." Westinghouse refused to honor the subpoena.

. . . .

NIOSH then filed this action in the district court seeking an order to enforce its subpoena. Following a hearing, the district court granted NIOSH's petition and ordered full enforcement of the subpoena. . . . Westinghouse filed this appeal. . . .

. . . .

[The court finds that Westinghouse had standing to assert its employee's privacy interests in this case and that the documents requested by NIOSH were relevant to an investigation within its statutory authority.]

IV

. . . .

Proliferation in the collection, recording and dissemination of individualized information has made the public, Congress and the judiciary increasingly alert to the threat such activity can pose to one of the most fundamental and cherished rights of American citizenship, falling within the right characterized by Justice Brandeis as "the right to be let alone." . . . Much of the concern has been with governmental accumulation of data and the ability of government officials to put information technology to uses detrimental to individual privacy, which have been facilitated by the spread of data banks and by the increasing storage in computers of sensitive information relating to the personal lives and activities of private citizens. . . .

. . . .

Although the full measure of the constitutional protection of the right to privacy has not yet been delineated, we know that it extends to two types of privacy interests: "One is the individual interest in avoiding disclosure of personal matters, and another is the interest in independence in making certain kinds of important decisions." (citation to *Whalen*.) The latter decisions have encompassed "matters relating to marriage, procreation, contraception, family relationships, and child rearing and education." The privacy interest asserted in this case falls within the first category referred to in *Whalen v. Roe*, the right not to have an individual's private affairs made public by the government.

There can be no question that an employee's medical records, which may contain intimate facts of a personal nature, are well within the ambit of materials entitled to privacy protection. Information about one's body and state of health is matter which the individual is ordinarily entitled to retain within the "private enclave where he may lead a private life." It has been recognized in various contexts that medical records and information stand on a different plane than other relevant material. For example, the Federal Rules of Civil Procedure impose a higher burden for discovery of reports of the physical and mental condition of a party or other person than for discovery generally. Medical files are the subject of a specific exemption under the Freedom of Information Act. 5 U.S.C. § 552(b) (6) (1976). This difference in treatment reflects a recognition that information concerning one's body has a special character. The medical information requested in this case is more extensive than the mere fact of prescription drug usage by identified patients considered in *Whalen v. Roe* and may be more revealing of intimate details. Therefore, we hold that it falls within one of the zones of privacy entitled to protection.

Westinghouse concedes that even material which is subject to protection must be produced or disclosed upon a showing of proper governmental interest. . . . In recognition that the right of an individual to control access to her or his medical history is not absolute, courts and legislatures have determined that public health or other public concerns may support access to facts an individual might otherwise choose to withhold. On this basis, disclosures regarding past medical history, present illness, or the fact of treatment have been required. The Court in *Whalen v. Roe* gave as illustrations the statutory reporting requirements relating to venereal disease, child abuse, injuries caused by deadly weapons and certification of fetal death. Generally, the reporting requirements which have been upheld have been those in which the government has advanced a need to acquire the information to develop treatment programs or control threats to public health.

. . . .

In the cases in which a court has allowed some intrusion into the zone of privacy surrounding medical records, it has usually done so only after finding that the societal interest in disclosure outweighs the privacy interest on the specific facts of the case. In *Detroit Edison Co. v. NLRB*, 440 U.S. 301, 313–17 (1979), the interests of the NLRB and the labor union in giving the union access to employees' scores in psychological aptitude tests to assist the union in processing a grievance were weighed against the strong interest of the Company and its employees in maintaining confidentiality. The Court held the NLRB had improperly compelled disclosure because "(t)he Board has cited no principle of national labor policy to warrant a remedy that would unnecessarily disserve (the Company's interest in test secrecy) and we are unable to identify one."

Thus, as in most other areas of the law, we must engage in the delicate task of weighing competing interests. The factors which should be considered in deciding whether an intrusion into an individual's privacy is justified are the type of record requested, the information it does or might contain, the potential for harm in any subsequent nonconsensual disclosure, the injury from disclosure to the relationship in which the record was generated, the adequacy of safeguards to prevent unauthorized disclosure, the degree of need for access, and whether there is an express statutory mandate, articulated public policy, or other recognizable public interest militating toward access.

Applying those factors in this case, we consider first that NIOSH was established as part of the comprehensive statutory scheme dealing with occupational health and safety embodied in the Occupational Safety and Health Act of 1970. In enacting that statute, Congress noted the "'grim current scene' . . . (i)n the field of occupational health," and sought, by passage of the statute, "to reduce the number and severity of work-related injuries and illnesses which, despite current efforts of employers and government, are resulting in ever-increasing human misery and economic loss." It was hoped and expected that NIOSH would "provide occupational health and safety research with the visibility and status it merits. . . ." Among the special "research, experiments, and demonstrations" which it is statutorily mandated to conduct are those "necessary to produce criteria . . . identifying toxic substances,"; those necessary to development of criteria "which will describe exposure levels that are safe for various periods of employment;" and those necessary "to explore new problems, including those created by new technology in occupational safety and health, which may require ameliorative action" beyond that provided for in the Act. The research activity in this case, a health hazard evaluation, requires that the Secretary determine "whether any substance normally found in the place of employment has potentially toxic effects in such concentrations as used or found. . . ."

Thus, the interest in occupational safety and health to the employees in the particular plant, employees in other plants, future employees and the public at large is substantial. It ranks with the other public interests which have been found to justify intrusion into records and information normally considered private.

Turning next to the degree of need for access, we have found in section III that NIOSH has shown a reasonable need for the entire medical file of the employees as requested. It seeks those records in order to be able to compare its findings of high levels of antibodies to HHPA and reduced pulmonary function with the comparable findings in the employees before they were exposed to the substances in the TC-74 area, and during the course of such exposure. Its need for all of the medical files requested in their complete form has also been satisfactorily demonstrated.

Westinghouse has not produced any evidence to show that the information which the medical records contain is of such a high degree of sensitivity that the intrusion could be considered severe or that the employees are likely to suffer any adverse effects from disclosure to NIOSH personnel. Most, if not all, of the information in the files will be results of routine testing, such as X-rays, blood tests, pulmonary function tests, hearing, and visual tests. This material, although private, is not generally regarded as sensitive. Furthermore, since Westinghouse's testing and NIOSH's examination of the records are both conducted for the purpose of protecting the individual employee from potential hazards, it is not likely that the disclosures are likely to inhibit the employee from undergoing subsequent periodic examinations required of Westinghouse employees.

Finally, we must consider whether there are effective provisions for security of the information against subsequent unauthorized disclosure. . . . Westinghouse argues that the security of the information in this case is inadequate. It stresses that the statute authorizes use of outside contractors for data processing and analysis, and contains neither means to police compliance with nondisclosure nor adequate sanctions for unwarranted disclosure. It also argues that removal by NIOSH of individual identifiers before disclosure to those parties is made will be inadequate, since only obvious identifiers, such as names and addresses, are deleted, but that identification may still be possible because more idiosyncratic identifiers will be included in the disclosed materials. For these reasons, Westinghouse conditioned its compliance with NIOSH's request for the records in issue on the provision by the government of written assurance that the contents of the employees' medical records will not be disclosed to third parties, a condition the government has refused to accept.

The district court . . . concluded that the "evidence indicates that NIOSH's procedures of safekeeping the records and of removing the names and addresses of the individuals in its compilation of published data represents sufficiently adequate assurance of non-disclosure by [NIOSH]." We see no reason to disturb this conclusion.

The applicable regulation expressly provides that unless otherwise specifically provided, "no disclosure will be made of information of a personal and private nature, such as information in personnel and medical files, . . . and any other information of a private and personal nature." Only aggregate data is included in the forms of the study distributed to employees and others. The excerpted data which is retained by NIOSH is maintained in locked cabinets, inside the Medical Section of the agency, in rooms locked during non-office hours. Material from small studies is not placed on computers; data from large studies is removed from the computer after six months. NIOSH has represented that no outside contractors are used for small studies, such as the one in issue here, and that when such contractors are used, they are bound to nondisclosure by their contract with NIOSH, as required by 5 U.S.C. § 552a(m). In the absence of any contrary evidence produced by Westinghouse, we cannot conclude that there are inadequate safeguards against disclosure.

Accordingly, we believe that the strong public interest in facilitating the research and investigations of NIOSH justify this minimal intrusion into the privacy which surrounds the employees' medical records, and that Westinghouse is not justified in its blanket refusal to give NIOSH access to them or to condition their disclosure on compliance with its unilaterally imposed terms.

V

. . . We recognize, however, that there may be information in a particular file which an employee may consider highly sensitive. Westinghouse has represented that the files are not limited to employment-related concerns but include records of the employees' personal consultations with the company physician and the physician's ministrations on a broad spectrum of health matters. Employees absent from work for medical reasons must clear through the medical department on their return. The medical records also contain reference to payments made under Westinghouse's comprehensive medical insurance program. Since the employees had no prior notice that their medical records might be subject to subsequent examination, they may have raised with the company physician medical matters unrelated to their employment which they consider highly confidential. We cannot assume that an employee's claim of privacy as to particular sensitive data in that employee's file will always be outweighed by NIOSH's need for such material.

Although Westinghouse has been permitted to assert the general claim of privacy on behalf of all of the employees, and has done so vigorously on the employees' behalf, each employee is entitled to make an individual judgment as to whether s/he regards the information so sensitive that it outweighs that employee's interest in assisting NIOSH in a health hazard investigation that may benefit the employee. We do not think it appropriate to permit Westinghouse to assert the claims of individual employees to privacy in particular documents. Each employee is uniquely capable of evaluating the degree of confidentiality which s/he attaches to discrete items of information in his or her file.

Westinghouse has suggested that the employees' privacy rights will not be adequately preserved unless their written consents are obtained. One district court has already conditioned the disclosure of personal identifiers on conducting a due process hearing. We believe that the requirement of securing written consent may impose too great an impediment to NIOSH's ability to carry out its statutory mandate. Although the number of employees involved in this particular investigation is not unwieldy, totalling no more than 100 employees, there may be other instances where the number of employees involved makes securing written consent difficult. Furthermore, there is the possibility that some employees will withhold consent either arbitrarily or because they do not understand the full nature of the investigation. Finally, some employees may withhold consent because they believe that is the course desired by their employer.

Under the circumstances, we believe the most appropriate procedure is to require NIOSH to give prior notice to the employees whose medical records it seeks to examine and to permit the employees to raise a personal claim of privacy, if they desire. The form of notice may vary in each case. . . . The touchstone should be provision for reasonable notice to as many affected individuals as can reasonably be reached; an opportunity for them to raise their objections, if any, expeditiously and inexpensively; preservation of confidentiality as to the objections and the material itself from unwarranted disclosure; and prompt disposition so that NIOSH's evaluation is not hampered. We are confident that the district court will be able to oversee this procedure which should, in the main, be self-executing by the parties.

. . . .

\* \* \*

## NATIONAL PROGRAM OF CANCER REGISTRIES
### 42 U.S.C. § 280e

(a) In general.

(1) Statewide cancer registries. The Secretary, acting through the Director of the Centers for Disease Control [and Prevention], may make grants to States, or may make grants or enter into contracts with academic or nonprofit organizations designated by the State to operate the State's cancer registry in lieu of making a grant directly to the State, to support the operation of population-based, statewide registries to collect, for each condition specified in paragraph (2) (A), data concerning —

(A) demographic information about each case of cancer;

(B) information on the industrial or occupational history of the individuals with the cancers, to the extent such information is available from the same record;

(C) administrative information, including date of diagnosis and source of information;

(D) pathological data characterizing the cancer, including the cancer site, stage of disease (pursuant to Staging Guide), incidence, and type of treatment; and

(E) other elements determined appropriate by the Secretary.

. . . .

(c) Eligibility for grants.

(1) In general. No grant shall be made by the Secretary under subsection (a) unless an application has been submitted to, and approved by, the Secretary. Such application shall be in such form, submitted in such a manner, and be accompanied by such information, as the Secretary may specify. No such application may be approved unless it contains assurances that the applicant will use the funds provided only for the purposes specified in the approved application and in accordance with the requirements of this section, that the application will establish such fiscal control and fund accounting procedures as may be necessary to assure proper disbursement and accounting of Federal funds paid to the applicant under subsection (a) of this section, and that the applicant will comply with the peer review requirements under sections 491 and 492 [42 USC § 289 and § 289a].

(2) Assurances. Each applicant, prior to receiving Federal funds under subsection (a), shall provide assurances satisfactory to the Secretary that the applicant will —

(A) provide for the establishment of a registry in accordance with subsection (a);

(B) comply with appropriate standards of completeness, timeliness, and quality of population-based cancer registry data;

(C) provide for the annual publication of reports of cancer data under subsection (a); and

(D) provide for the authorization under State law of the statewide cancer registry, including promulgation of regulations providing —

(i) a means to assure complete reporting of cancer cases (as described in subsection (a)) to the statewide cancer registry by hospitals or other facilities providing screening, diagnostic or therapeutic services to patients with respect to cancer;

(ii) a means to assure the complete reporting of cancer cases (as defined in subsection (a)) to the statewide cancer registry by physicians, surgeons, and all other health care practitioners diagnosing or providing treatment for cancer patients, except for cases directly referred to or previously admitted to a hospital or other facility providing screening, diagnostic or therapeutic services to patients in that State and reported by those facilities;

(iii) a means for the statewide cancer registry to access all records of physicians and surgeons, hospitals, outpatient clinics, nursing homes, and all other facilities, individuals, or agencies providing such services to patients which would identify cases of cancer or would establish characteristics of the cancer, treatment of the cancer, or medical status of any identified patient;

(iv) for the reporting of cancer case data to the statewide cancer registry in such a format, with such data elements, and in accordance with such standards of quality timeliness and completeness, as may be established by the Secretary;

(v) for the protection of the confidentiality of all cancer case data reported to the statewide cancer registry, including a prohibition on disclosure to any person of information reported to the statewide cancer registry that identifies, or could lead to the identification of, an individual cancer patient, except for disclosure to other State cancer registries and local and State health officers;

(vi) for a means by which confidential case data may in accordance with State law be disclosed to cancer researchers for the purposes of cancer prevention, control and research;

(vii) for the authorization or the conduct, by the statewide cancer registry or other persons and organizations, of studies utilizing statewide cancer registry data, including studies of the sources and causes of cancer, evaluations of the cost, quality, efficacy, and appropriateness of diagnostic, therapeutic, rehabilitative, and preventative services and programs relating to cancer, and any other clinical, epidemiological, or other cancer research; and

(viii) for protection for individuals complying with the law, including provisions specifying that no person shall be held liable in any civil action with respect to a cancer case report provided to the statewide cancer registry, or with respect to access to cancer case information provided to the statewide cancer registry.

* * *

## Wendy K. Mariner, *Mission Creep: Public Health Surveillance and Medical Privacy*
### 86 B.U. L. Rev. (forthcoming 2007)

* * *

## III.   FUNCTIONS OF SURVEILLANCE

Mandatory reporting laws are said to be for the purpose of protecting public health or preventing and controlling disease. . . . A closer look at surveillance programs, however, suggests that, in fact, they serve three more specific and immediate functions: outbreak investigation; ensuring essential medical care; and scientific research. . . .

### A.   Origins and Core Meanings: Outbreak Investigation

. . . Reporting systems were originally conceived and designed to prevent an epidemic of contagious disease. Reports to the health department included the patient's name and address, because of the possible need to contact the person. Timeliness was also a factor. Investigators would need to know that smallpox had been diagnosed within hours or days in order to find the source of infection and investigate whether and where it might have spread to protect other people from imminent infection. Although such outbreaks are rare, this remains a core public health function today.

Outbreak investigations are not limited solely to contagious diseases. They include investigating a source of poisoning, such as pesticides used in the environment, at least where there is no obvious cause. Where a public health agency has the responsibility for investigating the source of an illness that produces a serious injury or disability or death, the source must be identified immediately, and cannot be identified without interviewing the patient, there is ample reason for reporting the patient's identity to the health department. Thus, one useful criterion for characterizing data for outbreak investigation and epidemic control is that the data are needed right away to prevent imminent harm.

. . . If mandatory reporting systems were limited to data needed right away to prevent imminent harm, they would not bother to collect reports about the vast majority of cases, which are handled adequately by attending physicians. Nevertheless, case reporting systems typically insist on reports of every case, just to be sure no case is missed. . . . Yet, the required reports are still rarely submitted or reviewed more often than weekly. . . . Many health departments require physicians to telephone reports of disease cases that need immediate investigation, because ordinary weekly or monthly reports would come too late.

Traditional case reporting systems are not well suited to rapidly detecting epidemics or bioterrorist attacks using biological or chemical agents. New electronic syndromic surveillance systems offer more promise, although perhaps less for early warnings of terrorism and epidemics than for ordinary disease surveillance. Once installed in a location with electronic medical records, like a hospital emergency department, a computer program automatically scans medical records, logs the number of symptoms of interest without picking up personal information, and electronically transmits the totals to the tracking station, typically in a city or state health department. The tracking agency can review the data relatively promptly, often within 24 hours, and contact the hospital to see whether there is a dangerous outbreak.

Advantages of syndromic surveillance include speed and privacy. Most systems do not collect patient names or other identifying information. . . . Systems can be expensive, both to install the computer system and to hire people to monitor them. Because symptoms are common to many diseases, surveillance will produce many false positives and trigger costs to investigate ordinary cases of colds, influenza and other uncomplicated viral illnesses. Like sifting through billions of phone conversations, the task is to sift through billions of health records to find a genuine threat to public health.

. . . .

## B.  Assuring Essential Medical Care

Newborn genetic screening programs are designed to diagnose newborns with genetic anomalies causing severe developmental disabilities that could be prevented by beginning simple treatments soon after birth. [See Section G of this Chapter.] Almost all programs are modeled on phenylketonuria (PKU) screening, begun in the 1960's. By the mid 1970's, more than 40 states required PKU testing for newborns. These laws effectively require physicians to provide, and parents to accept, good medical care for an individual child. Indeed, proponents viewed mandatory PKU laws as enforcing both a legal and an ethical duty of parents to their children.

Newborn genetic screening laws, however, do not necessarily ensure treatment for the newborn. By itself, testing serves only a diagnostic function. The disability cannot be prevented without treatment. Screening laws that fail to assure treatment cannot serve the function of protecting children. . .

. . . Most experts agree that newborns should be tested for a condition that is reasonably serious, can be identified with a reliable test, and can be treated with relatively simple and effective measures. Between six and eight genetic and metabolic conditions meet these criteria.

. . . .

For conditions for which there is no treatment, the blood samples and linked information are used almost exclusively for research, such as testing experimental diagnostic assays to determine their sensitivity, specificity and reliability, estimating the incidence and prevalence of genetic conditions, and searching for risk factors. The screening program effectively creates a DNA bank. As more states expand their mandatory newborn screening laws to include these additional conditions, they may confront the question whether their power to protect children includes the power to create a DNA bank for future research.

. . . .

## C. Research

Data collected from surveillance are used for a variety of research studies. Cancer registries are perhaps the most salient example. In the mid-1930's, the Connecticut Medical Society began collecting information about patients with various cancers to see if they could identify cancer treatments that worked. . . . Since then, other organizations have initiated other programs with broader or narrower goals. Cancer registries typically collect detailed personally identifiable information, primarily to permit the registry to contact the patient periodically to update information. The data is ordinarily submitted by hospitals, clinics or physicians, either voluntarily or pursuant to a mandatory reporting law. Most registries receive multiple reports about the same person and deduplicate the reports by comparing names and dates of birth.

The National Cancer Institute (NCI) established its Surveillance, Epidemiology and End Results (SEER) program in 1973 [in 5 states and 6 cities], with a similar focus on analyzing methods of cancer treatment and outcomes (e.g., survival or death). Consistent with NCI's mission, SEER is primarily oriented toward medical research and uses research techniques. Most sites delegate the actual operation of the registry to a university, where researchers analyze the data and produce reports. They also follow cases annually to find out whether a patient remains alive and calculate survival rates. SEER publishes anonymous statistics on cancer annually, based on data as of about 28 months earlier.

The National Cancer Act was amended in 1992 to authorize the CDC to fund cancer registries in non-SEER states. The Cancer Registries Amendment Act requires, as a condition of eligibility for funding, that the data held by a CDC-funded cancer registry be made available for a wide range of research, both by the registry itself and by unrelated public or private entities. The difference between NCI and CDC registries is typical of the different methods the agencies use to collect data. NCI uses a representative sample of cancer cases to make estimates for the country, based on methods of research used in many other types of NCI studies. CDC prefers to collect data on every case of disease from case reports.

. . . Personal identifiers permit linking cancer registry data to other data bases such as the Behavioral Risk Factor Surveillance Survey, environmental health department records, Medicare and Medicaid health records, health insurance records, the National Death Index, death certificates and other vital statistics, geographic information systems, census data, registries of licensed practitioners (e.g., physicians, nurses, plumbers) and other specific populations (e.g., Vietnam Veterans registry). As information technology advances, the possible linkages are endless.

Several states have gone beyond authorizing the creation of cancer registries and have enacted laws or adopted regulations that either authorize medical providers to voluntarily report cancer cases to a registry or require such reporting without the patient's consent. In some states, advocacy groups lobbied state legislatures or health departments for a centralized source of information about a disease to try to explain unusually high rates of cancer in their communities or in response to fears of exposure to hazards from a local manufacturing plant. The more important factor appears to be the availability of federal grant funds to create or expand a registry. CDC prefers that registries be located in states that require the reporting of cancer cases by law.

. . . .

Arguably, any use of personally identifiable surveillance data — apart from outbreak investigation and newborn treatment — could qualify as research with human subjects. Cancer registries squarely present the question whether the state can demand access to an individual's personally identifiable information for use in research without consent. Since the Nuremberg Code was issued in 1947, research with human subjects has been deemed unethical and unlawful unless the subject voluntarily and knowledgeably consents. The consent requirement is intended to protect the individual's right of self-determination and the dignity of human beings recognized in all international declarations and covenants on human rights. . . . These foundational principles have been embodied in the common law, in regulations governing federally funded research known as the "Common Rule," and may have constitutional protection. All support the conclusion that the use of personal information without the subject's consent violates the subject's rights. Federal Common Rule regulations expressly specify that research with human subjects includes the use of personally identifiable information.

. . . .

. . . If a project is designed to obtain generalizable knowledge, rather than help an identifiable patient, it is research. In the public health context, this would mean that research includes projects that are designed to identify the incidence and prevalence of diseases, analyze data to see if there is a common risk factor for a disease, compare outcomes to see whether particular preventive or treatment measures work, and similar studies that are disseminated to other researchers or the public.

## Summary

It can be seen that different public health surveillance programs serve very different functions. To complicate matters, the same program can serve a different function at each of the levels of surveillance shown in Surveillance Data Flow Chart [below]. Although some infectious disease programs are designed for outbreak investigation at the first level, they may actually investigate very few outbreaks. And, at the second level, the data reported serves research functions almost exclusively. . . . State public health surveillance programs are third parties who collect data in the first level and then also redisclose it to fourth parties like CDC in the second level, who may in turn release it to fifth parties. A surveillance program may collect personally identifiable data at the first level for some purposes and uses, but not others, without patient consent. However, even if a surveillance program may collect that information without consent, that does not necessarily answer the question whether it can then further disclose the information to researchers without the person's consent for secondary and tertiary uses.

* * *

# SURVEILLANCE DATA FLOW CHART

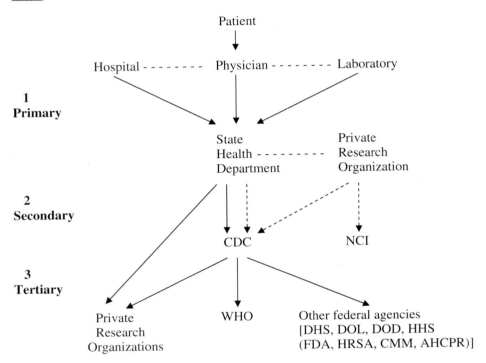

**Reporting**
**Disclosure**
**Level**

**1**
**Primary**

**2**
**Secondary**

**3**
**Tertiary**

Key:    - - - Dashed lines indicate contractual/grant relationship
           Arrows show direction of data reporting

Note:    In Level 1, provider reports of contagious disease cases sometimes go their local health department (if immediate response is needed), which then sends the report on to the state health department.

           Also, in Level 1, states sometimes contract with university researchers to receive data from providers for specific programs like cancer registries.

## NOTES AND QUESTIONS

**1.** *Westinghouse* illustrates one way that an administrative agency can obtain data to investigate health risks to a particular person or group of people. It is often cited for the factors it used to weigh the government's interest in obtaining medical information and the individual's interest in preventing disclosure to the government: "The factors which should be considered in deciding whether an intrusion into an individual's privacy is justified are the type of record requested, the information it does or might contain, the potential for harm in any subsequent nonconsensual disclosure, the injury from disclosure to the relationship in which the record was generated, the adequacy of safeguards to prevent unauthorized disclosure, the degree of need for access, and whether there is an express statutory mandate, articulated public policy, or other recognizable public interest militating toward access." *See, e.g., Middlebrooks v. Board of Health*, 710 So. 2d 891 (Ala. 1998) (state HIV case reporting statute, discussed *supra*). Although the U.S. Supreme Court has not had occasion to consider this six-factor balancing test, some of its elements can be discerned from the high court's earlier decisions. It remains unclear whether all of these factors should be considered and how much each should weigh. *Westinghouse* has also been cited as endorsing a public health exception to privacy, sometimes in *dictum. See, e.g., Sterling v. Borough of Minersville*, 232 F.3d 190, 195 (3d Cir. 2000) ("Public health or like public concerns may justify access to information an individual may desire to remain confidential"); *Fraternal Order of Police v. City of Philadelphia*, 812 F.2d 105, 110 (3d Cir. 1987) ("Disclosure may be required if the government interest in disclosure outweighs the individual's privacy interest"). Consider what is meant by public health in each of these cases.

NIOSH's request was a one-off demand for specific records, not for the continuing or perpetual submission of information, as in a surveillance program. NIOSH obtained employee records by issuing a subpoena to Westinghouse, which Westinghouse could and did contest, leaving it to a court to determine the legitimacy of NIOSH's demand. While the governing statute included NIOSH's authority to conduct certain investigations and research activities, NIOSH did not assume that it could automatically obtain medical records without a subpoena which would be subject to objection by the recipient or the workers whose information would be disclosed. Does this statutory structure authorize NIOSH to demand employee medical records without a subpoena? An agency's scope of authority to conduct research is governed by its own particular statute, so that it is difficult to generalize from one statute to another.

**2.** The NIOSH request in *Westinghouse* was prompted by the employees at risk; it was not spontaneously generated by the agency. How might this affect the court's view of the need for the information? Can NIOSH represent the employees? Companies may have little incentive to encourage investigations into workplace hazards. Is there greater justification for obtaining access to employee records than to patient records? Do patients have more bargaining power than employees? Are there any limits on when a company is entitled to assert the privacy interests of its employees? The "research activity" in this case appears to be directly for the benefit of existing Westinghouse employees. It also may provide information for former employees. Thus, it combined an investigation with a research study to find out what may have been causing ill health in employees.

**3.** As discussed in the Mariner article, the National Cancer Registries Amendments were enacted with the goal of building a national database of cancer cases. States are encouraged to create state registries by the offer of federal funding. The text of the statute included above states that applicants for funding must provide an assurance that, among other things, the applicant will "provide for the authorization under State law of the statewide cancer registry, including promulgation of regulations providing . . . a means to assure complete reporting of cancer cases . . . to the [registry] by hospitals or other facilities providing screening, diagnostic or therapeutic services to patients with respect to cancer . . . by physicians, surgeons, and all other health practitioners diagnosing or providing treatment for cancer patients . . ." How might those goals be accomplished? Must the information provided be personally identifiable? Section 208e(a) (1) (A) seeks data on "demographic information," which the CDC interprets to include a person's name, street address, city, county, state, zip code, census tract, race, sex, birth date, social security number, and industrial or occupational history. It would be difficult to study causes of specific cancers without being able to link individual cases to past exposures to cancer risks or to investigate whether particular treatments are effective without knowing how each patient treated fared. Cancer researchers generally assume that, to be useful for research, registries must contain identifiable information about each patient.

Does "authorization under State law" require that the data be collected or reported without the patient's knowledge or consent? Can Congress require the states to enact a mandatory reporting law as a condition of federal funding? *See* the discussion of conditions on federal spending in Section D, *supra*. Many states have adopted mandatory cancer reporting laws as the most efficient or desirable means of collecting the data. Would states that do not adopt a mandatory reporting law qualify for federal funding? If not, could the state claim that the condition was beyond the power of Congress to impose in order to obtain funding nonetheless? *See United States v. Am. Library Ass'n*, 539 U.S. 194 (2003); *New York v. United States*, 505 U.S. 144 (1992); *South Dakota v. Dole*, 483 U.S. 20 (1987). As a practical matter, it might be difficult to convince the CDC that a registry's data are "complete" in the absence of a law requiring that all cases be reported without patient consent. Could patients or physicians challenge the state's power to require reporting without consent? Would the law meet the *Westinghouse* balancing test? Does that test apply to the ongoing collection of data?

**4.** The Massachusetts Department of Public Health adopted the following regulation as part of its disease surveillance regulations after it determined that the text gave the Department the authority to receive the data, but did not require the Department to demand the information without patient consent:

Surveillance of Diseases Possibly Linked to Environmental Exposures, 105 MASS CODE REGS. 300.192

300.192: Surveillance of Diseases Possibly Linked to Environmental Exposures

The Department is authorized to collect from health care providers and other persons subject to 105 CMR 300.000 *et seq.,* and/or prepare data, as detailed in 105 CMR 300.190 and 105 CMR 300.191, on individuals evaluated for or diagnosed with the following diseases possibly linked to environmental exposures:

Amyotrophic Lateral Sclerosis (ALS)

Aplastic Anemia

Asthma

Autism Spectrum Disorder (ASD)

Multiple Sclerosis (MS)

Myelodysplastic Syndrome (MDS)

Scleroderma

Systemic Lupus Erythematosus

**5.** Cancer registries provide some data to study whether particular environmental hazards can cause specific cancers. Environmental and occupational health specialists and epidemiologists are especially supportive of such registries for that reason. In principle, information about industrial hazards could be obtained from industry. In practice, legislation compelling industry reporting has faced political opposition. Cancer registries may be the fallback option. However, cancer registries do not typically collect relevant data about a patient's occupational or geographic exposures, which would be needed for linking exposures to illness. Occupations are listed by category rather than employer and location. By the time they are diagnosed, many cancer patients are listed simply as retired. To investigate the relationship between health and environmental hazards, a different approach may be needed.

CDC is developing a national environmental health tracking system, providing grants to states to create their own state systems that could be linked to the CDC's National Electronic Disease Surveillance System (NEDSS). California passed legislation to study how best to create a system to track environmental exposures that affect health, CALIF. HEALTH & SAFETY CODE ch. 7 § 104324, and received a CDC grant in 2002 to develop its program. A working group, created to develop the system, recommended collecting data on the use and distribution of chemical, physical and biological hazards, rather than relying on patient medical records alone. *See* STRATEGIES FOR ESTABLISHING AN ENVIRONMENTAL HEALTH SURVEILLANCE SYSTEM IN CALIFORNIA: REPORT OF THE SB 702 WORKING GROUP xv (California Policy Research Center, 2004), *available at* www.ucop.edu/cprc (last visited Aug. 2006). The group also favored research studies on hazards and health outcomes, rather than physician reporting, to collect data, noting that "Physician case reporting has not generally proven to be fruitful or reliable outside the framework of infectious disease because of widespread underreporting and inconsistency of diagnostic criteria." *Id.* at 32.

The results of such studies may help researchers learn more about the causes of disease and where certain diseases are concentrated. Studies may also discover that certain racial, ethnic or age groups are more or less susceptible to chronic diseases. For examples, see L. Rosenstock, *The Environment as a Cornerstone of Public Health*, 111(7) ENVT'L HEALTH PERSP. A376 (2003). Policy makers could use the results for future policy decisions with respect to water purity and pollution, safe methods for handling toxic substances, or recommendations to physicians to offer tests for certain chemicals to patients who work in industries using those chemicals. Cities and states could use the information to change standards for construction, land use, zoning, and licensing certain businesses. It may also create baseline information about the kinds of risks that people who live or work in particular places may be subject to, which may interest their employers and insurers. Policymakers might be able to determine whether, for example, a large chemical spill is likely to add a small or large risk of cancer to people in that neighborhood. The cost of a large environmental tracking system may be quite high, however. A statewide California registry for Parkinson's and Alzheimer's diseases alone was estimated require at least $8.3 million to create and more than $1 million a year to operate. Where might a state obtain the necessary resources to pay for this and all its other disease surveillance programs?

**6.** For an interesting case involving claims that a survey of student behaviors and exposures to health risks violated the Family Educational Records Privacy Act, the Protection of Pupil Rights Amendment, and the United States Constitution, see *C. N. v. Ridgewood Board of Education*, 430 F.3d 159 (3d Cir. 2005).

**7.** In 2004, the National Institutes of Health considered developing a large research study to investigate whether and how genetic variations may interact with the physical environment, as well as behavioral and social factors, to produce disease. *See* DHHS, POLICY ISSUES ASSOCIATED WITH UNDERTAKING A LARGE U.S. POPULATION COHORT PROJECT ON GENES, ENVIRONMENT AND DISEASE, A DRAFT REPORT OF THE SECRETARY'S ADVISORY COMMITTEE ON GENETICS, HEALTH AND SOCIETY (May 2006), *available at* www4.od.nih.gov/oba/sacghs/reports/ LPS%20Public%20Comment%20Draft%20Report.pdf (last visited Aug. 2006). Hundreds of thousands of subjects could be needed to achieve statistical power for any results. The draft report recognized that the project was research with human subjects, because it would collect both biological specimens and personally identifiable information about individuals. A major policy question is whether it would be possible for prospective research subjects to validly consent to participate if future research uses of their specimens and data could not be predicted at the time of collection. Does the HIPAA Privacy Rule provide any guidance on this question? Would it apply to research conducted or funded by NIH? Does the Common Rule answer the question? For recent reviews of these issues, see Ellen Wright Clayton, *Informed Consent and Biobanks*, 33 J.L. MED. & ETHICS 15 (2005); Daniel S. Strouse, *Informed Consent to Genetic Research on Banked Human Tissue*, 45 JURIMETRICS 135 (2005).

* * *

# In the Matter of the Proposed Rules of the Department of Health Related to the Collection of Administrative Billing Data

www.oah.state.mn.us/cases/healthdata/
090015017.rr (Dec. 2, 2002)

Allan W. Klein, Administrative Law Judge.

\* \* \*

This Report is part of a rulemaking proceeding held pursuant to Minn. Stat. §§ 14.131 to 14.20 to hear public comment, determine whether the Department of Health . . . has fulfilled all relevant substantive and procedural requirements of law applicable to the adoption of the rules, evaluate whether the proposed rules are needed and reasonable. . . .

. . . .

## Nature of the Proposed Rules

1. The proposed rules establish requirements for the collection and use of administrative billing data created by health care providers to obtain payment from insurers (or other third-party payors). . . .

2. . . . Because the capacity exists for these codes to disclose private information about medical care received by individuals, detailed requirements for the handling and use of the data compiled are proposed in these rules. And because of the same privacy concerns, many citizens and groups are opposed to the adoption of these rules.

## Statutory Authority

. . . The statute states that [t]he commissioner may adopt rules to implement sections 62J.301 to 62J.452.

The purpose of those sections is set out in Minn. Stat. § 62J.301, subd. 2, which states . . . [that the] commissioner of health shall conduct data and research initiatives in order to monitor and improve the efficiency and effectiveness of health care in Minnesota.

The Department is obligated to perform a number of duties relating to the collection and use of data [relating to the following functions]:

(1) collect and maintain data which enable population-based monitoring and trending of the access, utilization, quality, and cost of health care services within Minnesota;

(2) collect and maintain data for the purpose of estimating total Minnesota health care expenditures and trends;

(3) collect and maintain data for the purposes of setting cost containment goals under section 62J.04, and measuring cost containment goal compliance;

(4) conduct applied research using existing and new data and promote applications based on existing research;

(5) develop and implement data collection procedures to ensure a high level of cooperation from health care providers and health plan companies, as defined in section 62Q.01, subdivision 4;

(6) work closely with health plan companies and health care providers to promote improvements in health care efficiency and effectiveness; and

(7) participate as a partner or sponsor of private sector initiatives that promote publicly disseminated applied research on health care delivery, outcomes, costs, quality, and management.

The proposed rules establish the collection and maintenance of information for a database to be used for research, cost containment, and improvement of health care. . . . Therefore, the Administrative Law Judge finds that the Board has statutory authority to adopt the proposed rules.

Generally speaking, an agency can adopt a rule if the agency shows that the rule is needed and reasonable, and the Legislature has authorized the adoption of the rule in statute. An agency cannot adopt a rule that conflicts with a statute, the Minnesota Constitution, or the United States Constitution.

. . . .

### Need for the Proposed Database

The need for the Department to be collecting this data at all was questioned by a large number of commentators. Many considered the existence of such a database of information to have no use other than to serve potential employers, the insurance industry, and others who wanted to obtain otherwise private data about individuals without having to ask for it. Other commentators acknowledged the benefits that could flow from researchers having access to a good database, but they did not believe that this outweighed the harm that would occur if private data were released.

Similar databases are already in existence at the federal level for recipients of Medicaid and Medicare. A collection of databases exists through a voluntary partnership between the federal Agency for Healthcare Research and Quality (AHRQ), thirty states, and the healthcare industry. Such databases are used for research into the effectiveness of treatment, quality of care from particular providers, and the reduction of health care costs. Recently, the findings of research performed with these databases, presented in nonscientific language, have been published to help consumers choose between health plans, medical providers, and long-term care facilities. This research benefits all consumers of healthcare by reducing costs, identifying appropriate and effective treatments, and ensuring the safety of treatments. The University of Minnesota described the database as the "proper tools and information" needed to allow "employers, employees and their families to become better consumers of health care."

. . . .

At the hearing, Dr. Harry Hull, the State Epidemiologist, discussed the need for the database. He stated:

Let me give you a few examples of how I and my staff would use this information:

The Minnesota Department of Health has a newborn screening program. Before a newborn baby leaves the hospital, a couple of drops of blood are taken and put on a piece of filter paper and they are tested for more than 20 genetic diseases. Now, these diseases are rare and the program is expensive, but because treatment of these diseases is so expensive, early identification of these individuals saves huge amounts of money for the state. There is a rare infectious disease called toxoplasmosis. It's a parasite that's passed from cats typically to pregnant women, and they sometimes pass it to their unborn babies. The question is, should we screen additionally for toxoplasmosis? It would be expensive to do so. This database could provide information on the frequency of the disease, the cost of treatment of the disease, and allow us to make a recommendation to the legislature for funding for additional testing.

Another example. It used to be that people on Medicare or citizens over 65 years of age could not be reimbursed for influenza immunizations. Dr. Marshall McBean, who is currently with the University of Minnesota School of Public Health, did a study using Medicare data and found out that the cost to Medicare for hospitalizations related to influenza was between $750,000,000 and a billion dollars per year. The result of that was that Medicare finally decided to reimburse the cost of influenza immunization to help keep our older population out of the hospital as a result of complications of influenza. We need similar data here to look at the total cost of influenza, so that we can evaluate whether or not expanded influenza immunization programs would be desirable.

Another example. The Minnesota legislature, when they revised the immunization law a year and a half ago, at our request (suggestion) stated that we needed to provide data on the cost effectiveness and the incidence of disease related to the vaccinations that we were proposing. We're currently looking at the possibility of adding varicella — that is chicken pox — to the school immunization law. Having statewide data on the frequencies of occurrences of this disease and the cost of treating this disease is vital to our providing the information that the people need to know to make a rational recommendation.

. . . .

The Department has shown that there are significant benefits in reducing costs to the public, improving treatment for patients, informing consumer choice in medical care, and preventing inadvertent harm when receiving medical care. Each of these reasons is a sufficient justification for establishing a database populated with billing data created for payment of medical services, so long as patient privacy can be protected.

*Consent*

. . . .

CCHC [Citizen's Council on Health Care] asserted that obtaining this information without individual consent exceeds the Department's statutory authority. . . .

The Department responded that obtaining the encounter data without consent is authorized by Minn. Stat. §§ 62J.321, subd. 1, and 144.335, subd. 3b.[20] Minn. Stat. § 62J.321, subd. 1, states:

> Subdivision 1. Data collection. (a) The commissioner shall collect data from health care providers, health plan companies, and individuals in the most cost-effective manner, which does not unduly burden them. The commissioner may require health care providers and health plan companies to collect and provide patient health records and claim files, and cooperate in other ways with the data collection process. The commissioner may also require health care providers and health plan companies to provide mailing lists of patients. Patient consent shall not be required for the release of data to the commissioner pursuant to sections 62J.301 to 62J.42 by any group purchaser, health plan company, health care provider; or agent, contractor, or association acting on behalf of a group purchaser or health care provider. Any group purchaser, health plan company, health care provider; or agent, contractor, or association acting on behalf of a group purchaser or health care provider, that releases data to the commissioner in good faith pursuant to sections 62J.301 to 62J.42 shall be immune from civil liability and criminal prosecution.

The general standards for access to health records are contained in Minn. Stat. § 144.335. Subdivision 3a generally requires patient consent before health records are to be released. But subdivision 3b of that statute states:

> Subd. 3b. Release of records to commissioner of health or health data institute. Subdivision 3a does not apply to the release of health records to the commissioner of health or the health data institute under chapter 62J, provided that the commissioner encrypts the patient identifier upon receipt of the data.

These statutes unambiguously grant the Department the authority to receive health records without the consent of the individual patient for the purposes of this rule [provided patient identifiers are encrypted]. . . .

*Fourth Amendment Considerations*

A related comment was that the proposed rules violated the Fourth Amendment prohibition against "unreasonable searches and seizures." . . . . Similar information to the administrative billing data that is collected under this rule is currently being collected by 44 states. The collection, maintenance, and appropriate handling of such data is governed by federal rule, 45 CFR § 500, *et seq.*, in addition to each individual state's rules. . . . No court has determined such data collection to be constitutionally prohibited. To the contrary, required data collection has been expressly found to be consistent with the constitutional exercise of a State's authority. . . .

*Constitutional Right to Privacy*

. . . .

The leading case on the issue of privacy regarding state-maintained databases containing medical information is *Whalen v. Roe.*

. . . .

As demonstrated by the number of public comments in this proceeding (and as recognized by both the Legislature and the Department), the nature of the information to be provided by this rule is traditionally kept private, and disclosure of the information poses a significant risk of harm to the person and that person's relationship with the medical professionals involved in creating that information. . . . The Department immediately addresses this potential for harm by encrypting the personally identifying data (names and addresses) and storing this information apart from the remaining data that is not personally identified. . . . The proposed rules use this data encryption, as well as physical isolation, designated employee access, use restrictions, and security audits as means of protecting the collected data. . . . The Department has shown the statutory authorization to collect this data and articulated valid public policy reasons for doing so. The showing of need, safeguards against release, express statutory authority, and articulated public interest meets the *Westinghouse* factors for assessing permissible intrusions into the private sphere. As with the Fourth Amendment issues discussed in the foregoing Findings, there has been no showing that the proposed rule infringes on a protected privacy right.

. . . .

IT IS HEREBY RECOMMENDED: That the proposed rules be adopted, except where noted above.

\* \* \*

## Wendy K. Mariner, *Medicine and Public Health: Crossing Boundaries*
### 10 J. HEALTH CARE L. & POL'Y 101 (2007)

\* \* \*

On December 14, 2005, the New York City Department of Health and Mental Hygiene adopted a new diabetes surveillance program. The new health code regulation requires medical laboratories to submit to the Health Department the results of every patient's blood sugar tests, together with the patient's name, date of birth, address, medical record number, physician, and other information. [Rules of the City of New York, Title 24: Department of Health and Mental Hygiene, Health Code of the City of New York, Title II, Control of Disease, Article 13, Clinical Laboratories, § 13.04. (24 RCNY Health Code Reg. § 13.04)] The report does not require the patient's consent. The Health Department will review the reports to see which patients are not controlling their blood sugar levels and will contact the physician (or perhaps the patient) to encourage the patient to change his or her behavior, by losing weight, eating better, taking medication and/or seeing a physician more often. Is this an innovative way to improve the health of several hundred thousand New Yorkers, a presumptuous invasion of privacy, or usurpation of the physician's role?

[The City] Commissioner of Health is enthusiastic about the new program, hoping it will reduce the number of people in New York City with uncontrolled . . . Type 2 diabetes.

Critics, on the other hand, worry that the program invades personal privacy. Physicians worry that the city will tell them how to treat their patients. Critics may also be concerned that what begins as a benevolent effort to encourage better medical care may mutate into requiring compliance with a medical regimen as a condition for Medicaid eligibility, private health insurance, public or private employment, or even a general duty to stay healthy. A disproportionate number of diabetics in New York City are Medicaid beneficiaries and/or disadvantaged minorities and the City would benefit financially from any reduction in the cost of their care. If the city or state can monitor a chronic condition like diabetes, why not heart disease, cancers, asthma, hypertension, low back pain, and other chronic conditions?

. . . .

The Health Department's reason for adopting the new program was set forth in its preface to the new ordinance:

> Diabetes, a life-long disease, has recently become epidemic in New York City (NYC) and is a major public health problem. The prevalence of diabetes in NYC has doubled in the past ten years. The NYC 2003 Community Health Survey (CHS) estimates that 9% (530,000) of adult New Yorkers and 20% of adults over 65 have diagnosed diabetes. People may have diabetes an average of 4–7 years before being diagnosed, and it is estimated that another 265,000 may have diabetes and not yet know it. Diabetes is now the fourth leading cause of death in New York City, moving up from 6th in 2002. This epidemic condition requires similar or greater urgency in public health response to that traditionally accorded to infectious disease monitoring and control.

. . . .

Beyond the commendable goal of improving health, taking action against diabetes may be financially necessary. The rise in diabetes appears to parallel rising pharmaceutical prices and possible reductions in state Medicaid budgets. The NYC Health Department says that in "New York State, 31% of diabetic patients in commercial managed care and 42% in Medicaid Managed Care have an A1C>9.0%," which is higher than the recommended level of less than 7%. The Health Department further argues that "tight blood sugar control" can reduce "by over 25%" the small blood vessel complications that lead to eye disease, kidney complications and peripheral nerve disorders. Thus, [it] concludes, "Keeping the average blood sugar (A1C) under 7.0% can prevent many diabetes-related complications and deaths."

This goal may prove difficult to achieve, since, as the department acknowledges, the CDC has found that "only 37% of US adults with diabetes have an A1C<7% and 20% have an A1C>9%." Moreover, blood sugar levels are not the only measure of diabetes control. . . .

. . . .

The New York City program was modeled after a genuine experiment currently being conducted in Vermont. Researchers created a research study — a randomized controlled trial funded by a grant from the National Institutes of Health — to test an information system for physicians and their patients. . . [P]atients were invited to become research subjects and only those who did not object were enrolled. . . .

. . .

What does the NYC health department intend to do with the reports it receives? First, it will enter all the data into a new diabetes registry, the New York City Hemoglobin A1C Registry. It plans to use that data "for public health surveillance and monitoring of trends of blood sugar control in people with diabetes." Specifically, it will "plan programs in the Diabetes Prevention and Control Program" and "measure outcomes of diabetes care". It plans to "report a roster of patients to clinicians, stratified by patient A1C levels, highlighting patients under poor control (e.g., A1C>9%) who may need intensified follow-up and therapy."

. . . .

There are at least three arguments that New York City does not have the legal authority to adopt or implement its diabetes reporting program. The first is that the health department's regulatory authority over clinical laboratories does not include the power to require the reporting of personally identifiable medical information. The second is that neither the State nor the City of New York has the power to require the reporting of such information in the absence of a credible threat posed by the patients whose information is reported to the health or safety of other people. The third is that, to the extent that the health department uses or discloses this information, it is engaged in research that requires the consent of the patient whose identifiable information is so used.

* * *

# NOTES AND QUESTIONS

**1.** In March 2003, after legislators and citizens strongly objected to the health care data collection rule at issue in the above administrative decision, the Minnesota Department of Health withdrew the rule. *See* www.news.mpr.org/features/s003/03/21_ap_healthdata/ (last visited August 2006). Objections were based primarily on concern for personal privacy. The records collected would identify individuals who had any type of medical condition, including stroke, abortion, sexually transmitted disease, and mental disorders, as well as treatment and medicines, such as Prozac, contraception, and high blood pressure medication. Insurance industry representatives also objected to the expense and burdensomeness of collecting the data.

The Department of Health relied on MINN. STAT. § 62J.321 (set out in the opinion above) as authority for obtaining patient records without consent. The objections to the proposed rule raise questions about the meaning of that statute. Did the administrative law judge interpret it correctly? If legislators were among those opposed to the rule, what might they have believed that the statute authorized? Do you agree with the administrative law judge's conclusion that neither the Fourth Amendment nor the Fourteenth Amendment required consent? How do the department's reasons for collecting the data compare with the reason for the compulsory reporting of controlled substances prescriptions or for compulsory reporting of contagious diseases? If health departments have the authority to adopt a rule like Minnesota proposed, would they still need those other reporting laws?

The Department also rejected the argument that patient consent should be required to obtain the desired data on the ground that not all patients would consent and the resulting data would not represent the entire spectrum of patients in the state. At the same time, the Department's ultimate proposed rule in effect limited the data collected to patients with private group health insurance and excluded data from health plans that covered beneficiaries of Medicaid, Medicare, and other government health benefit programs. What effect might that have on the comprehensiveness and utility of the data for the purposes sought by the Department? Would the Department have access to that data from other sources?

**2.** The Minnesota proposal is an example of increasingly wide-ranging data linkage systems. *See* www.ahcpr.gov/data/hcup/statesid.htm (last visited Aug. 2006). A report by the U.S. General Accounting Office (now the General Accountability Office) contains a good comprehensive description of the promise and peril of data linkage. GENERAL ACCOUNTING OFFICE, RECORD LINKAGE AND PRIVACY: ISSUES IN CREATING NEW FEDERAL RESEARCH AND STATISTICAL INFORMATION, GAO-01-126SP (April 2001), *available at* www.gao.gov/new.items/d1126sp.pdf. The GAO notes that it is less expensive to obtain data by record linkage than by collecting it from scratch, so to speak. Advances in computer technology permitting large data set transfer and storage, as well as manipulation using sophisticated statistical analyses, simplify and encourage both data mining and data linkage. Linked data creates new information that can be used "to describe or make inferences about a population of individuals, analyze patterns in the data, and evaluate or inform programs or policies." The privacy issues raised by such linkage include "whether consent to linkage was obtained; whether linkages required sharing identifiable data with other organizations; and whether 'deidentified' linked data are subject to reidentification risks when released for research or other purposes." Questions may also arise about the authority of specific government agencies to share data with other agencies. For example, if agency A is prohibited from sharing its data, but agency B is not, then agency A cannot give its data to agency B, but agency B can give its data to agency A. Agency A can then link the data from both agencies. The GAO report confirmed this practice: "OMB's Order Providing for the Confidentiality of Statistical Information limits sharing of personally identifiable survey data without respondent consent. However, while this may be relevant to specific linkages, we found that the examples of survey-archive linkage discussed in the previous chapter do not involve sharing *survey* data. Rather, in each instance, administrative data were transferred to the survey agency." *Id.*

Data linkage does not necessarily raise new privacy issues, but resolving them may be more complex, because linked data sets create new information, formerly innocuous information may become sensitive, and responsibility for protecting privacy is dispersed over more than one entity. Not surprisingly, researchers, especially those in health fields and government agencies, generally advocate linkage without consent, while consumer groups generally advocate consent to linkage. For a readable account of the comprehensive data bases, links and search systems created after September 11, 2001, see ROBERT O'HARROW JR., NO PLACE TO HIDE (2005). (For a discussion of responses to terrorism, see Chapter Eight.)

**3.** The New York City blood sugar (Hemoglobin A1C) registry described above represents a new and highly controversial type of surveillance program that is intended to encourage people to improve their own health. Is this an example of public health stepping up to contemporary problems or intruding into the physician's role? Is it an effective way to find people who need medical care or an unjustifiably paternalistic way to get people to take better care of themselves? (See the discussion of legal and ethical arguments for and against various types of health promotion policies in Chapter Six.) To analyze the state's power to adopt this type of program, the threshold question is whether it should be tested against the cases and decisions governing disease surveillance programs, or those governing informed consent to medical care, or those governing research with human subjects. The Mariner article goes on to examine the three arguments that the program fails to meet legal standards under each of those options. Can you flesh out those arguments and those in rebuttal? Which arguments are most persuasive?

Type 2 diabetes, like obesity (which is a risk factor for diabetes), is the sixth leading cause of death in the United States, and is also a risk factor for heart disease, the first major cause of death. Diabetes affects a growing number of Americans. Researchers at the National Institute of Diabetes and Digestive and Kidney Diseases estimated that 6.5% of Americans have been diagnosed with diabetes and another 2.8% are undiagnosed. Another 26% had higher than normal blood sugar levels, but not high enough to qualify as diabetes. Catherine C. Cowie et al., *Prevalence of Diabetes and Impaired Fasting Glucose in Adults in the U.S. Population: National Health and Nutrition Examination Survey,* 29 DIABETES CARE 1263 (2006). Perhaps equally important, especially in New York City, is the fact that a disproportionate number of Medicaid beneficiaries have diabetes. About 95% of diabetes cases are Type 2, which typically arises in adulthood, from an inability to use insulin properly, and is believed to result from poor nutrition. People with Type 2 diabetes sometimes suffer from the stigmatizing view that it is primarily a disease of elderly, obese people. Type 1 diabetes is a genetic condition that is usually diagnosed in childhood and typically well-controlled. The majority of research funding goes to Type 1. (A third form of gestational diabetes, in which placental hormones block insulin's effect in pregnancy, affects about 4% of pregnant women, but normally disappears after delivery.) For basic information on

Diabetes, see American Diabetes Assocation, www.diabetes.org (last visited Aug. 2006); and World Health Organization, Fact Sheet: Diabetes Mellitus (April 2002), *available at* www.who.int/mediacentre/factsheets/fs138/en/.

\* \* \*

## G.  GENETIC TESTING AND DNA- OR BIO-BANKING

### Patricia A. Roche, *Genetic Information and Testing, in* 1 Encyclopedia of Privacy
252, 252–56 (William G. Staples ed., 2007)

\* \* \*

Genetic testing can be defined as any technique that can be used to gain information about aspects of an individual that are influenced, caused by, or controlled by genes. Defined this broadly, it encompasses methodologies not reliant on laboratory analyses or technology, such as the compilation of a detailed family medical history. In common usage, however, genetic testing usually refers more narrowly to processes used to determine the structure of an individual's genes and includes molecular testing (examination of DNA or RNA), microscopic examination of chromosomes and biochemical tests that determine the presence or absence of gene products (proteins). . . . Depending upon the purpose of a genetic test and the surrounding circumstances, testing and the resultant information may have a profound impact on individual and family privacy or none at all. Perhaps most critical to this determination is the degree to which the identity of the individual who is being tested is linked to specimens and information throughout testing activities. These activities include the collecting of specimens or samples for testing, storage of samples (pre and post testing), the analysis itself, the storage of genetic information generated from the analysis (DNA banking) and disclosures of samples and data to third parties.

The informational value of a DNA sample can increase after the sample is collected from an individual because scientific breakthroughs in deciphering the genetic code and understanding the function of genes are continually being made. The scope of genetic tests now available illustrates the informational value of samples that have been collected and hints at the range of information that might be culled from them in the future. In health care genetic testing is used to identify predispositions to rare genetic diseases (*e.g.*, Huntington's Disease), to predict response to drugs, to estimate risks for developing common illnesses (*e.g.*, some cancers), and to determine carrier status for reproductive purposes. Outside of medicine it is employed to identify bodily remains, connect individuals to criminal acts, and determine paternity. It has been incorporated into genealogical research and is used for marketing nutritional supplements and skin-care products to consumers. In the future it may be used to identify predispositions to injury or to screen for cognitive abilities and other traits unrelated to health.

Of course, not all the genetic information produced from testing is highly private, powerful or sensitive; some genetic information is quite benign or obvious. But because much genetic information is highly personal, prolonged storage of, and easy accessibility to, identifiable samples (and genetic data) presents significant risks to individual privacy. . . .

. . . All states compel collection of samples from felony sex offenders, a majority of states extend their authority to include all convicted felons and approximately half of the states authorize collection from individuals convicted of misdemeanors. A few states go so far as to include those arrested on suspicion of committing a crime (*e.g.*, Texas). States contribute the genetic data generated under these laws to the Combined DNA Index System (CODIS), which is also the repository of genetic information about individuals convicted of violent crimes under federal law. CODIS is maintained by the Federal Bureau of Investigation and it enables federal, state, and local crime labs to exchange and compare DNA profiles electronically.

The type of genetic profiling authorized under these statutes involves decoding regions on the human genome that are sufficiently unique so as to be useful for identification purposes but which are not generally thought to contain information associated with any known physical or mental traits. . . . The constitutional challenges raised thus far in regard to such forensic testing have been based on the Fourth Amendment guarantees against unreasonable search and seizures and protection of personal security. The Supreme Court has yet to review and rule on the constitutionality of any of these statutes. But the federal circuit courts that have reviewed these Fourth Amendment claims have declined to find any of these statutes to be in violation of the U.S. Constitution.

Genetic testing conducted by governmental agents for entirely different purposes has also been challenged on constitutional grounds. In 1995 employees in a federally funded research laboratory brought a lawsuit against their employers claiming that they had been subjected to nonconsensual testing for several conditions including sickle cell trait and that the testing violated (in addition to some statutes) their rights to privacy as guaranteed by the constitutions of California and the United States. The trial court dismissed the plaintiffs' claims, but in *Norman-Bloodsaw v. Lawrence Berkeley Laboratory*, 135 F.3d 1260 (9th Cir. 1998), the circuit court reinstated the constitutional claims, recognizing that few subject areas are more personal and more likely to implicate privacy interests than one's health or genetic make-up. As a result the case went back to the trial court. Neither the California Supreme Court nor the U.S. Supreme Court has subsequently addressed or ruled on the privacy issues raised in the *Bloodsaw* case. Therefore, the relationship between constitutionally protected rights to privacy and secret or non-consensual genetic testing of governmental employees has yet to be authoritatively defined by any court.

. . . Under Executive Order 13145 [issued by President Clinton in February of 2000], federal employers are prohibited from discriminating against their employees on the basis of genetic information and are further prohibited (with a few exceptions) from disclosing genetic information about an employee or any member of a federal employee's family. . . .

In the 1970s states began enacting laws to protect individuals with specific genetic traits from being discriminated against on the basis of those traits. Typically, these statutes addressed sickle cell disease, thalessemia, Tay Sachs, and cystic fibrosis as the traits of concern and extended protection to individuals who either had these genetic conditions or were carriers of the conditions. For the most part these laws regulate how information regarding the traits could be used in the employment and insurance arenas; they do not restrict how the information might be acquired in the first place, nor do they restrict disclosures or sharing of information about these, (or any other genetic diseases) outside of employment or insurance. Consequently, they provide little in the way of privacy protections, even for those affected by one of the named conditions.

A second wave of genetic legislation that began across states in the early 1990s had the primary purpose of protecting economic interests that might be affected as a result of the expansion of genetic testing and thereby opportunities for genetic discrimination. These statutes mainly focused on regulating uses of genetic information in health insurance and employment and incorporate privacy protections to varying degrees. Wisconsin is credited with being the first state to generally ban genetic discrimination in employment and to ban genetic discrimination in health insurance. By 2000, a majority of states had enacted genetic anti-discrimination laws that apply to health insurance and employment practices. Commonly, these statutes regulate the extent to which an insurer or employer can request or require that individuals disclose genetic information to them or undergo testing that would generate genetic information. Thus, these laws are based on the notion that genetic information should be treated differently from other personal or health information but many states limit this policy of so called genetic exceptionalism to the realms of insurance or employment. . . .

States also determine the impact of statutory rules through the definitions that are employed within a statute. Here, the scope of definitions employed for genetic testing and genetic information affects the reach of protections that statutory rules provide. Some states, like New Mexico, define genetic information broadly to include: information about the genetic makeup of a person or members of a person's family, information resulting from genetic testing, genetic analysis, or DNA composition, information that an individual has participated in genetic research or information related to the use of genetic services. Other states define it more narrowly. For example, Maryland defines genetic testing as laboratory tests of human chromosomes or DNA, thus excluding any other methods by which genetic information can be generated.

Some states have taken a wide view towards protecting genetic privacy and regulate genetic testing regardless of where it occurs. For example, Illinois prohibits genetic testing by anyone (not just health insurers or employers) without the individual's informed and written consent. They also treat information derived from genetic testing as confidential and privileged and as a general rule permit releases of genetic information only to the individual tested or to persons specifically authorized in writing by that individual to receive the information.

. . . .

In order to thoroughly protect privacy, however, legislation should also address routine destruction of samples as well as routine destruction of genetic information that is maintained in an individually identifiable form, include stringent penalties and provide for strict enforcement. While some states provide statutory penalties, most often in the form of monetary fines for violations and grant enforcement authority to one or more state agencies, few require routine destruction of samples in order to guard against unauthorized testing.

The impact that state insurance laws described above can have on protecting privacy is further tempered by the Employee Retirement Income Security Act of 1974 (ERISA), a federal statute that removes some employee benefit plans (including health plans) from the reach of state insurance laws. Therefore individuals in states that have enacted such laws may not be protected by them, depending upon how they obtain their health insurance coverage. Several bills that would remedy this disparity have been introduced in Congress. . . but to date no federal law has been enacted that contains provisions comparable to these state insurance and employment laws.

[T]he Health Insurance Portability and Accountability Act of 1996 (HIPAA) provides some protection from discrimination on the basis of genetic information to individuals when they move from one health plan to another. However, it does not put restrictions on the collection of genetic information by insurers, prohibit insurers from requiring an individual to take a genetic test or limit the disclosure of genetic information by insurers and therefore lacks any privacy provisions.

[T]he HIPAA Privacy Rules [protect any] genetic information that fits the definition of health information . . .

. . . .

In regard to genetic information that would fall outside of medical record or health information laws (because of who holds the information or how it was created) individuals would need to look to common law for protection of genetic privacy. No court has yet applied any of the common law protections of generalized privacy interests to circumstances involving nonconsensual genetic testing, unauthorized disclosure of genetic test results to third parties, or publication of private genetic information.

* * *

# NOTES AND QUESTIONS

**1.** About 4 million babies are born each year in the United States. Almost all are tested for a variety of genetic conditions. In the 1960s, Dr. Robert Guthrie developed a bacterial assay for phenylketonuria (PKU), which became the model for all newborn screening in the country. A few drops of blood are taken from a newborn (usually from the heel) and placed on what became known as a Guthrie card. PKU is caused by a defective enzyme for metabolizing phenylalanine, a common amino acid in protein rich food, and results in severe neurological damage. In the 1950s, Horst Bickel, a German pediatrician, found that a special diet low in phenylalanine could reduce or prevent the development of mental retardation. Guthrie's test made it easy to identify newborns with PKU in time to start them on the diet that could prevent life-long damage. This success encouraged a search for other conditions that might be prevented by early intervention. PKU remains the paradigm condition for testing in a newborn because of the relative simplicity and accuracy of the diagnostic test, the need for immediate intervention to prevent severe illness or disability, and the availability of a relatively accessible intervention (the diet) that can prevent the condition. Even the test for PKU, however, produced false positives in the early years, and the special diet given to newborns mistakenly diagnosed with PKU caused neurological damage in those children. Norman Fost, *Genetic Diagnosis and Treatment: Ethical Considerations*, 147 AM. J. DISEASES CHILD. 1190 (1993). Adhering to the diet presents its own challenges, especially for adolescents. It can be more expensive than an ordinary diet. Is such a diet medical treatment? Do health insurance plans pay for such foods as a covered benefit? Who is responsible for providing this "treatment"?

**2.** PKU screening began as a voluntary test, but by the mid 1970's more than 40 states had laws requiring PKU testing for all newborns, some with religious exceptions. In addition to PKU, all states require testing for congenital hypothyroidism and classical galactosemia. Forty-eight states require testing for hemoglobinopathies (sickle cell), and at least 30 states require it for congenital adrenal hyperplasia, biotinidase deficiency, maple syrup urine disease, and homocystinuria. Most expert groups agree that at least the first six of these disorders should be identified by screening, because some form of treatment is available to prevent or ameliorate the condition when given or begun in infancy. Laws requiring newborn screening for specific conditions can be found at National Newborn Screening and Genetics Resources Center, genes-r-us.uthscsa.edu/ (last visited August 2006).

Currently, about 38 states require parents to be notified that screening tests will be done, but do not afford the parents the right to refuse. Another 10 states do not require notification or consent. Two states require parental consent. Several states, including Massachusetts, require consent only for pilot studies about conditions for which there is as yet either no satisfactory test or no effective treatment. For a description of newborn screening programs around the country, see GENERAL ACCOUNTING OFFICE, NEWBORN SCREENING — CHARACTERISTICS OF STATE PROGRAMS, GAO-03-449 (March 2003).

What is the justification for mandatory newborn screening laws? Parents have a common law obligation to provide life-saving and medically necessary medical care for their children. They also have an obligation to act in the best interest of their children. The state also has the *parens patriae* power to protect children in need of necessary medical care. Faden and others argue that parents have a moral obligation to determine whether their newborns have a genetic condition that can be treated, and that such testing should be required by law because there is no reasonable issue of judgment on the prospect of benefit to the child. Ruth R. Faden, *Parental Rights, Child Welfare, and Public Health: The Case of PKU Screening*, 72 AM. J. PUB. HEALTH 1396 (1982). Others argue that because newborn screening is simply another diagnostic test for the newborn's own benefit, it is not justified without parental consent unless effective treatment must begin in the newborn period to prevent significant disability. *See* Sheila Wildeman & Jocelyn Downie, *Genetic and Metabolic Screening of Newborns: Must Health Care Providers Seek Explicit Parental Consent?*, 9 HEALTH L.J. 61 (2001). Since almost all parents want to find out whether their children have a medical problem that can be prevented or treated and there may be some risks associated with false positive tests or the absence of effective treatment, Annas concludes that it is difficult to justify mandatory screening. George J. Annas, *Mandatory PKU Screening: The Other Side of the Looking Glass*, 72 AM. J. PUBLIC HEALTH 1401 (1982). Some parents may object to newborn screening for religious reasons. *See e.g., Douglas County Nebraska v. Anaya*, 269 Neb. 552 (2005). Are there any circumstances in which such objections would permit refusing a test? See the discussion in Chapter Two.

A state survey of screening programs found that only 22 states follow up to ensure that parents of newborns are notified of test results, advised about how to care for a child with a positive test, and confirm that treatment has begun. *See* Kenneth D. Mandl et al., *Newborn Screening Program Practices in the United States: Notification, Research and Consent*, 109 PEDIATRICS 269 (2002). How might this affect the justification for mandatory screening programs? How might it affect estimates of costs and benefits?

Is newborn screening a "public health activity"? How does the reason for newborn screening compare with the reason for laws requiring communicable diseases to be reported? What is done to the patient in each case? Are there other laws requiring adults to be tested for any genetic or medical condition? How does it compare with the New York City diabetes blood sugar test reporting law, discussed in Section F, *supra*?

**3.** Several groups have offered criteria for selecting conditions that should be identified in the neonatal period. *See* Jean-Louis Dhondt & Jean-Pierre Farriaux, *Impact of French Legislation on Neonatal Screening*, in HUMAN DNA: LAW AND POLICY 285, 286 (Bartha Maria Knoppers, ed. 1997). The essential elements common to all can be summarized as follows:

1 — the disease will result in severe morbidity (mental and physical) and/or mortality if not diagnosed in the neonatal period;

2 — clinical screening by simply physical examination is not totally effective to identify the disease;

3 — an effective treatment is available

4 — there is a significant improved prognosis with early treatment;

5 — there is a simple rapid, reliable, inexpensive screening test.

Are these criteria for physicians to use in determining whether to recommend testing or are they criteria for assessing the validity of statutory requirements for tests?

**4.** Genetic testing simply identifies a genetic condition or anomaly; it does not prevent or cure it. Unfortunately, more genetic conditions can be identified than can be prevented or treated. As technology advances, a recurring question is whether to require or even offer tests for conditions that cannot be treated or genetic variations about which little is known. The Institute of Medicine recommended against screening for conditions for which there is no beneficial treatment: "Newborn screening is not a trivial intervention and may raise important health and social issues. For example, detection of an affected child can disrupt the relationship between the parents and the newborn. Parents often experience guilt at having passed on a genetic disorder to their child. In addition, there may be social stigma, and such stigma may be increased if a reliable carrier screening test was available *before* pregnancy or birth." INSTITUTE OF MEDICINE, ASSESSING GENETIC RISKS: IMPLICATIONS FOR HEALTH AND SOCIAL POLICY (Lori Andrews et al., eds. 1994). Does routine screening for genetic conditions foster the idea that genetic variations are so abnormal that they should be prevented or fixed or that parents should not have children with genetic abnormalities? Would it encourage prospective parents to seek genetic enhancements for their future children? For an analysis of the prospects for and implications of genetic enhancement, see MAXWELL J. MEHLMAN, WONDERGENES: GENETIC ENHANCEMENT AND THE FUTURE OF SOCIETY (2003).

In 2005, the American College of Medical Genetics (ACMG) recommended that all newborns be screened for 29 diseases. *Newborn Screening: Toward a Uniform Screening Panel and System — Report for Public Comment*, 70 Fed. Reg. (March 8, 2005), *available at* www.mchb.hrsa.gov/screening (last visisted Aug. 2006). The report generated controversy, partly because the conditions newly recommended for screening cannot yet be prevented or treated and partly because its conclusions were based primarily on a survey of the opinions of practitioners and laypeople rather than scientific evidence. See Jeffrey R. Botkin et al., *Newborn Screening Technology: Proceed With Caution*, 117 PEDIATRICS 1793 (2006). The ACMG used an expansive definition of the benefits provided by the tests it recommended, concluding that screening produces a "benefit" if life-saving treatment is available for the condition, *or* if the test could provide information for the parents' future reproductive decisions, *or* if test "could be performed on a multiplex machine regardless of whether it had any proven benefits." *Id*. at 1794. Does this definition meet the standards required for the adoption of *mandatory* newborn testing?

**5.** Tandem mass spectronomy and DNA analysis now make it possible to screen a single blood sample for many genetic and metabolic conditions. The technology is less expensive than conducting independent analyses for each condition to be identified. In 2000, the American Academy of Pediatrics recognized that, "Pressure is mounting to employ new diagnostic capabilities despite possessing limited knowledge of their risk or benefit, or their analytic or clinical validity and utility." American Academy of Pediatrics Taskforce, *Newborn Screening: A Blueprint for the Future*, 106 PEDIATRICS 389 (2000). How might the use of such testing technology affect informed consent?

These technologies have also prompted business and political disputes over who should operate — and profit from — providing screening programs. For an interesting example, see *Neo Gen Screening, Inc. v. New England Newborn Screening Program*, 187 F.3d 24 (1st Cir.), *cert. denied*, 528 U.S. 1061 (1999).

New technology, combined with increased attention to genetics, may encourage the use of newborn screening programs as a resource for research that uses DNA samples. Are blood samples property? Who owns the blood samples retained by newborn screening programs? *See generally* ROBERT F. WEIR & R. S. OLICK, THE STORED TISSUE ISSUE: BIOMEDICAL RESEARCH, ETHICS AND LAW IN THE ERA OF GENOMIC MEDICINE (2004); Gary E. Marchant, *Property Rights and Benefit-Sharing for DNA Donors?*, 45 JURIMETRICS 153 (2005). Should researchers obtain the parents' consent to allow their children's blood samples to be used in a research study? In *Ande v. Rock*, 256 Wis. 2d 365, 647 N.W.2d 265 (Wis. App.), *reh'g denied*, 256 Wis. 2d 64 (2002), *cert. denied sub nom. Ande v. Fost,* 537 U.S. 1107 (2003), parents brought a medical malpractice action against researchers for failing to obtain their informed consent to a test for cystic fibrosis in their children and failing to notify them of the results. Their malpractice claim was dismissed because the researchers had no physician-patient relationship with the Andes or their children. The case illustrates how newborn screening blood samples can be and are used for biomedical research, especially for the majority of conditions for which there is no known or effective treatment. The Wisconsin court did not address the substance of any claim that the Andes should have been asked to donate their child's blood sample for the research, because they claimed no injury from the initial collection of blood. Might they have? *See* Ellen Wright Clayton et al., *Informed Consent for Genetic Research on Stored Tissue Samples*, 274 JAMA 1786 (1995) (discussing informed consent to donating tissue samples for genetic research and whether consent should be required for a later different research study using such samples). Might the Andes have brought a successful negligence claim against the researchers for failure to tell them the results of their child's test? The research protocol specified that parents would not be told, and the researchers apparently did not see the results of individual tests for the control group. Who would ordinarily be responsible for advising the parents of the results of a child's diagnostic test? It depends on whether the test was conducted as part of the child's medical care or solely for purposes of research.

**6.** Parents of children with a genetic or metabolic condition may have a special interest in encouraging newborn testing. Parents of children with Canavan's disease encouraged a research scientist to develop a genetic test for the disease, collecting tissue samples and medical histories from other families. Although a test was developed, disputes over patent rights divided the families, the investigator, his university, and its assignees. The parents, who had intended for the test to be widely used, affordable or free, objected to the university's royalty demands and brought an unsuccessful suit alleging unjust enrichment, conversion, lack of informed consent, fraudulent concealment, breach of fiduciary duty, and misappropriation of trade secrets. After a federal district court found that the families did not retain any property interest in their genetic information or tissue samples, *Greenberg v. Miami Children's Hospital, Inc.*, 264 F. Supp. 2d 1064 (S.D. Fla. 2003), the families reached a settlement with the university allowing certain universities to use the test royalty-free. Canavan Foundation and Miami Children's Hospital, Joint Press Release, (September 29, 2003), www.canavanfoundation.org/news2/09-03_miami.php (last visited Aug. 2006). Another group did retain control over their samples and information. One family created a foundation to collect tissue samples and genetic information about children with PXE (pseudox-anathoma elasticum) and provided the data to a researcher, who developed a genetic test for the disease. The founder participated in the research sufficiently to be named as a co-inventor on the resulting patent, which allowed the foundation to maintain some control over the use of the test. *See* Eliot Marshall, *Patient Advocate Named Co-Inventor on Patent for PXE Disease Gene*, 305 SCIENCE 1226 (2004), *available at* www.sciencemag.org/cgi/content/full/305/5688/1226a.

**7.** The former Office of Technology Assessment estimated that the United States saved $3.2 million for every 100,000 babies screened for PKU and congenital hypothyroidism, with a per case savings of $93,000. OFFICE OF TECHNOLOGY ASSESSMENT, HEALTHY CHILDREN: INVESTING IN THE FUTURE 107 (Feb. 1988). Most testing programs are funded by federal maternal and child health programs. Public Health Service Act § 1109 authorizes the Secretary of Health and Human Services to provide grants to state agencies for "screening, counseling or health care services to newborns and children having or at risk for heritable disorders." Subsection (e) of that section also states: "The participation by any individual in any program or portion thereof established or operated with funds received under this section shall be wholly voluntary and shall not be a prerequisite to eligibility for or receipt of any other service or assistance from, or to participation in, another Federal or State program." How does that subsection affect the laws of a state that receives federal funding to operate its newborn screening program? How does it compare with the federally-funded programs to create HIV reporting programs (discussed in Section D, *supra*) and cancer registries (discussed in Section F, *supra*)?

* * *

### Patricia A. Roche, *DNA and DNA Banking,* *in* 1 ENCYCLOPEDIA OF PRIVACY 174, 174–77 (William G. Staples ed., 2007)

* * *

DNA is the abbreviation for deoxyribonucleic acid, a molecule encoding genetic information found in the nucleus of all human cells, except mature red blood cells. It controls the structure, function and behavior of cells and determines individual hereditary characteristics. DNA banking involves the collection and storage of bodily specimens that contain DNA, the storage of strands of DNA extracted from such specimens, and the maintenance of databases of sequenced DNA. According to an inventory commissioned by the National Bioethics Advisory Committee in 1999, specimens of human material that contain DNA are collected from approximately 20 million individuals per year and stored in collections ranging in size from less than 200 specimens to more than 92 million. Given this proliferation of DNA banking, a significant part of the general public has or soon will have their DNA stored in a DNA repository. These repositories, sometimes referred to as DNA banks, tissue banks, gene banks or biobanks, . . . may be organized as a public, private, non-profit or commercial entity that exists for a discrete period of time, or indefinitely, depending upon its purposes. Some repositories store DNA as the unintended consequence of possessing bodily material that has been collected for other uses. Other repositories store bodily specimens (*e.g.*, blood, saliva, urine, sperm) specifically because the specimens contain human DNA. Of the dedicated DNA repositories only a few engage in DNA banking as an end in itself; most intentional DNA banking is undertaken to support activities such as biomedical research, law enforcement or genealogical research. The purpose, size, storage methods, longevity and corporate status of the entity can influence the kind and degree of privacy risks presented by its DNA banking and the extent to which its activities are regulated to reduce those risks.

Since DNA is present in most human cells, it would be impossible to conduct routine medical care and related laboratory services without collecting and banking DNA. For example, blood banks and clinical, diagnostic and pathology laboratories routinely collect and process tissue samples for a variety of diagnostic and therapeutic purposes with no intention of deriving genetic information from the samples. This incidental DNA banking does not in itself raise privacy issues beyond those associated with creating and maintaining personal medical information. Although federal and state privacy laws that govern medical record keeping and disclosures of health information undoubtedly apply to their activities, no additional legal restraints are placed on these entities merely because they are in possession of DNA samples. Most notably, institutions such as these are not required by federal or state law to destroy specimens after a particular time and therefore they may retain specimens (and any information linked to them) based on their storage capacity and internal policies. Consequently, the possibility, if not the probability, of unauthorized access and misuse of samples is presented by incidental DNA banking. Until the samples are either destroyed or stripped of individual identifiers, this possibility entails some risk to personal privacy.

. . . [S]ome companies bank DNA as a consumer service that is available to anyone who is able to pay the requisite fees. This service has been marketed to parents as a means of preserving their DNA or their children's DNA to make it available if needed for identifying missing persons or bodily remains. In this kind of DNA banking, samples must be maintained in an identifiable form, but there is no need for them to be linked to any personal information beyond identifiers and contact information. Assuming that storage facilities fulfill their contractual obligations to safeguard the samples against unauthorized access, any personal genetic information should remain encoded in the DNA, and banking under these conditions would appear to present minimal risk to personal privacy. Nevertheless, commercial DNA banking of this type is a new industry that is relatively unregulated in the United States. It presents unresolved legal issues, including the degree of privacy protections available to those who purchase banking services. For example, some banks offer to store samples for 20 years or longer. What happens to the contractual promises made to "depositors" in the event that a bank goes out of business, files for bankruptcy protection or merges with another entity is not clear. What such banks are legally obligated or permitted to do with samples that are unclaimed when the term of storage expires, or when storage fees are not paid has yet to be addressed by any state or federal statute or court ruling.

The concerns related to storing or banking DNA are compounded when banking is done for purposes related to genetic testing. An individual's entire genome is encoded in each DNA sample collected from that individual. Since DNA is relatively stable, there is no need to go back to an individual to collect additional samples every time a new procedure for deriving information from DNA becomes available. Therefore, possession and storage of a DNA sample presents an opportunity to access a wealth of information about that individual, including information that could not be anticipated at the point in time the sample was collected. . . . [O]nce steps are taken to preserve an individually identifiable sample for analysis, the risks to that individual's privacy can be significant. Given that an individual shares DNA to varying degrees with his or her genetic relatives, those privacy implications may extend to family members as well. The primary risk is that unauthorized testing of DNA might result in strangers knowing more about an individual's genetic makeup than that person might know herself or might want others to know. In response to these concerns, many states have enacted laws that regulate the circumstances under surrounding genetic testing. However, few of these laws even mention the collection or storage of DNA samples and instead focus on what constitutes adequate consent or authorization to conduct testing and to use or disclose test results. Moreover, these laws tend to be directed towards the behaviors of insurers or employers and do not usually create a general prohibition against secret or surreptitious collection and testing of DNA applicable to everyone.

### Biobanking for population research

In 1998, the Icelandic Parliament enacted the Act on a Health Sector Database, a law authorizing the collection and storage of the entire nation's health information and genetic material by a private biotechnology corporation and granting that company, deCODE Genetics, an exclusive license to exploit the data. This model of a national biobank ignited an ethical and legal debate about how biobanks of this type and magnitude should be regulated. Specific questions were raised about whether the planned methods for collection and storage of DNA samples and personal information will adequately protect the privacy of the hundreds of thousands of Icelanders involved. Much of the criticism of the Icelandic model focused on its use of presumed, open ended consent for inclusion of Icelanders' personal information in the databank as opposed to a voluntary, informed consent process. Doubts were also raised as to whether measures for protecting data, such as the use of encryption techniques, were sufficient to guard against breaches or disclosures of data.

In the wake of the controversies over Iceland's model for biobanking, planners of other large-scale gene banks (*e.g.*, in Estonia, the UK, Japan, and Quebec) are experimenting with different approaches with regard to the structure, protocols and oversight of their banks to protect the interests of individuals who contribute samples and information. Notable differences include the consent procedures that the banks will employ, the extent of personal information that will be passed on to researchers, and the measures that will be taken to prevent researchers from being able to determine whose DNA and information they receive.

The United States has not yet set up a national DNA bank to support genetic variation research that is comparable to the Icelandic project or the

UK Biobank. Nevertheless, DNA banking is being pursued by a significant number of non-profit as well as for-profit entities in the United States. Several of the for-profit banks function as brokers and intermediaries that facilitate research and don't actually conduct in-house research. This is significant because established laws and regulations for the protection of human subjects in research do not apply to a broker model of DNA banking. However, research laws, particularly the federal regulations known as the Common Rule (codified at 45 CFR 46) will generally apply to the researchers that purchase samples and data from these broker style banks. Therefore to satisfy concerns of their clients over compliance issues and to protect their own options to directly engage in research at a later time, some banks have chosen to design their protocols for collecting samples and information and for protecting the privacy of their donors to be consistent with the federal research regulations. Nevertheless, such compliance is voluntary and in the absence of a federal law imposing such rules on DNA banking or uniform state laws regulating these activities, the bank's policies would not be enforceable.

# Chapter 5

# TOBACCO, SMOKING, AND THE PUBLIC'S HEALTH

## A. INTRODUCTION

This chapter reviews the ongoing health problems associated with smoking and other uses of tobacco products and the various ways in which the local, state, and federal governments have attempted to reduce the impact of tobacco on the public's health.

The chapter begins with readings that suggest some of the reasons for the persistence of smoking, notwithstanding widespread knowledge of its hazards. Section B then explores contemporary evidence of those hazards, from which two government interests in reducing the use of tobacco can be inferred. The first is based on the growing list of illnesses and disabilities associated with tobacco use, particularly cigarette smoking. Despite the ever more convincing data on the direct connection between smoking and lung cancer, heart disease, and a great number of other serious health-threatening diseases, the rates of smoking, especially in various segments of the population, have only been reduced slightly in the last several decades, a reality that can be measured both in terms of the lives that will be lost as well as in the dollars that will be spent.

But the government's interest in reducing smoking and other uses of tobacco is further supported by growing evidence that smokers impose a heavy toll on those around them. The causal link between "passive smoking" and various risks to health has been longer in coming and is harder to document, but is growing in significance. Thus, governmental explanations for the regulation of the use of tobacco products can be justified, both politically and constitutionally, as an attempt to protect individuals from their own behavior, and also under the classic (and, for some, less controversial) "harm" rationale: protecting the broader public from the effects of smokers' behavior.

Of particular interest in evaluating the effectiveness of various public health strategies is the fact that some strategies for reducing smoking raise unique constitutional issues (explored in Section C). As local, state, and federal anti-smoking programs attempt to reduce smoking through educational campaigns and efforts to limit the advertising or promotion of tobacco — eschewing more draconian forms of tobacco regulation — they must surmount the more difficult constitutional barriers to government regulation of what is considered speech; somewhat ironically, lesser constitutional constraints would apply if the government were to more directly regulate or prohibit altogether the use of tobacco. Section C also considers the complicated issues of preemption that arise when various state and local efforts to reduce or eliminate tobacco use exceed and, arguably, conflict with, the efforts imposed by federal administrative and legislation limits on the sale or use of tobacco. State pre-emption of local government regulation is likewise given some attention in this connection.

Section D reviews several of the leading private lawsuits that have been brought by consumers of tobacco products against sellers and manufacturers of tobacco, as a vehicle for considering the role of private litigation in influencing public health policy. Finally, Section E briefly explores the shifts in the legal boundaries of "privacy" that accompany the growing perception of smoking as a *non*-private activity.

## RICHARD KLUGER, ASHES TO ASHES
### XI–XIX (1996)

\* \* \*

As the twentieth century wanes, we may marvel justifiably at the triumphs of the human intellect in the course of this span over the visitations of nature at its unkindest. We have largely overcome the savaging effects of infection and contagion, of extreme climates and turbulent weather, of famine and peril from other species. We have attacked the vastness of our planet's distances, even the force of gravity itself, while unlocking the earth's elemental secrets. We have generated creature comforts and pleasures on a scale undreamed of by our forebears and doubled our expected life span.

Yet, as if to reassure the overseers of the universe that we have not attained godlike status but remain in essence creatures of folly and victims of our darker natures, we have also ingeniously crafted fresh forms of misery and death-dealing. We have generated vile effluents with our life-enhancing technology, fouling soil, waters, and skies in ways only beginning to be understood. We have fashioned doomsday weaponry. We have promoted mindless tribal hatreds into genocide and rationalized it in the name of profane statecraft. And worst of all, if we are to credit the number of fatalities as calculated by public health authorities, twentieth-century man has embraced the cigarette and paid dearly for it.

The stated toll is horrific. Americans are said to die prematurely from diseases caused or gravely compounded by smoking at the rate of nearly half a million a year; a multiple of that figure is put forward as the world toll approaches several million. The number claimed has risen appallingly as the century has lengthened, population and wealth have grown, and social customs have turned more permissive. No one can make more than an informed guess at the total loss of life, but those decrying it most urgently assert that the mortality figure from smoking for the century as a whole rivals the multi-millions who have fallen in all its wars.

Yet there has been little outrage at the appalling statistics — only a dirge-like, loosely orchestrated, and inconstant chorus of protest over the continuing practice of the custom and, increasingly of late, restrictions on where it may be undertaken. At mid-century, nearly half the adult American population smoked; near the end of the century, despite massive indictment of the habit by medical science, more than a quarter of all Americans over eighteen continues to smoke — nearly 50 million people. And while overall consumption has declined somewhat, those who cling to the custom smoke more heavily than ever, an estimated twenty-seven cigarettes a day on average. Meanwhile, in Asia, Africa, and Eastern Europe, tobacco is a growth industry. There the cigarette is widely regarded as a sign of modernity, an emblem of advancement, fashion, *savoir-faire*, and adventure as projected in images beamed and plastered everywhere by its makers. And, in a case of supreme irony, not to say perversity, the more evidence accumulated by science on the ravaging effects of tobacco, the more lucrative the business has become and the wider the margin of profit.

Why should this be? Did mankind simply become putty in the hands of the master manipulators who ran the cigarette business? Were we so charmed by the iconography with which these marketing Svengalis enriched our popular culture — a fantasyland populated by heroically taciturn cowboys, sportive camels, and an array of young lovers, auto racers, and assorted *bons vivants* all vibrantly alive with pleasure — that we exonerated them from all charges of capital crimes?

Or have we been convinced by these merchants' unyielding insistence that peddling poison in the form of tobacco is no vice if (a) it is freely picked by its users and (b) its dangers have not yet been conclusively, to the last logarithm of human intellect, proven? Or perhaps our complicity in this man-made plague stems from our very familiarity with the subject; the product has become so ubiquitous and the case against it so clear that we are plain bored by the whole matter. Or perhaps it is the circumstances of death from smoking. The toll is slowly exacted, in the form of seven or eight years of lost life to the average smoker, who, like the rest of us, succumbs mostly to the degenerative diseases of old age: cancer, failing hearts, blocked arteries, dysfunctional lungs. Death from such causes comes singly, and usually at hospitals, not in spectacular conflagrations or crashes obliterating hundreds at a time and capturing the world's attention and sympathy. The smoker's death is banal, private, noticed only by family and friends, and, in the final analysis, self-inflicted.

Doubtless there is an element of plausibility in each of these explanations, but the persistent sway of the cigarette may be equally understood by dwelling not on the consequences of the habit, as its detractors naturally do, and why these people ought to have curtailed it, but on the reason for the phenomenon in the first place. Simply put, hundreds of millions worldwide have found smoking useful to them in myriad ways, subconscious or otherwise.

The proverbial visitor from a distant planet would likely find no earthling custom more pointless or puzzling than the swallowing of tobacco smoke followed by its billowy emission and accompanying odor. Told that the act neither warms nor cleanses the human interior, that it neither repels enemies nor attracts lovers, our off-planet visitor would be still more baffled. The utility of the exercise, he would be informed, is traceable to the changing pace, scale, and nature of daily living in this century. Lives used to be simpler and shorter, given over largely to the struggle for survival. But the technological marvels of our age have provoked attendant stresses from congested living and our often grating interdependence; from the irksome nature of our duties and lack of time to accomplish them; from a welter of conflicting values and emotions born of unattainable expectations and unmanageable frustrations; and from the often careening velocity of life. Many of us have lacked the inner resources to get through the battle and gain a little repose without help wherever and however we could find it, and no device, product, or pastime has been more readily seized upon for this purpose than the cigarette. It has been the preferred and infamous pacifier of the twentieth century, even as — or if — it has been our worst killer. Its users have found it their all-purpose psychological crutch, their universal coping device, and the truest, cheapest, most accessible opiate of the masses.

Let us consider, then, this protean usefulness of the cigarette, which, practically speaking, is the tobacco business in the United States, accounting for some 95 percent of the industry's revenues. The unique value of the cigarette to its users has resided in its perceived dual (and contradictory) role as both stimulant and sedative. Clinically, smoking has been found to speed up a number of bodily functions, most notably the flow of adrenaline, with its quickening effect on the beat of the heart, but the smoker when questioned will most often characterize the cigarette as a relaxant. This seeming paradox is the essence of the product's appeal, for in fact, the smoker uses it to meet both needs.

The smoker smokes when feeling up or in the dumps, when too harassed and overburdened or too unchallenged and idle, when threatened by the crowd at a party or when lonely in a strange place. A smoke is a reward for a job well done or consolation for a job botched. It can fuel the smoker for the intensity of life's daily confrontations yet seem to insulate him from the consuming effects of any given encounter. It defines and punctuates the periods of the smoker's day, and nothing helps as much in dealing on the telephone with trying people or unpleasant matters. The cigarette, in short, has been the peerless regulator of its user's moods, the merciful stabilizing force against the human tendency to over respond to the infinite stimuli that inescapably impinge upon us.

Abetting this admirable, if illusory, versatility of the cigarette have been its obvious virtues as an item of merchandise. It is remarkably convenient: small, portable, readily concealable though highly visible, for sale all over, easy to operate and swiftly disposable, a quick fit into respites throughout the day, usable — until recent years — almost anywhere indoors or out, interchangeable with any other brand of like strength, as blindfold tests have demonstrated (despite company claims of unique flavorfulness, smoothness, and goodness), and cheap. Even at ten or so cents apiece, or a bit over a penny per minute of enjoyment — or of relief, perhaps — the butt has ranked as one of life's least costly indulgences. . . .

Whatever its utility otherwise, smoking is essentially a physical and highly sensual experience. . . .

That smoking is equally a boon to the soul as to the body, few partakers would claim, but most believe it helps them think. Samuel Johnson, among the eighteenth century's more celebrated pipe-puffers, modestly praised the practice as "a thing which requires so little exertion and yet preserves the mind from total vacuity." Freud went a good deal further. "I owe to the cigar a great intensification of my capacity to work." This was written in his seventy-second year after thirty agonizing operations for cancer of the jaw, by which time the connection between the two was not likely lost on him. . . .

Is there clinical support for smoking as brain food? Some experimenters have found, though the evidence is equivocal at best, that nicotine, tobacco's psycho-activating ingredient, excites the brain waves, can increase vigilance in the performance of repetitive (one might say mindless) tasks, and may improve the processing of sensory stimuli — provided, that is, one keeps on smoking. Does any of this amount to a boost in productive mental energy? Some scientists have theorized that smoking creates an apparent heightening effect by neutralizing (one might say numbing) the edges of one's consciousness and thereby reducing distractions. Translation: Smoking may help you concentrate by emptying the mind of all but the subject of the moment.

In the even murkier realm of the subconscious, smoking has been arguably credited with filling needs and registering impulses not conceded or even guessed at by the smoker. The cigar-loving Freud contended that smoking was an oral autoerotic manifestation of inadequate breast-suckling, presumably in infancy, and likened it to thumb-sucking. Lesser sages have ascribed overeating to this same "orality," but the smoker is far busier with his fix if measured in mouth-hours. Some Freudian followers, licensed and otherwise, have hypothesized that cigars, cigarettes, and pipes are all phallic substitutes, or possibly supplements, and smoking a surrogate form of sexuality. Higher-minded cultural anthropologists have attributed to male smokers a yearning for the primal power of Man as Fire-Conqueror or for the magical potency of the fire-breathing shaman or, when not on those particular power trips, for the comforts of hearth and home evoked by their little portable tobacco furnaces. And many social commentators have concluded that smoking for women is both a badge of would-be equality with smoking men and a sanctioned outlet for the frustrated expression of combativeness and other impulses that men are allowed to vent but that are forbidden to the female of the species, always supposed the gentler and more nurturing of the two.

Nor to be minimized, either, has been the usefulness of smoking as coded defiance of authority, of the hand fate has dealt you, of sweet reason itself. It is most favored, in the first instance, by juvenile smokers as an initiator into the mysteries and empowerment of the adult world; the accompanying displeasures of nausea and dizziness assaulting the novice inhaler are tolerated as rites of passage and the price to be paid for partaking of forbidden fruit. . . .

For those millions enslaved by nicotine, the weightier charge that the addiction can ultimately prove lethal inspires a lot of fast talking and whistling by the graveyard. The catechism of the hopelessly habituated runs something like this: (1) Even if those busybody biostatisticians are right, only one of four smokers will die due, more or less, to smoking, so the odds are on my side. (2) Besides, you've got to die of something, so why not from a source of pleasure? (3) Anyway, it takes decades for the diseases linked to smoking to develop, and those years I might lose aren't exactly quality time, coming late in life when many human faculties and the yen for living are diminished. (4) Life is full of dangers — to live is to take risks of all sorts every day; I may get hit by a truck tomorrow. I'm here and want to enjoy myself to the fullest extent possible, and cigarettes help me do that. And (5), let's face it, I might have gone cuckoo a long while back without smoking or stressed out terminally, as they say. So, (6) if you don't mind — or even if you do — please get out of my face and tend to your own garden P.S. (7) When your number's up, it's up; you can't mess with your karma.

Why, given the enormity of the crimes against humanity with which it has been charged, the cigarette has not been outlawed or its ingredients and design modified by government command is thus explainable in the first place by the immense and continuing consumption of the product for all the above uses and excuses. It must then be added at once, without excessive moralizing, that the tobacco industry, understandably devoted to its own survival ahead of all others', has labored prodigiously to reassure its customers, disarm its foes, purchase allies in high places, and minimize government intrusion into its gravely suspect business. But the success of that industry cannot be facilely dismissed as greedy capitalism at its most predatory, for in many nations, capitalist and socialist alike, the manufacture and sale of tobacco products have been reserved as an operation of the state, carried out in the name of the public interest if not the public health. Among these nations have been China, Japan, the constituent states of the former Soviet Union, France, Spain, Italy, all the Eastern European countries before their liberation from totalitarian rule, Kenya, both Koreas, Taiwan, and Thailand.

Around the world, moreover, the pro-smoking cause is championed by millions dependent on the tobacco industry for their livelihood. Most numerous among these are the growers of what the industry claims is the most widely cultivated non-food plant on earth. In the United States, tobacco remains the most profitable cash crop on a per-acre basis, and in many places throughout Latin America, Africa, and Asia, where subsistence farming is the obligatory way of life for the masses, pending the creation of viable domestic industry, tobacco has been considered a godsend. . . .

Beyond growers, the ranks of those with a prominent vested interest in sustaining smoking are swollen by machinists operating state-of-the-art cigarette makers that spit out 10,000 units per minute; by distributors and vendors, including supermarket managers who hawk Marlboros by the carton, state-store operators in Burgundy pushing Gauloises by the pack, men on bikes traveling the Ugandan bush country, and street urchins in Calcutta selling smokes by the single stick; by Madison Avenue dream merchants dependent on the U.S. tobacco trade's more than $5 billion annual advertising and promotion outlay as well as by newspaper and magazine editors; by auto-racing drivers and their pit crews, dance troupes, and symphony orchestras perennially on the edge of extinction; by professional women tennis players (until recently); by museum directors, colleges, and social action groups, all gratefully accepting cigarette manufacturers' largesse without perceptible qualms of conscience. With such a mammoth and influential constituency in place, it is no surprise that would-be tobacco regulators are scarce in the political arena. Governments, furthermore, have themselves become addicted to the cigarette because of the taxes it harvests for them. Cigarettes are the most heavily taxed consumer product in the world. About twenty industrialized nations tax cigarettes more heavily than the U.S., some of them five times more. In China, they have been the largest source of capital formation for broadening the country's industrial base. Few politicians have been willing to forgo such revenues, as well as the votes and support of smokers and all those battening on the habit. Even the World Health Organization, a unit of the United Nations, has been hamstrung in its efforts to combat tobacco by the indifference of member-nation governments and the pressures applied by the private international goliaths, Philip Morris Companies, Inc., British-American Tobacco, RJR Nabisco, and Rothmans.

And so, near the end of the century, the debate over smoking rages on. The cigarette makers argue that the smoking of tobacco has persisted in civilized places for 500 years now, never without its loud detractors; that science may have incriminated the practice but has not found it guilty beyond a shadow of a doubt, and that, regardless of how definitive the findings to date, every smoker knows, whether from warning labels, public reports, media attention, or word of mouth, that there are risks attached. Antismoking activists respond that most smokers begin at an immature and suggestible age — 90 percent of them in the U.S. by the time they are twenty — when they are incapable of weighing the prospect of an early grave and believe they can break the habit at will; that the perceived benefits of smoking are in reality a delusion induced by a drug, which when consumed at the rate of 70,000 or so hits a year (twenty or twenty-five cigarettes a day x eight or ten puffs each x 365 days) causes deeply conditioned behavior and a corrosive effect on human tissue, and that the medical case is proven, except to the extent that science is only just beginning to grasp the precise mechanics by which all diseases assault the body's intricate defense and immune systems. That tobacco smoke is a ruthless pathological agent provocateur, there remains no doubt. The question, then, is whether cigarette merchants are businessmen basically like any other, selling a product judged to be highly hazardous long after its usefulness to millions was well established, and are now sorely abused by "health fascists" and moralizing busybodies, or are they moral lepers preying on the ignorant, the miserable, the emotionally vulnerable, and the genetically susceptible?

* * *

# NICKY, NICKY. IT'S ALL ABOUT LITTLE NICKY, ISN'T IT?

For centuries, people have chewed and smoked tobacco, which comes from the plant nicotiana tabacum. The reason tobacco is used by so many people is because it contains a powerful drug known as nicotine.

When tobacco is smoked, nicotine is absorbed by the lungs and quickly moved into the bloodstream, where it is circulated throughout the brain. All of this happens very rapidly. In fact, nicotine reaches the brain within eight seconds after someone inhales tobacco smoke. Nicotine can also enter the bloodstream through the mucous membranes that line the mouth (if tobacco is chewed) or nose (if snuff is used), and even through the skin.

Nicotine affects the entire body. Nicotine acts directly on the heart to change heart rate and blood pressure. It also acts on the nerves that control respiration to change breathing patterns. In high concentrations, nicotine is deadly, in fact one drop of purified nicotine on the tongue will kill a person. It's so lethal that it has been used as a pesticide for centuries.

So why do people smoke? Because nicotine acts in the brain where it can stimulate feelings of pleasure. . . . Your brain is made up of billions of nerve cells. They communicate by releasing chemical messengers called neurotransmitters. Each neurotransmitter is like a key that fits into a special "lock," called a receptor, located on the surface of nerve cells. When a neurotransmitter finds its receptor, it activates the receptor's nerve cell.

The nicotine molecule is shaped like a neurotransmitter called acetylcholine. Acetylcholine and its receptors are involved in many functions, including muscle movement, breathing, heart rate, learning, and memory. They also cause the release of other neurotransmitters and hormones that affect your mood, appetite, memory, and more. When nicotine gets into the brain, it attaches to acetylcholine receptors and mimics the actions of acetylcholine.

Nicotine also activates areas of the brain that are involved in producing feelings of pleasure and reward. Recently, scientists discovered that nicotine raises the levels of a neurotransmitter called dopamine in the parts of the brain that produce feelings of pleasure and reward. Dopamine, which is sometimes called the pleasure molecule, is the same neurotransmitter that is involved in addictions to other drugs such as cocaine and heroin. Researchers now believe that this change in dopamine may play a key role in all addictions. This may help explain why it is so hard for people to stop smoking.

Nicotine is as addictive as heroin or cocaine. If someone uses nicotine again and again, such as by smoking cigarettes or cigars or chewing tobacco, his or her body develops a tolerance for it. When someone develops tolerance, he or she needs more drug to get the same effect. Eventually, a person can become addicted. Once a person becomes addicted, it is extremely difficult to quit. People who start smoking before the age of 21 have the hardest time quitting, and fewer than 1 in 10 people who try to quit smoking succeed.

When nicotine addicts stop smoking they may suffer from restlessness, hunger, depression, headaches, and other uncomfortable feelings. These are called "withdrawal symptoms" because they happen when nicotine is withdrawn from the body.

Withdrawal may be bad, but long-term smoking can be much worse. It raises your blood pressure, dulls your senses of smell and taste, reduces your stamina, and wrinkles your skin. More dangerously, long-term smoking can lead to fatal heart attacks, strokes, emphysema, and cancer. . . . But even when faced with risk of death, many people keep using tobacco because they are so addicted to nicotine.

Source: NATIONAL INSTITUTE ON DRUG ABUSE/NATIONAL INSTITUTE OF HEALTH, THE BRAIN'S RESPONSE TO NICOTINE, found at www.drugabuse. gov/mom (last visited December 2006)

## B.  THE HEALTH CONSEQUENCES OF SMOKING AND TOBACCO

### 1. The Effects of Smoking Tobacco

SURGEON GENERAL, U.S. DEPARTMENT OF HEALTH & HUMAN SERVICES, EXECUTIVE SUMMARY, THE HEALTH CONSEQUENCES OF SMOKING
8–17 (2004)

\* \* \*

Forty years after the first Surgeon General's report in 1964, the list of diseases and other adverse effects caused by smoking continues to expand. Epidemiologic studies are providing a comprehensive assessment of the risks faced by smokers who continue to smoke across their life spans. Laboratory research now reveals how smoking causes disease at the molecular and cellular levels. Fortunately for former smokers, studies show that the substantial risks of smoking can be reduced by successfully quitting at any age. The evidence reviewed in this and prior reports of the Surgeon General leads to the following major conclusions: (1) Smoking harms nearly every organ of the body, causing many diseases and reducing the health of smokers in general; (2) Quitting smoking has immediate as well as long-term benefits, reducing risks for diseases caused by smoking and improving health in general; (3) Smoking cigarettes with lower machine-measured yields of tar and nicotine provides no clear benefit to health; (4) The list of diseases caused by smoking has been expanded to include abdominal aortic aneurysm, acute myeloid leukemia, cataract, cervical cancer, kidney cancer, pancreatic cancer, pneumonia, periodontitis, and stomach cancer.

. . . .

The publication of the first Surgeon General's report on smoking and health in January of 1964 was a landmark and pivotal event in the history of public health. By that time, there was a rapidly accumulating amount of evidence on the dangers of smoking, and it was inevitable that action would follow the publication of a comprehensive expert report with the powerful conclusion that smoking causes disease. Since 1964, there has been a broad societal shift in the acceptability of tobacco use and in the public's knowledge about the accompanying health risks. In 1963, per capita annual adult consumption in the United States peaked at 4,345 cigarettes, a figure that included both smokers and nonsmokers. By 2002, per capita annual consumption in this country had declined to 1,979 cigarettes, the lowest level since before the start of World War II. In 1964, the majority of men smoked and an increasing number of women were becoming smokers. Today, there are more former smokers than current smokers, and each year over half of all daily smokers try to quit. In 1964, smoking a cigarette was viewed as a "rite of passage" by almost all adolescents. Today, only about half of all high school seniors have ever smoked a cigarette and less than one in four is a current smoker, the lowest level since researchers started monitoring smoking rates among high school seniors in the mid-1970s.

In 1964, smoking was permitted almost everywhere, and even the U.S. Public Health Service had logo ashtrays on its conference tables. Today, secondhand tobacco smoke is widely accepted as a public health hazard and levels of exposure among nonsmokers have declined dramatically over the last decade. In fact, there is an unprecedented level of activity to achieve clean indoor air quality at both the local and state levels. More communities and states are considering and adopting laws that are even more comprehensive in the range of venues they cover. . . .

Smoking remains the leading preventable cause of disease and death in the United States, resulting in more than 440,000 premature deaths each year. In 1964, the list of diseases known to be caused by smoking was short: chronic bronchitis and cancers of the lung and larynx. Each subsequent Surgeon General's report has expanded the understanding of the magnitude of the health consequences of tobacco use. According to this 2004 report, the number of diseases caused by smoking has continued to increase. . . . [T]he burden of tobacco use on the physical and economic health of this country remains staggering. Since the release of the 1964 Surgeon General's report on smoking and health, more than 12 million Americans have died prematurely due to smoking. Currently, estimates of annual smoking attributable economic costs in the United States are over $157 billion.

Some may view the progress achieved in the country since 1964 as evidence that the problem has been solved. Unfortunately, the data indicate that future reductions in the morbidity, mortality, and economic costs of tobacco use will require a continuing and sustained effort. Since 1965, the overall proportion of adults in this country who are current smokers has been reduced by half; however, the rate of decline in adult smoking prevalence has slowed in recent years. Equally disturbing, the rates of smoking among some racial and ethnic minority populations and among less educated Americans remain high. Although the percentage of high school seniors who are current smokers has been reduced from 36.5 percent in 1997 to 24.4 percent in 2003, the trends in youth smoking over the last few years indicate that the rate of decline is slowing appreciably. Although the level of secondhand tobacco smoke that nonsmokers are exposed to has declined significantly in the last decade, the decline has been greater among adults than among children, who are largely exposed at home. Currently, levels of exposure to this known human carcinogen are more than twice as high among nonsmoking children than among nonsmoking adults. Finally, while the knowledge that smoking can adversely affect health has become widespread among the general public, the grave health risks remain poorly understood.

. . . .

One major topic in need of more research is to complete the understanding of the mechanisms by which tobacco-related diseases are caused. A greater understanding of these causal mechanisms should have implications for disease prevention that extend to agents other than smoking. This report reviews the association between smoking and cancer, cardiovascular diseases, respiratory diseases, reproductive effects, and other health consequences, and defines a variety of specific research questions and issues related to the biologic mechanisms by which the multiple toxic agents in tobacco products and tobacco smoke cause specific adverse health outcomes. For example, the lung remains the primary site for elevated tobacco-related cancer risk; however, during the past 40 years, the type of lung cancer caused by smoking has changed for reasons still unknown. Similarly, as the evidence that smoking damages the heart and circulatory system and is a primary preventable cause of heart disease and stroke continues to expand, important research questions remain about how smoking interacts with other cardiovascular risk factors and accelerates the atherosclerotic disease process. With respect to these and the other research questions, the public health message remains the same: Smoking greatly increases the risk of many adverse health effects. Therefore, never start smoking or quit as soon as possible.

For several organ sites, there is a need for more evidence regarding the possible causal role of smoking on cancer risk. For prostate and colorectal cancers, the evidence is suggestive but not sufficient to determine a possible causal relationship. For breast cancer, even though there is no evidence overall for a causal role of smoking, on a genetic basis some evidence suggests that some women may be at an increased risk if they smoke. For other sites such as the liver, confounding exposures to other risk factors have made the evaluation of the risk of smoking very complex, but this report finds the evidence to be suggestive of causation. There should be further research on those sites where the evidence is suggestive but not yet sufficient to warrant a causal conclusion.

. . . [O]verall, smokers are less healthy than nonsmokers. Most often the risks of smoking are discussed with respect to a specific cancer, to heart disease, or to respiratory disease risk. Unfortunately, because smoking is such a powerful cause of disease, most smokers suffer from adverse health effects in many parts of their bodies at once. Additionally, before a death from one of the diseases caused by smoking, which is often quite premature, many smokers live for years with a diminished quality of life from the burden of chronic and disabling health effects (*e.g.*, reduced breathing capacity, poor heart functioning, greater susceptibility to lung infections, visual loss due to cataracts, and others). More research emphasis needs to be placed on the broad health consequences of smoking — namely, how smoking has a negative impact on many aspects of the body at the same time, and how these multiple adverse health effects combine to produce an overall reduced quality of life and greater health care costs prior to causing premature death. Recently, preliminary estimates indicated that for every premature death caused each year by smoking, there were at least 20 smokers living with a smoking-related disease.

This report highlights the diversity of the health effects caused by smoking, and how dramatically smoking affects the risk of the leading causes of death in this country (e.g., cancer, heart disease, respiratory disease). These findings emphasize that tobacco prevention and control should be key elements in a national prevention strategy for all of these major causes of death. Additionally, there is great disparity in tobacco-related disease and death among populations and the need to address the research gaps that exist for many special populations. Research is needed not only on disease outcome but also on the development of more effective strategies to reach and involve high risk populations (e.g., race/ethnicity, low income, low education, the unemployed, blue-collar and service workers, and heavily addicted smokers).

Finally, more research is needed on how changing tobacco products, as well as pharmaceutical products, have affected and could continue to affect health. In this report, one major conclusion finds that cigarettes with lower machine-measured yields of tar and nicotine (i.e., low-tar/nicotine cigarettes) have not produced a lower risk of smoking-related diseases. Yet there are rapidly growing numbers of modified tobacco products characterized as Potentially Reduced Exposure Products (PREPS). Research has demonstrated that with the expectation of reducing risk, many smokers switched to low machine-measured tar/nicotine cigarettes, and may thus have been deterred from quitting. Therefore, it is critically important that the health risks of the emerging PREPS be evaluated comprehensively and quickly to avoid a replication of that unfortunate low-tar/nicotine cigarette experience. Research on the biologic mechanisms by which the multiple toxic agents in tobacco products and tobacco smoke cause specific adverse health outcomes can help establish an important scientific foundation for evaluating the potential health effects of PREPS. Similarly, the public health and policy implications of changes in manufactured cigarettes, other tobacco-containing products, and pharmaceutical products will require the continued attention of public health researchers and policymakers.

As the world enters this new millennium, it is faced with many new public health challenges even as many of the old risks to good health remain. During the last 40 years, people have become increasingly more aware of the adverse health consequences of tobacco use. Currently, tobacco use is the leading cause of preventable illness and death in this nation, in the majority of other high-income nations, and increasingly in low- and middle-income nations. Unfortunately, the high rates of tobacco-related illnesses and deaths will continue until tobacco prevention and control efforts worldwide are commensurate with the harm caused by tobacco use. At the start of the last century, lung cancer was a very rare disease. Now lung cancer is the leading cause of cancer deaths in both men and women in this country. Our success in reducing tobacco use during the last 40 years has led to a reversal in the epidemic of lung cancer among men; nationwide, rates of lung cancer deaths among men have declined since the early 1990s. In California, where there has been a comprehensive tobacco control program in place since 1989, reductions in rates of tobacco-related disease and deaths already have been observed. If we apply what we know works, we can make lung cancer a rare disease again by the end of this century.

\* \* \*

## SURGEON GENERAL, U.S. DEPARTMENT OF HEALTH & HUMAN SERVICES, THE IMPACT OF SMOKING ON DISEASE AND THE BENEFITS OF SMOKING REDUCTION, THE HEALTH CONSEQUENCES OF SMOKING
### 858–72 (2004)

\* \* \*

Smoking caused an estimated total of 263,600 deaths in males and 176,500 deaths in females in the United States each year from 1995–1999. For men aged 35 years and older, annual smoking attributable deaths (SAM) were 105,700 for cancers, 87,600 for cardiovascular diseases (CVDs), and 53,700 for respiratory diseases. For women aged 35 years and older, the annual SAM was 53,900 for cancers, 55,000 for CVDs, and 44,300 for respiratory diseases. Among adults, the most smoking attributable deaths were from lung cancer (124,800), ischemic heart disease (IHD) (82,000), and chronic airways obstruction (64,700).

Smoking during pregnancy was estimated to result in 560 deaths in infant boys and 410 deaths in infant girls annually. Excluding adult deaths from secondhand smoke, the estimated SAM was responsible for a total annual years of preventable lost life (YPLL) of 3,319,000 for males and 2,152,600 for females.

The annual SAM will likely remain fairly stable if trends in smoking prevalence among adults do not decrease substantially. Adult smoking prevalence rates have decreased over the past few years, but the prevalence of smoking among adolescents increased from 1992 until 1997. However, youth smoking has also decreased more recently. Yet, the burden of disease attributable to smoking is driven by those with long-term previous exposures, so unless smoking cessation among current smokers increases quite rapidly, SAM is not expected to decline substantially for many years. . . .

. . . .

Until the early 1990s, only a few estimates of the cost of smoking had been made in the United States. Estimates of the costs of smoking received increased attention in the 1990s when the states were estimating damages for purposes of lawsuits. . . . Published studies on the medical costs of smoking have used a number of approaches to estimate costs, including PAR calculations, model-based approaches, incidence-based measures of present and future costs attributable to smoking, indirect costs of human capital lost from disability and premature deaths, and net social costs. These studies have produced a wide range of estimates, depending on methodologies, assumptions incorporated into models, data sets used, and other methodological issues. One key issue is the comparison of the net versus the gross costs of smoking to society. Net costs would include consideration of the economic benefits of taxes, agricultural revenue, ancillary economic activity, and the "costs" of longer lives among nonsmokers that might offset the medical care costs of smokers or their lost productivity while they are alive.

. . . .

In the United States, direct medical costs for the detection, treatment, and rehabilitation of persons with smoking attributable clinical diseases have been the primary outcome variable in the cost models. These smoking attributable costs have been consistently estimated at 6 to 8 percent of the total annual expenditures for health care, with an estimated upper bound as high as 14 percent. Indirect morbidity and mortality costs are defined as the costs for excess sickness and disability days for smoking-linked illnesses, as well as lost productivity due to premature death from the effect of smoking on longevity.

. . . .

. . . [E]conomists have used econometric models to estimate the net effects of prolonged life on health and social support systems, considering not only the costs of smoking but of potential economic gains from smoking. For example, Barendregt and colleagues (1997) concluded that successful smoking cessation and health promotion activities would produce positive economic outcomes (referred to as gross outcomes) in the short run. Barendregt and colleagues, however, did not consider the higher contribution made by longer living nonsmokers to pension and tax systems in making their calculations.

Manning and colleagues (1989) estimated the lifetime, discounted costs that smokers impose on others. Instead of total economic costs, the study focused on only those financial costs that are external to the smokers and their family members; that is, costs paid by insurance companies, the state, or public agencies in caring for smokers and borne by nonsmokers because these are the costs relevant to tax policy. Results indicate that nonsmokers subsidize smokers' medical care and group life insurance while smokers subsidize nonsmokers' pension and nursing home payments because of their shorter life expectancy. The net external financial costs that smokers impose on nonsmokers are positive at a 5 percent discount rate ($0.15 per pack), but the excise tax revenue from cigarettes at the time of the analysis exceeded those external costs. The costs of lung cancer deaths caused by involuntary smoking and deaths caused by smoking-related fires were not included in this estimate because they were considered internal costs (costs to the individual or to his/her family unit). Costs related to maternal smoking were also omitted. With all lives lost to involuntary smoking and to smoking-related fires defined as external costs, the total external cost per pack was estimated at $0.38 in 1986 dollars. This may be an uncertain estimate of net external costs due to imperfect data sources and unquantifiable confounding factors. In addition, there was no consideration of annoyance, pain and suffering, or other non-economic costs. This same study found that the range of costs produced by various authors varied between net external savings of $0.17 per pack to costs of $2.36 per pack. . . .

In an extensive review by the World Bank, the gross health care costs of smoking for high-income countries ranged from 0.10 to 1.1 percent of the gross domestic product, and most of the net-versus-gross cost studies showed net costs for smoking.

The value of longevity and quality of life may be difficult to economically quantify. However, at least one study has discussed the issue of compression of morbidity when smoking is reduced. Using a cross-sectional study of Dutch nationals, Nusselder and colleagues (2000) found that a nonsmoking population spends fewer years with disability than a reference population of smokers and nonsmokers. The nonsmokers had lower mortality risks, but they also had a lower incidence of disability and a higher level of recovery from disability. This status resulted in reduced average time lived with disability (−0.9 years for men aged 30 years and −1.1 years for women) and increased average time lived without disability (2.5 years for men and 1.9 years for women). Thus, with a nonsmoking population the length of life as well as the length of a disability-free life will be extended. This extension will then compress the disability for nonsmokers into a shorter period toward death; smokers, with lengthier periods of disability, will suffer earlier mortality, but they will also have more disability and certainly more medical care expenditures while disabled when compared with nonsmokers. Although the disability suffered by former smokers will be less than that of current smokers, mortality and disability risks will still be higher among former smokers than among lifetime nonsmokers.

. . . .

. . . Previously described studies do not describe all dimensions of the impact of smoking and smoking attributable disease. For example, the pain and suffering, decreased quality of life, and related psychosocial aspects of physical illness are not measured. Prevalence-based, cost-of-illness calculations do not account for economic factors such as Social Security disbursements, pension claims, changes in the demand for health specialties related to the treatment of smoking-related illnesses, and the employment by or monetary dividends from the tobacco industry. Smoking can cause costs without impacting mortality or even morbidity among smokers. For example, the health or mortality of a smoking spouse may have an effect on nursing home admission rates for the nonsmoking spouse; in addition, lost income to family members who must care for smokers with prolonged disabilities is not usually measured. These are actually direct costs rather than indirect or human capital losses. Costs to employers for absenteeism, lost productivity, higher insurance premiums for smokers and liability incurred for exposing nonsmokers to passive smoke may also be included as an economic cost of smoking.

Several studies have reviewed these economic issues and ongoing controversies that primarily involve the net-versus-gross cost of tobacco on society. This controversy, however, ignores the main burden — that of health — when it dwells on the "benefits" of smoking that result from premature death. Generally, however, it appears that direct costs attributable to smoking comprise 6 to 9 percent of the total national health care budget. Cost estimates have tended to increase over time, reflecting improvements in methodology, increases in medical expenditures for smoking-related diseases because of inflation and/or technology, and expansion of the list of diseases caused by smoking.

Further research on the economic costs of nursing home care is needed as the impact of smoking on admissions to and utilization of nursing homes is not well described. There are also insufficient data on the costs from passive smoking-related illnesses. Indirect costs need more research at the national level, and costs to employers resulting from smoking by their employees should also be the subject of additional research.

. . . .

Regardless of the methodological issues around the estimation methods, cigarette smoking remains the leading single cause of preventable mortality in the United States. . . . These estimates are not biased strongly by confounding factors, even though smokers, compared with nonsmokers, tend to have different profiles for a number of lifestyle-related risk factors for disease and may have different costs for even the same condition. Economic disease burden estimates have been used to provide a more compelling argument as to the costs of smoking to governments and society in general, thus adding information that can be used to support comprehensive tobacco use prevention and control programs.

. . . Smoking remains the leading preventable cause of premature death in the United States. The burden of smoking attributable mortality will remain at current levels for several decades. Comprehensive programs that reflect the best available science on tobacco use prevention and smoking cessation have the potential to reduce the adverse impact of smoking on population health. Meeting the Healthy People 2010 goals for current smoking prevalence reductions to 12 percent among persons aged 18 years and older and to 16 percent among youth aged 14 through 17 years will prevent an additional 7.1 million premature deaths after 2010. Without substantially stronger national and state efforts, it is unlikely that this health goal can be achieved. However, even with more modest reductions in tobacco use, significant additional reductions in premature death can be expected.

* * *

## 2.   The Effects of Smoking on Others

### SURGEON GENERAL, U.S. DEPARTMENT OF HEALTH & HUMAN SERVICES, EXECUTIVE SUMMARY, THE HEALTH CONSEQUENCES OF INVOLUNTARY EXPOSURE TO TOBACCO SMOKE (2006)

\* \* \*

This report returns to involuntary smoking, the topic of the 1986 Surgeon General's report. Since then, there have been many advances in the research on secondhand smoke, and substantial evidence has been reported over the ensuing 20 years. This report uses the revised language for causal conclusions that was implemented in the 2004 Surgeon General's report. Each chapter provides a comprehensive review of the evidence, a quantitative synthesis of the evidence if appropriate, and a rigorous assessment of sources of bias that may affect interpretations of the findings. The reviews in this report reaffirm and strengthen the findings of the 1986 report. With regard to the involuntary exposure of nonsmokers to tobacco smoke, the scientific evidence now supports the following major conclusions:

— Secondhand smoke causes premature death and disease in children and in adults who do not smoke.

— Children exposed to secondhand smoke are at an increased risk for sudden infant death syndrome (SIDS), acute respiratory infections, ear problems, and more severe asthma. Smoking by parents causes respiratory symptoms and slows lung growth in their children.

— Exposure of adults to secondhand smoke has immediate adverse effects on the cardiovascular system and causes coronary heart disease and lung cancer.

— The scientific evidence indicates that there is no risk-free level of exposure to secondhand smoke.

— Many millions of Americans, both children and adults, are still exposed to secondhand smoke in their homes and workplaces despite substantial progress in tobacco control.

— Eliminating smoking in indoor spaces fully protects nonsmokers from exposure to secondhand smoke. Separating smokers from nonsmokers, cleaning the air, and ventilating buildings cannot eliminate exposures of nonsmokers to secondhand smoke.

### Toxicology of Secondhand Smoke

— More than 50 carcinogens have been identified in sidestream and secondhand smoke.

— The evidence is sufficient to infer a causal relationship between exposure to secondhand smoke and its condensates and tumors in laboratory animals.

— The evidence is sufficient to infer that exposure of nonsmokers to secondhand smoke causes a significant increase in urinary levels of metabolites of the tobacco-specific lung carcinogen 4-(methylnitrosamino)-1-(3-pyridyl)-1-

butanone (NNK). The presence of these metabolites links exposure to second-hand smoke with an increased risk for lung cancer.

— The mechanisms by which secondhand smoke causes lung cancer are probably similar to those observed in smokers. The overall risk of secondhand smoke exposure, compared with active smoking is diminished by a substantially lower carcinogenic dose.

. . . .

### Assessment of Exposure to Secondhand Smoke

— Current heating, ventilating, and air conditioning systems alone cannot control exposure to secondhand smoke.

— The operation of a heating, ventilating, and air conditioning system can distribute secondhand smoke throughout a building.

. . . .

— Smoking increases indoor particle concentrations.

### Prevalence of Exposure to Secondhand Smoke

— The evidence is sufficient to infer that large numbers of nonsmokers are still exposed to secondhand smoke.

— Exposure of nonsmokers to secondhand smoke has declined in the United States since the 1986 Surgeon General's report. . . .

— The evidence indicates that the extent of secondhand smoke exposure varies across the country.

— Homes and workplaces are the predominant locations for exposure to secondhand smoke.

— Exposure to secondhand smoke tends to be greater for persons with lower incomes.

— Exposure to secondhand smoke continues in restaurants, bars, casinos, gaming halls, and vehicles.

### Reproductive and Developmental Effects from Exposure to Secondhand Smoke

The evidence is sufficient to infer a causal relationship between:

> — exposure to secondhand smoke and sudden infant death syndrome.

> — maternal exposure to secondhand smoke during pregnancy and a small reduction in birth weight

The evidence is suggestive but not sufficient to infer a causal relationship between:

> — maternal exposure to secondhand smoke during pregnancy and preterm delivery.

— prenatal and postnatal exposure to secondhand smoke and childhood cancer.

— prenatal and postnatal exposure to secondhand smoke and childhood leukemias.

— prenatal and postnatal exposure to secondhand smoke and childhood lymphomas.

— prenatal and postnatal exposure to secondhand smoke and childhood brain tumors.

The evidence is inadequate to infer the presence or absence of a causal relationship between:

— maternal exposure to secondhand smoke and female fertility or fecundability. No data were found on paternal exposure to secondhand smoke and male fertility or fecundability.

— maternal exposure to secondhand smoke during pregnancy and spontaneous abortion.

— exposure to secondhand smoke and neonatal mortality.

— exposure to secondhand smoke and congenital malformations.

— exposure to secondhand smoke and cognitive functioning among children.

— exposure to secondhand smoke and behavioral problems among children.

— exposure to secondhand smoke and children's height/growth.

— maternal exposure to secondhand smoke during pregnancy and childhood cancer.

— exposure to secondhand smoke during infancy and childhood cancer.

— prenatal and postnatal exposure to secondhand smoke and childhood cancers other than the types mentioned above.

## Respiratory Effects in Children from Exposure to Secondhand Smoke

— The evidence is sufficient to infer a causal relationship between secondhand smoke exposure from parental smoking and lower respiratory illnesses in infants and children.

— The increased risk for lower respiratory illnesses is greatest from smoking by the mother.

— The evidence is sufficient to infer a causal relationship between parental smoking and middle ear disease in children, including acute and recurrent otitis media and chronic middle ear effusion.

— The evidence is suggestive but not sufficient to infer a causal relationship between parental smoking and the natural history of middle ear effusion.

— The evidence is inadequate to infer the presence or absence of a causal relationship between parental smoking and an increase in the risk of adenoidectomy or tonsillectomy among children.

— The evidence is sufficient to infer a causal relationship between parental smoking and cough, phlegm, wheeze, and breathlessness among children of school age.

— The evidence is sufficient to infer a causal relationship between parental smoking and ever having asthma among children of school age.

. . . .

— The evidence is inadequate to infer the presence or absence of a causal relationship between parental smoking and the risk of immunoglobulin E-mediated allergy in their children.

— The evidence is sufficient to infer a causal relationship between maternal smoking during pregnancy and persistent adverse effects on lung function across childhood.

— The evidence is sufficient to infer a causal relationship between exposure to secondhand smoke after birth and a lower level of lung function during childhood.

## Cancer Among Adults from Exposure to Secondhand Smoke

— The evidence is sufficient to infer a causal relationship between secondhand smoke exposure and lung cancer among lifetime nonsmokers. This conclusion extends to all secondhand smoke exposure, regardless of location.

— The pooled evidence indicates a 20 to 30 percent increase in the risk of lung cancer from secondhand smoke exposure associated with living with a smoker.

— The evidence is suggestive but not sufficient to infer a causal relationship between secondhand smoke and breast cancer.

— The evidence is suggestive but not sufficient to infer a causal relationship between secondhand smoke exposure and a risk of nasal sinus cancer among nonsmokers.

— The evidence is inadequate to infer the presence or absence of a causal relationship between secondhand smoke exposure and a risk of nasopharyngeal carcinoma among nonsmokers.

— The evidence is inadequate to infer the presence or absence of a causal relationship between secondhand smoke exposure and the risk of cervical cancer among lifetime nonsmokers.

## Cardiovascular Diseases from Exposure to Secondhand Smoke

— The evidence is sufficient to infer a causal relationship between exposure to secondhand smoke and increased risks of coronary heart disease morbidity and mortality among both men and women.

— Pooled relative risks from meta-analyses indicate a 25 to 30 percent increase in the risk of coronary heart disease from exposure to secondhand smoke.

— The evidence is suggestive but not sufficient to infer a causal relationship between exposure to secondhand smoke and an increased risk of stroke.

— Studies of secondhand smoke and subclinical vascular disease, particularly carotid arterial wall thickening, are suggestive but not sufficient to infer a causal relationship between exposure to secondhand smoke and atherosclerosis.

## Respiratory Effects in Adults from Exposure to Secondhand Smoke

— The evidence is sufficient to infer a causal relationship between secondhand smoke exposure and odor annoyance.

— The evidence is sufficient to infer a causal relationship between secondhand smoke exposure and nasal irritation.

— The evidence is suggestive but not sufficient to conclude that persons with nasal allergies or a history of respiratory illnesses are more susceptible to developing nasal irritation from secondhand smoke exposure.

— The evidence is suggestive but not sufficient to infer a causal relationship between secondhand smoke exposure and acute respiratory symptoms, including cough, wheeze, chest tightness, and difficulty breathing among persons with asthma.

— The evidence is suggestive but not sufficient to infer a causal relationship between secondhand smoke exposure and acute respiratory symptoms, including cough, wheeze, chest tightness, and difficulty breathing among healthy persons.

— The evidence is suggestive but not sufficient to infer a causal relationship between secondhand smoke exposure and chronic respiratory symptoms.

— The evidence is suggestive but not sufficient to infer a causal relationship between short-term secondhand smoke exposure and an acute decline in lung function in persons with asthma.

— The evidence is inadequate to infer the presence or absence of a causal relationship between short-term secondhand smoke exposure and an acute decline in lung function in healthy persons.

— The evidence is suggestive but not sufficient to infer a causal relationship between chronic second-hand smoke exposure and a small decrement in lung function in the general population.

— The evidence is inadequate to infer the presence or absence of a causal relationship between chronic secondhand smoke exposure and an accelerated decline in lung function.

— The evidence is suggestive but not sufficient to infer a causal relationship between secondhand smoke exposure and adult-onset asthma.

— The evidence is suggestive but not sufficient to infer a causal relationship between secondhand smoke exposure and a worsening of asthma control.

— The evidence is suggestive but not sufficient to infer a causal relationship between secondhand smoke exposure and risk fro chronic obstructive pulmonary disease.

— The evidence is inadequate to infer the presence or absence of a causal relationship between secondhand smoke exposure and morbidity in persons with chronic obstructive pulmonary disease.

### Control of Secondhand Smoke Exposure

— Workplace smoking restrictions are effective in reducing secondhand smoke exposure.

— Workplace smoking restrictions lead to less smoking among covered workers.

— Establishing smoke-free workplaces is the only effective way to ensure that secondhand smoke exposure does not occur in the workplace.

— The majority of workers in the United States are now covered by smoke-free policies.

— The extent to which workplaces are covered by smoke-free policies varies among worker groups, across states, and by sociodemographic factors. Workplaces related to the entertainment and hospitality industries have notably high potential for secondhand smoke exposure.

— Evidence from peer-reviewed studies shows that smoke-free policies and regulations do not have an adverse economic impact on the hospitality industry.

— Evidence suggests that exposure to secondhand smoke varies by ethnicity and gender.

— In the United States, the home is now becoming the predominant location for exposure of children and adults to secondhand smoke.

— Total bans on indoor smoking in hospitals, restaurants, bars, and offices substantially reduce secondhand smoke exposure, up to several orders of magnitude with incomplete compliance, and with full compliance, exposures are eliminated.

— Exposures of nonsmokers to secondhand smoke cannot be controlled by air cleaning or mechanical air exchange.

\* \* \*

# NOTES AND QUESTIONS

**1.** The 2004 Surgeon General's Report, two excerpts from which appear *supra*, is lengthy and much is lost in its excessive detail and science-speak, but its overall findings are clear and convincing: Smoking causes cancer, heart disease, stroke, respiratory diseases of various kinds, a myriad of health problems for unborn babies, infants, and children, and potentially damages virtually every organ of the body. For a summary of some of the same information in a more concise form, see the various fact sheets prepared by the CDC and the sources cited by the CDC at www.cdc.gov/tobacco/ (last visited December 2006). For a summary of some of the same information in a more concise form, see the various fact sheets prepared by the CDC and the sources cited by the CDC at www.cdc.gov/tobacco/ (last visited December 2006).

For recent data on the number of people who smoke in the United States, see *State-Specific Prevalence of Current Cigarette Smoking Among Adults — United States, 2003*, 53 MORBIDITY/MORTALITY WKLY REP. 1035 (2004) found at www.cdc.gov/mmwr (last visited December 2006).

**2.** The various effects on non-smokers who are exposed to tobacco smoke were first addressed in a Surgeon General's report in 1986, but, oddly, this subject was not addressed (or even mentioned) in the 2004 report. The 2006 report, however, was unequivocal in its conclusion "secondhand smoke" is a major health hazard and still another reason to reduce smoking.

What is "secondhand smoke"? As described by one expert:

> Secondhand smoke (SHS) is the toxic waste of tobacco combustion, emitted from the combination of tobacco smoke from the burning end of cigarettes, pipes, and cigars, and exhaled smoke from smokers. The widespread practice of smoking in buildings exposes nonsmoking occupants to combustion by-products under conditions where airborne contaminant removal is slow and uncertain. Over the past two decades, medical science has shown that nonsmokers suffer many of the diseases of active smoking when the breathe SHS.
>
>     . . . .
>
> Epidemiological studies around the world have investigated whether passive smoke causes elevations in lung cancer, heart disease, and other diseases. These secondhand smoke epidemiological studies generally assess exposure using surrogate exposure variables such as spousal smoking. They also often suffer from the lack of a truly unexposed control group. These problems tend to obscure risks. Nevertheless, the epidemiological studies of passive smoking provide convincing evidence of the detection of an effect at environmental levels of exposure. The most powerful evidence of effect is the existence of dose-response relationships: of the 30 world studies of passive smoking and lung cancer extant in 1992, 14 reported a test for exposure-response, and 10 were statistically significant at the 95 percent confidence level. The probability of ten or more studies reaching this level by chance alone is less then one in ten billion . . .

REPACE ASSOCIATES, INC., FACT SHEET OF SECONDHAND SMOKE (2005) (found at www.repace.com/ (last visited December 2006).

According to estimates by the CDC:

> . . . Secondhand smoke contains a complex mixture of more than 4,000 chemicals, more than 50 of which are cancer-causing agents (carcinogens). Secondhand smoke is associated with an increased risk for lung cancer and coronary heart disease in nonsmoking adults. Because their lungs are not fully developed, young children are particularly susceptible to secondhand smoke. Exposure to secondhand smoke is associated with an increased risk for sudden infant death syndrome (SIDS), asthma, bronchitis, and pneumonia in young children.

> — An estimated 3000 lung cancer deaths and 35,000 coronary heart disease deaths occur annually among adult nonsmokers in the United States as a result of exposure to secondhand smoke.

> — Each year, secondhand smoke is associated with an estimated 8000–26,000 new asthma cases in children.

> — Annually an estimated 150,000–300,000 new cases of bronchitis and pneumonia in children aged less than 18 months (7500–15,000 of which will require hospitalization) are associated with secondhand smoke exposure in the United States.

> — Approximately 60% of people in the United States have biological evidence of secondhand smoke exposure.

> — Among children aged less than 18 years, an estimated 22% are exposed to secondhand smoke in their homes, with estimates ranging from 11.7% in Utah to 34.2% in Kentucky.

Source: www.cdc.gov/tobacco/factsheets/secondhand (last visited Dec. 2006).

For similar estimates and additional analysis of the effects of "secondhand smoke," see INTERNATIONAL AGENCY FOR RESEARCH ON CANCER, MONOGRAPHS ON THE EVALUATION OF CARCINOGENIC RISKS TO HUMANS: TOBACCO SMOKE AND INVOLUNTARY SMOKING (IARC 2002); CALIFORNIA ENVIRONMENTAL PROTECTION AGENCY, HEALTH EFFECTS OF EXPOSURE TO ENVIRONMENTAL TOBACCO SMOKE (1997).

In January of 2006, the California Air Resources Board declared "secondhand smoke" a toxic air pollutant, claiming that recent studies had indicated that secondhand smoke exposure in the general environment — most of the data summarized *supra* refers to harm from exposure to *indoor* tobacco smoke — and increased the risk of breast cancer in young women. As such, "secondhand smoke" must be treated under California law as comparable to benzene, diesel exhaust, and arsenic. For more information, see www. arb.ca.gov/ (last visited February 2006).

Note the importance of assessing the impact of "secondhand smoke" in the cases that are discussed in this chapter. Many of the recent efforts to regulate smoking, such as the prohibitions on smoking in various public places are essentially efforts to protect the non-smoking public from smokers — not to protect the smokers themselves. In this respect they are grounded in familiar public health law notions.

**3.** The evidence regarding the health consequences of smoking provides an interesting demonstration of the inherent problems facing epidemiologists and other experts when they attempt to assess the causal linkage between morbidity and mortality and various potential risks such as smoking. In the 2004 Surgeon General's Report, the authors established four levels of causation: "proven to cause the disease;" "may cause the disease;" "there is not enough proof that smoking does or does not cause the disease;" and "probably does not cause the disease." In making these determinations, a panel of experts (the final determinations of the panel were made by majority vote) reviewed the available literature and considered a number of questions including:

— Do multiple high-quality studies show a consistent association between smoking and disease?

— Are the measured effects large enough and statistically strong?

— Does the evidence show that smoking occurs before the disease occurs (i.e., a temporal association)?

— Is the relationship between smoking and disease coherent or plausible in terms of known scientific principles, biologic mechanisms, and observed patterns of disease?

Note that all of these questions call for a mix of good scientific research, expert opinion about that research, data analysis, and — particularly when the state of knowledge becomes relevant to policymaking — value-laden judgment. In some cases, lung cancer, for example, the evidence is overwhelming: There is no doubt that smoking tobacco is a direct and primary cause of lung cancer in smokers. In other cases, any assessment of a causal link must be made with some qualification. Research may be limited and the results may be hard to interpret. Direct measures of effect may be difficult to obtain, especially if there are many causes for a disease or if exposure to a potential cause may result in the disease in some but not all of those who are exposed. For that matter, it may be both scientifically and ethically impossible to engage in the kind of controlled clinical trial that might provide the most probative evidence. Studying the health effects of "secondhand" smoke is particularly problematic, even more so than studying the effects of smoking on smokers.

For additional and more specific analysis of the health risks of smoking and for references to the studies that the Surgeon General's Report claims to assess, see the database collected by the Surgeon General and containing more than 1600 articles on smoking and its consequences, at www.cdc.gov/tobacco (last visited December 2006).

**4.** The 2004 Surgeon General's Report highly recommends that efforts be made to educate the public and reduce the number of people who smoke or otherwise use tobacco products. But even if we are able — and willing — to fund more and better programs to prevent smoking, do anti-tobacco programs really work? According to the report, the answer is that they do, sometimes, but not always or as well as one would hope:

A comprehensive review of programs in California, Massachusetts, Oregon, Arizona, and Florida by Siegel [in 2002] covers both the positive effects of such programs on smoking prevalence and the negative effects that follow reduced support from the states. . . .

[S]ubstantial declines in the per capita use of cigarettes and in adult smoking prevalence in California through the 1990s were associated with a comprehensive program implemented in 1988. During the first years of the program (1989–1993), adult prevalence declined 1.1 percentage points per year in California, compared with 0.6 percentage points per year in the rest of the United States. Adult smoking prevalence is now 17.2 percent in California, compared with the median of 23.3 percent for all states. Moreover, there is now evidence to suggest that this reduction has contributed to a decline in the tobacco-related disease burden over time. During 1988–1997, age-adjusted incidence rates for lung cancer declined 14 percent in California, compared with only 2.7 percent in non-California cancer surveillance regions. In an analysis of trends in mortality from heart disease between 1989 and 1997, there were 33,300 fewer deaths from heart disease than expected in California compared with the rest of the United States. However, lung cancer mortality will change slowly in response to population smoking prevalence changes. . . . Cardiovascular mortality changes will be much more rapid, and these changes appear to be closely associated with program activity level.

In Massachusetts, a comprehensive tobacco control program implemented in 1992 was associated with a decline of 0.43 percentage points per year in adult smoking prevalence between 1992 and 1999. In Arizona, state-specific surveys following implementation of a comprehensive program in 1994 indicate that adult prevalence declined from an estimated 23 percent to approximately 20 percent between 1996 and 1999. In Oregon, adult smoking prevalence declined from 23.4 percent in 1996 to 21.4 percent in 1999 after implementation of the 1996 tobacco control program. These changes, although modest, compare favorably with the 0.03 annual percentage point increase in adult prevalence in comparison states during approximately the same period.

SURGEON GENERAL 2004 REPORT, *supra,* at 874–76.

California has been particularly aggressive in attempting to reduce smoking and limit the other uses of tobacco. For information on programs in California, see www.dhs.ca.gov/tobaccco (last visited December 2006).

For a good series of articles evaluating the effectiveness of various anti-smoking campaigns, particularly those that are targeted towards children, see Matthew Farrelly, et al., *Getting to the Truth: Evaluating National Tobacco Counter-marketing Campaigns*, 92 AM. J. PUB. HEALTH 901 (2002); Anne Landman, et al., *Tobacco Industry Youth Smoking Prevention Programs: Protecting the Industry and Hurting Tobacco Control*, 92 AM. J. PUB. HEALTH 917 (2002). Both articles conclude that the putative "anti-smoking campaigns" that are conducted by the tobacco industry often result in *increases* in smoking by children.

# C.   THE CONSTITUTIONAL AUTHORITY TO REGULATE SMOKING AND TOBACCO USE

We begin this section with a case that raises issues touched on earlier — the constitutionally-based sharing of power between the federal and state governments — in the particular context of tobacco regulation. We turn next to similar questions under state law, implicating the distribution of regulatory power between state and local governments. Throughout both topics are important issues of constitutional and statutory interpretation, and of one ("higher") government's pre-emption of power otherwise exercisable by a "lower" government. We then turn from these "structural" questions to a particularized constitutional tension in tobacco control: the claim of merchants to First Amendment protection for promotion of their products, against the efforts of public health authorities who seek to limit what they deem to be pernicious messages. Finally, we return to a structural-power issue, this time "horizontal" rather than "vertical": the legal dimensions of the Food and Drug Administration's initiative to regulate tobacco on the basis of disputed statutory power to do so.

## AUSTIN v. TENNESSEE
### 179 U.S. 343 (1900)

Brown, Justice.

\* \* \*

It is charged that the act in question [a state law criminalizing the sale or importation into Tennessee of cigarettes for sale or distribution] is an infringement upon the exclusive power of Congress to regulate commerce between the states. This is the sole question presented for our determination.

We are not disposed to question the general principle that the states cannot, under the guise of inspection or revenue laws, forbid or impede the introduction of products, and more particularly of food products, universally recognized as harmless or otherwise burden foreign or interstate commerce by regulations adopted under the assumed police power of the state, but obviously for the purpose of taxing such commerce or creating discriminations in favor of home producers or manufacturers. . . . "If, therefore, a statute purporting to have been enacted to protect the public health, the public morals, or the public safety has no real or substantial relation to those objects, or is a palpable invasion of rights secured by the fundamental law, it is the duty of the courts to so adjudge, and thereby give effect to the Constitution."

[The Tennessee Supreme Court had upheld Austin's conviction, ruling that the law's enforcement against him did not violate the commerce clause for two reasons: cigarettes were not "legitimate articles of commerce," and Austin's sale of cigarettes was "not the sale of an original package." The Court addressed both rationales. Of the first, it said:]

. . . Whatever product has from time immemorial been recognized by custom or law as a fit subject for barter or sale, particularly if its manufacture has been made the subject of Federal regulation and taxation, must, we think, be recognized as a legitimate article of commerce although it may to a certain extent be within the police power of the states. Of this class of cases is tobacco. From the first settlement of the colony of Virginia to the present day tobacco has been one of the most profitable and important products of agriculture and commerce, and while its effects may be injurious to some, its extensive use over practically the entire globe is a remarkable tribute to its popularity and value. We are clearly of opinion that it cannot be classed with diseased cattle or meats, decayed fruit, or other articles, the use of which is a menace to the health of the entire community. Congress, too, has recognized tobacco in its various forms as a legitimate article of commerce by requiring licenses to be taken for its manufacture and sale, imposing a revenue tax upon each package of cigarettes put upon the market, and by making express regulations for their manufacture and sale, their exportation and importation. Cigarettes are but one of the numerous manufactures of tobacco, and we cannot take judicial notice of the fact that it is more noxious in this form than in any other. Whatever might be our individual views as to its deleterious tendencies, we cannot hold that any article which Congress recognizes in so many ways is not a legitimate article of commerce. . . .

[The Court then analogized tobacco to intoxicating liquors and reviewed its cases approving the states' authority to regulate the latter, up to and including the prohibition of intrastate sales. The Court said of those cases:]

These cases recognize the fact that intoxicating liquors belong to a class of commodities which, in the opinion of a great many estimable people, are deleterious in their effects, demoralizing in their tendencies, and often fatal in their excessive indulgence; and that, while their employment as a medicine may sometimes be beneficial, their habitual and constant use as a beverage, whatever it may be to individuals, is injurious to the community. It may be that their evil effects have been exaggerated, and that, though their use is usually attended with more or less danger, it is by no means open to universal condemnation. It is, however, within the power of each state to investigate the subject and to determine its policy in that particular. If the legislative body comes deliberately to the conclusion that a due regard for the public safety and morals requires a suppression of the liquor traffic, there is nothing in the commercial clause of the Constitution, or in the 14th Amendment to that instrument, to forbid its doing so. While, perhaps, it may not wholly prohibit the use or sale of them for medicinal purposes, it may hedge about their use as a general beverage such restrictions as it pleases. Nor can we deny to the legislature the power to impose restrictions upon the sale of noxious or poisonous drugs, such as opium and other similar articles, extremely valuable as medicines, but equally baneful to the habitual user.

Cigarettes do not seem until recently to have attracted the attention of the public as more injurious than other forms of tobacco; nor are we now prepared to take judicial notice of any special injury resulting from their use or to indorse the opinion of the supreme court of Tennessee that "they are inherently bad and bad only." At the same time we should be shutting our eyes to what is constantly passing before them were we to affect an ignorance of the fact that a belief in their deleterious effects, particularly upon young people, has become very general, and that communications are constantly finding their way into the public press denouncing their use as fraught with great danger to the youth of both sexes. Without undertaking to affirm or deny their evil effects, we think it within the province of the legislature to say how far they may be sold, or to prohibit their sale entirely, after they have been taken from the original packages or have left the hands of the importer, provided no discrimination be used as against such as are imported from other states, and there be no reason to doubt that the act in question is designed for the protection of the public health.

We have had repeated occasion to hold, where state legislation has been attacked as violative either of the power of Congress over interstate commerce, or of the 14th Amendment to the Constitution, that, if the action of the state legislature were as a *bona fide* exercise of its police power, and dictated by a genuine regard for the preservation of the public health or safety, such legislation would be respected, though it might interfere indirectly with interstate commerce.

. . . .

We are therefore of opinion that although the state of Tennessee may not wholly interdict commerce in cigarettes it is not, in the language of Chief Justice Taney in *The License Cases,* "bound to furnish a market for [them], nor to abstain from the passage of any law which it may deem necessary or advisable to guard the health or morals of its citizens, although such law may discourage importation, or diminish the profits of the importer, or lessen the revenue of the general [federal] government."

[The Court next turned to the second basis of the Tennessee court's affirmance of Austin's conviction: its conclusion that because Austin's conviction was for sale of cigarettes not in their "original packages," the law's application to him was insulated from the reach of the commerce clause:]

There is no reason to doubt the good faith of the legislature of Tennessee in prohibiting the sale of cigarettes as a sanitary measure, and if it be inoperative as applied to sales by the owner in the original packages, of cigarettes manufactured in and brought from another state, we are remitted to the inquiry whether a paper package of 3 inches in length and 1 1/2 inches in width, containing ten cigarettes, is an original package protected by the Constitution of the United States against any interference by the state while in the hands of the importer? This we regard as the vital question in the case.

The whole law upon the subject of original packages is based upon a decision of this court, in *Brown v. Maryland,* in which a statute of Maryland, requiring all importers of foreign articles, "by bale or package," or of intoxicating liquors, and other persons selling the same, "by wholesale, bale or package, hogshead, barrel or tierce," to take out a license, was held to be repugnant to that provision of the Constitution forbidding states from laying a duty upon imports, as well as to that declaring that Congress should have power to regulate commerce with foreign nations. . . .

. . . .

The real question in this case is whether [in determining whether or not packaging is "original"] the size of the package in which the importation is actually made is to govern; or, the size of the package in which bona fide transactions are carried on between the manufacturer and the wholesale dealer residing in different states. We hold to the latter view. The whole theory of the exemption of the original package from the operation of state laws is based upon the idea that the property is imported in the ordinary form in which, from time immemorial, foreign goods have been brought into the country. These have gone at once into the hands of the wholesale dealers, who have been in the habit of breaking the packages and distributing their contents among the several retail dealers throughout the state. It was with reference to this method of doing business that the doctrine of the exemption of the original package grew up. But taking the words "original package" in their literal sense, a number of so-called original package manufactories have been started through the country, whose business it is to manufacture goods for the express purpose of sending their products into other states in minute packages, that may at once go into the hands of the retail dealers and consumers, and thus bid defiance to the laws of the state against their importation and sale. In all the cases which have heretofore arisen in this court the packages were of such size as to exclude the idea that they were to go directly into the hands of the consumer, or be used to evade the police regulations of the state with regard to the particular article. No doubt the fact that cigarettes are actually imported in a certain package is strong evidence that they are original packages within the meaning of the law; but this presumption attaches only when the importation is made in the usual manner prevalent among honest dealers, and in a bona fide package of a particular size. Without undertaking to determine what is the proper size of an original package in each case, evidently the doctrine has no application where the manufacturer puts up the package with the express intent of evading the laws of another state, and is enabled to carry out his purpose by the facile agency of an express company and the connivance of his consignee. . . .

     . . . .

The defendant purchased from the American Tobacco Company, at its factory, in Durham, North Carolina, a lot of cigarettes manufactured by that company at that factory, and thereby it put into pasteboard boxes, in quantities of ten cigarettes to each box; that each of these boxes, known as packages, was separately stamped and labeled, as prescribed by the United States revenue statute; that after defendant's purchase the American Tobacco Company piled upon the floor of its warehouse, in Durham, North Carolina, the number of boxes or packages sold, and, having done so, notified the Southern Express Company to come and get then, and said company, by its agent, took them from the floor and placed them in an open basket already and previously in the possession of the Southern Express Company, and in that basket had them transported by express to the defendant's town in Tennessee, and there an agent of the same express company took the basket to defendant's place of business and lifted from it on to the counter of the defendant the lot of detached boxes or packages of cigarettes, and thereupon took a receipt and departed with the empty basket. Thereafter the defendant sold one of these boxes or packages without breaking it, and for that sale he stands convicted.

And yet we are told that each one of these packages is an original package, and entitled to the protection of the Constitution . . . as a separate and distinct importation. We can only look upon it as a discreditable subterfuge. . . . If there be any original package at all in this case we think it is the basket, and not the paper box. . . .

There is doubtless fair ground for dispute as to whether the use of cigarettes is not hurtful to the community, and therefore it would be competent for a state, with reference to is own people, to declare, under penalties, that cigarettes should not be manufactured within its limits . . . . [Yet if we were to accept defendant's argument] . . . citizens of Tennessee may, under the commerce clause . . . bring into that State from other States cigarettes in unlimited quantities, and sell them. . . . [We reject the view that] . . . the reserved power of the state to protect the health of its people, by reasonable regulations, has application only in respect of articles manufactured within its own limits, and that an open door exists for the introduction into the State, against its will, of all kinds of property which may be fairly regarded as injurious in their use to health. . . .

* * *


# D.A.B.E. v. CITY OF TOLEDO
## 393 F.3d 692 (6th Cir. 2005)

Martin, Judge.

* * *

The City of Toledo has regulated smoking in public places since 1987, when it enacted the original Clean Indoor Air Ordinance. In early 2003, the City Council formed a task force to consider strengthening the ordinance in order to protect employees and non-smoking patrons from the harmful effects of secondhand smoke. After holding numerous meetings and public hearings, the City Council unanimously repealed the 1987 Clean Indoor Air Ordinance and enacted a new Clean Indoor Air Ordinance, No. 509-03.

Ordinance No. 509-03 regulates the ability to smoke in public places, such as retail stores, theaters, courtrooms, libraries, museums, health care facilities, and — most relevant to the instant case — restaurants and bars. [Proprietors of restaurants and bars were the plaintiffs-appellants in this case.] In enclosed public places, smoking is generally prohibited except in a "separate smoking lounge" that is designated for the exclusive purpose of smoking and that satisfies the following criteria:

(1) it cannot constitute more than thirty percent of the total square footage of space to which the public is invited;

(2) it must be completely enclosed on all sides by floor-to-ceiling walls;

(3) it must have a separate ventilation system not used by the non-smoking portion of the establishment;

(4) it must not incorporate the sole path to or from the restrooms, to or from the non-smoking portion of the establishment, or into or out of the building or waiting areas; and

(5) it cannot be located in an area where employees are required to work.

The ordinance provides for a 120-day exemption within which an establishment may construct a smoking lounge meeting these requirements.

Various interested parties attempted to seek repeal of the amended ordinance by referendum, but the referendum failed for lack of the requisite number of valid signatures. Appellants then filed suit against the City of Toledo seeking declaratory and injunctive relief. They challenged the ordinance on two grounds: first, that it constitutes a regulatory taking of their property in violation of the Fifth and Fourteenth Amendments; and second, that it is preempted by a state law that regulates smoking in places of public assembly but that does not apply to restaurants, bowling alleys and bars.

[The federal district court dismissed the appellants' complaint, ruling that the ordinance was not a regulatory taking, did not conflict with the state statute discussed below, and was accordingly not preempted by it. This appeal followed.]

## A. Regulatory Taking Claim

The Takings Clause of the Fifth Amendment, made applicable to the States through the Fourteenth Amendment, provides that private property shall not "be taken for public use, without just compensation." The Supreme Court has recognized two categories of takings: regulatory and physical. Furthermore, their attack on the ordinance is limited to a facial challenge, which requires them to prove that the "mere enactment" of the ordinance constitutes a taking of their property. According to the Supreme Court, the test to be applied in considering facial challenges such as this one is "fairly straightforward." Under that test, "[a] statute regulating the uses that can be made of property effects a taking if it denies an owner economically viable use of his [property]."

The evidence presented in this case fails to establish that, on its face, the Clean Indoor Air Ordinance denies appellants "economically viable use" of their respective properties. Appellants have submitted affidavits alleging that they have lost — or fear they will lose — customers as a result of the ordinance, because smoking is an activity in which many customers wish to engage while patronizing their establishments. Even if true, however, those allegations are simply not enough to satisfy appellants' burden of proof.

. . . [T]here is nothing on the face of the Clean Indoor Air Ordinance that prevents the "beneficial use" of appellants' property. To the contrary, the ordinance has absolutely no effect on any aspect of appellants' businesses other than to restrict the areas in which appellants' patrons may smoke. Second, the ordinance does not "categorically prohibit" smoking inside appellants' establishments; it "merely regulates the conditions under which" smoking is permitted. We recognize that the construction of separate smoking lounges in most cases will require some financial investment, but an ordinance does not effect a taking merely because compliance with it "requires the expenditure of money." Finally, for obvious reasons, the ordinance does not "purport to regulate alternative uses" of appellants' respective properties. . . .

## B. Preemption Claim

Appellants' second argument is that the Clean Indoor Air Ordinance conflicts with — and, therefore, is preempted by Section 3791.031(A) of the Ohio Revised Code.

A state statute takes precedence over a local ordinance when (1) the ordinance is in conflict with the statute, (2) the ordinance is an exercise of police power, rather than of local self-government, and (3) the statute is a general law.

"In determining whether an ordinance is in 'conflict' with general laws, the test is whether the ordinance permits or licenses that which the statute forbids or prohibits, and vice versa." To the extent that the statute does not address or apply to an item or issue, however, an ordinance regulating the excluded item or issue does not conflict with the statute, even if it deals with the same general subject matter. . . . "The law in Ohio on 'conflict' is stringent. Preemption is not really demonstrated." [citation to Ohio supreme court decision omitted.]

In this case, Section 3791.031 regulates indoor smoking throughout the State of Ohio within "places of public assembly." It explicitly provides, however, that "[r]estaurants, food service establishments, dining rooms, cafes, cafeterias, or other rooms used primarily for the service of food, as well as bowling alleys and places licensed by the division of liquor control to sell intoxicating beverages for consumption on the premises, are not places of public assembly." As discussed, the City of Toledo's Clean Indoor Air Ordinance prohibits smoking in all public places, including restaurants and bars, except in separate smoking lounges.

Appellants argue that because smoking is allowed in their establishments under state law but not under the ordinance, there is a conflict that renders the ordinance preempted by state law. The City argues, by contrast, that the statute "simply does not regulate the establishments" that are subject to the ordinance and, therefore, municipalities within the State of Ohio are free to regulate smoking within these establishments in the exercise of their "home rule" authority. See Ohio Const. art. XVIII, § 3 ("Municipalities shall have authority to exercise all powers of local self-government and to adopt and enforce within their limits such local policy, sanitary and other similar regulations, as are not in conflict with general laws.")

. . . [B]y stating that certain types of establishments — such as restaurants, bars, bowling alleys, etc. — "are not places of public assembly," the legislature indicated not that these establishments were immune to smoking-related regulation, but that they simply did not fall within the ambit of the statute.

Our independent research reveals that other courts that have considered whether smoking-related ordinances are preempted by state law have reached similar conclusions. . . .

In an attempt to overcome this persuasive authority supporting the City's position, appellants point to the case . . . in which a New Jersey trial court held that a local ordinance prohibiting smoking in "restaurants, bars, cabarets, and taverns" in an attempt to protect the public from the deleterious effects of smoking was preempted by a state law that did not prohibit smoking in restaurants, but merely "encourage[d] restaurants to establish non-smoking areas." That case, however, is significantly distinguishable from the present one. The statute . . . [therein]provided that any guidelines suggested by political subdivisions such as municipalities would "in no case . . . be mandatory." The court also found it significant that the statute explicitly stated that its provisions "shall supersede" any municipal ordinance concerning smoking in restaurants except ordinances that are enacted "for purposes of protecting life and property from fire." . . . Because none of the factors that compelled . . . [that] court's decision is present here, that case fails to undermine our conclusion that Section 3791.031 does not preempt the City of Toledo's Clean Indoor Air Ordinance.

\* \* \*

# LORILLARD TOBACCO v. REILLY
## 533 U.S. 525 (2001)

O'Connor, Justice.

\* \* \*

In November 1998, Massachusetts, along with over 40 other States, reached a landmark agreement with major manufacturers in the cigarette industry. The signatory States settled their claims against these companies in exchange for monetary payments and permanent injunctive relief. At the press conference covering Massachusetts' decision to sign the agreement, then-Attorney General Scott Harshbarger announced that as one of his last acts in office, he would create consumer protection regulations to restrict advertising and sales practices for tobacco products. He explained that the regulations were necessary in order to "close holes" in the settlement agreement and "to stop Big Tobacco from recruiting new customers among the children of Massachusetts."

[The "master settlement agreement" is summarized and explained later in this chapter.]

In January 1999, pursuant to his authority to prevent unfair or deceptive practices in trade, the Massachusetts Attorney General (Attorney General) promulgated regulations governing the sale and advertisement of cigarettes, smokeless tobacco, and cigars. The purpose of the cigarette and smokeless tobacco regulations is "to eliminate deception and unfairness in the way cigarettes and smokeless tobacco products are marketed, sold and distributed in Massachusetts in order to address the incidence of cigarette smoking and smokeless tobacco use by children under legal age . . . [and] in order to prevent access to such products by underage consumers." The similar purpose of the cigar regulations is "to eliminate deception and unfairness in the way cigars and little cigars are packaged, marketed, sold and distributed in Massachusetts [so that] . . . consumers may be adequately informed about the health risks associated with cigar smoking, its addictive properties, and the false perception that cigars are a safe alternative to cigarettes . . . [and so that] the incidence of cigar use by children under legal age is addressed . . . in order to prevent access to such products by underage consumers." The regulations have a broader scope than the master settlement agreement, reaching advertising, sales practices, and members of the tobacco industry not covered by the agreement. The regulations place a variety of restrictions on outdoor advertising, point-of-sale advertising, retail sales transactions, transactions by mail, promotions, sampling of products, and labels for cigars.

The cigarette and smokeless tobacco regulations being challenged before this Court provide: . . . "Except as otherwise provided . . . it shall be an unfair or deceptive act or practice for any person who sells or distributes cigarettes or smokeless tobacco products through a retail outlet located within Massachusetts to engage in any of the following retail outlet sales practices: . . . (c) Using self-service displays of cigarettes or smokeless tobacco products; (d) Failing to place cigarettes and smokeless tobacco products out of the reach of all consumers, and in a location accessible only to outlet personnel. . . . (5) [I]t shall be an unfair or deceptive act or practice for any manufacturer, distributor or retailer to engage in any of the following practices: (a) Outdoor advertising, including advertising in enclosed stadiums and advertising from within a retail establishment that is directed toward or visible from the outside of the establishment, in any location that is within a 1000 foot radius of any public playground, playground area in a public park, elementary school, or secondary school; (b) Point-of-sale advertising of cigarettes or smokeless tobacco products any portion of which is placed lower than five feet from the floor of any retail establishment which is located within a one thousand foot radius of any public playground, playground area in a public park, elementary school or secondary school, and which is not an adult-only retail establishment."

[The regulations concerning cigar sales and the definition of advertising are then set out by the Court.]

Before the effective date of the regulations, February 1, 2000, members of the tobacco industry sued the Attorney General in the United States District Court for the District of Massachusetts [claiming] that many of the regulations violate the Commerce Clause, the Supremacy Clause, the First and Fourteenth Amendments, and [various federal statutes]. . . .

In its first ruling, the District Court considered the Supremacy Clause claim that the FCLAA [Federal Cigarette Labeling and Advertising Act] pre-empts the cigarette advertising regulations. The FCLAA prescribes the health warnings that must appear on packaging and in advertisements for cigarettes. The FCLAA contains a pre-emption provision that prohibits a State from imposing any "requirement or prohibition based on smoking and health . . . with respect to the advertising or promotion of . . . cigarettes." The FCLAA's pre-emption provision does not cover smokeless tobacco or cigars.

The District Court explained that the central question for purposes of pre-emption is whether the regulations create a predicate legal duty based on smoking and health. The court reasoned that to read the pre-emption provision to proscribe any state advertising regulation enacted due to health concerns about smoking would expand Congress' purpose beyond a reasonable scope and leave States powerless to regulate in the area. The court concluded that restrictions on the location of advertising are not based on smoking and health and thus are not pre-empted by the FCLAA. The District Court also concluded that a provision that permitted retailers to display a black and white "tombstone" sign reading "Tobacco Products Sold Here," was pre-empted by the FCLAA.

In a separate ruling, the District Court considered the claim that the Attorney General's regulations violate the First Amendment. Rejecting petitioners' argument that strict scrutiny should apply, the court applied the four-part test of *Central Hudson* for commercial speech. The court reasoned that the Attorney General had provided an adequate basis for regulating cigars and smokeless tobacco as well as cigarettes because of the similarities among the products. The court held that the outdoor advertising regulations, which prohibit outdoor advertising within 1000 feet of a school or playground, do not violate the First Amendment because they advance a substantial government interest and are narrowly tailored to suppress no more speech than necessary. The court concluded that the sales practices regulations, which restrict the location and distribution of tobacco products, survive scrutiny because they do not implicate a significant speech interest. The court invalidated the point-of-sale advertising regulations, which require that indoor advertising be placed no lower than five feet from the floor, finding that the Attorney General had not provided sufficient justification for that restriction. The District Court's ruling with respect to the cigar warning requirements and the Commerce Clause is not before this Court.

The United States Court of Appeals [held] the court held that the outdoor advertising regulations do not violate the First Amendment. . . . The Court of Appeals reversed the District Court's invalidation of the point-of-sale advertising regulations. . . . The Court of Appeals also held that the sales practices regulations are valid under the First Amendment. . . .

As for the argument that smokeless tobacco and cigars are different from cigarettes, the court expressed some misgivings about equating all tobacco products, but ultimately decided that the Attorney General had presented sufficient evidence with respect to all three products to regulate them similarly. The Court of Appeals' decision with respect to the cigar warning requirements and the Commerce Clause is not before this Court.

. . . .

## II

Before reaching the First Amendment issues, we must decide to what extent federal law pre-empts the Attorney General's regulations. . . .

### A

[The Court notes that that the supremacy clause (Art. VI, cl. 2) is the constitutional basis of federal preemption; that its "relatively clear and simple mandate has generated considerable discussion" by the Court, which is surely an understatement; and that pre-emption may arise in several different ways: from (1) "express" Congressional language pre-empting state and local activity in a given area; (2) by implication, where the "depth and breath" of a congressional scheme "occupies the legislative field"; or (3) by implication "because of a conflict a with a congressional enactment."]

In the FCLAA, Congress has crafted a comprehensive federal scheme governing the advertising and promotion of cigarettes. The FCLAA's pre-emption provision provides:

> . . . No statement relating to smoking and health, other than the statement required by this title, shall be required on any cigarette package [and] no requirement or prohibition based on smoking and health shall be imposed under State law with respect to the advertising or promotion of any cigarettes the packages of which are labeled in conformity with the provisions of this chapter. . . .

The FCLAA's pre-emption provision does not cover smokeless tobacco or cigars.

In these cases, our task is to identify the domain expressly pre-empted . . . because "an express definition of the pre-emptive reach of a statute . . . supports a reasonable inference . . . that Congress did not intend to pre-empt other matters". . . . [W]e "wor[k] on the assumption that the historic police powers of the States [a]re not to be superseded by the Federal Act unless that [is] the clear and manifest purpose of Congress."

. . . In the pre-emption provision, Congress unequivocally precludes the requirement of any additional statements on cigarette packages beyond those provided in § 1333. Congress further precludes States or localities from imposing any requirement or prohibition based on smoking and health with respect to the advertising and promotion of cigarettes. Without question, the second clause is more expansive than the first; it employs far more sweeping language to describe the state action that is pre-empted. We must give meaning to each element of the pre-emption provision. We are aided in our interpretation by considering the predecessor pre-emption provision and the circumstances in which the current language was adopted.

In 1964, the ground-breaking Report of the Surgeon General's Advisory Committee on Smoking and Health concluded that "[c]igarette smoking is a health hazard of sufficient importance in the United States to warrant appropriate remedial action." In 1965, Congress enacted the FCLAA as a proactive measure in the face of impending regulation by federal agencies and the States. The purpose of the FCLAA was twofold: to inform the public adequately about the hazards of cigarette smoking, and to protect the national economy from interference due to diverse, non-uniform, and confusing cigarette labeling and advertising regulations with respect to the relationship between smoking and health. The FCLAA prescribed a label for cigarette packages: "Caution: Cigarette Smoking May Be Hazardous to Your Health." The FCLAA also required the Secretary of Health, Education, and Welfare (HEW) and the Federal Trade Commission (FTC) to report annually to Congress about the health consequences of smoking and the advertising and promotion of cigarettes.

Section 5 of the FCLAA included a pre-emption provision in which Congress spoke precisely and narrowly. . . . As we have previously explained, "on their face, [the pre-emption] provisions merely prohibited state and federal rule-making bodies from mandating particular cautionary statements. . . ."

. . . In the intervening years [between 1965 and 1969], Congress received reports and recommendations from the HEW Secretary and the FTC. The HEW Secretary recommended that Congress strengthen the warning, require the warning on all packages and in advertisements, and publish tar and nicotine levels on packages and in advertisements. The FTC made similar and additional recommendations. The FTC sought a complete ban on radio and television advertising, a requirement that broadcasters devote time for health hazard announcements concerning smoking, and increased funding for public education and research about smoking. The FTC urged Congress not to continue to prevent federal agencies from regulating cigarette advertising. In addition, the Federal Communications Commission (FCC) had concluded that advertising which promoted the use of cigarettes created a duty in broadcast stations to provide information about the hazards of cigarette smoking.

In 1969, House and Senate committees held hearings about the health effects of cigarette smoking and advertising by the cigarette industry. The bill that emerged from the House of Representatives strengthened the warning and maintained the pre-emption provision. The Senate amended that bill, adding the ban on radio and television advertising, and changing the pre-emption language to its present form. . . . The final result was the Public Health Cigarette Smoking Act of 1969, in which Congress, following the Senate's amendments, made three significant changes to the FCLAA. First, Congress drafted a new label that read: "Warning: The Surgeon General Has Determined That Cigarette Smoking Is Dangerous to Your Health." Second, Congress declared it unlawful to advertise cigarettes on any medium of electronic communication subject to the jurisdiction of the FCC. Finally, Congress enacted the current pre-emption provision, which proscribes any "requirement or prohibition based on smoking and health . . . imposed under State law with respect to the advertising or promotion" of cigarettes. The new [provision] did not pre-empt regulation by federal agencies, freeing the FTC to impose warning requirements in cigarette advertising. The new pre-emption provision, like its predecessor, only applied to cigarettes, and not other tobacco products.

In 1984, Congress again amended the FCLAA in the Comprehensive Smoking Education Act. The purpose of the Act was to "provide a new strategy for making Americans more aware of any adverse health effects of smoking, to assure the timely and widespread dissemination of research findings and to enable individuals to make informed decisions about smoking." The Act established a series of warnings to appear on a rotating basis on cigarette packages and in cigarette advertising, and directed the Health and Human Services Secretary to create and implement an educational program about the health effects of cigarette smoking.

The FTC has continued to report on trade practices in the cigarette industry. In 1999, the first year since the master settlement agreement, the FTC reported that the cigarette industry expended $8.24 billion on advertising and promotions, the largest expenditure ever. Substantial increases were found in point-of-sale promotions, payments made to retailers to facilitate sales, and retail offers such as buy one, get one free, or product giveaways. Substantial decreases, however, were reported for outdoor advertising and transit advertising. Congress and federal agencies continue to monitor advertising and promotion practices in the cigarette industry.

The scope and meaning of the current pre-emption provision become clearer once we consider the original pre-emption language and the amendments to the FCLAA. Without question, "the plain language of the pre-emption provision in the 1969 Act is much broader." Rather than preventing only "statements," the amended provision reaches all "requirement[s] or prohibition[s] . . . imposed under State law." And, although the former statute reached only statements "in the advertising," the current provision governs "with respect to the advertising or promotion" of cigarettes. Congress expanded the pre-emption provision with respect to the States, and at the same time, it allowed the FTC to regulate cigarette advertising. Congress also prohibited cigarette advertising in electronic media altogether. Viewed in light of the context in which the current pre-emption provision was adopted, we must determine whether the FCLAA pre-empts Massachusetts' regulations governing outdoor and point-of-sale advertising of cigarettes.

### B

The Court of Appeals . . . concentrated its analysis on whether the regulations are "with respect to" advertising and promotion. . . . The Court of Appeals also reasoned that the Attorney General's regulations are a form of zoning, a traditional area of state power; therefore the presumption against pre-emption applied.

. . . .

Turning first to the language in the pre-emption provision relied upon by the Court of Appeals, we reject the notion that the Attorney General's cigarette advertising regulations are not "with respect to" advertising and promotion. . . . [T]here is no question about an indirect relationship between the regulations and cigarette advertising because the regulations expressly target cigarette advertising.

Before this Court, the Attorney General focuses on a different phrase in the pre-emption provision: "based on smoking and health." The Attorney General argues that the cigarette advertising regulations are not "based on smoking and health," because they do not involve health-related content in cigarette advertising but instead target youth exposure to cigarette advertising. [W]e cannot agree with the Attorney General's narrow construction of the phrase.

. . . In the 1969 amendments, Congress not only enhanced its scheme to warn the public about the hazards of cigarette smoking, but also sought to protect the public, including youth, from being inundated with images of cigarette smoking in advertising. In pursuit of the latter goal, Congress banned electronic media advertising of cigarettes. And to the extent that Congress contemplated additional targeted regulation of cigarette advertising, it vested that authority in the FTC.

The context in which Congress crafted the current pre-emption provision leads us to conclude that Congress prohibited state cigarette advertising regulations motivated by concerns about smoking and health. Massachusetts has attempted to address the incidence of underage cigarette smoking by regulating advertising much like Congress' ban on cigarette advertising in electronic media. At bottom, the concern about youth exposure to cigarette advertising is intertwined with the concern about cigarette smoking and health. Thus the Attorney General's attempt to distinguish one concern from the other must be rejected.

The Attorney General next claims that the State's outdoor and point-of-sale advertising regulations for cigarettes are not pre-empted because they govern the location, and not the content, of advertising. . . . But the content/location distinction cannot be squared with the language of the pre-emption provision, which reaches all "requirements" and "prohibitions" "imposed under State law." A distinction between the content of advertising and the location of advertising in the FCLAA also cannot be reconciled with Congress' own location-based restriction, which bans advertising in electronic media, but not elsewhere. We are not at liberty to pick and choose which provisions in the legislative scheme we will consider. . . .

Moreover, any distinction between the content and location of cigarette advertising collapses once the implications of that approach are fully considered. . . . We believe that Congress wished to ensure that "a State could not do through negative mandate (*e.g.*, banning all cigarette advertising) that which it already was forbidden to do through positive mandate (*e.g.*, mandating particular cautionary statements)." . . .

. . . .

In sum, we fail to see how the FCLAA and its pre-emption provision permit a distinction between the specific concern about minors and cigarette advertising and the more general concern about smoking and health in cigarette advertising, especially in light of the fact that Congress crafted a legislative solution for those very concerns. We also conclude that a distinction between state regulation of the location as opposed to the content of cigarette advertising has no foundation in the text of the pre-emption provision. Congress pre-empted state cigarette advertising regulations like the Attorney General's because they would upset federal legislative choices to require specific warnings and to impose the ban on cigarette advertising in electronic media in order to address concerns about smoking and health. Accordingly, we hold that the Attorney General's outdoor and point-of-sale advertising regulations targeting cigarettes are pre-empted by the FCLAA.

C

Although the FCLAA prevents States and localities from imposing special requirements or prohibitions "based on smoking and health" "with respect to the advertising or promotion" of cigarettes, that language still leaves significant power in the hands of States to impose generally applicable zoning regulations and to regulate conduct. . . . For instance, the FCLAA does not restrict a State or locality's ability to enact generally applicable zoning restrictions. We have recognized that state interests in traffic safety and esthetics may justify zoning regulations for advertising. . . . Although Congress has taken into account the unique concerns about cigarette smoking and health in advertising, there is no indication that Congress intended to displace local community interests in general regulations of the location of billboards or large marquee advertising, or that Congress intended cigarette advertisers to be afforded special treatment in that regard. . . .

The FCLAA also does not foreclose all state regulation of conduct as it relates to the sale or use of cigarettes. The FCLAA's pre-emption provision explicitly governs state regulations of "advertising or promotion." Accordingly, the FCLAA does not pre-empt state laws prohibiting cigarette sales to minors. To the contrary, there is an established congressional policy that supports such laws; Congress has required States to prohibit tobacco sales to minors as a condition of receiving federal block grant funding for substance abuse treatment activities.

In Massachusetts, it is illegal to sell or distribute tobacco products to persons under the age of 18. Having prohibited the sale and distribution of tobacco products to minors, the State may prohibit common inchoate offenses that attach to criminal conduct, such as solicitation, conspiracy, and attempt. States and localities also have at their disposal other means of regulating conduct to ensure that minors do not obtain cigarettes.

. . . .

## III

By its terms, the FCLAA's pre-emption provision only applies to cigarettes. Accordingly, we must evaluate the smokeless tobacco and cigar petitioners' First Amendment challenges to the State's outdoor and point-of-sale advertising regulations. The cigarette petitioners did not raise a pre-emption challenge to the sales practices regulations. Thus, we must analyze the cigarette as well as the smokeless tobacco and cigar petitioners' claim that certain sales practices regulations for tobacco products violate the First Amendment.

## A

For over 25 years, the Court has recognized that commercial speech does not fall outside the purview of the First Amendment. Instead, the Court has afforded commercial speech a measure of First Amendment protection "commensurate" with its position in relation to other constitutionally guaranteed expression. In recognition of the "distinction between speech proposing a commercial transaction, which occurs in an area traditionally subject to government regulation, and other varieties of speech," we developed a framework for analyzing regulations of commercial speech that is "substantially similar" to the test for time, place, and manner restrictions. The analysis contains four elements:

At the outset, we must determine whether the expression is protected by the First Amendment. For commercial speech to come within that provision, it at least must concern lawful activity and not be misleading. Next, we ask whether the asserted governmental interest is substantial. If both inquiries yield positive answers, we must determine whether the regulation directly advances the governmental interest asserted, and whether it is not more extensive than is necessary to serve that interest." [citation to *Central Hudson*]

Petitioners urge us to reject this analysis and apply strict scrutiny. They are not the first litigants to do so. Admittedly, several Members of the Court have expressed doubts about the *Central Hudson* analysis and whether it should apply in particular cases. But here we see no need to break new ground. *Central Hudson* provides an adequate basis for decision.

Only the last two steps of the four-part analysis are at issue here. The Attorney General has assumed for purposes of summary judgment that petitioners' speech is entitled to First Amendment protection. With respect to the second step, none of the petitioners contests the importance of the State's interest in preventing the use of tobacco products by minors.

The third step concerns the relationship between the harm that underlies the State's interest and the means identified by the State to advance that interest. It requires that[:]

> the speech restriction directly and materially advanc[e] the asserted governmental interest. This burden is not satisfied by mere speculation or conjecture; rather, a governmental body seeking to sustain a restriction on commercial speech must demonstrate that the harms it recites are real and that its restriction will in fact alleviate them to a material degree.

We do not, however, require that "empirical data come . . . accompanied by a surfeit of background information. . . . [W]e have permitted litigants to justify speech restrictions by reference to studies and anecdotes pertaining to different locales altogether, or even, in a case applying strict scrutiny, to justify restrictions based solely on history, consensus, and simple common sense."

The last step of the analysis "complements" the third step, "asking whether the speech restriction is not more extensive than necessary to serve the interests that support it." We have made it clear that "the least restrictive means" is not the standard; instead, the case law requires a reasonable "fit between the legislature's ends and the means chosen to accomplish those ends . . . [and] a means narrowly tailored to achieve the desired objective." Focusing on the third and fourth steps, we first address the outdoor advertising and point-of-sale advertising regulations for smokeless tobacco and cigars. We then address the sales practices regulations for all tobacco products.

B

The outdoor advertising regulations prohibit smokeless tobacco or cigar advertising within a 1000-foot radius of a school or playground. The District Court and Court of Appeals concluded that the Attorney General had identified a real problem with underage use of tobacco products, that limiting youth exposure to advertising would combat that problem, and that the regulations burdened no more speech than necessary to accomplish the State's goal. The smokeless tobacco and cigar petitioners take issue with all of these conclusions.

1

The smokeless tobacco and cigar petitioners . . . maintain that although the Attorney General may have identified a problem with underage cigarette smoking, he has not identified an equally severe problem with respect to underage use of smokeless tobacco or cigars. The smokeless tobacco petitioner emphasizes the "lack of parity" between cigarettes and smokeless tobacco. The cigar petitioners catalog a list of differences between cigars and other tobacco products, including the characteristics of the products and marketing strategies. The petitioners finally contend that the Attorney General cannot prove that advertising has a causal link to tobacco use such that limiting advertising will materially alleviate any problem of underage use of their products.

In previous cases, we have acknowledged the theory that product advertising stimulates demand for products, while suppressed advertising may have the opposite effect. The Attorney General relies in part on evidence gathered by the Food and Drug Administration (FDA) in its attempt to regulate the advertising of cigarettes and smokeless tobacco. [*See FDA v. Brown & Williamson infra.*] The FDA promulgated the advertising regulations after finding that the period prior to adulthood is when an overwhelming majority of Americans first decide to use tobacco products, and that advertising plays a crucial role in that decision. (We later held that the FDA lacks statutory authority to regulate tobacco products.) Nevertheless, the Attorney General relies on the FDA's proceedings and other studies to support his decision that advertising affects demand for tobacco products.

. . . .

In its rulemaking proceeding, the FDA considered several studies of tobacco advertising and trends in the use of various tobacco products. The Surgeon General's report and the Institute of Medicine's report found that "there is sufficient evidence to conclude that advertising and labeling play a significant and important contributory role in a young person's decision to use cigarettes or smokeless tobacco products."

. . . .

The FDA also made specific findings with respect to smokeless tobacco. The FDA concluded that "[t]he recent and very large increase in the use of smokeless tobacco products by young people and the addictive nature of these products has persuaded the agency that these products must be included in any regulatory approach that is designed to help prevent future generations of young people from becoming addicted to nicotine-containing tobacco products.". . .

Researchers tracked a dramatic shift in patterns of smokeless tobacco use from older to younger users over the past 30 years. In particular, the smokeless tobacco industry boosted sales tenfold in the 1970's and 1980's by targeting young males. . . .

The Attorney General presents different evidence with respect to cigars. There was no data on underage cigar use prior to 1996 because the behavior was considered "uncommon enough not to be worthy of examination." In 1995, the FDA decided not to include cigars in its attempted regulation of tobacco product advertising, explaining that "the agency does not currently have sufficient evidence that these products are drug delivery devices. . . . FDA has focused its investigation of its authority over tobacco products on cigarettes and smokeless tobacco products, and not on pipe tobacco or cigars. . . .

More recently, however, data on youth cigar use has emerged. The National Cancer Institute concluded in its 1998 Monograph that the rate of cigar use by minors is increasing and that, in some States, the cigar use rates are higher than the smokeless tobacco use rates for minors. . . .

Studies have also demonstrated a link between advertising and demand for cigars. After Congress recognized the power of images in advertising and banned cigarette advertising in electronic media, television advertising of small cigars "increased dramatically in 1972 and 1973," "filled the void left by cigarette advertisers," and "sales . . . soared." In 1973, Congress extended the electronic media advertising ban for cigarettes to little cigars. In the 1990's, cigar advertising campaigns triggered a boost in sales.

Our review of the record reveals that the Attorney General has provided ample documentation of the problem with underage use of smokeless tobacco and cigars. In addition, we disagree with petitioners' claim that there is no evidence that preventing targeted campaigns and limiting youth exposure to advertising will decrease underage use of smokeless tobacco and cigars. On this record and in the posture of summary judgment, we are unable to conclude that the Attorney General's decision to regulate advertising of smokeless tobacco and cigars in an effort to combat the use of tobacco products by minors was based on mere "speculation [and] conjecture."

2

Whatever the strength of the Attorney General's evidence to justify the outdoor advertising regulations, however, we conclude that the regulations do not satisfy the fourth step of the *Central Hudson* analysis. The final step, the "critical inquiry in this case," requires a reasonable fit between the means and ends of the regulatory scheme. The Attorney General's regulations do not meet this standard. The broad sweep of the regulations indicates that the Attorney General did not "carefully calculat[e] the costs and benefits associated with the burden on speech imposed" by the regulations.

The outdoor advertising regulations prohibit any smokeless tobacco or cigar advertising within 1000 feet of schools or playgrounds. In the District Court, petitioners maintained that this prohibition would prevent advertising in 87% to 91% of Boston, Worcester, and Springfield, Massachusetts. The 87% to 91% figure appears to include not only the effect of the regulations, but also the limitations imposed by other generally applicable zoning restrictions. The Attorney General disputed petitioners' figures but "concede[d] that the reach of the regulations is substantial." Thus, the Court of Appeals concluded that the regulations prohibit advertising in a substantial portion of the major metropolitan areas of Massachusetts.

The substantial geographical reach of the Attorney General's outdoor advertising regulations is compounded by other factors. "Outdoor" advertising includes not only advertising located outside an establishment, but also advertising inside a store if that advertising is visible from outside the store. The regulations restrict advertisements of any size and the term advertisement also includes oral statements.

In some geographical areas, these regulations would constitute nearly a complete ban on the communication of truthful information about smokeless tobacco and cigars to adult consumers. The breadth and scope of the regulations, and the process by which the Attorney General adopted the regulations, do not demonstrate a careful calculation of the speech interests involved.

First, the Attorney General did not seem to consider the impact of the 1000-foot restriction on commercial speech in major metropolitan areas. The Attorney General apparently selected the 1000-foot distance based on the FDA's decision to impose an identical 1000-foot restriction when it attempted to regulate cigarette and smokeless tobacco advertising. But the FDA's 1,000-foot regulation was not an adequate basis for the Attorney General to tailor the Massachusetts regulations. The degree to which speech is suppressed — or alternative avenues for speech remain available — under a particular regulatory scheme tends to be case specific. And a case specific analysis makes sense, for although a State or locality may have common interests and concerns about underage smoking and the effects of tobacco advertisements, the impact of a restriction on speech will undoubtedly vary from place to place. The FDA's regulations would have had widely disparate effects nationwide. Even in Massachusetts, the effect of the Attorney General's speech regulations will vary based on whether a locale is rural, suburban, or urban. The uniformly broad sweep of the geographical limitation demonstrates a lack of tailoring.

In addition, the range of communications restricted seems unduly broad. For instance, it is not clear from the regulatory scheme why a ban on oral communications is necessary to further the State's interest. Apparently that restriction means that a retailer is unable to answer inquiries about its tobacco products if that communication occurs outdoors. Similarly, a ban on all signs of any size seems ill suited to target the problem of highly visible billboards, as opposed to smaller signs. To the extent that studies have identified particular advertising and promotion practices that appeal to youth, tailoring would involve targeting those practices while permitting others. As crafted, the regulations make no distinction among practices on this basis.

. . . Even on the premise that Massachusetts has demonstrated a connection between the outdoor advertising regulations and its substantial interest in preventing underage tobacco use, the question of tailoring remains. . . .

The State's interest in preventing underage tobacco use is substantial, and even compelling, but it is no less true that the sale and use of tobacco products by adults is a legal activity. We must consider that tobacco retailers and manufacturers have an interest in conveying truthful information about their products to adults, and adults have a corresponding interest in receiving truthful information about tobacco products. . . . As the State protects children from tobacco advertisements, tobacco manufacturers and retailers and their adult consumers still have a protected interest in communication. . . .

In some instances, Massachusetts' outdoor advertising regulations would impose particularly onerous burdens on speech. For example, we disagree with the Court of Appeals' conclusion that because cigar manufacturers and retailers conduct a limited amount of advertising in comparison to other tobacco products, "the relative lack of cigar advertising also means that the burden imposed on cigar advertisers is correspondingly small." If some retailers have relatively small advertising budgets, and use few avenues of communication, then the Attorney General's outdoor advertising regulations potentially place a greater, not lesser, burden on those retailers' speech. Furthermore, to the extent that cigar products and cigar advertising differ from that of other tobacco products, that difference should inform the inquiry into what speech restrictions are necessary.

In addition, a retailer in Massachusetts may have no means of communicating to passersby on the street that it sells tobacco products because alternative forms of advertisement, like newspapers, do not allow that retailer to propose an instant transaction in the way that onsite advertising does. The ban on any indoor advertising that is visible from the outside also presents problems in establishments like convenience stores, which have unique security concerns that counsel in favor of full visibility of the store from the outside. It is these sorts of considerations that the Attorney General failed to incorporate into the regulatory scheme.

We conclude that the Attorney General has failed to show that the outdoor advertising regulations for smokeless tobacco and cigars are not more extensive than necessary to advance the State's substantial interest in preventing underage tobacco use. . . . We believe that a remand is inappropriate in these cases because the State had ample opportunity to develop a record with respect to tailoring (as it had to justify its decision to regulate advertising), and additional evidence would not alter the nature of the scheme before the Court.

A careful calculation of the costs of a speech regulation does not mean that a State must demonstrate that there is no incursion on legitimate speech interests, but a speech regulation cannot unduly impinge on the speaker's ability to propose a commercial transaction and the adult listener's opportunity to obtain information about products. After reviewing the outdoor advertising regulations, we find the calculation in these cases insufficient for purposes of the First Amendment.

Massachusetts has also restricted indoor, point-of-sale advertising for smokeless tobacco and cigars. Advertising cannot be "placed lower than five feet from the floor of any retail establishment which is located within a one thousand foot radius of" any school or playground. . . .

We conclude that the point-of-sale advertising regulations fail both the third and fourth steps of the *Central Hudson* analysis. . . . As outlined above, the State's goal is to prevent minors from using tobacco products and to curb demand for that activity by limiting youth exposure to advertising. The 5-foot rule does not seem to advance that goal. Not all children are less than 5 feet tall, and those who are certainly have the ability to look up and take in their surroundings.

. . . .

Massachusetts may wish to target tobacco advertisements and displays that entice children, much like floor-level candy displays in a convenience store, but the blanket height restriction does not constitute a reasonable fit with that goal. . . .

### D

The Attorney General also promulgated a number of regulations that restrict sales practices by cigarette, smokeless tobacco, and cigar manufacturers and retailers. Among other restrictions, the regulations bar the use of self-service displays and require that tobacco products be placed out of the reach of all consumers in a location accessible only to salespersons. The cigarette petitioners do not challenge the sales practices regulations on pre-emption grounds.

Petitioners devoted little of their briefing to the sales practices regulations, and our understanding of the regulations is accordingly limited by the parties' submissions. As we read the regulations, they basically require tobacco retailers to place tobacco products behind counters and require customers to have contact with a salesperson before they are able to handle a tobacco product.

The cigarette and smokeless tobacco petitioners contend that "the same First Amendment principles that require invalidation of the outdoor and indoor advertising restrictions require invalidation of the display regulations at issue in this case." The cigar petitioners contend that self-service displays for cigars cannot be prohibited because each brand of cigar is unique and customers traditionally have sought to handle and compare cigars at the time of purchase.

We reject these contentions. Assuming that petitioners have a cognizable speech interest in a particular means of displaying their products, these regulations withstand First Amendment scrutiny.

Massachusetts' sales practices provisions regulate conduct that may have a communicative component, but Massachusetts seeks to regulate the placement of tobacco products for reasons unrelated to the communication of ideas. . . . We conclude that the State has demonstrated a substantial interest in preventing access to tobacco products by minors and has adopted an appropriately narrow means of advancing that interest. (citation to *O'Brien v. United States*).

Unattended displays of tobacco products present an opportunity for access without the proper age verification required by law. Thus, the State prohibits self-service and other displays that would allow an individual to obtain tobacco products without direct contact with a salesperson. It is clear that the regulations leave open ample channels of communication. The regulations do not significantly impede adult access to tobacco products. Moreover, retailers have other means of exercising any cognizable speech interest in the presentation of their products. We presume that vendors may place empty tobacco packaging on open display, and display actual tobacco products so long as that display is only accessible to sales personnel. As for cigars, there is no indication in the regulations that a customer is unable to examine a cigar prior to purchase, so long as that examination takes place through a salesperson.

We conclude that the sales practices regulations withstand First Amendment scrutiny. The means chosen by the State are narrowly tailored to prevent access to tobacco products by minors, are unrelated to expression, and leave open alternative avenues for vendors to convey information about products and for would-be customers to inspect products before purchase.

. . . .

## IV

We have observed that "tobacco use, particularly among children and adolescents, poses perhaps the single most significant threat to public health in the United States." From a policy perspective, it is understandable for the States to attempt to prevent minors from using tobacco products before they reach an age where they are capable of weighing for themselves the risks and potential benefits of tobacco use, and other adult activities. Federal law, however, places limits on policy choices available to the States.

In these cases, Congress enacted a comprehensive scheme to address cigarette smoking and health in advertising and pre-empted state regulation of cigarette advertising that attempts to address that same concern, even with respect to youth. The First Amendment also constrains state efforts to limit advertising of tobacco products, because so long as the sale and use of tobacco is lawful for adults, the tobacco industry has a protected interest in communicating information about its products and adult customers have an interest in receiving that information.

To the extent that federal law and the First Amendment do not prohibit state action, States and localities remain free to combat the problem of underage tobacco use by appropriate means. . . .

[Note: There were four separate concurring opinions, agreeing with some, but not all of the majority analysis set out above.]

\* \* \*

# FDA v. BROWN & WILLIAMSON TOBACCO CORP.
## 529 U.S. 120 (2000)

O'Connor, Justice.

\* \* \*

. . . In 1996, the Food and Drug Administration (FDA), after having expressly disavowed any such authority since its inception, asserted jurisdiction to regulate tobacco products. The FDA concluded that nicotine is a "drug" within the meaning of the Food, Drug, and Cosmetic Act (FDCA or Act), and that cigarettes and smokeless tobacco are "combination products" that deliver nicotine to the body. Pursuant to this authority, it promulgated regulations intended to reduce tobacco consumption among children and adolescents. The agency believed that, because most tobacco consumers begin their use before reaching the age of 18, curbing tobacco use by minors could substantially reduce the prevalence of addiction in future generations and thus the incidence of tobacco-related death and disease.

Regardless of how serious the problem an administrative agency seeks to address, however, it may not exceed its authority "in a manner that is inconsistent with the administrative structure that Congress enacted into law." And although agencies are generally entitled to deference in the interpretation of statutes that they administer, a reviewing "court, as well as the agency, must give effect to the unambiguously expressed intent of Congress." [citing *Chevron U.S.A., Inc.*]. In this case, we believe that Congress has clearly precluded the FDA from asserting jurisdiction to regulate tobacco products. Such authority is inconsistent with the intent that Congress has expressed in the FDCA's overall regulatory scheme and in the tobacco-specific legislation that it has enacted subsequent to the FDCA. In light of this clear intent, the FDA's assertion of jurisdiction is impermissible.

The FDCA grants the FDA, as the designee of the Secretary of Health and Human Services (HHS), the authority to regulate, among other items, "drugs" and "devices." The Act defines "drug" to include "articles (other than food) intended to affect the structure or any function of the body." It defines "device," in part, as "an instrument, apparatus, implement, machine, contrivance, . . . or other similar or related article, including any component, part, or accessory, which is . . . intended to affect the structure or any function of the body." The Act also grants the FDA the authority to regulate so-called "combination products," which "constitute a combination of a drug, device, or biological product." The FDA has construed this provision as giving it the discretion to regulate combination products as drugs, as devices, or as both.

On August 11, 1995, the FDA published a proposed rule concerning the sale of cigarettes and smokeless tobacco to children and adolescents. The rule, which included several restrictions on the sale, distribution, and advertisement of tobacco products, was designed to reduce the availability and attractiveness of tobacco products to young people. A public comment period followed, during which the FDA received over 700,000 submissions [the most in its history].

On August 28, 1996, the FDA issued a final rule [and] determined that nicotine is a "drug" and that cigarettes and smokeless tobacco are "drug delivery devices," and therefore it had jurisdiction under the FDCA to regulate tobacco products as customarily marketed — that is, without manufacturer claims of therapeutic benefit. First, the FDA found that tobacco products "affect the structure or any function of the body" because nicotine "has significant pharmacological effects." Specifically, nicotine "exerts psychoactive, or mood-altering, effects on the brain" that cause and sustain addiction, have both tranquilizing and stimulating effects, and control weight. Second, the FDA determined that these effects were "intended" under the FDCA because they "are so widely known and foreseeable that [they] may be deemed to have been intended by the manufacturers," [and because] consumers use tobacco products "predominantly or nearly exclusively" to obtain these effects, and the statements, research, and actions of manufacturers revealed that they "have designed cigarettes to provide pharmacologically active doses of nicotine to consumers." Finally, the agency concluded that cigarettes and smokeless tobacco are "combination products" because, in addition to containing nicotine, they include device components that deliver a controlled amount of nicotine to the body."

Having resolved the jurisdictional question, the FDA next explained the policy justifications for its regulations, detailing the deleterious health effects associated with tobacco use. It found that tobacco consumption was "the single leading cause of preventable death in the United States." According to the FDA, "[m]ore than 400,000 people die each year from tobacco-related illnesses, such as cancer, respiratory illnesses, and heart disease." The agency also determined that the only way to reduce the amount of tobacco-related illness and mortality was to reduce the level of addiction, a goal that could be accomplished only by preventing children and adolescents from starting to use tobacco. The FDA found that 82% of adult smokers had their first cigarette before the age of 18, and more than half had already become regular smokers by that age. It also found that children were beginning to smoke at a younger age, that the prevalence of youth smoking had recently increased, and that similar problems existed with respect to smokeless tobacco. The FDA accordingly concluded that if "the number of children and adolescents who begin tobacco use can be substantially diminished, tobacco-related illness can be correspondingly reduced because data suggest that anyone who does not begin smoking in childhood or adolescence is unlikely ever to begin."

Based on these findings, the FDA promulgated regulations concerning tobacco products' promotion, labeling, and accessibility to children and adolescents. The access regulations prohibit the sale of cigarettes or smokeless tobacco to persons younger than 18; require retailers to verify through photo identification the age of all purchasers younger than 27; prohibit the sale of cigarettes in quantities smaller than 20; prohibit the distribution of free samples; and prohibit sales through self-service displays and vending machines except in adult-only locations. The promotion regulations require that any print advertising appear in a black-and-white, text-only format unless the publication in which it appears is read almost exclusively by adults; prohibit outdoor advertising within 1,000 feet of any public playground or school; prohibit the distribution of any promotional items, such as T-shirts or hats, bearing the manufacturer's brand name; and prohibit a manufacturer from sponsoring any athletic, musical, artistic, or other social or cultural event using its brand name. The labeling regulation requires that the statement, "A Nicotine-Delivery Device for Persons 18 or Older," appear on all tobacco product packages.

The FDA promulgated these regulations pursuant to its authority to regulate "restricted devices." The FDA construed § 353(g) [of the FDCA] as giving it the discretion to regulate "combination products" using the Act's drug authorities, device authorities, or both, depending on "how the public health goals of the act can be best accomplished." Given the greater flexibility in the FDCA for the regulation of devices, the FDA determined that "the device authorities provide the most appropriate basis for regulating cigarettes and smokeless tobacco." Under § 360j(e) the agency may "require that a device be restricted to sale, distribution, or use . . . upon such other conditions as [the FDA] may prescribe in such regulation, if, because of its potentiality for harmful effect or the collateral measures necessary to its use, [the FDA] determines that there cannot otherwise be reasonable assurance of its safety and effectiveness." The FDA reasoned that its regulations fell within [its authority] because they related to the sale or distribution of tobacco products and were necessary for providing a reasonable assurance of safety.

Respondents, a group of tobacco manufacturers, retailers, and advertisers, filed suit in United States District Court for the Middle District of North Carolina challenging the regulations. . . .

The Court of Appeals for the Fourth Circuit reversed [the lower court's ruling], holding that Congress has not granted the FDA jurisdiction to regulate tobacco products. . . .

We granted the federal parties' petition for certiorari to determine whether the FDA has authority under the FDCA to regulate tobacco products as customarily marketed.

## II

The FDA's assertion of jurisdiction to regulate tobacco products is founded on its conclusions that nicotine is a "drug" and that cigarettes and smokeless tobacco are "drug delivery devices." Again, the FDA found that tobacco products are "intended" to deliver the pharmacological effects of satisfying addiction, stimulation and tranquilization, and weight control[;] because those effects are foreseeable to any reasonable manufacturer, consumers use tobacco products to obtain those effects, and tobacco manufacturers have designed their products to produce those effects. As an initial matter, respondents take issue with the FDA's reading of "intended," arguing that it is a term of art that refers exclusively to claims made by the manufacturer or vendor about the product. That is, a product is not a drug or device under the FDCA unless the manufacturer or vendor makes some express claim concerning the product's therapeutic benefits. We need not resolve this question, however, because assuming, *arguendo*, that a product can be "intended to affect the structure or any function of the body" absent claims of therapeutic or medical benefit, the FDA's claim to jurisdiction contravenes the clear intent of Congress.

Because this case involves an administrative agency's construction of a statute that it administers, our analysis is governed by *Chevron U.S.A., Inc.* Under *Chevron,* a reviewing court must first ask "whether Congress has directly spoken to the precise question at issue." If Congress has done so, the inquiry is at an end; the court "must give effect to the unambiguously expressed intent of Congress." But if Congress has not specifically addressed the question, a reviewing court must respect the agency's construction of the statute so long as it is permissible.

. . . .

[W]e find that Congress has directly spoken to the issue here and precluded the FDA's jurisdiction to regulate tobacco products.

## A

Viewing the FDCA as a whole, it is evident that one of the Act's core objectives is to ensure that any product regulated by the FDA is "safe" and "effective" [terms defined in the Act] for its intended use. This essential purpose pervades the FDCA. . . . Thus, the Act generally requires the FDA to prevent the marketing of any drug or device where the "potential for inflicting death or physical injury is not offset by the possibility of therapeutic benefit."

In its rulemaking proceeding, the FDA quite exhaustively documented that "tobacco products are unsafe," "dangerous," and "cause great pain and suffering from illness." It found that the consumption of tobacco products presents "extraordinary health risks" and that "tobacco use is the single leading cause of preventable death in the United States." . . .

These findings logically imply that, if tobacco products were "devices" under the FDCA [as the FDA found in its rulemaking proceeding], the FDA would be required to remove them from the market. Consider, first, the FDCA's provisions concerning the misbranding of drugs or devices. The Act prohibits "[t]he introduction or delivery for introduction into interstate commerce of any food, drug, device, or cosmetic that is adulterated or misbranded." In light of the FDA's findings, two distinct FDCA provisions would render cigarettes and smokeless tobacco misbranded devices. . . . Given the FDA's conclusions concerning the health consequences of tobacco use, there are no directions that could adequately protect consumers. . . . Thus, were tobacco products within the FDA's jurisdiction, the Act would deem them misbranded devices that could not be introduced into interstate commerce. . . .

Second, the FDCA requires the FDA to place all devices that it regulates into one of three classifications. The agency relies on a device's classification in determining the degree of control and regulation necessary to ensure that there is "a reasonable assurance of safety and effectiveness." The FDA has yet to classify tobacco products. Instead, the regulations at issue here represent so-called "general controls," which the Act entitles the agency to impose in advance of classification. Although the FDCA prescribes no deadline for device classification, the FDA has stated that it will classify tobacco products "in a future rulemaking" as required by the Act. Given the FDA's findings regarding the health consequences of tobacco use, the agency would have to place cigarettes and smokeless tobacco in Class III because, even after the application of the Act's available controls, they would "presen[t] a potential unreasonable risk of illness or injury." As Class III devices, tobacco products would be subject to the FDCA's pre-market approval process. Under these provisions, the FDA would be prohibited from approving an application for pre-market approval without "a showing of reasonable assurance that such device is safe under the conditions of use prescribed, recommended, or suggested in the proposed labeling thereof." In view of the FDA's conclusions regarding the health effects of tobacco use, the agency would have no basis for finding any such reasonable assurance of safety. Thus, once the FDA fulfilled its statutory obligation to classify tobacco products, it could not allow them to be marketed.

The FDCA's misbranding and device classification provisions therefore make evident that were the FDA to regulate cigarettes and smokeless tobacco, the Act would require the agency to ban them. In fact, based on these provisions, the FDA itself has previously taken the position that if tobacco products were within its jurisdiction, "they would have to be removed from the market because it would be impossible to prove they were safe for their intended us[e]." . . .

Congress, however, has foreclosed the removal of tobacco products from the market. A provision of the United States Code currently in force states that "[t]he marketing of tobacco constitutes one of the greatest basic industries of the United States with ramifying activities which directly affect interstate and foreign commerce at every point, and stable conditions therein are necessary to the general welfare." 7 U.S.C. § 1311(a). More importantly, Congress has directly addressed the problem of tobacco and health through legislation on six occasions since 1965. [A list of statutes is omitted.] When Congress enacted these statutes, the adverse health consequences of tobacco use were well known, as were nicotine's pharmacological effects. Nonetheless, Congress stopped well short of ordering a ban. Instead, it has generally regulated the labeling and advertisement of tobacco products, expressly providing that it is the policy of Congress that "commerce and the national economy may be . . . protected to the maximum extent consistent with" consumers "be[ing] adequately informed about any adverse health effects.". . . [T]he collective premise of these [specifically tobacco-related] statutes [enacted subsequently to and independently of the FDCA,] is that cigarettes and smokeless tobacco will continue to be sold in the United States. A ban of tobacco products by the FDA would therefore plainly contradict congressional policy.

The FDA apparently recognized this dilemma and concluded, somewhat ironically, that tobacco products are actually "safe" within the meaning of the FDCA. In promulgating its regulations, the agency conceded that "tobacco products are unsafe, as that term is conventionally understood." Nonetheless, the FDA reasoned that, in determining whether a device is safe under the Act, it must consider "not only the risks presented by a product but also any of the countervailing effects of use of that product, including the consequences of not permitting the product to be marketed." Applying this standard, the FDA found that, because of the high level of addiction among tobacco users, a ban would likely be "dangerous." In particular, current tobacco users could suffer from extreme withdrawal, the health care system and available pharmaceuticals might not be able to meet the treatment demands of those suffering from withdrawal, and a black market offering cigarettes even more dangerous than those currently sold legally would likely develop. The FDA therefore concluded that, "while taking cigarettes and smokeless tobacco off the market could prevent some people from becoming addicted and reduce death and disease for others, the record does not establish that such a ban is the appropriate public health response under the act."

It may well be, as the FDA asserts, that "these factors must be considered when developing a regulatory scheme that achieves the best public health result for these products." But the FDA's judgment that leaving tobacco products on the market "is more effective in achieving public health goals than a ban," is no substitute for the specific safety determinations required by the FDCA's various operative provisions. Several provisions in the Act require the FDA to determine that the product itself is safe as used by consumers. That is, the product's probable therapeutic benefits must outweigh its risk of harm. In contrast, the FDA's conception of safety would allow the agency, with respect to each provision of the FDCA that requires the agency to determine a product's "safety" or "dangerousness," to compare the aggregate health effects of alternative administrative actions. This is a qualitatively different inquiry.

Thus, although the FDA has concluded that a ban would be "dangerous," it has not concluded that tobacco products are "safe" as that term is used throughout the Act.

. . . .

A straightforward reading of [the FDCA] dictates that the FDA must weigh the probable therapeutic benefits of the device to the consumer against the probable risk of injury. Applied to tobacco products, the inquiry is whether their purported benefits — satisfying addiction, stimulation and sedation, and weight control — outweigh the risks to health from their use. To accommodate the FDA's conception of safety, however, one must read "any probable benefit to health" to include the benefit to public health stemming from adult consumers' continued use of tobacco products, even though the reduction of tobacco use is the raison d'etre of the regulations. In other words, the FDA is forced to contend that the very evil it seeks to combat is a "benefit to health." This is implausible.

The FDA's conception of safety is also incompatible with the FDCA's misbranding provision. . . .

. . . .

The dissent contends that our conclusion means that "the FDCA requires the FDA to ban outright 'dangerous' drugs or devices," and that this is a "perverse" reading of the statute. This misunderstands our holding. The FDA, consistent with the FDCA, may clearly regulate many "dangerous" products without banning them. Indeed, virtually every drug or device poses dangers under certain conditions. What the FDA may not do is conclude that a drug or device cannot be used safely for any therapeutic purpose and yet, at the same time, allow that product to remain on the market. Such regulation is incompatible with the FDCA's core objective of ensuring that every drug or device is safe and effective.

Considering the FDCA as a whole, it is clear that Congress intended to exclude tobacco products from the FDA's jurisdiction. A fundamental precept of the FDCA is that any product regulated by the FDA — but not banned — must be safe for its intended use. Various provisions of the Act make clear that this refers to the safety of using the product to obtain its intended effects, not the public health ramifications of alternative administrative actions by the FDA. That is, the FDA must determine that there is a reasonable assurance that the product's therapeutic benefits outweigh the risk of harm to the consumer. According to this standard, the FDA has concluded that, although tobacco products might be effective in delivering certain pharmacological effects, they are "unsafe" and "dangerous" when used for these purposes. Consequently, if tobacco products were within the FDA's jurisdiction, the Act would require the FDA to remove them from the market entirely. But a ban would contradict Congress' clear intent as expressed in its more recent, tobacco-specific legislation. The inescapable conclusion is that there is no room for tobacco products within the FDCA's regulatory scheme. If they cannot be used safely for any therapeutic purpose, and yet they cannot be banned, they simply do not fit.

## B

In determining whether Congress has spoken directly to the FDA's authority to regulate tobacco, we must also consider in greater detail the tobacco-specific legislation that Congress has enacted over the past 35 years. At the time a statute is enacted, it may have a range of plausible meanings. Over time, however, subsequent acts can shape or focus those meanings. The "classic judicial task of reconciling many laws enacted over time, and getting them to 'make sense' in combination, necessarily assumes that the implications of a statute may be altered by the implications of a later statute." This is particularly so where the scope of the earlier statute is broad but the subsequent statutes more specifically address the topic at hand.

[The opinion then reviews the Federal Cigarette Labeling and Advertising Act and a number of other federal laws that require that health warnings appear on all packaging and in all print and outdoor advertisements, prohibit the advertisement of tobacco products in the electronic media, require the Secretary of HHS to report every three years to Congress on research findings concerning "the addictive property of tobacco," and make States' receipt of certain federal block grants contingent on their making it unlawful "for any manufacturer, retailer, or distributor of tobacco products to sell or distribute any such product to any individual under the age of 18."]

In adopting each statute, Congress has acted against the backdrop of the FDA's consistent and repeated statements that it lacked authority under the FDCA to regulate tobacco absent claims of therapeutic benefit by the manufacturer. In fact, on several occasions over this period, and after the health consequences of tobacco use and nicotine's pharmacological effects had become well known, Congress considered and rejected bills that would have granted the FDA such jurisdiction. Under these circumstances, it is evident that Congress' tobacco-specific statutes have effectively ratified the FDA's long-held position that it lacks jurisdiction under the FDCA to regulate tobacco products. . . .

. . . .

Taken together, these actions by Congress over the past 35 years preclude an interpretation of the FDCA that grants the FDA jurisdiction to regulate tobacco products. We do not rely on Congress' failure to act — its consideration and rejection of bills that would have given the FDA this authority — in reaching this conclusion. Indeed, this is not a case of simple inaction by Congress that purportedly represents its acquiescence in an agency's position. To the contrary, Congress has enacted several statutes addressing the particular subject of tobacco and health, creating a distinct regulatory scheme for cigarettes and smokeless tobacco. . . .

Under these circumstances, it is clear that Congress' tobacco-specific legislation has effectively ratified the FDA's previous position that it lacks jurisdiction to regulate tobacco. . . . As a result, Congress' tobacco-specific statutes preclude the FDA from regulating tobacco products as customarily marketed.

. . . .

By no means do we question the seriousness of the problem that the FDA has sought to address. The agency has amply demonstrated that tobacco use, particularly among children and adolescents, poses perhaps the single most significant threat to public health in the United States. Nonetheless, no matter how "important, conspicuous, and controversial" the issue, and regardless of how likely the public is to hold the Executive Branch politically accountable, an administrative agency's power to regulate in the public interest must always be grounded in a valid grant of authority from Congress. . . . Reading the FCDA as a whole, as well as in conjunction with Congress' subsequent tobacco-specific legislation, it is plain that Congress has not given the FDA the authority that it seeks to exercise here. For these reasons, the judgment of the Court of Appeal . . . is affirmed.

[A dissent by Justices Breyer, Stevens, Souter, and Ginsburg argued strongly in favor of upholding the FDA's asserted jurisdiction over tobacco. First, the key statutory language confers regulatory authority over articles "intended to affect the structure or any function of the body." Read literally this language embraces tobacco products, since both manufacturers and smokers are well aware of, and desire, the "mood-stabilizing effects [achieved] through the interaction of the chemical nicotine and the cells of the central nervous system." A broad reading, moreover, is counseled by the legislative history surrounding the enactment of these terms in 1938. Second, the basic purpose of the statute — protection of public health — supports an interpretation that includes tobacco as regulated subject matter. Third, recall the majority's view that the FDCA would require the FDA to *ban* tobacco if it had any jurisdiction at all, and therefore that the agency's proposed (mere) *regulation* of tobacco establishes that tobacco simply doesn't "fit" under FDCA at all (and hence is beyond the agency's reach). The dissent claims that this view is wrong: It misreads the agency's statutory discretion to choose remedies short of imposing a ban. Fourth, Congress' later tobacco-specific enactments, properly read, have no implications one way or the other for the jurisdictional issue, but rather simply leave that question unaddressed and undisturbed for resolution under the FDCA itself. And finally, the agency's reversal (in the 1990s) of its prior disclaimers of jurisdiction over tobacco was fully justified, in the dissent's view, by new information regarding the manufacturers' "intent" to affect smokers' physiology; by mounting scientific consensus about tobacco's dangers; and by a shift in regulatory philosophy — entirely permissible in connection with agency interpretations of their statutes — under a new government administration.]

\* \* \*

# NOTES AND QUESTIONS

**1.** *Austin v. Tennessee* is essentially the equivalent of the *Jacobson* decision: It clearly recognizes the power of the states to regulate or, should they choose to do so, prohibit the sale, possession, or use of tobacco products. It is more complicated than *Jacobson* in that the Court is concerned with defining the line between the congressional authority to regulate interstate commerce and the states' authority to regulate items of commerce once they have entered the state. Observe, though, that in drawing this line the Court seeks to reconcile the preservation of both powers, each in its designated activity-realm, and refrains from any assumption that the federal commerce power operates to strip states of their pre-existing authority in matters of public health. Once having determined that the activity-realms are different, the Court regards the state's decision to regulate tobacco (at least in the manner that Tennessee has done) as a constitutional given. For that matter, the case could be cited as implying, as well, that the federal government has plenary authority over tobacco products while they remain in, and insofar as they implicate, interstate commerce.

At the time of *Austin,* the Supreme Court had a somewhat limited view of the congressional authority to regulate interstate commerce: Congress could only regulate commercial activities that were, in the most literal sense, interstate in nature, and all commercial activities were defined as either intrastate or interstate. If an activity were an intrastate activity, the state could regulate it; if it were an interstate activity, only the Congress could regulate it. Each activity was either one or the other, hence the significance in pre-*Austin* cases of the determination that items potentially subject to state regulation were still in their original interstate shipping package. Since the mid-1930s, the Court has greatly expanded its view of the congressional authority to regulate interstate commerce. For the most part, mechanical definitions of interstate commerce such as the "package" rule have been abandoned. Activities are no longer categorized as *either* interstate or intrastate. If there is a rational basis for concluding that an intrastate activity has some effect on interstate commerce, Congress can choose to regulate that activity or, conversely, can regulate interstate commerce so as to have some desirable effect on the intrastate activity. *See, e.g., Katzenbach v. McClung,* 379 U.S. 274 (1964).

The Court has in recent years indicated that there may be some enhanced judicial role in determining whether the Congress has exceeded its commerce authority, but these cases appear to be more in the nature of a marginal shift in judicial attitudes than a re-working of the broad, basic principles that have been followed for nearly 70 years. *See, e.g., United States v. Lopez,* 514 U.S. 549 (1995).

In any event, as the cases discussed *infra* illustrate, there has been little debate over the extent of the federal government's constitutional authority to tax, regulate, or prohibit tobacco products; the economic effects on interstate commerce of the sale of cigarettes and other tobacco products would be easy to document. For that matter, smoking and other tobacco uses could be easily linked to interstate commerce. The notable exceptions are those otherwise constitutional exercises of federal authority that implicate the First Amendment, *i.e.,* efforts to limit advertising as discussed in *Lorillard.* In these situations, the constitutional analysis may be somewhat more complicated. Nonetheless, for the most part, however, the cases examining federal power have involved statutory and administrative law issues.

**2.** For a good survey of state laws regulating the sale and use of tobacco, see CDC, *State Laws on Tobacco Control — United States, 1998,* 48 Morbidity/Mortality Wkly Rep. 21-62 (1999); *see also* American Lung Association, State of Tobacco Control: 2005 (2006) found at www.lungaction.org/reports/tobacco-control05.html (last visited December 2006) (including laws on maintenance of smoke-free environments, youth access to tobacco, statewide spending on tobacco prevention and control, and cigarette taxes).

**3.** As demonstrated by *D.A.B.E.*, there have been many challenges to the various local laws that attempt to regulate or prohibit smoking. These cases are usually a matter of statutory (and sometimes state constitutional) interpretation and will differ from jurisdiction to jurisdiction. For a recent case closely following the facts and analysis in *D.A.B.E.*, see *American Lithuanian Naturalization Club, Athol, Mass., Inc. v. Board of Massachusetts*, 446 Mass. 310, 844 N.E.2d 231 (2006).

The most successful challenges have been those that argue that the local government is exercising powers that are reserved for the general (meaning state) government or that the local law has been preempted by the state legislature. For a counter-illustration to *D.A.B.E.*, see *Entertainment Industry Coalition v. Tacoma-Pierce County Health Dep't*, 153 Wash. 2d 657, 105 P.3d 985 (2005) (local ordinance that prohibited smoking in all indoor areas preempted by similar, but more permissive statewide law that allowed some businesses to establish segregated "smoking areas". Later that year, however, the state enacted by public referendum a new statewide law, which provides a "cutting edge" illustration of how far states may go in regulating the permissible sites for smoking in public. *See* Wash. Rev. Code § 70.160.011.

**4.** The more complicated preemption issues involve the extent to which various federal laws preempt state or local laws that attempt to regulate smoking or the use or sale of tobacco. In *Lorillard* the Supreme Court had to determine the extent to which the federal FCLAA legislation enacted in the 1960s (and amended several times thereafter) preempted state anti-tobacco laws — at least the advertising and sales practice laws that the Massachusetts attorney general attempted to implement in 2001 that are the subject of this litigation. (Note that the attorney general undertook the tobacco initiative, and determined its content, under very general state consumer-protection statutes. That is, there was no specific legislative mandate to do so; the campaign arose administratively). The FCLAA required the now-familiar warning labels on cigarettes and other tobacco advertising, and limiting advertisement of cigarettes and most other forms of tobacco (but not cigars and smokeless products) on electronic media.

*Lorillard* gives a broad reading to the preemptive language of the FCLAA that stated that "no requirement or prohibition . . . with respect to the advertising or promotion of cigarettes. . . ." could be enacted under state law. As a consequence, it invalidated most of Massachusetts' proposed regulations with respect to cigarettes — but not as applied to cigars or smokeless tobacco products. *Lorillard* did allow that the state could impose some limits on cigarette advertising, despite the preemption language of the FCLAA; the Court refers to "zoning restrictions," presumably restrictions that apply to all advertising in certain locales, such as generally-applicable limits on outdoor billboards. The opinion also notes that the state is still free to regulate conduct that is not within the definition of "promotion and advertising" in the FCLAA preemption. As an illustration, the Court specifically held that Massachusetts laws prohibiting the sale of cigarettes to minors are not preempted. The open question — not asked or answered by the opinion — is whether the state could exercise its otherwise legitimate police powers to regulate or prohibit altogether the sale of cigarettes to adults as well. Is there an argument that the FCLAA preempts this type of legislation? Or, to ask a more practical and relevant question, can the FCLAA preemption act as a bar to a state effort to ban cigarette smoking in public places or indoors, as was attempted in the D.A.B.E. case? The tobacco industry could argue that the federal legislation requires labels on cigarettes and prohibits some form of advertising — restrictions that anticipate that, within these restrictions, tobacco products and their use would be permitted. Is that enough to infer preemption?

**5.** Since the FCLAA preemption applied only to cigarettes, and because Massachusetts was attempting to regulate cigars and smokeless tobacco products as well, the *Lorillard* decision also addressed the First Amendment problem that arises when government attempts to impose restrictions on the advertising or promotion of otherwise legal commercial goods.

As set out in the opinion, the basic "commercial speech" principles were first enunciated in *Central Hudson Gas & Electric Corp. v. Public Serv.Comm'n*, 447 U.S. 557 (1980). Since then, the application of the *Central Hudson* principles has not been without controversy. *See, e.g., Liquormart, Inc. v. Rhode Island*, 517 U.S. 484 (1996). But as applied in *Lorillard* and most other post-*Central Hudson* "commercial speech" cases, the Court first decides whether the commercial speech is not misleading or fraudulent and whether it concerns a lawful activity. (Note that with noncommercial speech, neither of these elements would disqualify the speech from First Amendment protections.) If commercial speech is not misleading and concerns lawful activities, the Court essentially applies a type of "mid-level scrutiny," imposing on the government the burden to show that its purpose is substantial, that the purpose is directly advanced by the regulation, and that the regulation is no more extensive than necessary to achieve its purpose. In this regard, *Lorillard* is a good textbook illustration of the rigors of this "mid-level scrutiny," but also of how it differs from the more demanding "close scrutiny" applied in other First Amendment cases.

The result, however, is not without irony. Had Massachusetts decided to ban the sale, use, or possession of tobacco in more draconian ways (and assuming such legislation is not preempted by federal legislation), the Court would have applied a more deferential "rationality" standard to the state's ban. Having decided to only limit the advertising of tobacco products, not limit or prohibit their use or sale, Massachusetts must meet a more demanding constitutional burden. This is true because the more limited regulation on advertising affects an activity that is constitutionally protected, whereas a more far-reaching limit on the product's use or sale does not. This is fairly straightforward constitutional logic, but it may not make as much sense in political or public debates where constitutional logic and common sense are not always equated.

The *Lorillard* opinion also makes passing reference to *United States v. O'Brien*, 391 U.S. 367 (1968). The *O'Brien* "expressive conduct" doctrine allows the government to regulate conduct that also involves some elements of speech or expression, again under a form of judicial review that is somewhat more demanding than "rationality," but less rigorous than "close scrutiny." Essentially, so long as the court finds that the government's purpose is to regulate the conduct and not the speech and the impact on the speech is "incidental," the *O'Brien* test will be satisfied. In *Lorillard,* the Court used this analysis to uphold some of the Massachusetts laws that limited the manner in which tobacco products can be displayed and other related sales practices; apparently the Court was not prepared to regard these practices as "commercial speech." *O'Brien* may be applied in other cases where the regulated activity has elements of both conduct and expression and the courts are unwilling to make a determination that the activity is exclusively one or the other.

For a (somewhat) related case, see *R.J. Reynolds Tobacco, Co. v. Shewry,* 384 F.3d. 1126 (9th Cir. 2004) (upholding the power of the State of California to impose a surtax on the sale of cigarettes and use the revenues to fund anti-tobacco advertising; the court holds that this is not a regulation of speech, but merely an otherwise constitutional funding of governmental speech).

**6.** The *FDA* decision (which actually preceded the decision in *Lorillard*) analyzes the impact of the FCLAA and other federal laws on a different and even more complex issue: the jurisdictional limits on the FDA's authority. The FDA proposed issuing regulations that would ban the sale of cigarettes and other tobacco products to people under 18 years of age, impose drastic limits on advertising, and impose other measures that would limit access of minors to tobacco products — but not outright ban the sale or use of tobacco.

According to Justice O'Connor, the proposed regulations were beyond the authority of the FDA. Again speaking for a closely (5-4) divided Court, O'Connor found that the FDA legislation gives the agency the authority to determine whether a drug or device is safe for its intended use. In doing so, the agency must weigh the benefits of the drug or device against its risks. According to O'Connor's view of the meaning of the FDCA, when the agency makes findings such as those made by the FDA with regard to tobacco products, the FDA has no choice but to remove those products from the market. There is essentially no medicinal benefit from the use of tobacco that out weighs the inherently dangerous effects of its use. No amount of disclosure or other warnings can help the consumer avoid the risks to achieve the minimal benefit. Thus, under O'Connor's interpretation of the FDA's authority, the FDCA statutes would require the agency to prohibit — rather than allow it to regulate — tobacco products under its own factual findings.

Note that the FDA made a somewhat-strained argument that regulation was preferable to prohibition because of the immediate effects of a total prohibition on the existing nicotine-addicted population. The Court rejected the logic of this position.

O'Connor then went on to read other federal legislation — particularly the FCLAA and its subsequent amendments — as anticipating that cigarettes and other products would be available to adults, even if subject to various forms of state and federal regulation of their advertising or promotion, and of the terms and conditions of their sale (*e.g.,* limits on package size). Because of these laws, O'Connor found that Congress could not have intended to give the FDA the authority to prohibit cigarettes or other tobacco products, even if the FDA legislation, read alone, might allow that authority. In fact, O'Connor relies on these legislative efforts to regulate tobacco to conclude that the FDA has been given no authority to prohibit or regulate tobacco in any manner whatsoever.

The strongest rhetorical support for O'Connor's argument comes from the language of 7 U.S.C. § 1311(a), the preamble to the tobacco growers' subsidy program enacted in 1938, which describes "the marketing of tobacco" as "one of the greatest basic industries of the United States" (although that legislation has since been repealed). More substantial support comes from the FCLAA and other federal laws, as discussed in *Lorillard,* requiring various warnings to be attached to cigarettes and their advertising, and banning advertising in electronic media. Congress clearly wanted to regulate tobacco, but to allow for its sale to and use by adults. From this O'Connor argues, it can be inferred that Congress did not want to allow the sale and use of tobacco products under one set of laws, and allow a federal agency to prohibit their sale altogether under another.

O'Connor's logic is a little strained, especially in light of the evolving understanding of the risks of smoking and tobacco use. Further, it is at least possible that even if Congress did not want to prohibit smoking when it enacted the tobacco advertising limits in the 1960s, it nonetheless accepted the possibility that the FDA, in the future, could find that the dangers of smoking are even greater than was then understood. Congress could have anticipated that the FDA could in the future enact regulations that impose even greater regulatory controls. It is also possible that when Congress enacted the regulatory legislation if the 1960s, no one was concerned with the FDA's authority — one way or the other. Justice Breyer makes this point in his dissent. Justice Breyer also gives an account of the critical and still-operative text of the FDCA, and the legislative history surrounding its enactment in 1938, that at the very least suggests the "enacting" Congress did not contemplate a narrow vision of FDA jurisdiction. This point highlights an interpretive question fascinating in itself: Should a judge be interested in the understanding of a law held by the particular legislature that enacted it? Or in the understanding arguably evinced by successive, later institutional versions of that body, over many decades? Which approach does O'Connor take?

Perhaps O'Connor's best argument is one based on common sense. Regulating cigarettes and other tobacco products under legislation that is generally considered an effort to protect the public from unsafe drugs and medical devices is a bit of an interpretative stretch, and apparently one that a majority of the Supreme Court was unwilling to make in this case. No one seems to question whether Congress could, as a constitutional matter, regulate or even prohibit the sale or use of tobacco, presumably under Congress' plenary authority to regulate interstate commerce. The question is whether Congress has exercised that power or not. In *FDA,* the Court's answer is "no" or, at least, not at this time. For a strongly-worded and closely-argued disagreement, read the dissenting opinion by Justice Breyer in its entirety. Whatever you make of the merits of the outcome reached by the majority and explained by O'Connor, Breyer's application of the tools of statutory interpretation — text, legislative history, purpose, and deference to administrative agencies — is compelling reading.

**7.** Hidden in these cases is an important and sobering political insight. In many, though, as we have seen, not all cases, the enactment of state laws preempts further actions by city and local governments. Federal laws such as the FCLAA are enacted to regulate the sale or use of tobacco, but by implication or, in some cases, by explicit caveat, that regulation preempts further or additional efforts by local or state legislation, or by administrative action by the FDA or other federal agencies. Is the creation and enforcement of these layers of preemption merely an attempt, as O'Connor claims in *Lorillard*, to insure that legal requirements are uniform? Or are the lawyers and lobbyists of tobacco interests managing to turn today's loss into tomorrow's victory? More broadly, do you think these sorts of decisions — essentially "fixing" the limits on the regulatory requirements imposed on tobacco to no more than those that are specifically enacted at one point in time by one level of government — should be decided this way? After all, tobacco is a classic case of a problem about which we learn more and more as time goes by. Yet new solutions frequently are preempted by decades-old legal provisions. Is that unfortunate? Is it accidental?

It's very unlikely that this is an accident. It's more likely that the lawyers and lobbyists for tobacco interests knew that accepting limited regulation on their advertising and promotion in 1969 was a more than acceptable trade-off for a prohibition, one that would, in the future, bar so many other attacks on their clients. But did the public know that they were making such a deal? Did the legislators who authored it? Or were they more focused on the immediate albeit limited effects of the legislation?

## D.  LITIGATION AND ITS EFFECT ON PUBLIC POLICY CONCERNING SMOKING AND TOBACCO USE

This section addresses, first, the use of tort litigation by individuals seeking damages from tobacco companies for their smoking-related harms. In doing so it further illuminates the impact of (and some paths around) the pre-emptive provisions of the federal labeling laws. The material then turns to the "Master Settlement Agreement" (MSA) designed to end the litigation that states brought against the companies during the 1990s to recover for their expenditure of public funds on medical care necessitated by tobacco use. Litigation over the meaning and enforcement of the MSA itself followed, perhaps inevitably.

In addition to the specifics of legal doctrine (tort law, contract law, issues of federalism) and public health impact, consider these materials as a window on legal process as it affects powerful interests. Spurred by (and sometimes spurring) changes in social attitudes and scientific knowledge, litigation and legal policymaking resolve some issues — yet they also beget additional ones, which in turn generate further litigation and policymaking. The process moves onward — perhaps, on occasion, even forward.

# CARTER v. BROWN & WILLIAMSON TOBACCO CORP.
778 So. 2d 932 (Fla.), *cert. denied*, 533 U.S. 950 (2001)

Harding, Justice.

\* \* \*

Grady Carter smoked cigarettes for forty-four years, from 1947 until January 1991. Initially, Carter smoked unfiltered Lucky Strike cigarettes (a product of the American Tobacco Company or ATC, Brown & Williamson's predecessor), and in 1972, he changed to another company's product. According to Carter's testimony, he became concerned about his health on January 29, 1991, when he coughed and spit up blood. Carter, concerned that "something was bad wrong with me," consulted a family medical dictionary, which gave two possible explanations for spitting up blood: lung cancer and tuberculosis. Carter immediately called and made an appointment with Dr. Gary Decker for February 4, 1991. On January 29, 1991, Carter quit smoking.

On February 4, 1991, Dr. Decker took chest x-rays and told Carter that he had observed a spot or abnormality on his lung. According to Dr. Decker, this spot could be indicative of several things, including cancer or tuberculosis. Since Dr. Decker was not a lung specialist, he referred Carter to Dr. Bruce Yergin, a pulmonary specialist. Dr. Decker further expressed that Carter probably needed to see Dr. Yergin immediately. Carter saw Dr. Yergin the very next day.

When Carter first visited Dr. Yergin on February 5, 1991, Dr. Yergin examined the chest x-rays and observed a large left upper lobe mass lesion, which he indicated in his report was "highly suggestive of a neoplasm ['most suspicious' for a lung tumor]." Dr. Yergin also noted his impressions of this first visit in Carter's file, which read: "left upper lobe nodule, COPD (chronic obstructive pulmonary disease), chronic bronchitis, cigarette abuse — 65 pack years." Based on his initial examination of Carter's x-rays, Dr. Yergin testified that he did not tell Carter that he had lung cancer because "many different things can mimic other things on the chest x-ray" and it would have been "absolutely" incorrect to tell Carter that he had lung cancer during the initial visit. Dr. Yergin also testified that on February 5, 1991, he did not know what the nodule was; the nodule could have been tuberculosis or slowly resolving pneumonia and additional tests were necessary in order to make an accurate diagnosis.

On February 12, 1991, Dr. Yergin performed numerous tests, including a bronchoscopy, during which a tissue sample was taken from the lung. The bronchoscopy pathology report showed that Carter had lung cancer and Dr. Yergin told Carter that he had lung cancer on February 14, 1991. Ultimately, Carter had surgery to remove the cancer.

Carter and his wife filed suit against the American Tobacco Company on February 10, 1995, asserting claims for negligence and strict liability. The Carters later amended their case to reflect the merger of ATC and Brown & Williamson. The allegations in the complaint were predicated solely on Carter's smoking Lucky Strikes from 1947 until 1972. Prior to trial, the trial court ruled that whether or not the action was barred by the statute of limitations was an issue for the jury to decide. The jury subsequently determined that the action was not barred by the statute of limitations and awarded a verdict in favor of the Carters on both claims.

Brown & Williamson appealed to the First District Court of Appeal, which reversed the jury's verdict and remanded the case with the instruction that it be dismissed due to the claim being barred by the statute of limitations. . . . The court also held that if it were not for its decision regarding the statute of limitations, the court would have reversed and remanded the case for a new trial because the Carters were allowed to introduce testimony and evidence at trial which alluded to information that was preempted by the 1969 Federal Cigarette Labeling and Advertising Act. . . .

. . . .

## II. Analysis

. . . [Florida law] states that "[a]n action for injury to a person founded on the design, manufacture, distribution, or sale of personal property . . . shall be commenced . . . [w]ithin four years." The Florida statute of limitations law further provides that "[a]ctions for products liability," as described above, "must be begun within the period described in this chapter [four years], with the period running from the time the facts giving rise to the cause of action [a] were [actually] discovered [by the claimant] or [b] should have been discovered [by the claimant] with the exercise of due diligence. . . ."

Lung cancer caused by smoking is a latent or "creeping disease." . . . In products liability actions involving latent or creeping diseases, we agree with the test [that the] action accrues . . . only when the accumulated effects of the deleterious substance manifest themselves [to the claimant], in a way which supplies some evidence of causal relationship to the manufactured product."

. . . [W]e also agree . . . that the question of when the statute of limitations begins to run in this type of case is "generally treated as [a] fact question for a jury to resolve, and therefore inappropriate for resolution on a summary judgment or directed verdict.". . .

. . . .

In the present case, we acknowledge that a jury could reasonably conclude that Carter knew or should have known, on either January 29, 1991 (when Carter coughed and spit up blood) or February 4, 1991 (when Dr. Decker told Carter that he observed a spot on his lung and that this spot could be related to several things including cancer or tuberculosis), that the effects of smoking cigarettes manifested themselves to Carter in a way which supplied some evidence of a causal relationship to the cigarettes. However, we cannot agree that a jury could not reasonably fail to do so. Given that Dr. Decker gave Carter at least two possible explanations for the spot, one of which was tuberculosis based on Carter's recent contact with someone who had that disease, a reasonable person could conclude that the spot was not related to smoking or cancer. Because conflicting reasonable inferences can be drawn from the record, this issue was a question of fact for the jury to resolve.

. . . .

If it were not for its decision regarding the statute of limitations, the district court's holding would have been to reverse and remand the case for a new trial because the Carters were allowed to introduce testimony and evidence at trial which alluded to evidence that was preempted by the 1969 Federal Cigarette Labeling and Advertising Act. . . .

In 1965, Congress passed the Federal Cigarette Labeling and Advertising Act, which required all cigarette packages to contain the warning: "Caution: Cigarette Smoking May Be Hazardous to Your Health." Four years later, Congress enacted the Public Health Cigarette Smoking Act of 1969, which amended the 1965 Act to require the following warning: "The Surgeon General Has Determined That Cigarette Smoking is Dangerous to Your Health." The 1969 Act included the following provision: "(b) No requirement or prohibition based on smoking and health shall be imposed under State law with respect to the advertising or promotion of any cigarettes the packages of which are labeled in conformity with the provisions of this Act."

In *Cipollone v. Liggett,* the United States Supreme Court was asked to consider whether state common law actions filed against tobacco companies for failure to warn, breach of warranty, fraudulent misrepresentation, and conspiracy were preempted by either the 1965 or 1969 Acts. A plurality of the United States Supreme Court held that the 1965 Act only preempted state and federal rulemaking bodies from mandating particular cautionary statements and did not preempt state-law damages actions. However, the Court came to a different conclusion regarding the 1969 Act. The plurality addressed each of the claims separately. First, the plurality held that the 1969 Act expressly preempts post-1969 failure-to-warn claims that cigarette "advertising or promotions should have included additional, or more clearly stated, warnings." The plurality added that the "[1969] Act does not, however, preempt petitioner's claims that rely solely on respondent's testing or research practices or other actions unrelated to advertising or promotion." Next, the plurality concluded that express warranty claims were not preempted by the 1969 Act because liability for express warranty is not imposed under state law but rather by the warrantor's express actions. The plurality also concluded that the 1969 Act does not preempt fraudulent misrepresentation claims because fraudulent misrepresentation claims are based on a state law duty not to deceive rather than a state law duty "based on smoking and health." Finally, the plurality concluded that the 1969 Act does not preempt conspiracy to defraud claims because such claims are based on a duty not to conspire to commit fraud rather than a duty "based on smoking and health."

. . . .

Prior to trial, Brown & Williamson sought partial summary judgment as to any claim that post-1969 cigarette warning labels were inadequate. In response, the Carters argued that the 1969 Act only preempted claims regarding ATC's post-1969 *advertising or promotions,* but that according to the language of *Cipollone* itself, the 1969 Act does not preempt their claims that rely solely on ATC's "testing or research practices or other actions unrelated to advertising or promotion." The Carters also attached a number of so-called advocacy statements of the cigarette industry to its motion, as well as the affidavit of Professor Richard Polley. Polley stated in the affidavit that "in numerous instances, major cigarette manufacturers conducted public relations campaigns, including but not limited to purchasing newspaper space for making public statements [and] issuing press releases." Polley stated that such mass communications are not considered advertising or promotion, as the statements did not contain the cautionary labels which were federally required on all advertisements or promotions. In its order denying the motion for partial summary judgment, the trial court cited to Polley's affidavit and concluded that "a genuine issue of material fact" exists regarding the general usage of the terms "advertising or promotions." Brown & Williamson argues that this decision paved the way for the Carters to introduce a proposed package insert.

. . . Based on Polley's affidavit, we cannot conclude that the trial court erred in denying Brown & Williamson's motion for partial summary judgment. More importantly, any such error on this issue would be harmless, as our review of the record reveals that the Carters' claims were clearly limited to injuries which allegedly resulted from the defendant's failure to provide adequate warnings *prior* to 1969, as explained below.

. . . .

During the trial, the Carters' counsel asked Dr. Feingold about a proposed package insert which Dr. Feingold stated should have been prepared by the cigarette industry, and in particular, ATC. The defense objected, arguing that the package insert was preempted by the 1969 Act. The Carters' counsel argued at sidebar that the insert was only being offered to support the Carters' pre-1969 claims. The trial court overruled the defense's objection and permitted the introduction of the insert, but assured the defense that the jury would be specifically instructed regarding which dates to be considered by them with respect to warnings. . . .

. . . Even assuming that some of the information in the proposed insert was not available until after 1969, we do not find that this prejudiced Brown & Williamson, as this information was not the focus of Dr. Feingold's testimony. Hence, we disapprove the district court's analysis and conclusion on this issue.

. . . .

Brown & Williamson [also] asserts that the district court correctly ruled that the Carters were improperly allowed to submit proof of a cause of action they never alleged. The district court found that the Carters' use of the so-called Brown & Williamson documents during the trial, as well as expert testimony concerning the documents, in effect amounted to an unpleaded claim against Brown & Williamson in its own right rather than against Brown & Williamson as successor to ATC. Again, we disagree.

The evidence in question consisted of documentary and testimonial evidence showing research conducted by Brown & Williamson, the British American

Tobacco Company, and the Battelle Institute in the 1950s through the 1970s. The story behind how this evidence came to light is most peculiar, but fortunately the tale is one that we need not tell nor address. [The court then cites to various outside sources. See the references in the Note at end of this chapter.] The evidence allegedly revealed that Brown & Williamson and its affiliates had conducted research on the dangers of smoking and learned as early as 1963 that nicotine was addictive.

During the trial, the Carters presented the testimony of ATC officials, including a former CEO and a former research director, who testified that ATC never conducted any tests to determine whether smoking was harmful or whether nicotine was addictive. The Carters argue that the Brown & Williamson documents were relevant to establish the state of the art pertaining to possible risks associated with smoking, i.e., that had ATC conducted testing, it would have learned of the harmful nature of smoking. However, the district court below concluded that "the focus placed on the objectionable documents was less on what Brown & Williamson, and therefore other manufacturers, knew, and more on Brown & Williamson's alleged failure to disclose all that it knew, an allegation not attributable to ATC by virtue of its position in the industry."

. . . .

Florida courts have recognized that "[a] manufacturer has the duty to possess expert knowledge in the field of its product." . . . If ATC had not merged with Brown & Williamson, there would be no question that the evidence would have been admissible, as the evidence was relevant to establish that the risks of cigarette smoking that were discovered by one cigarette manufacturer were scientifically discoverable by other cigarette manufacturers. The question is therefore whether this evidence was more prejudicial than probative due to the merger. Certainly the corporate acquisition of ATC by Brown & Williamson is fortuitous; however, we do not find that this fact alone rendered the evidence inadmissible. First, after concluding that the evidence would have been admissible absent the merger, we do not believe that the Carters should be disadvantaged merely because of the corporate acquisition. Second, the trial court instructed the jury that Plaintiffs Grady and Mildred Carter do not raise claims based on the conduct of Brown & Williamson Tobacco Corporation. Their claims are based solely on the conduct of the American Tobacco Company, prior to the time that it merged with the Brown and Williamson Tobacco Corporation in 1995. . . . Based on the record in this case, we conclude that the trial court did not err in permitting the evidence.

We hold that the district court erred in its decision that the statute of limitations had run on the Carters' claims. Additionally, we find that evidence presented at trial was not preempted by the Federal Cigarette Labeling and Advertising Act. Finally, we find no merit to Brown & Williamson's argument that the Carters were allowed to proceed on an unpleaded claim. Accordingly, we quash the district court's decision in this case.

* * *

# HAGLUND v. PHILLIP MORRIS, INC.
### 446 Mass. 744, 847 N.E.2d 315 (2006)

Marshall, Chief Justice.

* * *

We determine in this case whether a cigarette manufacturer in a wrongful death action predicated on breach of the warranty of merchantability may assert as an affirmative defense that the decedent smoker's use of cigarettes was "unreasonable.". . .

Following the death from lung cancer of her husband, Stephen C. Haglund (decedent), a long-time smoker, Brenda Haglund filed a wrongful death product liability action against Philip Morris Incorporated (Philip Morris) . . . In denying all liability, Philip Morris asserted, among other things, that the decedent's decision to begin and continue smoking its cigarettes constituted "unreasonable use" pursuant to our holding in [*Correia v. Firestone Tire*]. The plaintiff moved for summary judgment to preclude assertion of the *Correia* defense, arguing that the *Corriea* defense should, as a matter of law, be unavailable because a cigarette is an inherently dangerous product that causes injury when used for its ordinary purpose. . . .

We affirm the judge's denial of the motion to strike and reverse the judgment of dismissal. As we explain more fully below, the *Correia* defense presumes that the product at issue is, in normal circumstances, reasonably safe and capable of being reasonably safely used, and therefore that the consumer's unreasonable use of the product he knows to be defective and dangerous is appropriately penalized. Here, however, both Philip Morris and the plaintiff agree that cigarette smoking is inherently dangerous and that there is no such thing as a safe cigarette. Because no cigarette can be safely used for its ordinary purpose, smoking, there can be no nonunreasonable use of cigarettes. Thus the defense, which serves to deter unreasonable use of products in a dangerous and defective state, will, in the usual course, be inapplicable.

However, we also agree with Philip Morris that, in certain conceivable scenarios, an individual consumer's behavior may be so overwhelmingly unreasonable in light of the consumer's knowledge about, for example, a specific medical condition from which he suffers, that the *Correia* defense may be invoked. The jury determines unreasonable use from the specific factual context of each case, and we are loathe to foreclose assertion of the defense as a matter of law in every cigarette-related product liability action. Because the plaintiff's motion for summary judgment on the *Correia* defense was brought early in the litigation, we reverse the judgment of dismissal to afford the parties the opportunity to develop more fully the evidence supporting their claims and defenses.

We summarize the relevant background.

1. *Background.* The decedent was born on July 22, 1948, and began smoking in 1973. The plaintiff alleged that, initially, the decedent smoked only Philip Morris's Marlboro brand cigarettes, through which he became addicted to nicotine. She also alleged that the decedent tried several times to quit smoking cigarettes. The decedent died as a result of lung cancer on May 10, 2000.

The plaintiff filed the present wrongful death action . . . in March, 2001; it was transferred to Worcester County in November, 2001, pursuant to a joint motion to sever and suspend case processing. . . . In relevant part, the plaintiff claimed the decedent used cigarettes "exactly as intended and foreseen" by the defendant, that his death was the "direct result" of his addiction to smoking Marlboro cigarettes, that Marlboro cigarettes were defectively designed because, in 1973, when the decedent began smoking, Philip Morris could have implemented, but did not, "a safer reasonable alternative design: a non-addictive cigarette through nicotine extraction," and that "[a] cigarette without nicotine would be non-addictive and would [have] enable[d] the smoker to quit smoking at will, or reduce use below disease threshold levels."

In its answer, Philip Morris denied all liability. It stated that "nicotine in cigarette smoke is addictive and that cigarette smoking is addictive," that "nicotine plays an important role in cigarette smoking," that "it can be very difficult to quit smoking," that "the technology exists to reduce, but not completely remove, the nicotine content in tobacco," and that such technology existed prior to 1973, when the decedent began smoking. Philip Morris also averred that the risks of cigarette smoking are widely known, that individual decisions whether and how much to smoke vary from individual to individual, that no consensus exists in the scientific community about what constitutes a safer alternative cigarette design, and that the company's attempt to market a reduced nicotine cigarette proved unsuccessful. Philip Morris interposed forty affirmative defenses, including, as its thirty-fourth defense, the *Correia* defense that is at the heart of this appeal.

On September 1, 2004, the plaintiff sought summary judgment to preclude Philip Morris from asserting the *Correia* defense. The grounds for preclusion were, first, that the defense is inapplicable where the product, cigarettes, "are the only consumer product in existence which when used exactly as intended, and in the complete absence of any mishaps, causes injury. . . . The plaintiff "concede[d] and . . . stipulate[d]" in her summary judgment motion that, "if [Philip Morris] is permitted to assert the defense in this case, the Defendant will prevail on the basis of this defense." . . .

. . . .

2. *Discussion.* We have not previously been asked to address the question posed by the plaintiff: whether the *Correia* defense is unavailable as a matter of law to cigarette product liability claims based on a theory of breach of the implied warranty of merchantability. Because the defense is part of a comprehensive scheme of warranty liability, we begin with an overview of the relevant law.

a. *Implied warranty of merchantability.* The plaintiff's claim for breach of the implied warranty of merchantability is governed principally by G.L. c. 106, § 2-314(20(c). We have previously noted that, as a matter of social policy, the warranty of merchantability imposes a "special responsibility" on the seller toward "*any* member of the consuming public who may be injured" by its product (emphasis added). Warranty liability is "fully as comprehensive as the strict liability theory of recovery that has been adopted by a great many other jurisdictions." . . . The stringent responsibility placed on sellers under our warranty scheme is justified on the ground that:

> [T]he public has the right to and does expect, in the case of products which it needs and for which it is forced to rely upon the seller, that reputable sellers will stand behind their goods; that public policy demands that the burden of accidental injuries caused by products intended for consumption be placed upon those who market them, and be treated as a cost of production against which liability insurance can be obtained; and that the consumer of such products is entitled to the maximum of protection at the hands of someone, and the proper persons [to] afford it are those who market them. . . .

A seller breaches its warranty obligation when a product that is "defective and unreasonably dangerous," for the "[o]rdinary purposes" for which it is "fit" causes injury. "Ordinary purposes" refers to a product's intended and foreseeable uses. "Fitness" is a question of degree that primarily, although not exclusively, concerns reasonable consumer expectations. Both "ordinary purposes" and "fitness" are concepts that demand close attention to the actual environment in which the product is used. The plaintiff in a design liability warranty case must prove that, at the time he was injured, he was "using the product in a manner that the defendant seller, manufacturer, or distributor reasonably could have foreseen." (citations omitted)

Warranty liability may be premised either on the failure to warn, or, as here, on defective design. In determining warranty liability in the latter case, the relevant inquiry focuses on the product's features, not the seller's conduct. Although the manufacturer is not expected to design against "bizarre, unforeseeable accidents," the manufacturer will be liable if its "conscious design choices" fail to anticipate the reasonably foreseeable risks of "ordinary" use. Thus, warranty liability may be imposed even where the product was properly designed, manufactured, or sold; conformed to industry standards; and passed regulatory muster, and even where the consumer used the product negligently. . . . The plaintiff need only convince the jury that a safer alternative design was feasible, not that any manufacturer in the industry employed it or even contemplated it. The . . . test is one of feasibility. The "plaintiff's case is not automatically defeated merely because the alternative design was not being used at the material time." To determine the adequacy of a product's design, the jury must weigh multiple factors, including "the gravity of the danger posed by the challenged design, the likelihood that such danger would occur, the mechanical feasibility of a safer alternative design, the financial cost of an improved design, and the adverse consequences to the product and to the consumer that would result from an alternative design." We have recognized that the balance struck by the jury is ultimately a judgment about the "social acceptability" of the design.

b. *The* Correia *defense.* As our summary above indicates, warranty liability poses weighty burdens on manufacturers to safeguard consumers. Warranty liability, however, is not "absolute." Tempering the manufacturer's burden is the duty of the consumer "to act reasonably with respect to a product which he knows to be defective and dangerous." A user who "unreasonably proceeds to use a product which he knows to be defective and dangerous" violates his "only duty" under our warranty law and thereby forfeits the law's protection. When the consumer's knowing use of a product in a dangerous and defective condition is unreasonable, the consumer's own conduct has become the proximate cause of his injuries, and he can recover nothing from the seller.

The defense is applicable only after a plaintiff has proved the case-in-chief. A defendant must then demonstrate that the plaintiff "subjectively knew that the product was defective and dangerous, and that, despite that subjective belief, the plaintiff's use of the product was objectively unreasonable, and that the plaintiff's conduct was a cause of the injury." The plaintiff's subjective knowledge of a product's defect need not be technically specific; "it is enough to show that the plaintiff knew the product was defective in some way, rather than showing that it knew the technical elements of the defect." The defense may apply even where the plaintiff's unreasonable use of the product was foreseeable.

Against the standards we have just summarized, we now examine whether, as the plaintiff argues, the defense should be foreclosed as a matter of law to defendants in tobacco product liability warranty claims.

   c. *Cigarettes and warranty liability.* The plaintiff's rationale for opposing the *Correia* defense as an affirmative defense is that "[c]igarettes are the only consumer product in existence which when used exactly as intended, and in the complete absence of any mishaps, cause injury." . . .

The manufacture, marketing, and sale of cigarettes are, indisputably, legitimate, for-profit business enterprises. The United States Congress has declared the marketing of tobacco to be "one of the greatest basic industries of the United States." [citation to the *Williamson* case] We may take judicial notice that, as a for-profit enterprise and a publicly traded company, Philip Morris seeks to manufacture, market, and sell cigarettes to the general adult public in a manner intended to attract and retain as many consumers as possible. Philip Morris does not dispute that its efforts to market and sell its cigarettes to the broad general adult public is anything other than robust.

At the same time, and as Philip Morris readily admits, cigarettes are a product that cannot be used safely for the "ordinary purposes" for which they are fit, namely, smoking. The record discloses two inherent dangers of smoking cigarettes that Philip Morris does not deny. First, cigarette smoking poses serious health risks. . . .

The second danger of cigarette smoking is that the nicotine in cigarettes is addictive. An addiction is an "[h]abitual psychological and physiological dependence on a substance or practice which is beyond voluntary control." A reasonable inference from Philip Morris's acknowledgment that the nicotine in cigarettes makes smoking addictive is that its product was consciously designed to induce cigarette dependency in the ordinary smoker, regardless whether any individual smoker becomes addicted to cigarettes.

Because the product cannot be used safely in its ordinary-use environment, cigarette merchandising is incompatible with the *Correia* defense in most circumstances. The purpose of our warranty laws, as we have shown, is to encourage safe products in the stream of commerce. The duty of the consumer is "to act reasonably with respect to a product which he knows to be defective and dangerous." But in the case of cigarette use, the consumer cannot fulfil that duty, because no nonunreasonable use of cigarettes, as they are currently designed, is possible. The social policy that animates the defense — to encourage reasonable use of products by consumers — cannot be accomplished. The legislative intent of our warranty laws would be sidestepped were the manufacturer of cigarettes permitted routinely to escape all liability merely by proving that the plaintiff was an ordinary consumer who used its products in a manner readily foreseeable.

Philip Morris argues that consumers often elect to use products that may cause harm as a "byproduct" of normal use and for which the defense presumptively is available. One can become addicted to the sugar in candy, it points out, or contract skin cancer by using suntan oil. Guns are dangerous; aspirin taken for a headache can reduce the tendency of blood to clot. These are false analogies. The fallacy in Philip Morris's argument is that in none of these examples, or others it offers, is any reasonable use of the product whatsoever foreclosed by the nature of the product itself. Sugar, suntan oil, guns, and aspirin are not inherently addictive to the general public or incapable of being used reasonably. The *Correia* defense is available for warranty claims for these products because the defense serves an actual purpose: to deter a consumer from knowingly using a product in a defective and dangerous (as opposed to its ordinary) condition. The consumer has a choice of using a product reasonably or unreasonably, and the defense penalizes the consumer for unreasonable use. It does not presume that the only safe use of a product is nonuse, a position urged on us by Philip Morris but which runs contrary to our entire scheme of commerce.

We have examined the numerous warranty cases cited to us by the parties in which the defense was invoked and there is none where the defendant conceded that reasonable use of the product was impossible. . . .

Nor do we conclude, in the circumstances of this case, that the plaintiff's stipulation of knowing unreasonable use to be fatal. On the record before us, the plaintiff's stipulation restates the obvious: that cigarettes cannot be used safely and therefore that cigarette use is unreasonable. The stipulation that the decedent was aware of the well-publicized health risks of cigarettes merely places him in the same position as the ordinary consumer or potential consumer of cigarettes. Without more, it is insufficient to justify dismissal of the defective design warranty claim.

Our conclusion does not, as Philip Morris claims, eviscerate the *Correia* defense. We agree with the defendant that the "key to the defense is not the care, knowledge, or intent of the manufacturer, but the duty of the user to act reasonably concerning a product known to be defective and dangerous." But where the defendant merchant affirmatively invites the consumer to use a product that cannot safely be used for its ordinary purposes, then public policy demands that the merchant bear the burden of reasonably foreseeable injuries that result from that invitation. If Philip Morris chooses to market an inherently dangerous product, it is at the very least perverse to allow the company to escape liability by showing only that its product was used for its ordinary purpose.

We agree with Philip Morris, however, that a defendant in a cigarette product liability warranty claim should not be entirely foreclosed from asserting the defense as a matter of law. We are persuaded by Philip Morris's argument that, in certain situations, a consumer's use of cigarettes may be so overwhelmingly unreasonable as to make the imposition of warranty liability on the merchant fundamentally unfair. When a consumer, for example, begins smoking cigarettes knowing that she has a particular medical condition, such as emphysema that is exacerbated by smoking, the *Correia* defense may be appropriately invoked. To succeed in interposing the defense in such circumstances, the defendant must demonstrate that the plaintiff knew of her particular medical condition and the risks smoking posed to that specific condition at the time she began smoking. The defendant need not show that the consumer had a medical expert's knowledge of the risk; it is enough for the defendant to demonstrate that the plaintiff knew that smoking would exacerbate her specific illness.

The record before us contains no evidence that the decedent's use of cigarettes was overwhelmingly unreasonable in the manner we have described above. However, the plaintiff brought her summary judgment motion early in the litigation, when neither side had full opportunity for discovery. At that stage, the judge properly denied the motion to strike the defense, but she terminated the case prematurely. We do not foreclose the plaintiff from renewing, at a later time and on a more fully developed record, her motion to preclude the *Correia* defense.

. . . .

For the reasons stated above, we affirm the judge's denial of the motion to strike but reverse the judgment of dismissal. The case is remanded to the Superior Court for further proceedings consistent with this opinion.

* * *

# NOTES AND QUESTIONS

**1.** As illustrated by the *Carter* decision, there have been many private lawsuits by smokers claiming that they have been injured by smoking tobacco products, based on a variety of theories. Prior to the 1990s, virtually all such efforts were unsuccessful, either because of a failure to prove causation or due to some variation on the argument that "everybody knows smoking is unhealthy and anyone who smokes is choosing to accept the consequent risks."

In the 1990s, however, private litigants began to meet with occasional success, at least where they were seeking damages for injuries prior to the 1960s, when the first Surgeon General's Report confirmed and publicized the health risks of smoking. Also pivotal were the revelations in the 1990s that smoking was, in fact, far more dangerous than had been previously believed and that the nicotine levels in cigarettes were being enhanced by the tobacco manufacturers, despite claims to the contrary. Some of these revelations came out during discovery in the *Cipollone* litigation, described *infra*; but public and political attention was particularly galvanized when a Congressman released documents that a former employee of Brown & Williamson, a British-American tobacco company, had stolen from his employer, revealing that the tobacco companies' knowledge of the enhanced risks of smoking and of the addictive properties of nicotine was far more extensive than they had claimed — even in their courtroom statements. The results were devastating to the tobacco companies' public and judicial standing. As noted in *Carter*, the "Brown & Williamson documents" have played an evidentiary role in many subsequent lawsuits. For a good description of the disclosure of those documents, see S.A. Glantz, et al., *Looking Through a Keyhole at the Tobacco Industry: The Brown & Williamson Documents*, 274 JAMA 219 (1995); S.A. GLANTZ, ET AL., THE CIGARETTE PAPERS (1996) (available online at www.ark.cdlib.org/ (last visited December 2006). To view the documents and other related papers, see www.library.ucsf.edu/tobacco (last visited December 2006) (The University of California at San Francisco library acts as an official repository of documents that have been released incident to various lawsuits or as part of the settlement agreement between the states and the tobacco industry, described *infra*).

In *Cipollone v. Liggett Group*, 505 U.S. 504 (1992), a plurality of the Supreme Court addressed the pre-emptive impact of the FCLAA and other federal laws on smokers' state-law-based claims against tobacco companies. As summarized in *Carter,* the Court found that the 1964 federal legislation preempted only agency regulatory action imposing additional or variant "warnings," but did not preempt private litigation based on state common law theories. The language of the 1969 amendments to the FCLAA, however, pre-empted many privately common law claims as well — those relating to advertising, package warnings, and other matters that are the subject of the federal legislation — but not claims based on express warranties, fraudulent behavior, and other activities unrelated to advertising and promotion.

For other, more recent cases that have attempted to determine which sorts of privately initiated lawsuits survive federal preemption, see *Rivera v. Phillip Morris, Inc.*, 395 F.3d 1142 (9th Cir. 2005) (Nevada state strict liability cause of action survives federal preemption, but plaintiffs face various difficult problems of proof); *Burton v. R.J. Reynolds, Tobacco Co.*, 397 F.3d 906 (10th Cir. 2005) (plaintiff's action for failure to warn and failure to test may proceed, but no action for fraudulent concealment; compensatory but not punitive damages available to plaintiff). *See also Grisham v. Phillip Morris U.S.A.*, 403 F.3d 631 (9th Cir. 2005) (discussion of the elements of proof under California state law in cases brought by private litigants).

**2.** *Haglund* is potentially a significant decision for two reasons: It is based on a calim that the defendants violated their duty under an implied warranty of merchantability — a claim that may not be preempted by the FCLAA; and it allows the plaintiff to overcome what is often the most difficult barrier to lawsuits brought by smokers against tobacco manufacturers: the plaintiff-smoker's knowledge of the risks of smoking. As described in the text of the opinion, typically a defendant in a suit based on product liability or a related cause of action can claim that the plaintiff(s) knew of the defect or "unreasonable risk" but used the product anyway. That "unreasonable risk" defense (as recognized in the *Correia* decision in Massachusetts), however, is not available where there is no "*non*unreasonable" (the court's word) use of the product; that is, the product is inherently dangerous even if used as intended by the manufacturer. The implications of that limitation on the "unreasonable use" defense are potentially far-reaching.

On the other hand, the significance of *Haglund* is premised on the particular doctrine of product liability alleged by the plaintiff and applicable in Massachusetts, breach of the "implied warranty of merchantability." The Massachusetts court expressly distinguishes this theory from "the strict liability theory of recovery that has been adopted by a great many other jurisdictions'" the latter appears to be more common, and may not lend itself to the doctrinal twist implemented by the Massachusetts court.

Assume that you are in a jurisdiction that embraces the Massachusetts approach for smokers claiming injury, at least in some cases. Consider application of the Massachusetts approach — including its treatment of the "unreasonable risk" defense — in similar actions brought against (a) manufacturers of high-fat foods, (b) guns, or (c) other potential risks to the public's health. Are such cases essentially the same as *Haglund,* or are there legally significant differences? Phrased otherwise, if you find *Haglund* well-reasoned, is that because you favor rejection of the "unreasonable risk" defense generally, or because you think tobacco is particularly dangerous and should be regarded differently from other potential public health risks? (See related discussion of private litigation against food manufacturers in Chapter Six and against gun sellers and manufacturers in Chapter Seven.)

**3.** For a good, recent example of a successful private lawsuit and the award of punitive damages of over $79 million to the family of a deceased smoker, see *Williams v. Philip Morris, Inc.*, 340 Ore. 35, 127 P.3d 1165 (2006) (reviewing the efforts of the defendants to defraud the public concerning the health effects of smoking and the addictive properties of nicotine, and rejecting a constitutional challenge to the size of the punitive damage award) In November of 2006, the Supreme Court heard argument on this case. *See* 126 S. Ct. 2329 (2006).

Obviously such private lawsuits are even more significant if they involve multiple plaintiffs. In *Castano v. American Tobacco Co.*, 84 F.3d 734 (5th Cir. 1996), the plaintiffs were initially successful in obtaining a motion for class certification on behalf of all smokers and nicotine dependent persons and their families against all American tobacco companies. As such, the litigation would have been the largest class action ever attempted in federal court. The court of appeals held that the multi-state class was improperly certified because the district court's inquiry did not include consideration of how the trial on the merits would be conducted, and the class independently failed the "superiority requirement," (the requirement that a class action be superior to alternative forms of adjudication).

For another, similar effort, see *Philip Morris, Inc. v. Angeletti*, 358 Md. 689, 752 A.2d 200 (2000) (certification of class action denied). *See also SEIU Health & Welfare Fd. v. Philip Morris, Inc.*, 249 F.3d 1068 (D.C. Cir. 2001), *cert. denied*, 534 U.S. 994 (2001) (RICO suits by labor unions and by foreign countries denied).

For additional citations and other references concerning privately initiated lawsuits against tobacco manufacturers, see ACTION ON SMOKING AND HEALTH, www.ash.org/ (last visited December 2006). For a compendium of lawsuits and an accounting of awards that have actually paid, see www.tobacco. neu.edu/ (last visited December 2006).

None of these privately initiated lawsuits fits neatly into the usual concept of "public health." Their significance in the present context lies in their potential impact on the tobacco industry. While few of the individual lawsuits and none of the multiple-party lawsuits have been successful in obtaining damages from the tobacco companies, obviously any large scale award would affect the profitability and, possibly, the financial stability of the complex of industries that produces and sells cigarettes and other tobacco products. While it is unlikely that it would happen, if the award of damages were great enough — the amount paid by the tobacco companies would have to be measured in tens of billions of dollars to really affect their stability — the net result could have a more widespread effect on the availability of tobacco in the United States than any of the governmental "public health" measures that have been undertaken thus far.

**4.** In 1999 the U.S. Attorney General filed suit against cigarette manufacturers and related organizations claiming that they had engaged in a fraudulent pattern of covering up the dangers of tobacco use and had disguised their efforts to market cigarettes to minors. In large part, these allegations were based on the "tobacco papers" that had been discovered during the privately initiated lawsuits discussed *supra*. The government argued that under the federal RICO [anti-racketeering] legislation the courts could order both injunctive relief and disgorgement of all profits from the allegedly unlawful activities — essentially asking for hundreds of billions of dollars in damages. In 2000, the district court dismissed most of the other claims, but allowed the government to proceed on the RICO claim. In the Spring of 2005, the D.C. Circuit issued an opinion holding that disgorgement of profits is not available under the RICO legislation, and holding that the government could seek only injunctive relief, essentially gutting the government's case. *See United States v. Philip Morris USA, Inc.,* 396 F.3d 1190 (D.C. Cir.), *cert. denied,* 126 S. Ct. 478 (2005). Following that decision, the attorney general announced that if the government were successful in pursuing the remaining viable causes of action, it would seek $140 million from the defendants, claimed to be the cost to the government of pursuing the lawsuit. The attorney general also announced that the government would seek $10 billion in damages from the defendants and use those damages to fund an anti-smoking campaign — a vastly lower figure than the $140 billion in damages it had earlier sought. For an explanation, see 2005 WL 1830815 (unreported opinion of the district court). Separately, the federal government was pursuing an appeal of the circuit court ruling concerning disgorgement. For updates, see www. usdoj.gov/civil/cases/tobacco2/ (last visited November 2006). For the latest decision in this extended litigation (an extended discourse on the history of malfeasance by the industry, see *United States v. Philip Morris USA, Inc.,* F. Supp. 2d. __ (D.D.C. 2006).

# A Brief Summary of the 1998 Master Settlement Agreement Between the States and Tobacco Manufacturers

As the evidence mounted in the 1990s revealing that the manufacturers of tobacco products knew much more about the dangers of smoking and the addictive properties of nicotine than they had previously claimed, a number of individual states initiated lawsuits against the tobacco companies, essentially asking for the recovery of the states' Medicaid funds spent for smoking-related health care. Some of the states' lawsuits were based on common law equity theories, others on claims of fraud or antitrust violations. Many of these claims did not survive even initial judicial examination, but some were still active and before the courts in 1996 when some of the larger tobacco companies began negotiating with several of the states with the intention of striking some sort of settlement. At that same time, there were many privately initiated lawsuits before the courts; and the FDA was pursuing the regulatory efforts that culminated in the *FDA* decision.

The first round of settlement negotiations was brokered with the help of various congressional leaders who had anticipated that federal legislation would be necessary to codify the ultimate agreement. Ultimately, the various parties, alternately blaming each other, the political climate, and the uncertainty of various pending lawsuits, were unable to agree on anything. The negotiations that resulted in the final agreement in 1998 began in 1997 as some of the states' lawsuits became more promising and, in fact, in three states (Florida, Mississippi, and Texas), multi-billion dollar settlements had been completed between the individual states and the larger tobacco companies. Authored by the attorneys general of Washington State and several other key states, and the "Big Four of tobacco:" the Philip Morris, RJR Nabisco, Brown & Williamson, and Lorillard companies, a settlement agreement was finalized in November of 1998. Eventually all of the states that had not previously settled individual lawsuits, signed on to the agreement (and under the terms of the agreement, other tobacco companies were allowed to join as well).

The key terms of the agreement are described below:

## Financial payments to the states

The tobacco companies agreed to make annual payments to the states in perpetuity, estimated to total over $206 billion at least through the year 2025 (and to continue as long as the companies exist); these payments were intended to compensate states for the Medicaid-related costs of the states' smokers. In addition, they agreed to pay $1.5 billion in attorney fees to private lawyers who had represented the states. (Additional one-time payments for anti-tobacco programs are described below.)

The tobacco companies make their annual payments into a fund based on an initial schedule of payments, adjusted each year by 3 percent or the Consumer Price Index, whichever is greater, but subject to "volume adjustments," *i.e.*, the payments of each tobacco company rise or fall if their sales increase or decrease. There is also an allowance for adjustments if federal legislation is enacted affecting these obligations and if other tobacco companies join in the settlement agreement (which many have). The states receive their payments from a master fund; each state's share is based on a formula reflecting its efforts in resolving the initial lawsuits and reaching the settlement (*i.e.*, some states, such as the State of Washington, receive a larger proportional share because of the lead role of the state's attorney general in the negotiations.)

## Limits on advertising and promotion

The tobacco companies agreed to various advertising limits, including a ban on transit and billboard signs, bans on advertising at sporting events, and prohibitions on product placement in movies and videos and on merchandise bearing cigarette brand logos.

The companies agreed not to oppose proposed state or local laws intended to limit youth access or consumption of tobacco products; or to oppose legislation banning the manufacture or sale of cigarettes in packs less than 20.

The companies agreed to stop using Joe Camel and other cartoons in advertising and promotion, packaging, or labeling.

They agreed to stop hiding what they knew about the health effects of tobacco products, and to release secret documents concerning those effects, and to shut down the research institute that had produced tobacco-friendly research. (For references to the current sources of the secret documents, see websites *infra*.)

The companies agreed to provide $250 million ($25 million a year for the first ten years) for a foundation dedicated to reducing youth smoking and $1.5 billion for national anti-smoking advertisement campaign. (This foundation is the American Legacy Foundation, described *infra* in *American Legacy Foundation v. Lorrilard Tobacco*.)

## Terms related to the maintenance of market share and regulation of non-participating tobacco companies

Under the terms of the settlement, if the combined market share of the settling tobacco companies is reduced below what it was in 1997 in any particular state (prior to the settlement), the financial obligations of the tobacco companies are reduced by a percentage determined by a complicated formula set out in the settlement agreement — unless the state in question enacts a "qualifying statute," a state law that would impose a tax or other charges on the sale of cigarettes by companies that are not parties to the settlement that would effectively neutralize any price advantage. (The settlement anticipates that the payments by the tobacco companies will require all participating companies to raise the price of their products in order to make the payments to the states.) In fact, most domestic and many foreign tobacco companies have joined in the settlement.

## Terms related to the settlement of past and future lawsuits

Under the terms of the settlement, the states and local governments are precluded from pursuing lawsuits for past or future actions by the tobacco companies, or anyone else involved in the production, marketing, or sale of tobacco products, except for criminal violations, and except for civil actions brought to enforce the provisions of the settlement.

Why would the tobacco companies agree to these restrictions and, in particular, to make payments, in perpetuity, to the states, especially payments that may total hundreds of billions of dollars? What do they gain from doing so?

The answer is *not* that they feared losing the state-initiated lawsuits. The answer has more to do with the indirect and direct effects of the settlement on the future of the tobacco companies and their business. The states now have a very good reason not to unduly hinder tobacco sales, through taxes that might ultimately reduce demand or through other measures. The more tobacco products that are sold, the more money each state will get. If a state decides to reduce the sale or use of tobacco, fine. The obligations of the companies are reduced accordingly. For that matter, if the sales of a particular company changes, the payments by that company are changed accordingly. Each state must be aware of the implications for its own treasury.

So long as the tobacco companies can raise their prices to cover their obligations to pay the states, they don't really lose money; rather they maintain their current, rather profitable status and that status is secured into the future. Moreover, one major category of litigant — the states — has settled all past and future lawsuits. Not a bad deal, eh?

For additional information on the Master Settlement Agreement, see www.atga.wa/gov/tobacco (Washington Attorney General's website, last visited December 2006); www.naag.org/document (national association of attorneys general's website; last visited December 2006); www. library.ucsf.edu/tobacco (for papers released as a result of the settlement; last visited December 2006); www.tobacco.neu.edu/msa (website of the Tobacco Control Resource Center, Inc.; last visited December 2006).

For a good discussion of the role of non-participating tobacco companies and the "qualifying statute provisions," see Richard Daynard, *The Non-Participating Manufacturer Adjustment, Qualifying Statutes, and the Model Statute in Exhibit T of the MSA*, THE MULTISTATE MASTER SETTLEMENT AGREEMENT AND THE FUTURE OF STATE AND LOCAL TOBACCO CONTROL (1999) (available on the Tobacco Control Resource Center website *supra*).

## STATE TOBACCO-PREVENTION SPENDING vs. STATE TOBACCO REVENUES

[All amounts are in millions of dollars per year, except where otherwise indicated]
Despite receiving massive amounts of annual revenue from tobacco taxes and the state tobacco lawsuit settlements with the cigarette companies, the vast majority of states are still failing to invest even the minimum amounts recommended by the U.S. Centers for Disease Control and Prevention (CDC) to prevent and reduce tobacco use and minimize related health harms and costs.

| State | Annual Smoking Caused Health Costs | FY 2006 Tobacco Prevention Spending | CDC Minimum Prevention Spending Target | Tobacco Prevention Spending % of CDC Minimum | Tobacco Prevention Spending Rank (1= high) | FY 2006 State Tobacco Settlement Revenues (est.) | FY 2006 State Tobacco Tax Revenues (est.) | Total Annual State Revenues From Tobacco (est.) | Tobacco Prevention Spending % of Tobacco Revenue |
|---|---|---|---|---|---|---|---|---|---|
| States Total | $89+ billion | $551.0 | $1.6 billion | 34.4% | -- | $7,179 | $14,105 | $21,283.9 | 2.6% |
| Alabama | $1.38 bill. | $0.325 | $26.7 | 1.2% | 44 | $97.8 | $133.2 | $231.0 | 0.1% |
| Alaska | $156 | $5.7 | $8.1 | 70.5% | 12 | $20.7 | $62.9 | $83.6 | 6.8% |
| Arizona | $1.18 bill. | $23.1 | $27.8 | 83.1% | 6 | $89.2 | $274.0 | $363.2 | 6.4% |
| Arkansas | $748 | $17.5 | $17.9 | 97.7% | 5 | $50.1 | $144.4 | $194.5 | 9.0% |
| California | $8.41 bill. | $79.7 | $165.1 | 48.3% | 16 | $772.5 | $1,033.4 | $1,805.9 | 4.4% |
| Colorado | $1.21 bill. | $27.0 | $24.5 | 110.0% | 2 | $83.0 | $205.4 | $288.4 | 9.4% |
| Connecticut | $1.50 bill. | $0.04 | $21.2 | 0.2% | 45 | $112.4 | $271.2 | $383.6 | 0.0% |
| Delaware | $262 | $9.2 | $8.6 | 106.6% | 3 | $23.9 | $70.4 | $94.4 | 9.7% |
| DC | $224.1 | $0.0 | $7.5 | 0.0% | 51 | $36.7 | $20.8 | $57.5 | 0.0% |
| Florida | $5.82 bill. | $1.0 | $78.4 | 1.3% | 43 | $391.6 | $437.6 | $829.2 | 0.1% |
| Georgia | $2.07 bill. | $3.1 | $42.6 | 7.3% | 39 | $148.5 | $228.7 | $377.3 | 0.8% |
| Hawaii | $309 | $5.8 | $10.8 | 53.8% | 14 | $36.4 | $80.5 | $116.9 | 5.0% |
| Idaho | $294 | $0.544 | $11.0 | 4.9% | 42 | $22.0 | $50.5 | $72.4 | 0.8% |
| Illinois | $3.78 bill. | $11.0 | $64.9 | 16.9% | 34 | $281.7 | $724.6 | $1,006.3 | 1.1% |
| Indiana | $1.91 bill. | $10.8 | $34.8 | 31.1% | 27 | $123.5 | $334.2 | $457.7 | 2.4% |
| Iowa | $937 | $5.6 | $19.3 | 28.9% | 30 | $52.6 | $92.1 | $144.8 | 3.9% |
| Kansas | $854 | $1.0 | $18.1 | 5.5% | 41 | $50.5 | $121.2 | $171.7 | 0.6% |
| Kentucky | $1.38 bill. | $2.7 | $25.1 | 10.8% | 37 | $106.6 | $141.9 | $248.5 | 1.1% |
| Louisiana | $1.35 bill. | $8.0 | $27.1 | 29.5% | 29 | $136.5 | $141.3 | $277.8 | 2.9% |
| Maine | $554 | $14.2 | $11.2 | 126.9% | 1 | $46.6 | $138.8 | $185.4 | 7.7% |
| Maryland | $1.80 bill. | $9.2 | $30.3 | 30.4% | 28 | $136.8 | $263.2 | $400.0 | 2.3% |
| Massachusetts | $3.26 bill. | $4.3 | $35.2 | 12.1% | 36 | $244.4 | $419.8 | $664.2 | 0.6% |
| Michigan | $3.13 bill. | $0.0 | $54.8 | 0.0% | 51 | $263.4 | $1,196.4 | $1,459.8 | 0.0% |
| Minnesota | $1.90 | $22.1 | $28.6 | 77.2% | 9 | $184.9 | $369.3 | $554.2 | 4.0% |
| Mississippi | $662 | $20.0 | $18.8 | 106.4% | 4 | $121.0 | $53.9 | $174.9 | 11.4% |
| Missouri | $1.96 bill. | $0.0 | $32.8 | 0.0% | 51 | $137.7 | $107.0 | $244.7 | 0.0% |
| Montana | $255 | $6.8 | $9.4 | 72.6% | 11 | $25.7 | $89.1 | $114.8 | 5.9% |
| Nebraska | $494 | $3.0 | $13.3 | 22.5% | 32 | $36.0 | $70.4 | $106.4 | 2.8% |
| Nevada | $520 | $4.2 | $13.5 | 31.2% | 26 | $36.9 | $125.2 | $162.1 | 2.6% |
| New Hampshire | $519 | $0.0 | $10.9 | 0.0% | 51 | $40.3 | $137.2 | $177.5 | 0.0% |
| New Jersey | $2.92 bill. | $11.5 | $45.1 | 25.5% | 31 | $234.0 | $817.9 | $1,051.9 | 1.1% |
| New Mexico | $425 | $6.0 | $13.7 | 43.8% | 19 | $36.1 | $62.7 | $98.7 | 6.1% |
| New York | $7.52 bill. | $43.4 | $95.8 | 45.3% | 18 | $772.4 | $972.5 | $1,744.9 | 2.5% |
| North Carolina | $2.26 bill. | $15.0 | $42.6 | 35.2% | 23 | $141.2 | $153.7 | $294.9 | 5.1% |
| North Dakota | $228 | $3.1 | $8.2 | 38.0% | 22 | $22.2 | $19.8 | $42.0 | 7.4% |
| Ohio | $4.02 bill. | $47.2 | $61.7 | 76.4% | 10 | $304.9 | $1,009.1 | $1,314.0 | 3.6% |
| Oklahoma | $1.07 bill. | $8.9 | $21.8 | 40.8% | 21 | $62.7 | $298.4 | $361.1 | 2.5% |
| Oregon | $1.02 bill. | $3.5 | $21.1 | 16.3% | 35 | $69.5 | $238.0 | $307.5 | 1.1% |
| Pennsylvania | $4.78 bill. | $32.9 | $65.6 | 50.2% | 15 | $347.8 | $1,032.9 | $1,380.7 | 2.4% |
| Rhode Island | $466 | $2.1 | $9.9 | 21.2% | 33 | $43.5 | $140.5 | $184.0 | 1.1% |
| South Carolina | $1.00 bill. | $0.0 | $23.9 | 0.0% | 51 | $71.2 | $29.0 | $100.2 | 0.0% |
| South Dakota | $252 | $0.707 | $8.7 | 8.1% | 38 | $21.1 | $26.8 | $47.9 | 1.5% |
| Tennessee | $1.99 bill. | $0.0 | $32.2 | 0.0% | 51 | $147.7 | $115.6 | $263.3 | 0.0% |
| Texas | $5.36 bill. | $7.0 | $103.2 | 6.8% | 40 | $501.2 | $548.5 | $1,049.7 | 0.7% |
| Utah | $322 | $7.2 | $15.2 | 47.3% | 17 | $26.9 | $57.7 | $84.6 | 8.5% |
| Vermont | $215 | $4.9 | $7.9 | 61.9% | 13 | $24.9 | $50.7 | $75.6 | 6.5% |
| Virginia | $1.92 bill. | $12.8 | $38.9 | 32.9% | 24 | $123.8 | $159.2 | $282.9 | 4.5% |
| Washington | $1.80 bill. | $27.2 | $33.3 | 81.6% | 7 | $124.3 | $417.1 | $541.3 | 5.0% |
| West Virginia | $636 | $5.9 | $14.2 | 41.7% | 20 | $53.6 | $102.0 | $155.6 | 3.8% |
| Wisconsin | $1.86 bill. | $10.0 | $31.2 | 32.1% | 25 | $125.4 | $298.3 | $423.7 | 2.4% |
| Wyoming | $125 | $5.9 | $7.4 | 79.9% | 8 | $15.0 | $15.8 | $30.8 | 19.2% |

Source: www.tobaccofreekids.org/reports/settlements/2006/spendingrevenues (last visited February 2006)

# AMERICAN LEGACY FOUNDATION v. LORILLARD TOBACCO CO.
### 886 A.2d 1 (Del. Ct. Chan. 2005)

Lamb, Vice Chancellor.

\* \* \*

This litigation arises out of the historic 1998 tobacco settlement between the nation's largest tobacco companies and 46 of the states' attorneys general. In the settlement, the tobacco companies agreed to fund a foundation charged with creating programs to reduce youth tobacco product usage in the United

States. As part of its mission, the foundation created a series of television and radio ads under the brand "the truth."

. . . .

The defendant is Lorillard Tobacco Company, the oldest tobacco company in the United States and a Delaware corporation. The plaintiff is American Legacy Foundation ("ALF"), a Delaware non-profit corporation formed pursuant to the terms of the Master Settlement Agreement (the "MSA"), a 1998 agreement whereby the nation's largest tobacco companies settled lawsuits brought against them by the attorneys general of 46 states. The MSA requires that the tobacco signatories make collective Base Fund Payments of $25,000,000 per year for nine years. The MSA also requires the tobacco signatories to make collective payments in the amount of $250,000,000 in 1999 and $300,000,000 per year for the next four years for ALF's National Public Education Fund ("NPEF"). These funds have been used by ALF to produce its ad campaigns.

ALF's mission, as originally stated in the MSA and later incorporated into ALF's bylaws, is to educate America's youth about the dangers of tobacco products and to reduce the usage of tobacco products by young people. To fulfill its mission, ALF launched an advertising campaign universally known as "the truth" campaign. This campaign involved various television and radio ads aimed at young people that portray the negative side of tobacco products. To make sure that its ads were effective in reaching young people, ALF purposefully made them edgier and more confrontational than regular television and radio ads. Many ads could be described as "in your face" and "eye-catching."

The funding provided to ALF pursuant to the MSA did not come without restrictions. A majority of ALF's funding was earmarked for the public's education (i.e., advertising), and the content of that advertising is made subject to both requirements and prohibitions. The MSA required that the advertising concern only the "addictiveness, health effects, and social costs related to the use of tobacco products." The MSA also prohibited the advertising from being a personal attack or a vilification of tobacco company employees or tobacco companies.

The relationship between ALF and the tobacco companies got off to a rocky start. In July 2001, Lorillard threatened litigation against ALF because of a radio ad that mentions Lorillard by name and implies that cigarettes contain dog urine. Lorillard initially threatened claims of defamation and unfair business practices against ALF, but later changed its position to assert that ALF's ads were a breach of the MSA.

In a January 18, 2002 letter, Lorillard notified ALF that it intended to bring suit for a breach of the MSA. Lorillard could not, however, bring suit at that time due to a 30-day notice provision of the MSA. ALF, as a non-signatory to the MSA, was not similarly bound. Thus, after a Lorillard spokesman indicated that Lorillard might sue ALF in 46 different states, ALF sued first, filing this action in Delaware on February 13, 2002.

In its complaint, ALF seeks a declaratory judgment that its advertisements do not violate Section VI(h) of the MSA. ALF also seeks injunctive relief on the theory that the continuing threat of litigation from Lorillard, especially the possibility that it may need to defend itself in multiple jurisdictions, threatened irreparable harm to its ability to continue its day-to-day operations.

Lorillard counterclaims that ALF's advertisements violate Section VI(h) of the MSA. . . .

This opinion is the fourth in a series of opinions concerning the litigation between these parties. In *Lorillard I,* the court held that ALF's claims would be litigated in Delaware. In *Lorillard II,* the court granted partial summary judgment in favor of Lorillard, finding that the MSA could be enforced against ALF even though it did not sign the agreement. In *Lorillard III,* the court granted a motion to compel certain documents, and denied a motion to compel other documents, all of which related to the contested advertisements.

Now, after years of litigation and several months before trial, both parties move for summary judgment, neither party contending that there is a material issue of fact.

## C.   The Dispute

Section VI(h) of the MSA is at the center of the dispute between Lorillard and ALF. That section, titled "Foundation Activities," states, in relevant part, as follows:

> The Foundation shall not engage in, nor shall any of the Foundation's money be used to engage in, any political activities of lobbying, including, but not limited to, support of or opposition to candidates, ballot initiatives, referenda or other similar activities. The National Public Education Fund shall be used only for public education and advertising regarding the addictiveness, health effects, and social costs related to the use of tobacco products and shall not be used for any personal attack on, or vilification of, any person (whether by name or business affiliation), company, or governmental agency, whether individually or collectively.

The parties argue about three separate clauses in this provision:(1) the anti-vilification and personal attack clause; (2) the restriction of ALF to addressing the "addictiveness, health effects, and social costs related to the use of tobacco products" (the "three criteria clause"); and (3) the funding of ALF's advertisements. . . .

## 1.   Vilification And Personal Attack

The fundamental argument between the parties is the meaning of the word "vilification" and the phrase "personal attack." ALF defines vilification as "advertising that strikes out at tobacco companies or their employees with extreme intensity and contains untruthful information." ALF defines a personal attack as "advertising that is hostile or aggressive in tone and addresses subjects that are strictly private-individual characteristics unrelated to the person's public role.". . . In contrast, Lorillard defines "vilification" and "personal attack" with less forceful terminology. Lorillard defines vilification as "the use of words or visuals that have the tendency to degrade, disparage, or lessen the standing of another." Lorillard defines personal attack as "a negative depiction or hostile criticism of another." Lorillard argues that under these definitions, ALF has violated Section VI(h) of the MSA.

## 2.    The Addictiveness, Health Effects, And Social Costs Related To The Use Of Tobacco Products

ALF argues that all of the ads in question address the addictiveness, health effects, and social costs related to the use of tobacco products. ALF also maintains that Lorillard has challenged whether some of the ads meet this standard. . . .

## 3.    The Funding Of ALF's Ads

ALF argues that Section VI(h) treats the two sources of funds differently. It maintains that the first sentence relates to its Base Fund and that the second sentence relates to the NPEF. ALF claims that "the Base Fund, unlike the NPEF, is not subject to the constraints of either the three-criteria clause or the vilification/personal attack clause." Thus, according to ALF, "as a matter of law, advertisements funded out of the Base Fund cannot violate those clauses." . . .

## D.    The Ads

For purposes of this motion, the parties stipulate that a determination of whether ALF has violated Section VI(h) of the MSA is confined to a select group of 20 ads. The parties chose this group of ads nearly a year ago, each side designating 10 ads. For the past year, the parties have conducted extensive discovery about those ads.

During the discovery process, ALF sought information from Lorillard that would prove or disprove the truth of the ads. Lorillard refused to provide the information, claiming that the truthfulness of the ads was not relevant to the court's analysis of the MSA as a contractual agreement. Indeed, Lorillard has not pointed to one fact in ALF's ads which has not been publicly admitted by either Lorillard or one of the other signatories to the MSA. For the purposes of this motion, if the court determines that truthfulness is relevant, Lorillard concedes that the court can assume all of the contested ads are true. ALF maintains now that truth matters, although there is evidence of a memo written by its CEO that truth is not a defense to vilification.

The ads are as follows, categorized by campaign:

In *Shredder,* two youths stand outside of an urban corporate building with a large machine described as the "Shredder 2000," which appears to be a large wood chipper. The building is identified only as a major tobacco company, although in reality it is Philip Morris's headquarters. The youths use megaphones to address employees in the building, asking them if there are "a lot of embarrassing reports lying around the office." One of the youths then tells the employees that they "need" the Shredder 2000 to handle reports from the tobacco industry that say "today's teenager is tomorrow's potential regular customer." He then runs to the back of Shredder 2000 and throws what appears to be a report into the chipper. The report is instantly shredded. The youths also point out that the reports do not even need to be removed from where they are, shredding a file cabinet, a briefcase, and a computer. The ad concludes with a voice over that says "Shredder 2000-now available in regular and king-size."

In *Hypnosis,* three youths driving a truck "somewhere in tobacco suburbia" ask various passers-by where tobacco company executives live. Eventually, they find their way to a suburban housing development. The setting is at night and the houses have their interior lights on. Inside the van, the youths marvel at the size of the large homes, saying that working in an industry that kills over a thousand people a day pays "pretty well." Then they cue a pre-recorded tape linked to a public address system on top of the truck. On the tape, a woman's voice speaks in hypnotic monotone. The following are examples of what the voice says: "I am a good person;" "Selling a product that kills people makes me uncomfortable;" "I realize that cigarettes are addictive;" and "Tomorrow I will look for a new job." The ad ends with a youth announcing that they are "just trying to help."

In *Body Bags,* an unmarked truck pulls up "outside a major tobacco company." A group of youths rush to the back of the truck, where the door opens. They begin to pull large bags out of the truck. The bags are marked in large block lettering "BODY BAGS." The youths stack the bags on the sidewalk next to the tobacco company building while employees inside watch. The bags line two sides outside of the building. Then, using a megaphone, a youth asks the employees inside if they know how many people tobacco kills every day. The answer is 1,200 people, according to the ad. The body bags represent each person killed everyday (i.e. 1,200 body bags). The ad ends with youths posting signs on poles that read: "Every day 1200 people die from tobacco."

     . . . .

*Dog Walker,* a radio ad, begins with the ringing of a telephone. A woman answers "Good afternoon, Lorillard." The caller asks to speak to someone about a "business idea." The caller announces that he is a professional dog walker and has noticed the waste of quality dog urine when dogs pee on fire hydrants and flowerbeds. He offers to collect the dog urine and sell it to the tobacco companies because, as he says, "dog pee is full of urea, one of the chemicals that [tobacco companies] put in cigarettes." He offers the woman samples from a Chihuahua, a Golden Retriever, and even, as he describes it, "high-test" pee from a Rottweiler. She then transfers the caller to someone else, who hangs up on him at the mention of a "pee proposal."

     . . . .

In *Ammonia Soul Train,* a group of youths are dancing in what appears to be a game show backdrop. One of the youths has a microphone and is presumably a game show host. He introduces two other youths as "contestants." There is a "scrambleboard" in the background that contains several jumbled letters that do not spell a word. The host asks the contestants to unscramble letters and make a word that is a chemical used to clean floors and that tobacco companies add to cigarettes to increase the impact of nicotine. The contestants successfully rearrange the letters to spell "ammonia."

. . . .

In *Choice,* the ad presents a close-up of a woman looking directly at the camera and not talking. She does not move during the entire ad, except for involuntary human movements like blinking. In a voiceover, a female narrator, presumably the woman on screen, says the following: "My name is Linda. I smoked for 21 years and I am dying of emphysema. The tobacco companies say smoking is an adult choice. Today I am dying because of a choice I made when I was sixteen. I am not going to get better. I am going to die."

As the narrator says "I am going to die," the woman's face fades away and the viewer is left looking at a blank white screen.

. . . .

ALF's ad campaign was modeled on an earlier campaign in Florida that successfully reduced tobacco usage among young people. The campaigns were alike in that they marketed their ads under the brand "the truth." Indeed, the first employee hired by ALF was the director of Florida's campaign, Chuck Wolfe, who was hired as Executive Vice President and Chief Operating Officer. Under Wolfe's direction, ALF retained Crispin, Porter & Bogusky, the primary advertising agency for the Florida truth campaign. As Wolfe testified in his deposition, he went to work for ALF in order to expand Florida's successful campaign to a national scale.

The key difference between the Florida campaign and ALF's campaign for the purposes of this litigation is that ALF is subject to the contractual provisions in the MSA. . . .

. . . .

As ALF knew, *Demon Awards,* a Florida truth campaign ad, was the reason that the tobacco companies sought a prohibition against vilification and personal attack in the MSA. In *Demon Awards,* tobacco wins the award for Most Deaths in a Single Year, beating out other contestants like murder, suicide, and illegal drugs. *Demon Awards* is a parody of such glamorous award ceremonies as the Oscars and the Emmys and it features tobacco industry executives applauding when tobacco is nominated for its gruesome award. The audience also includes Hitler and Stalin, who join in the applause.

. . . .

### III

Summary judgment shall be granted when there is no genuine issue as to any material fact and the moving party is entitled to judgment as a matter of law. . . .

"The principles of contract interpretation in Delaware are well settled. In construing the meaning of written contracts, the court's first obligation to the parties is to determine the nature and scope of the contractual rights and obligations they created and to enforce those rights and obligations in accordance with law." . . .

When a highly sophisticated company like Lorillard and a group of 46 of the nation's attorneys general sign a contract that includes two critical phrases, "personal attack" and "vilification," that have no accepted blackletter legal definition, the court presumes that there was an implicit agreement by the parties to avoid the use of legal terms of art. For example, the parties could have easily replaced "vilification" with a well defined legal term that approximates its meaning taken from the torts of libel, slander, or defamation. Each of those torts has a settled legal definition that would have allowed the parties to brief an extensive list of cases in support of their argument. Instead, the parties are left with legally undefined terms that they attempt to define by resort to meanings found in various dictionaries. Each party cites no less than three dictionaries in support of its definition of "vilification." The same is true of personal attack.

While dictionary definitions are helpful and instructive, they are not precedent and this court need not rely on them, especially when, as in this case, there are sufficient usages in legal opinions to inform the court as to whether the advertisements in question violate the MSA. . . .

"The primary rule of construction is [that] where the parties have created an unambiguous integrated written [contract] . . . the language of that contract . . . will control."

. . . .

In summary, the state and federal case law, as well as law reviews, support a view of vilification that is consistent with Delaware law. First, on a textual level, the words of vilification are stronger than disparagement. Second, on a contextual level, the term "vilification" is most often used to describe situations that implicate serious social issues, such as race or gender relations.

. . . .

. . . [F]or the purposes of the MSA, the court begins with the use of vilification in Delaware case law. As summarized above, Delaware courts have used "vilification" in conjunction with words like blasphemy, licentiousness, hatred, contempt, and ridicule. "Vilification" has also been used in two related cases that concerned an alleged fraud by swindlers who perhaps should have been put in jail. From these sources, it is clear that Delaware law regards vilification as stronger (i.e. more contemptuous or malicious) than disparaging someone.

. . . .

The court notes that the truthfulness of the ads, while not a complete defense to Lorillard's claims, is pertinent to the issues here. ALF has maintained from the beginning of this litigation that all of the facts in the ads are true. And, in a procedural maneuver, Lorillard has decided not to contest ALF's position for purposes of this motion. Lorillard's position that the truthfulness of the ad does not factor into the court's decision is incorrect. For example, if someone were to call someone else a thief, the court should look at the record evidence of whether the person had been arrested or convicted of being a thief before determining whether the accusation might be vilifying.

Lorillard's status as a tobacco company does not preclude it from being vilified, but any alleged violation of the anti-vilification clause of the MSA should be analyzed in context. For example, if ALF's ad campaigns contained only the federally-mandated warning that cigarette smoking is dangerous to your health, would Lorillard seriously claim that the ads violate the anti-vilification clause of the MSA? How would Lorillard argue that such an ad campaign lessened its standing in society when millions of people see that warning label everyday? More to the point, how could ALF carry out its mission of educating the public about the "health effects and social costs related to the use of tobacco products" without mentioning the increased risk of disease and death due to tobacco use? . . .

Although it refuses to admit as much, ALF's actions indicate that it agrees that Lorillard can be vilified. Indeed, ALF acknowledges that *Demon Awards* was the single reason why the tobacco companies negotiated Section VI(h)'s anti-vilification clause.

That being said, the court notes one final item about the tone of the ads. The parties take wildly divergent positions as to whether tone should be part of this court's analysis. ALF maintains that tone is a critical part of the analysis, citing the key adjective modifiers in its definitions, such as *abusive* language, *vicious* statements, *hostile* comments, and *bitter* words. Without the modifying adjectives, ALF contends, the nouns themselves cannot be vilification. . . .

At the other end of the spectrum, Lorillard takes the position that tone does not matter, only the words do. . . .

. . . [I]n its analysis of the ads, the court will take into account tone. However, tone will not necessarily provide an ad with a safe harbor. For example, *Demon Awards* is a parody of an awards show and a parody does have an element of humor. But the element of humor can be lost in the socially offensive comparison to murder and suicide. If, on the other hand, an ad is substantially humorous, but does mention that tobacco kills 1,200 people per day, that ad is most likely not a violation of the anti-vilification clause.

[The court then reviews each of the 20 ads to determine if any of them contravene the anti-vilification clause of the MSA.]

The youths in *Shredder* refer to tobacco industry reports targeting potential teenager consumers, calling the reports "embarrassing." Lorillard contends that the discussion of the reports focuses on the employees' behavior and not on tobacco products. Lorillard claims that *Shredder* has "the tendency to disparage and lessen the standing . . . of tobacco companies generally." While *Shredder* may be critical of tobacco companies and their employees, it does not rise to the level of vilification. Nothing in the ad lessens the standing of the tobacco companies any more than the existence of the reports themselves. Simply making the public aware of the reports and expressing a characterization or opinion does not constitute a violation of the MSA.

Additionally, the criticism implied by the youths' statements is offset by the humor involved in shredding various ridiculously oversized objects, like a briefcase and a file cabinet. Indeed, the "shredder" in the ad is clearly a wood chipper and not a shredder. These facts all point to the inescapable conclusion that *Shredder* is a humorous ad accentuated by the absurdity of shredding unshreddable objects.

In *Hypnosis,* youths drive a truck around late at night, apparently attempting to hypnotize tobacco company executives by playing recordings such as "I am a good person." Lorillard argues that *Hypnosis* sends the message that "tobacco executives are greedy and are bad people." They argue that *Hypnosis* "crosses well into the realm of negative depiction, negative criticism, and disparagement of tobacco company employees." Even though *Hypnosis* may be negative and may be critical, it is not vilifying. Calling someone greedy is not equivalent to calling someone a racist or a sexual abuser of children or a rapist. The negative implication that the sleeping executives are bad people is too far removed from a direct, confrontational attack to be considered vilification.

The message in *Hypnosis* is also toned down by the use of humor. For example, the youths go through a drive-thru window of a fast food restaurant and, instead of ordering food, they asked whether tobacco executives live in the area. Clearly, if the youths were intent on actually hypnotizing tobacco company executives, they would have researched where they live and driven straight there. Asking a fast food worker where tobacco company executives live is merely a comical diversion intended to grab a television viewer's attention.

Thus, *Hypnosis* does not violate the anti-vilification clause of the MSA.

In *Dog Walker,* a telephone caller asks a tobacco employee if the company is interested in buying dog urine to add to its supply of urea for the manufacture of cigarettes. Lorillard contends that *Dog Walker* "ridicules Lorillard's employees and casts them in a negative light." Lorillard's entire argument about this ad is focused on the use of the term "dog urine." Lorillard concedes that another ALF advertisement which states that cigarettes contain urea is not vilifying. What Lorillard does take issue with in *Dog Walker* is the implication that cigarettes contain dog urine. This is a minor point, especially because the ad does not expressly state that cigarettes contain dog urine. The caller merely gives the impression that a tobacco company could extract urea from dog urine and put it into cigarettes. Apparently, urea is common to both dog urine and cigarettes. The fact that the ad illustrates this point does not make the ad vilifying.

In addition, the tone of the ad is irreverent, especially when the caller offers Lorillard different breeds of urine. Just the fact that the caller offers high-test Rottweiler pee shows the comical side of the ad. If urea is present in dog urine, why would it matter if the urine were high-test or from a specific breed? The caller's offer is clearly meant as a joke that could not be taken seriously by any reasonable listener.

Thus, *Dog Walker* does not violate the anti-vilification clause of the MSA.

. . . .

After a review of the remaining 15 ads at issue, the court finds that none of them violate the anti-vilification clause of the MSA.

. . . .

Even the ads that involve tobacco industry employees do not constitute vilification. None of the ads subject the employees to the type of contemptuous language contained in other case law discussing vilification. There are no scurrilous and vitriolic attacks. There is no cruel slander. There is no social ostracism. There is no public ridicule, traduction, or calumny. Although the employees may be described, either explicitly or implicitly, as liars, greedy executives, or authors of embarrassing documents, the ads do not vilify them.

## C.   Legal Definitions Of Personal Attack

. . . .

A comprehensive review of case law, law reviews, and dictionaries demonstrates that there is no blackletter law definition of "personal attack." What is clear is that there is a range of meanings for "personal attack," both in the legal and nonlegal contexts.

. . . .

The court concludes that the term "personal" in the MSA's "personal attack" consists of two parts. The first part concerns the target's private characteristics, such as, for an individual, amorality. The second part concerns the specific identification of the target.

[The court then reviews each of the 20 ads to determine if any of them violated the personal attack prohibition of Section VI(h) of the MSA and concluded that none of them do.]

## 6.   ALF's thetruth.com Website

The court next turns to ALF's website, which allows users to send "pissed off" libs. Unlike the children's game [presumably "Mad Libs"] in which kids innocently insert wrong words, creating ridiculous stories, the pissed off libs of ALF's website appear designed to create negative messages for tobacco company executives. For example, one pissed off lib contained the statement "It's bad enough that you ____ at Lorillard. . . ." The same pissed off lib ended with the statement "May the lord have mercy on your pathetic ____." These emails were then sent to specific executives of tobacco companies.

Lorillard argues that the pissed off libs functioned to provide web surfers with an easy and convenient way to send vulgar, profane, and vilifying emails to tobacco company executives. As proof, it cites many emails received by tobacco company employees that contain all manner of expletives and gross anatomy in the blank spaces listed above. ALF maintained during the summary judgment hearing that it was not responsible for the filled-in content of the emails, arguing that it was protected by the Communications Decency Act.

The court finds that the emails generated by thetruth.com website constitute "personal attack" as it is used in Section VI(h) of the MSA. They are attacks because they go far beyond simple criticism. One of the example sentences of the boilerplate form provided by ALF states "It's bad enough that you . . . knew that smoking cigarettes caused cancer, and kept selling them anyway, but to be deceptive about what you knew and . . . try to cover it up is just plain ____." Even without any of the filled-in vulgarities from the numerous examples provided by Lorillard, this sentence is an attack on the recipient of the email. The sentence explicitly refers to covering up cigarettes' link to cancer, as well as making money from selling a product with known harmful effects. This content is not criticism. It is a scathing indictment of a person and a person's employment.

Moreover, the court finds that ALF is also responsible for the entire content of the emails, including any filled-in expletives, scatological references, and criminal insinuations. ALF created the website, designed its format, and provided web surfers with an easy method of ranting at tobacco company executives. All the web surfers had to do was fill in some dirty words and click the send button. The court rejects ALF's claim that it is not responsible for what web surfers entered into the emails. . . . Any argument about the Communications Decency Act is irrelevant in this context, in which ALF is contractually bound not to utter certain communications that would violate the MSA.

. . . .

Although the website violates Section VI(h) of the MSA, the court declines to award Lorillard any relief because the violation was *de minimis*. Very soon after the emails were received by its employees, Lorillard put in place technology that effectively blocked further communications from ALF's website. The evidence reflects that Lorillard expended less than $1000 to block the emails. Additionally, the pissed off libs function of the website has since been removed, so no more emails are being sent. For these reasons, the court will not award damages or injunctive relief connected to ALF's violation of Section VI(h) of the MSA.

## D. Funding ALF's Ad Campaign

Lorillard also argues that ALF cannot escape the vilification and personal attack prohibition by using the Base Fund to fund its ads. ALF, on the other hand, argues that the Base Fund is separate from the NPEF and therefore not subject to the vilification and personal attack clause. ALF maintains that ads paid for by the Base Fund are immune from contractual liability under Section VI(h).

The court need not resolve the issue of funding the ads at this time [as] none of the contested ads violate Section VI(h), so the issue of what effect the method of funding has on the court's analysis is moot.

Nevertheless, it would appear as if ALF's position might constitute a violation of the implied covenant of good faith and fair dealing that inheres in every contract. Although ALF may be technically correct that the prohibitions on the substance of the ads applies only to the NPEF, the MSA clearly reflects an understanding that the NPEF pays for ads and the Base Fund pays for ALF's administrative costs. Thus, ALF's gambit of using payment out of the Base Fund as a defense for Lorillard's claim that certain ads violate Section VI(h) would seem to deprive Lorillard of the bargain reflected in the structure of the MSA.

## E.    The Three Criteria Clause

While ALF maintains that the three criteria clause remains part of this litigation, Lorillard appears to concede the issue. Lorillard does not brief its position on the three criteria clause, most likely because it cannot seriously argue that the ads do not address the "addictiveness, health effects, and social costs related to the use of tobacco products."

* * *

# NOTES AND QUESTIONS

**1.** As noted in the discussion in the text of the Master Settlement Agreement, a number of states were pursuing or considering lawsuits against the tobacco companies prior to the negotiations that led to the agreement; most of them focused on the possible recovery of Medicaid expenditures for tobacco-related illnesses. The agreement essentially mooted those lawsuits. In Canada, however, one of the provinces successfully sued tobacco manufacturers under a (Canadian) federal statute allowing for recovery of the province's health expenditures attributable to tobacco-related illness (which are substantial since each province pays for a wide range of medical care for all its citizens). *See British Columbia v. Imperial Tobacco Canada Ltd*, 2005 S.C.C. 49. So far, efforts to reverse that decision have been unsuccessful.

**2.** The Master Settlement Agreement is an intriguing document with an intriguing history and, just as likely, an intriguing future as well. Most experts assumed that the states would spend their tobacco payments on smoking abatement or, at least, pay for their smoking-related health care costs with the new-found money. But there is nothing in the settlement that requires the funds to be spent for any particular program or to be spent at all. In fact, as the years have distanced the annual revenue received from it origins, many of the states have realized that the income from the settlement agreement is just that — a source of revenue and one that is not generated by any direct form of taxation. It is money that can be spent for anything. People who buy tobacco are paying more for their cigarettes and other tobacco products, but that is part of what they pay the seller, not a tax they pay the state — a fine point of economics but an important point of politics.

As with so many other highly publicized arrangements, the real implications of the MSA may lie in its details. How will the various adjustments work out in practice? Will the tobacco companies really pay nearly $250 billion or will they find some provision of the settlement that allows them to avoid some portion of their future payments? Note that the payments and their renegotiations take place out of the public's eye.

Also consider this: Will the states really be willing to carry out the enforcement provisions that are included in the MSA at some distant point down the road? For instance, what if the state attorney general wants to enforce part of the settlement, but the legislature is happy with the status quo — and the state's share of the revenues? What if public health officials think that the tobacco industry has transgressed some of the settlement's prohibitions, but the state budget officials prefer to accept the settlement payments and ignore the possible violation of the settlement?

For that matter, will the states grow so accustomed to this non-tax revenue that they will openly or tacitly back off from any future efforts that would reduce the number of smokers — and the number of tobacco dollars — in the state?

**3.** While there are a number of reasons to question whether the settlement was really an arms-length transaction, it appears that some of the provisions of the settlement have enforced and with some rigor. The funding of the American Legacy Foundation was originally viewed with some suspicion. Would this nonprofit "educational" foundation do little more than soft-sell the harms of smoking and tobacco use, harms that were already well-publicized? Would it become the successor to the sad history of the American Tobacco Institute? If the *American Legacy* litigation is an indication of what the organization is doing, it appears that the tobacco companies have been required to fund their own worst enemy. The ads depicted in the decision are hardly subtle. Note, however, as discussed *supra*, such negative ads may be pleasing to those who oppose smoking and tobacco use, but they have never been particularly effective in convincing smokers to stop smoking.

A request for a re-argument in the *American Legacy* case was denied in an unpublished opinion in August of 2005. In October of 2005, one of the ads produced by "the truth" campaign called *Shards O' Glass* was awarded an Emmy for being the Most Outstanding Public Service Announcement of 2005 by the National Television Academy (after being shown during the 2005 Super Bowl).

## E.   THE IMPACT OF SHIFTING NORMS ON THE CONCEPT OF "PRIVATE" CONDUCT

This section briefly introduces the ways that changing social attitudes about tobacco may alter the legal boundaries of behavior that, not long ago, would have been considered "private" and, as such, insulated from government regulation. As you read the materials, consider carefully the interests of the community that may (or may not) justify such "intrusions," and think about application of your views to other examples. More broadly, is law the proper tool for advancing public health goals in this context?

### MIAMI v. KURTZ
653 So. 2d 1025 (Fla. 1995)

Overton, Justice.

\* \* \*

. . . [T]he district court . . . certified . . . the following question as one of great public importance:

DOES ARTICLE I, SECTION 23 OF THE FLORIDA CONSTITUTION PROHIBIT A MUNICIPALITY FROM REQUIRING JOB APPLICANTS TO REFRAIN FROM USING TOBACCO OR TOBACCO PRODUCTS FOR ONE

YEAR BEFORE APPLYING FOR, AND AS A CONDITION FOR BEING CONSIDERED FOR EMPLOYMENT, EVEN WHERE THE USE OF TOBACCO IS NOT RELATED TO JOB FUNCTION IN THE POSITION SOUGHT BY THE APPLICANT?

. . . .

The record establishes the following unrefuted facts. To reduce costs and to increase productivity, the City of North Miami adopted an employment policy designed to reduce the number of employees who smoke tobacco. In accordance with that policy decision, the City issued Administrative Regulation 1-46, which requires all job applicants to sign an affidavit stating that they have not used tobacco or tobacco products for at least one year immediately preceding their application for employment. The intent of the regulation is to gradually reduce the number of smokers in the City's work force by means of natural attrition. Consequently, the regulation only applies to job applicants and does not affect current employees. Once an applicant has been hired, the applicant is free to start or resume smoking at any time. Evidence in the record, however, reflects that a high percentage of smokers who have adhered to the one year cessation requirement are unlikely to resume smoking.

Additional evidence submitted by the City indicates that each smoking employee costs the City as much as $4611 per year in 1981 dollars over what it incurs for non-smoking employees. The City is a self-insurer and its taxpayers pay for 100% of its employees' medical expenses. In enacting the regulation, the City made a policy decision to reduce costs and increase productivity by eventually eliminating a substantial number of smokers from its work force. Evidence presented to the trial court indicated that the regulation would accomplish these goals.

The respondent in this case, Arlene Kurtz, applied for a clerk-typist position with the City. When she was interviewed for the position, she was informed of Regulation 1-46. She told the interviewer that she was a smoker and could not truthfully sign an affidavit to comply with the regulation. The interviewer then informed Kurtz that she would not be considered for employment until she was smoke-free for one year. Thereafter, Kurtz filed this action seeking to enjoin enforcement of the regulation and asking for a declaratory judgment finding the regulation to be unconstitutional.

. . . [T]he trial judge recognized that Kurtz has a fundamental right of privacy under [the state constitution]. The trial judge noted that Kurtz had presented the issue in the narrow context of whether she has a right to smoke in her own home. While he agreed that such a right existed, he concluded that the true issue to be decided was whether the City, as a governmental entity, could regulate smoking through employment. Because he found that there is no expectation of privacy in employment and that the regulation did not violate any provision of either the Florida or the federal constitutions, summary judgment was granted in favor of the City.

The Third District Court of Appeal reversed. . . .

Florida's constitutional privacy provision provides as follows:

Right of privacy: Every natural person has the right to be let alone and free from governmental intrusion into his private life except as otherwise provided herein. This section shall not be construed to limit the public's right of access to public records and meetings as provided by law.

This right to privacy protects Florida's citizens from the government's uninvited observation of or interference in those areas that fall within the ambit of the zone of privacy afforded under this provision. Unlike the implicit privacy right of the federal constitution, Florida's privacy provision is, in and of itself, a fundamental one that, once implicated, demands evaluation under a compelling state interest standard. The federal privacy provision, on the other hand, extends only to such fundamental interests as marriage, procreation, contraception, family relationships, and the rearing and educating of children. (citations omitted)

Although Florida's privacy right provides greater protection than the federal constitution, it was not intended to be a guarantee against all intrusion into the life of an individual. First, the privacy provision applies only to government action, and the right provided under that provision is circumscribed and limited by the circumstances in which it is asserted. Further, "[d]etermining 'whether an *individual* has a legitimate expectation of privacy in any given case must be made by considering all the circumstances, especially objective manifestations of that expectation.' " Thus, to determine whether Kurtz, as a job applicant, is entitled to protection . . . we must first determine whether a governmental entity is intruding into an aspect of Kurtz's life in which she as a "legitimate expectation of privacy." If we find in the affirmative, we must then look to whether a compelling interest exists to justify that intrusion and, if so, whether the least intrusive means is being used to accomplish the goal.

In this case, we find that the City's action does not intrude into an aspect of Kurtz' life in which she has a legitimate expectation of privacy. In today's society, smokers are constantly required to reveal whether they smoke. When individuals are seated in a restaurant, they are asked whether they want a table in a smoking or non-smoking section. When individuals rent hotel or motel rooms, they are asked if they smoke so that management may ensure that certain rooms remain free from the smell of smoke odors. Likewise, when individuals rent cars, they are asked if they smoke so that rental agencies can make proper accommodations to maintain vehicles for non-smokers. Further, employers generally provide smoke-free areas for non-smokers, and employees are often prohibited from smoking in certain areas. Given that individuals must reveal whether they smoke in almost every aspect of life in today's society, we conclude that individuals have no reasonable expectation of privacy in the disclosure of that information when applying for a government job and, consequently, that Florida's right of privacy is not implicated under these unique circumstances.

In reaching the conclusion that the right to privacy is not implicated in this case, however, we emphasize that our holding is limited to the narrow issue presented. Notably, we are not addressing the issue of whether an applicant, once hired, could be compelled by a government agency to stop smoking.

Equally as important, neither are we holding today that a governmental entity can ask any type of information it chooses of prospective job applicants.

Having determined that Kurtz has no legitimate expectation of privacy in revealing that she is a smoker under the Florida constitution, we turn now to her claim that the regulation violates her rights under the federal constitution. As noted, the federal constitution's implicit privacy provision extends only to such fundamental interests as marriage, procreation, contraception, family relationships, and the rearing and educating of children. Clearly, the "right to smoke" is not included within the penumbra of fundamental rights protected under that provision. . . . On these facts, the City's policy cannot be deemed so irrational that it may be branded arbitrary. In fact, under the special circumstances supported by the record in this case, we would find that the City has established a compelling interest to support implementation of the regulation. As previously indicated, the record reflects that each smoking employee costs the City as much as $4611 per year in 1981 dollars over what it incurs for nonsmoking employees; that, of smokers who have adhered to the one year cessation requirement, a high percentage are unlikely to resume smoking; and that the City is a self-insurer who pays 100% of its employees' medical expenses. We find that the elimination of these costs, when considered in combination with the other special circumstances of this case, validates a compelling interest in the City's policy of gradually eliminating smokers from its work force. We also find that the City is using the least intrusive means in accomplishing this compelling interest because the regulation does not prevent current employees from smoking, it does not affect the present health care benefits of employees, and it gradually reduces the number of smokers through attrition. Thus, we find the regulation to be constitutional under both the federal and Florida constitutions.

For the reasons expressed, we answer the question in the negative, finding that Florida's constitutional privacy provision does not afford the applicant, Arlene Kurtz, protection because she has no reasonable expectation of privacy under the circumstances of this case. Accordingly, we quash the district court's decision, and we remand this case with directions that the district court of appeal affirm the trial court judgment.

. . . .

Justice, dissenting.

As the majority itself notes, job applicants are free to return to tobacco use once hired. I believe this concession reveals the anti-smoking policy to be rather more of a speculative pretense than a rational governmental policy. Therefore I would find it unconstitutional under the right of due process.

The privacy issue is more troublesome, to my mind. There is a "slippery-slope" problem here because, if governmental employers can inquire too extensively into off-job-site behavior, a point eventually will be reached at which the right of privacy clearly will be breached. An obvious example would be an inquiry into the lawful sexual behavior of job applicants in an effort to identify those with the "most desirable" lifestyles. Such an effort easily could become the pretext for a constitutional violation. The time has not yet fully passed, for example, when women job applicants have been questioned about their plans for procreation in an effort to eliminate those who may be absent on family leave. I cannot conceive that such an act is anything other than a violation of the right of privacy when done by a governmental unit.

Health-based concerns like those expressed by the City also present a definite slippery slope to the courts. The time is fast approaching, for example, when human beings can be genetically tested so thoroughly that susceptibility to particular diseases can be identified years in advance. To my mind, any governmental effort to identify those who might eventually suffer from cancer or heart disease, for instance, itself is a violation of bodily integrity guaranteed by [the state constitution]. Moreover, I cannot help but note that any such effort comes perilously close to the discredited practice of eugenics.

The use of tobacco products is more troubling, however. While legal, tobacco use nevertheless is an activity increasingly regulated by the law. If the federal government, for instance, chose to regulate tobacco as a controlled substance, I have no trouble saying that this act alone does not undermine anyone's privacy right. However, regulation is not the issue here because tobacco use today remains legal. The sole question is whether the government may inquire into off-job-site behavior that is legal, however unhealthy it might be. In light of the inherently poor fit between the governmental objective and the ends actually achieved, I am more inclined to agree with the district court that the right of privacy has been violated here. I might reach a different result if the objective were better served by the means chosen.

\* \* \*

# NOTES AND QUESTIONS

**1.** *Miami v. Kurtz* raises a series of interesting questions and answers only one relatively narrow one: Are there constitutional infirmities in a governmental policy that requires job applicants to refrain from smoking for one year prior to their application? As a matter of federal constitutional law, the answer is clearly no; there is no fundamental or otherwise constitutionally protected interest affected by such a policy and the policy is clearly within the bounds of the "rationality" standard typically applied in such cases. Nor is there, according to the *Miami* court, a violation of Florida state constitutional limits on government action. Nor is this a violation of any federal prohibition on discrimination (*e.g.*, this is not a discrimination based on disability).

The court's federal constitutional analysis seems forthrightly to engage the question whether personal *use* of tobacco off the job can be disqualifying for employment. Its treatment of the *state* constitutional claim, however, is somewhat more limited, and seems incomplete. The court treats the state-constitutional "privacy" violation as arising only from the forced *disclosure* of personal tobacco use (Ms. Kurtz is required to "reveal" her usage-status by signing a statement). But is this the question certified for resolution by the district court? (Hint: No). Assume Ms. Kurtz (or another claimant) raised no objection to the disclosure itself, or was "seen" smoking before her job interview, rendering the disclosure unimportant. Couldn't she still argue — wasn't she *in fact* arguing — that the rule, if enforced, violates her state constitutional "privacy" because of its impact on her non-working life, irrespective of the disclosure issue? The state constitutional analysis, unlike the federal one, sheds no light on this question.

The question explored here is constitutional, and thus constrains only "state" action. But it is worth noting in passing that the *Miami* rule does not violate any federal statutory prohibition on discrimination. Thus, absent any such statute (state or federal), it would appear that a private employer could adopt such a policy as well.

Consider other possibilities: Could an employer, public or private simply refuse to employ someone who smokes? At the other end of the spectrum, could an employer hire a smoker but offer more expensive (or less extensive) health benefits? Would it make any difference if a particular smoker claimed only to smoke in the privacy of his or her own home?

Given the lack of legal limits on employer discretion, it should not be surprising that many private and public employers are imposing some sort of incentive or penalty on their employees who smoke.

**2.** What other sorts of actions should be considered within the bounds of legal behavior? In what other ways can individuals or groups choose to discriminate, in the broader sense of the term, *i.e.,* distinguish or treat differently smokers and non-smokers? Obviously the government has to stay within constitutional limits, but as outlined in this chapter, those limits allow for a great deal of discretion. As *Kurtz* demonstrates, in most circumstances those constitutional limits are inapplicable to private behavior and most anti-discrimination or anti-harassment laws limits only certain kinds of actions. Can I refuse to sell my home to a smoker? Can my private club exclude smokers? Can public or nonprofit agencies only provide discretionary services to nonsmokers? Can universities limit enrollment or deny financial aid to smokers? The list goes on and on. What is at stake here? How do you measure the benefits of such actions? What are the costs?

**3.** Consider the following editorial:

> The World Health Organization (WHO), the health branch of the United Nations, has announced that it will no longer hire smokers. Its spokeswoman said, "As a matter of principle, WHO does not want to recruit smokers." The "principle," according to the spokeswoman, is: "WHO tries to encourage people to try and lead a healthy life."

> By this action WHO has transformed its war against smoking to a war against smokers. On its new job application, WHO asks applicants if they are smokers. If the applicant answers "yes," the application will be discarded.

> With the hanging of the "No Smokers Need Apply" sign on its door, WHO has joined a long line of bigots who would not hire people of color, members of religious minorities, or disabled or gay people because of who they are or what they lawfully do.

> To outlaw discriminatory hiring practices, both state and federal governments have passed a series of anti-discrimination laws that all share an underlying basis: The only legitimate job requirements are

those that are related to the applicant's ability to do the work, as long as they do not endanger others.

In the language of the law, employers may impose bona fide occupational requirements. Thus, it is one thing to ban smoking in the workplace but quite another to ban employees who smoke away from the workplace. What WHO's new policy says is that it will not hire any member of a group that constitutes 25 percent of adults in the United States — no matter how well qualified, dedicated and caring they are — because of activities away from the workplace that have no impact on their job performance.

Under WHO's policy, if Franklin Roosevelt, Winston Churchill, Albert Einstein and Adolf Hitler applied for a job, only Hitler, the sole nonsmoker in the group (and someone who would not allow anyone to smoke near him), would be eligible for consideration.

The organization's "principled" stand could, and logically should, be applied to other unhealthful activities. While WHO would be the first to note that smoking is the leading cause of premature deaths, there is no reason this policy should not be applied to the second- and third-leading causes and to various other unhealthful activities in which so many engage. And, of course, if WHO succeeds in eliminating smoking, some other activity will take its place as the number-one cause of premature death. WHO's logical next step in amending its application form is to ask for the height and weight of applicants so it can discard the applications of obese people.

In adopting this policy, WHO is not acting in its capacity as a health care organization but rather as an employer. And the principle that it argues for is that employers can impose job requirements based on what its employees do off the job. One can only imagine WHO's reaction to a tobacco company that requires all its employees to smoke or a gun company that requires them all to keep a gun and ammunition in their homes. The position that WHO has adopted would neatly support such ludicrous employment requirements.

I imagine that the health organization sees itself as leading the way in encouraging other companies to adopt similar oppressive and arbitrary job requirements. In doing so it encourages the most coercive form of social control short of outlawing smoking. Other than the very rich, people must work, and WHO's position is that smokers should not be allowed to work.

The proper response to such an oppressive condition of employment is for federal and state governments to adopt laws that prohibit job discrimination based on activities that employees engage in outside the workplace that have no impact on job performance. Several states have already adopted such laws, and WHO's actions demonstrate the need for them in every jurisdiction.

Leonard Glantz, *Smoke Got In Their Eyes,* BOSTON GLOBE, December 18, 2005, at B7.

Is Professor Glantz' comparison between the practices of employers such as WHO concerning smokers and more traditional forms of discrimination based on race, disability, or gender, valid — either as a factual matter or as a matter of law? Are there *bona fide* reasons for excluding smokers? How would you respond to his observation that once smokers are eliminated from employment because smoking is the leading cause of death, employers may then attempt to exclude obese people or people with chronic disease?

# Appendix to Chapter Four: World Health Assembly Resolution 56.1

\* \* \*

To achieve the objective of this Convention . . . the Parties shall be guided . . . by the principles set out below:

. . . .

Every person should be informed of the health consequences, addictive nature, and mortal threat posed by tobacco consumption and exposure to tobacco smoke and effective legislative, executive, administrative or other measures should be contemplated at the appropriate governmental level to protect all persons from exposure to tobacco smoke.

. . . .

## Article 5: General obligations

1. Each Party shall develop, implement, periodically update, and review comprehensive multi-sectoral national tobacco control strategies, plans and programs in accordance with this Convention and the protocols to which it is a Party.

2. Towards this end, each Party shall, in accordance with its capabilities [adopt] appropriate policies for preventing and reducing tobacco consumption, nicotine addiction, and exposure to tobacco smoke.

. . . .

## Article 6: Price and tax measures to reduce the demand for tobacco

1. The Parties recognize that price and tax measures are an effective and important means of reducing tobacco consumption by various segments of the population, in particular young persons.

2. . . . [E]ach Party should take account of its national health objectives concerning tobacco control and adopt or maintain, as appropriate, measures which may include:

— implementing tax policies and, where appropriate, price policies, on tobacco products so as to contribute to the health objectives aimed at reducing tobacco consumption; and

— prohibiting or restricting, as appropriate, sales to and/or importations by international travelers of tax- and duty-free tobacco products.

## Article 7: Non-price measures to reduce the demand for tobacco

The Parties recognize that comprehensive non-price measures are an effective and important means of reducing tobacco consumption. . . .

## Article 8: Protection from exposure to tobacco smoke

Parties recognize that scientific evidence has unequivocally established that exposure to tobacco smoke causes death, disease and disability. Each Party shall adopt and implement in areas of existing national jurisdiction as determined by national law and actively promote at other jurisdictional levels the adoption and implementation of effective legislative, executive, administrative and/or other measures, providing for protection from exposure to tobacco smoke in indoor workplaces, public transport, indoor public places and, as appropriate, other public places.

## Article 9: Regulation of the contents of tobacco products

The Conference of the Parties, in consultation with competent international bodies, shall propose guidelines for testing and measuring the contents and emissions of tobacco products, and for the regulation of these contents and emissions. Each Party shall, where approved by competent national authorities, adopt and implement effective legislative, executive and administrative or other measures for such testing and measuring, and for such regulation.

## Article 10: Regulation of tobacco product disclosures

1. Each Party shall, in accordance with its national law, adopt and implement effective legislative, executive, administrative or other measures requiring manufacturers and importers of tobacco products to disclose to governmental authorities information about the contents and emissions of tobacco products. Each Party shall further adopt and implement effective measures for public disclosure of information about the toxic constituents of the tobacco products and the emissions that they may produce.

## Article 11: Packaging and labeling of tobacco products

1. Each Party shall, within a period of three years after entry into force of this Convention for that Party, adopt and implement, in accordance with its national law, effective measures to ensure that:

— tobacco product packaging and labeling do not promote a tobacco product by any means that are false, misleading, deceptive or likely to create an erroneous impression about its characteristics, health effects, hazards or emissions, including any term, descriptor, trademark, figurative or any other sign that directly or indirectly creates the false impression that a particular tobacco product is less harmful than other tobacco products. These may include terms such as "low tar," "light," "ultra-light," or "mild"; and

— each unit packet and package of tobacco products and any outside packaging and labeling of such products also carry health warnings describing the harmful effects of tobacco use, and may include other appropriate messages. . . .

2. Each unit packet and package of tobacco products and any outside packaging and labeling of such products shall, in addition to the warnings specified in paragraph 1(b) of this Article, contain information on relevant constituents and emissions of tobacco products as defined by national authorities.

3. Each Party shall require that the warnings and other textual information specified in paragraphs 1 (b) and paragraph 2 of this Article will appear on each unit packet and package of tobacco products and any outside packaging and labeling of such products in its principal language or languages.

## Article 12: Education, communication, training and public awareness

Each Party shall promote and strengthen public awareness of tobacco control issues, using all available communication tools, as appropriate.

## Article 13: Tobacco advertising, promotion and sponsorship

Each party shall undertake a comprehensive ban of all tobacco advertising, promotion, and sponsorship. This shall include, subject to the legal environment and technical means available to that Party, a comprehensive ban on cross-border advertising, promotion and sponsorship originating from its territory. . . .

A Party that is not in a position to undertake a comprehensive ban due to its constitution or constitutional principles shall apply restrictions on all tobacco advertising, promotion and sponsorship. This shall include, subject to the legal environment and technical means available to that Party, restrictions or a comprehensive ban on advertising, promotion and sponsorship originating from its territory with cross-border effects. . . .

As a minimum, and in accordance with its constitution or constitutional principles, each Party shall:

— prohibit all forms of tobacco advertising, promotion and sponsorship that promote a tobacco product by any means that are false, misleading or deceptive or likely to create an erroneous impression about its characteristics, health effects, hazards or emissions;

— require that health or other appropriate warnings or messages accompany all tobacco advertising and, as appropriate, promotion and sponsorship;

— restrict the use of direct or indirect incentives that encourage the purchase of tobacco products by the public;

— require, if it does not have a comprehensive ban, the disclosure to relevant governmental authorities of expenditures by the tobacco industry on advertising, promotion and sponsorship not yet prohibited. . . .

— undertake a comprehensive ban or, in the case of a Party that is not in a position to undertake a comprehensive ban due to its constitution or constitutional principles, restrict tobacco advertising, promotion and sponsorship on radio, television, print media and, as appropriate, other media, such as the internet, within a period of five years; and

— prohibit, or in the case of a Party that is not in a position to prohibit due to its constitution or constitutional principles, restrict tobacco sponsorship of international events, activities and/or participants therein.

. . . .

## Article 14: Demand reduction measures concerning tobacco dependence and cessation

Each Party shall develop and disseminate appropriate, comprehensive and integrated guidelines based on scientific evidence and best practices, taking into account national circumstances and priorities, and shall take effective measures to promote cessation of tobacco use and adequate treatment for tobacco dependence.

Towards this end, each Party shall endeavor to:

— design and implement effective programs aimed at promoting the cessation of tobacco use in such locations as educational institutions, health care facilities, workplaces and sporting environments;

— include diagnosis and treatment of tobacco dependence and counseling services on cessation of tobacco use in national health and education programs, plans and strategies, with the participation of health workers, community workers and social workers as appropriate;

— establish in health care facilities and rehabilitation centers programs for diagnosing, counseling, preventing and treating tobacco dependence; and

— collaborate with other Parties to facilitate accessibility and affordability for treatment of tobacco dependence . . . .

## Article 15: Illicit trade in tobacco products

Each Party shall adopt and implement effective legislative, executive, administrative or other measures to ensure that all unit packets and packages of tobacco products and any outside packaging of such products are marked to assist Parties in determining the origin of tobacco products [and] assist Parties in determining the point of diversion and monitor, document and control the movement of tobacco products and their legal status. . . .

Each Party shall require that the packaging information or marking specified in paragraph 2 of this Article shall be presented in legible form and/or appear in its principal language or languages.

With a view to eliminating illicit trade in tobacco products, each Party shall:

— monitor and collect data on cross-border trade in tobacco products;

. . . .

— enact or strengthen legislation, with appropriate penalties and remedies, against illicit trade in tobacco products, including counterfeit and contraband cigarettes;

. . . .

— adopt measures as appropriate to enable the confiscation of proceeds derived from the illicit trade in tobacco products.

. . . .

The Parties shall, as appropriate and in accordance with national law, promote cooperation between national agencies, as well as relevant regional and international intergovernmental organizations as it relates to investigations, prosecutions, and proceedings, with a view to eliminating illicit trade in tobacco products. . . .

## Article 16: Sales to and by minors

Each Party shall adopt and implement effective legislative, executive, administrative or other measures at the appropriate government level to prohibit the sales of tobacco products to persons under the age set by domestic law, national law or eighteen. These measures may include:

— requiring that all sellers of tobacco products place a clear and prominent indicator inside their point of sale about the prohibition of tobacco sales to minors and, in case of doubt, request that each tobacco purchaser provide appropriate evidence of having reached full legal age;

— banning the sale of tobacco products in any manner by which they are directly accessible, such as store shelves;

— prohibiting the manufacture and sale of sweets, snacks, toys, or any other objects in the form of tobacco products which appeal to minors; and

— ensuring that tobacco vending machines under its jurisdiction are not accessible to minors and do not promote the sale of tobacco products to minors.

Each Party shall prohibit or promote the prohibition of the distribution of free tobacco products to the public and especially minors.

Each Party shall endeavor to prohibit the sale of cigarettes individually or in small packets which increase the affordability of such products to minors.

The Parties recognize that in order to increase their effectiveness, measures to prevent tobacco product sales to minors should, where appropriate, be implemented in conjunction with other provisions contained in this Convention.

When signing, ratifying, accepting, approving, or acceding to the Convention or at any time thereafter, a Party may, by means of a binding written declaration, indicate its commitment to prohibit the introduction of tobacco vending machines within its jurisdiction or, as appropriate, to a total ban on tobacco vending machines. . . .

Each Party shall adopt and implement effective legislative, executive, administrative, or other measures, including penalties against sellers and distributors, in order to ensure compliance with the obligations contained in paragraphs 1-5 of this Article.

Each Party should, as appropriate, adopt and implement effective legislative, executive, administrative, or other measures to prohibit the sales of tobacco products by persons under the age set by domestic law, national law or eighteen.

. . . .

## Article 18: Protection of the environment and the health of persons

In carrying out their obligations under this Convention, the Parties agree to have due regard to the protection of the environment and the health of persons in relation to the environment in respect of tobacco cultivation and manufacture within their respective territories.

\* \* \*

For the full text of Resolution 56.1, see www.who.int/tobacco/framework/final_text/ (last visited December 2006). See also the website of the Framework Convention Alliance at www.fctc.org/ (last visited December 2006).

Resolution 56.1 went into effect in February of 2005. As of October 2005, of the 168 countries that helped draft the original accord, 160 had ratified. In October 2005, China, one of the largest consumers of tobacco products in the world announced that it had ratified the agreement and was implementing a plan to limit the construction of new cigarette factories and take various steps to limit the availability of tobacco products. As of December 2006, however, the United States remained one of the few nations that had not agreed to ratify the resolution. The provisions of the original accord called for all of the nations that ratify the treaty by November 2005 to re-convene and begin negotiations on means for implementing the agreement. Presumably the United States will take no direct role in those future proceedings.

# Chapter 6

# HEALTH PROMOTION AND EDUCATION: ENCOURAGING HEALTHY PERSONAL BEHAVIOR

## A.  INTRODUCTION

In the United States, as in most of the industrialized West, the primary causes of death are chronic diseases, specifically heart disease, stroke, and cancers. As the threat of infectious diseases declined in the twentieth century, largely as a result of successful public health interventions to clean up the country's supplies of water, food, and industrial hazards, chronic diseases gained more prominence. Public health agencies began to consider how to organize programs to reduce mortality and morbidity from chronic diseases, perhaps encouraged by Canada's Lalonde Report,[1] which brought attention to the ways individuals may affect their own health by using illicit drugs like heroin, cocaine or marijuana, drinking alcohol, smoking cigarettes, driving without seatbelts, cycling without a helmet, eating a poor diet, getting little exercise, or engaging in promiscuous unprotected sex. Because chronic diseases often result from complex and in many cases still unknown factors, including the environment, one's genetic heritage, personal behavior, and social determinants like wealth, occupation, and education, preventing chronic diseases is even more complicated than preventing infectious diseases. By the end of the twentieth century, however, chronic disease prevention was firmly on the public health agenda, generally referred to as "health promotion."

To date, the majority of public health promotion policies that seek statutory or judicial changes focus on the risks posed by specific personal behaviors, perhaps because laws addressing other types of risks are more politically controversial.

This chapter considers examples of laws intended primarily to change personal behavior and to improve health in the indefinite future, rather than to prevent imminent death or injury. To be sure, the ultimate goal of most public health legislation is saving lives or at least preventing "premature death," that is, death at an abnormally early age. Still, the adverse effects of many behavioral risks to health lie far in the future. Preventing or reducing the risk may require preventive measures long before anyone could become ill or disabled. The lag between the time for intervention and the materialization of

---

[1] MARC LALONDE, A NEW PERSPECTIVE ON THE HEALTH OF CANADIANS (April 1974) (policy paper initiated by the Canadian Minister of Health, Michael Lalonde, presenting a new direction for health policy in Canada emphasizing prevention and health promotion, rather than curative medical care, and focusing on the environment, human biology, lifestyle, and health care organization), www.hc-sc.gc.ca/hcs-sss/com/lalonde/index_e.html (last visited Jan. 2007)

any harm creates some conceptual problems for applying several legal principles. Equally difficult questions arise from the fact that most, though not all, healthful changes in personal behavior benefit the person herself rather than protecting other people from harm.

All public health policy making, but especially that targeted at individual behavior and life style, raises the following questions:

- How does society decide what counts as a public health risk that should be prevented or reduced?

- Which, if any, legal measures should be adopted to prevent such risks?

A wide range of laws might prevent public health risks: criminal prohibitions, financial incentives (taxes, surcharges), tort liability, product standards, environmental controls or workplace standards by an administrative agency. Although each measure has specific statutory or doctrinal requirements, some of which may be debatable or elusive, those standards may be clearer than the policy or ethical rationale underlying the policy choice. The focus of this chapter is on the policy and doctrinal justifications for measures that reward or penalize individual behavior that affects health.

Section B offers some background for thoughtful answers to these questions, with an examination of the justifications for different measures intended to encourage or compel healthy behavior. The motivation underlying laws that regulate personal behavior, rather than things like products or environmental conditions, may be grounded in moral or health concerns or both. For this reason, this section should be read in light of the materials on legislating morality in Chapter Two. This section also provides an introduction to the sometimes dramatically different ways in which different people perceive risk. The case of *Christ's Bride* illustrates such different perceptions and how moral reasoning may affect risk perception.

Section C examines different contemporary approaches by states to prevent or regulate the use of controlled substances by pregnant women, school children, motor vehicle drivers, and patients with severe illness. In the first and last case, the policy questions underlying the statute at issue are whether the risk justifies the imposition of criminal sanctions and whether a different approach would be more effective from the public health perspective. Yet the policy implications are hidden within statutory interpretation and, in *Gonzales v. Raich*, implicate the sometimes shifting jurisdictional boundaries between the state and federal governments in our federal system. Both *Ferguson* and *Earls* reveal the unsettled scope and limits of constitutional protection against unreasonable searches and seizures, in the form of drug testing.

Section D uses contemporary concerns with obesity as a case study in defining a public health problem, examining possible sources of risk, and evaluating the likely effectiveness and justifications for alternative legal interventions, such as a fat tax, restrictions on food and beverages available in public schools, mandatory nutrition disclosures, public education curricula, and tort liability of the food industry. The so-called obesity epidemic and the responses it have parallels in the history of tobacco regulation and litigation.

Yet, because obesity is such a multi-faceted condition, it may be more emblematic of future public health problems than tobacco.

# B.   DEFINING RISKS TO PUBLIC HEALTH AND JUSTIFICATIONS FOR THEIR CONTROL

## Daniel I. Wikler, *Persuasion and Coercion for Health: Ethical Issues in Government Efforts to Change Life-Styles*
### 56 MILBANK MEMORIAL FUND Q. 303 (1978)

* * *

What should be the government's role in promoting the kinds of personal behavior that lead to long life and good health? Smoking, overeating, and lack of exercise increase one's chances of suffering illness later in life, as do many other habits. Education, exhortation, and other relatively mild measures may not prove effective in inducing self-destructive people to change their behavior. In this essay, I seek to identify the moral principles underlying a reasoned judgment on whether stronger methods might justifiably be used, and, if so, what limits ought to be observed.

. . . .

## Goals of Health Behavior Reform

. . . .

### Health as a Goal in Itself: Beneficence and Paternalism

Much of the present concern for the reform of unhealthy life-styles stems from concern over the health of those who live dangerously. . . . There are several steps that might immediately be justified: the government could make the effects of unhealthy living habits known to those who practice them, and sponsor research to discover more of these facts. . . .

Considerably more debate, however, would arise over a decision to use stronger methods. For example, a case in point might be a government "fat tax," which would require citizens to be weight and taxed if overweight. The surcharges thus derived would be held in trust, to be refunded with interest if and when the taxpayers brought their weight down. This pressure would, under the circumstances, be a bond imposed by the government upon its citizens, and thus can be fairly considered as coercive.

The two signal properties of this policy would be its aim of improving the welfare of obese taxpayers, and its presumed unwelcome imposition on personal freedom. (Certain individual taxpayers, of course, might welcome such an imposition, but this is not the ordinary response to penalties.) The first property might be called "beneficence," and it is generally a virtue. But the second property becomes paternalism; and its status as a virtue is very much in doubt. . . .

What is good about some paternalistic interventions is that people are helped, or saved, from harm. Citizens who have to pay a fat tax, for example, may lose weight, become more attractive, and live longer. In the eyes of many, these possible advantages are more than offset by the chief fault of paternalism, its denying persons the chance to make their own choices concerning matters that affect them. Self-direction, in turn, is valued because people usually believe themselves to be the best judges of what is good for them, and because the choosing is considered a good in itself. These beliefs are codified in our ordinary morality in the form of a moral right to noninterference so long as one does not adversely affect the interests of others. . . .

At the same time, the case for paternalistic intervention on at least some occasions seems compelling. There may be circumstances in which we lose, temporarily or permanently, our capacity for competent self-direction, and thereby inflict harm upon ourselves that serves little purpose. Like Ulysses approaching the Sirens, we may hope that others would then protect us from ourselves. This sort of consideration supports our imposed guardianship of children and of the mentally retarded. Although these persons often resent our paternalistic control, we reason that we are doing what they would want us to do were their autonomy not compromised. Paternalism would be a benefit under the sort of social insurance policy that a reasonable person would opt for if considered in a moment of lucidity and competence.

. . . .

## Paternalism: Theoretical Problems

There are a number of reasons to question the general argument for paternalism in the coercive eradication of unhealthful personal practices. First, the analogy between the cases of children and the retarded, where paternalism is most clearly indicated, and of risk-taking adults is misleading. If the autonomy of adults is compromised in one or more of the ways just mentioned, it might be possible to restore that autonomy by attending to the sources of the involuntariness; the same cannot ordinarily be done with the children or the retarded. Thus, adults who are destroying their health because of ignorance may be educated; adults acting under constraint may be freed. If restoration of autonomy is a realistic project, then paternalistic interference is unjustified. The two kinds of interventions are aimed at the same target, *i.e.*, harmful behavior not freely and competently chosen. But they accomplish the result differently. Paternalistic intervention blocks the harm; education and similar measures restore the choice. . . .

It remains true, however, that autonomy sometimes cannot be restored. It may be impossible to reach a given population with the information they need; or, once reached, the persons in question may prove ineducable. Psychological compulsions and social pressures may be even harder to eradicate. In these situations, the case for paternalistic interference is relatively strong, yet even here there is reason for caution. Persons who prove incapable of absorbing the facts about smoking, for example, or who abuse drugs because of compulsion or addiction, may retain a kind of second-order autonomy. They can be told that they appear unable to accept scientific truth, or that they are addicted; and they can then decide to reconsider the facts or to seek a cure. . . .

A second reason for doubting the justifiability of paternalistic interference concerns the subjectivity of the notion of harm. The same experience may be seen as harmful by one person and as beneficial by another. . . . Most of us subscribe to the pluralistic ethic, for better or for worse, which has as a central tenet the proposition that there are multiple distinct, but equally valid, concepts of the good and of the good life. It follows that we must use personal preferences and tastes to determine whether our health-related practices are detrimental.

. . . It is common to feel that one's own preferences reflect values that reasonable people adopt; one can hardly regard oneself as unreasonable. To the extent that government planners employ their own concepts of good in attempting to change health practices for the public's benefit, the social insurance rationale for paternalism is clearly inapplicable.

A third reason for criticism of paternalism is the vagueness of the notion of decision-making disability. The conscientious paternalist intervenes only when the self-destructive individual's autonomy is compromised. It is probably impossible, however, to specify a compromising condition. To be sure, there are cases in which the lack of autonomy is evident, such as that of a child swallowing dangerous pills in the belief that they are candy. But the sorts of practices that would be the targets of coercive campaigns to reform health-related behavior are less dramatic and their involuntary quality much less certain. . . .

. . . .

The difficulty for the paternalist at this point is plain. The desire to interfere only with involuntary risk-taking leads to designating individuals for intervention whose behavior proceeds from externally-instilled values. Pluralism commits the paternalist to use the persons' own values in determining whether a health-related practice is harmful. What is needed is some way of determining individuals' "true" personal values; but if these cannot be read off from their behavior, how can they be known?

In certain individual cases, a person's characteristic preferences can be determined from wishes expressed before losing autonomy, as was Ulysses' desire to be tied to the mast. But this sort of data is hardly likely to be available to government health planners. The problem would be at least partially solved if we could identify a set of goods that is basic and appealing, and that nearly all rational persons value. Such universal valuation would justify a presumption of involuntariness should an individual's behavior put these goods in jeopardy. . . .

The crucial question for health planners is whether *health* is one of these primary goods. Considered alone, it certainly is: it is valued for its own sake; and it is a means to almost all ends. Indeed, it is a necessary good. No matter how eccentric a person's values and tastes are, no matter what kinds of activities are pleasurable, it is impossible to engage in them unless alive. . . .

But the significance of health as a primary good should not be overestimated. The health planner may attempt to argue for coercive reform of health-destructive behavior with a line of reasoning that recalls Pascal's wager. Since death, which precludes all good experience, must receive an enormously negative valuation, contemplated action that involves risk of death will also receive a substantial negative value after the good and bad consequences have been considered. And this will hold true even if the risk is small, since even low probability multiplied by a very large quantity yields a large quantity. Hence anyone who risks death by living dangerously must, on this view, be acting irrationally. . . .

This argument, or something like it, may lie behind the willingness of some to endorse paternalistic regulation of the life-styles of apparently competent adults. It is, however, invalid. Its premises may sometimes be true, and so too may its conclusion, but the one does not follow from the other. Any number of considerations can suffice to show this. For example, time factors are ignored. An act performed at age 25 that risks death at age 50 does not threaten every valued activity. It simply threatens the continuation of those activities past the age of 50. The argument also overlooks an interplay between the possible courses of action: if every action that carries some risk of death or crippling illness is avoided, the enjoyment of life decreases. . . . The less value a person places on continued life, the more rational it is to engage in activities that may brighten it up, even if they involve the risk of ending it. . . .

. . . .

The trouble for a government policy of life-style reform is that a given intervention is more likely to be tailored to practices and habits than to people. Although we may someday have a fat tax to combat obesity, it would be surprising indeed to find one that imposed charges only on those whose obesity was due to involuntary factors. It would be difficult to reach agreement on what constituted diminished voluntariness; harder still to measure it; and perhaps administratively impractical to make the necessary exceptions and adjustments. . . . Perhaps the firmest conclusion one may draw from all this is that a thoroughly reasoned moral rationale for a given kind of intervention can be very difficult to carry out.

## Paternalism: Problems in Practice

Even if we accept the social insurance rationale for paternalism in the abstract, then, there are theoretical reasons to question its applicability to the problem of living habits that are injurious to health. . . .

First, there is the distinct possibility that the government takes over decision-making power from partially-incompetent individuals may prove even less adept at securing their interests that they would have been if left alone. Paucity of scientific data may lead to misidentification or risk factors. The primitive state of the art in health promotion and mass-scale behavior modification may render interventions ineffective or even counterproductive. And the usual run of political and administrative tempests that affect all public policy may result in the misapplication of such knowledge as is available in these fields. . . .

Second, there is some possibility that what would be advertised as concern for the individual's welfare (as that person defines it) would turn out to be simple legal moralism, i.e., an attempt to impose the society's or authorities' moral prescriptions upon those not following them. In Knowles' call for life-style reform (1976) the language is suggestive:

> The next major advances in the health of the American people will result from the assumption of individual responsibility for one's own health. This will require a change in lifestyle for the majority of Americans. The cost of sloth, gluttony, alcoholic overuse, reckless driving, sexual intemperance, and smoking is now a national, not an individual responsibility.

All save the last of these practices are explicitly *vices;* indeed, the first two — sloth and gluttony — use their traditional names. . . . Skiing and football produce injuries as surely as sloth produces heart disease; and the decision to postpone childbearing until the thirties increases susceptibility to certain cancers in women. If it is the unhealthiness of "sinful" living habits that motivates the paternalist toward reform, then ought not other acts also be targeted on occasions when persons exhibit lack of self-direction? . . . If enthusiasm for paternalistic intervention slackens in these latter cases, it may be a signal for reexamination of the motives.

A third problem is the involuntariness of some self-destructive behavior may make paternalistic reform efforts ineffective. To the extent that the unhealthy behavior is not under the control of the individual, we cannot expect the kind of financial threat involved in a "fat tax" to exert much influence. Paradoxically, the very conditions under which paternalistic intervention seems most justified are those in which many of the methods available are least likely to succeed. . . .

Although the discussion above has focused on the problems attendant to a paternalistic argument for coercive health promotion programs, I have implicitly outlined a positive case for such interventions as well. A campaign to reform unhealthy habits of living will be justified, in my view, so long as it does not run afoul of the problems I have mentioned. . . . Health-promotion programs that are only very mildly coercive, such as moderate increases in cigarette taxes, require very little justification; non-coercive measures such as health education require none at all. And the case for more intrusive measures would be stronger if greater and more certain benefits could be promised. . . .

[The author proceeds to examine two other possible goals of health behavior reform:]

## Fair Distribution of Burdens

[One argument is that the healthy should not have to pay for costs incurred by risk-takers.] In the view of these persons, those who indulge in self-destructive practices and present their medical bills to the public are free riders in an economy kept going by the willingness of others to stay fit and sober. . . .

   . . . .

This sort of argument presupposes a certain theory of justice. . . . A number of considerations lead to the conclusion that the fairness argument as a justification of coercive intervention, despite initial appearances, is anything but straightforward. Underlying this argument is an empirical premise that may well prove untrue of at least some unhealthy habits: that those who take chances with their health *do* place a significant financial burden upon society. It is not enough to point to the costs of medical care for lung cancer and other diseases brought on by individual behavior. [O]ne must also determine what the individual would have died of had he not engaged in the harmful practice, and subtract the cost of the care which that condition requires. There is no obvious reason to suppose that the diseases brought on by self-destructive behavior are costlier to treat than those that arise from "natural causes."

Skepticism over the burden placed on society by smokers and other risk-takers is doubly reinforced by consideration of the non-medical costs and benefits that may be involved. It may turn out, for all we know prior to investigation, that smoking tends to cause few problems during a person's productive years and then to kill the individual before the need to provide years of social security and pension payments. From this perspective, the truly burdensome individual may be the unreasonably fit senior citizen who lives on for 30 years after retirement, contributing to the bankruptcy of the social security system, and using up savings that would have reverted to the public purse via inheritance taxes had an immoderate life-style brought an early death. . . .

A second doubt concerning the claim that the burdens of unhealthy behavior are unfairly distributed also involves an unstated premise. The risk taker, according to the fairness argument, should have to suffer not only the illness that may result from the behavior but also the loss of freedom attendant to the coercive measures used in the attempt to change the behavior. What, exactly, is the cause cited by those complaining of the financial burdens placed upon society by the self-destructive? It is not simply the burden of caring and paying for care of these persons when they become sick. Many classes of persons impose such costs on the public besides the self-destructive. For example, diabetics, and others with hereditary dispositions to contract diseases, incur unusual and heavy expenses, and these are routinely paid by others. Why are these costs not resisted as well?

One answer is that there *is* resistance to these other costs, which partly explains why we do not yet have a national health insurance system. But even those willing to pay for the costs of caring for diabetics, or the medical expenses of the poor, may still bridle when faced by the needs of those who have compromised their own health. . . . One possible reason to distinguish the costs of the person with a genetic disease from those of the person with a life-style-induced disease is simply that one can be prevented and the other cannot. . . .

But this is not the argument we seek. The medical costs incurred by diseases caused by unhealthy life-styles may be preventable, if our behavior-modifying methods are effective; but . . . [i]f costs must be reduced, perhaps they should be reduced some other way (*e.g.*, by lessening the quality of care provided for all); or perhaps costs should not be lowered and those feeling burdened should be made to tolerate the expense. The fact that money could be saved by intruding into the choice of life-styles of the self-destructive does not *itself* show that it would be particularly fair to do so.

If intrusion is to be justified on the grounds that unhealthy lifestyles impose unfair financial burdens on others, then, something must be added to the argument. That extra element, it seems, is *fault.* . . .

The argument thus depends crucially on the premise that the person who engages in an unhealthy life-style is responsible for the costs of caring for the illness that it produces. . . . Since responsibility was brought into the argument in hopes of contrasting life-style-related diseases from others, it seems to involve the actions of choice and voluntariness. If the chronic diseases resulting from life-style were not the result of voluntary choices, then there could be no assignment of responsibility in the sense in which the term is being used. . . . Since much self-destructive behavior is the result of suggestion, constraint, compulsion, and other factors, the applicability of the fairness argument is limited.

Even if the behavior leading to the illness is wholly voluntary, there is not necessarily any justification for intervention *by the state.* The only parties with rights to reform life-styles on these grounds are those who are actually being burdened by the costs involved. A wealthy man who retained his own medical facilities would not justifiably be a target of any of these interventions, and a member of a prepaid health plan would be liable to intervention primarily from others in his payment pool. He would then, of course, have the option of resigning and continuing his self-destructive ways; or he might seek out an insurance scheme designed for those who wish to take chances but who also want to limit their losses. . . . Measures undertaken by the government and applied indiscriminately to all who indulge in a given habit may thus be unfair to some (unless other justification is provided). . . .

This objection may lose force should there be a national health insurance program in which membership would be mandatory. Indeed, it might be argued that existing federal support of medical education, research, and service answers this objection now. But this only establishes another ground for disputing the responsibility of the self-destructive individual for the costs of his medical care. To state this objection, two classes of acts must be distinguished: the acts constituting the life-style that causes the disease and creates the need for care; and the acts of imposing financial shackles upon an unwilling public. Unless the acts in the first group are voluntary, the argument for imposing behavior change does not get off the ground. Even if voluntary, those acts in the second class might not be. . . . If the financial arrangement is mandatory, then the individual may not have *chosen* that his acts should have these effects on others. The situation will have been this: an individual is compelled by law to enter into financial relationships with certain others as a part of an insurance scheme; the arrangement causes the individual's acts to have effects on others that the others object to; and so they claim the right to coerce the individual into desisting from those acts. It seems difficult to assign to this individual responsibility for the distribution of financial burdens. . . .

    . . . .

There is, however, a response that would seem to have more chance of success: allowing those with unhealthy habits to pay their own way. Users of cigarettes and alcohol, for example, could be made to pay an excise tax, the proceeds of which would cover the costs of treatment for lung cancer and other resulting illnesses. Unfortunately, these costs would also be paid by users who are not abusers: those who drink only socially would be forced to pay for the excesses of alcoholics. Alternatively, only those contracting the illnesses involved could be charged; but it would be difficult to distinguish illnesses resulting from an immoderate life-style from those due to genetic or environmental causes. . . .

This kind of policy has its good and bad points. Chief among the favorable ones is that it allows a maximum retention of liberty in a situation in which liberty carries a price. Under such a policy, those who wished to continue their self-destructive ways without pressure could continue to do so, provided that they absorbed the true costs of their practices themselves. Should they not wish to shoulder these costs, they could submit to the efforts of the government to induce changes in their behavior. . . .

The negative side of this proposal stems from the fact that under its terms the only way to retain one's liberty is to pay for it. This, of course, offers very different opportunities to rich and poor. . . . Only the poor would be forced to submit to loss of privacy, loss of freedom from pressure, and regulation aimed at behavior change. Such liberties are what make up full citizenship, and one might hold that they ought not to be made contingent on one's ability to purchase them.

. . . .

. . . The central difficulty for the fairness argument, mentioned above, is that much of the self-destructive behavior that burdens the public is not really the fault of the individual; various forces, internal and external, may conspire to produce such a behavior independently of the person's will. Conversely, a problem for the paternalist is that much of the harm from which the individual would be "protected" may be the result of free, voluntary choices, and hence beyond the paternalist's purview. The best reason to be skeptical of the first rationale, then, is doubt over the *presence* of voluntariness; the best reason to doubt the second concerns the *absence* of voluntariness. Whatever weighs against the one will count for the other.

. . . .

## Public Welfare

Aside from protecting the public from unfair burdens imposed by those with poor health habits, there may be social benefits to be realized by inducing immoderates to change their behavior. Health behavior change may be the most efficient way to reduce the costs of health care in this country, and the benefits derived may give reason to create some injustices. Further, life-style reform could yield some important collective benefits. A healthier work force means a stronger economy, for example, and the availability of healthy soldiers enhances national security. . . .

. . . .

## Means of Health Behavior Reform

Two questions arise in considering the ethics of government attempts to bring about healthier ways of living. The first question is: Should coercion, intrusion, and deprivation be used as methods for inducing change? The other question is: How do we decide whether a given health promotion is coercive, intrusive, or inflicts deprivations? These questions are independent of each other. . . .

. . . .

. . . What is the difference between persuasion and manipulation? Can offers and incentives be coercive, or is coerciveness a property only of threats? . . .

## Health Education

Health education seems harmless. Education generally provides information and this generally increases our power, since it enhances the likelihood that our decisions will accomplish our ends. . . .

. . . .

The main threat of coerciveness in health education programs, in my opinion, lies in the possibility that such programs may turn from providing information to manipulating attitude and motivation. Education, in the sense of providing information, is a means of inducing belief and knowledge. A review of the literature indicates, however, that when health education programs are evaluated, they are not judged successful or unsuccessful in proportion to their success in *inducing belief*. Rather, evaluators look at *behavior change*, the actions which, they hope, would stem from those beliefs. If education programs are to be evaluated favorably, health educators may be led to take a wider view of their role. This would include attempts to motivate the public to adopt healthy habits, and this might have to be supplied by covert appeals to other interests ("smokers are unpopular," and so on). Suggestion and manipulation may replace information as the tools used by the health educators to accomplish their purpose. Indeed, health education may call for actual and deliberate *mis*information: directives may imply or even state that the scientific evidence in favor of a given health practice is unequivocal even when it is not.

A fine line has been crossed in these endeavors. Manipulation and suggestion go well beyond providing information to enhance rational decision making. These measures bypass rational decision-making faculties and thereby inflict a loss of personal control. Thus, health education, except when restricted to information, requires some justification. . . .

## Incentives, Subsidies, and Taxes

. . . .

Generally speaking, justification is required only for coercive measures, not for incentives. However, the distinction is not as clear as it first appears. Suppose, for example, that the government wants to induce the obese to lose weight, and that a mandatory national health insurance plan is about to go into effect. The government's plan threatens the obese with higher premiums unless they lose their excess weight. Before the plan is instituted, however, someone objects that the extra charges planned for eager eaters make the program coercive. No adequate justification is found. Instead of calling off the program, however, some subtle changes are made. The insurance scheme is announced with higher premiums than had been originally planned. No extra charges are imposed on anyone; instead, discounts are offered to all those who avoid overweight. Instead of coercion, the plan now uses positive incentives; and this does not require the kind of justification needed for the former plan. Hence the new program is allowed to go into effect.

The effect of the rate structure in the two plans is, of course, identical: The obese would pay the higher rate, the slender the lower one. It seems that the distinction between coercion and incentive is merely semantic. But this is the wrong conclusion. . . . Ultimately, I believe, the judgment required for the obesity measure would require us to decide what a fair rate would have been for the insurance; any charges above that fair rate would be coercive, and any below, incentive. . . . [T]his shows that one cannot judge the coerciveness of a few structure merely by checking it for surcharges. . . .

. . . .

## Regulative Measures

. . . A different way of effecting a reform is to deprive self-destructive individuals of the means needed to engage in their unhealthy habits. Prohibition of the sale of cigarettes would discourage smoking at least as effectively as exhortations not to smoke or insurance surcharges for habitual tobacco use. Yet, these regulative measures are surely as coercive, although they do not involve direct interaction with the individuals affected. They are merely one more way of intervening in an individual's decision to engage in habits that may cause illness. As such, they are clearly in need of the same or stronger justification as those involving threats, despite the argument that these measures are taken only to combat an unhealthy *environment*, and thus cannot be counted as coercing the persons who have unhealthy ways of living. . . . What distinguishes these "environmental" causes of illness from, say, carcinogens in the water supply, is the active connivance of the victims. "Shielding" the "victims" from these external forces must involve making them behave in a way they do not choose. This puts regulative measures in the same category as those applied directly to the self-destructive individuals.

## Conclusions

. . . It is apparent that more is needed than a simple desire on the part of government to promote health and/or reduce costs. When the measures taken are intrusive, coercive, manipulative, and/or inflict deprivations — in short, when they are of the sort many might be expected to dislike — the moral justification required may be quite complex. The principles that would be used in making a case for these interventions may have limited scope and require numerous exceptions and qualifications; it is unlikely that they can be expressed as simple slogans such as "individuals must be responsible for their own health" or "society can no longer afford self-destructiveness."

. . . .

Inherent in the subject matter is a danger that reform efforts, however rationalized and advertised, may become "moralistic," in being an imposition of the particular preferences and values of one (powerful) group upon another. Workers in medicine and related fields may naturally focus on the medical effects of everyday habits and practices, but others may not. From this perspective, trying to induce the public to change its style of living would represent an enormous expansion of the medical domain, a "medicalization of life." The parochial viewpoint of the health advocate can reach absurd limits. . . .

When the motivation behind life-style reform is concern for taxpayers rather than for self-destructive individuals, problems of a different kind are posed. Insistence that individuals are "responsible" for their own health may stem from a conflation of two different phenomena: an individual's life-style playing a causal role in producing illness, and that individual being at fault and accountable for his or her life-style and illness. The former may be undeniable, but the latter may be very difficult to prove. Unless difficulties in this sort of view are acknowledged, attention may be diverted from the various external causes of dangerous health-related behavior, resulting in a lessening of willingness to aid the person whose own behavior has resulted in illness.

# CHRIST'S BRIDE MINISTRIES, INC. v. SOUTHEASTERN PENNSYLVANIA TRANSPORTATION AUTHORITY
## 148 F.3d 242 (3d Cir. 1998)

Roth, Judge.

* * *

Southeastern Pennsylvania Transportation Authority (SEPTA) refused to display an advertisement stating that "Women Who Choose Abortion Suffer More & Deadlier Breast Cancer." We must decide in this appeal whether, in doing so, SEPTA violated the First Amendment rights of the advertiser, Christ's Bride Ministries, Inc. (CBM). . . .

SEPTA is an "agency and instrumentality" of the Commonwealth of Pennsylvania. It operates buses, subways, and regional rail lines in and around the City of Philadelphia. SEPTA contracts with a licensee, Transportation Display's Inc. (TDI), for the construction and sale of advertising space in its stations and in and on its vehicles. TDI and SEPTA are the defendants in this case.

The plaintiff, CBM, began a public service campaign in 1995 to inform the public of what it believes to be the increased risk of breast cancer for women who have had abortions. . . .

CBM contacted SEPTA in late November 1995 about placing posters in the Philadelphia area transit system. . . . In December 1995, [Bradley] Thomas [president of CBM] sent a draft poster to TDI for review by [TDI] and SEPTA. The poster stated "Women Who Choose Abortion Suffer More & Deadlier

Breast Cancer." The district court described the poster as "graphically designed with bold white lettering on a background of black and bright red, except that the word 'deadlier' was written in red." The poster also included a 1-800 number for information which connected callers not with CBM but with an organization called the American Rights Coalition (ARC).

SEPTA requested that the poster better identify the sponsor, CBM. CBM complied and added a description of CBM: "Christ's Bride Ministries, Inc. is a charitable, religious, educational, non-profit 501(c)(3) organization. CBM, P.O. Box 22 Merrifield, VA 22116. (703) 598-2226." SEPTA then approved the posters for display.

On January 15, 1996, the posters went up. TDI put two of them next to over-head clocks in Suburban Station in Philadelphia, and 24 others in subway and railroad stations in Philadelphia and its suburbs. SEPTA immediately began receiving what it described as "numerous" complaints about the poster, which included "rider protest" and "criticism" by "women's health organizations" and "local government officials." . . .

After the posters were installed, TDI faxed to CBM a contract, which Thomas signed and returned to TDI, also via fax. The contract was signed by Robert Meara of TDI and dated January 22, 1996. The monthly charge for the signs on the clocks was $642.60, while the monthly charge for the 24 other posters was $2400. There were "terms and conditions" on the back of the con-tract, including one that stated "if the Transportation Facility concerned should deem such advertising objectionable for any reason, TDI shall have the right to terminate the contract and discontinue the service without notice."

In early February, SEPTA received a copy of a letter written by Dr. Philip Lee, Assistant Secretary of Health in the United States Department of Health and Human Services [which said:] "It has recently come to my attention that the Metro Transit System has posted more than 1,100 free public service ads from the Christ's Bride Ministries. The ad states: 'Women who choose abortion suffer more & deadlier breast cancer. Information: 1-800-634-2224.' This ad is unfortunately misleading, unduly alarming, and does not accurately reflect the weight of the scientific literature."

Dr. Lee went on to state that in his opinion the studies showing a link between breast cancer and abortion suffered from methodological weaknesses, that there was no consensus on the purported relationship between breast cancer and abortion, and that Dr. Lee knew of no evidence supporting the claim that abortion causes "deadlier" breast cancer. Dr. Lee also complained that callers to the 1-800 number were referred to an article in the Journal of the National Cancer Institute, describing a study that suggested a positive correlation between induced abortions and breast cancer. Dr. Lee noted that although the article did appear in the Journal, the Journal also published an editorial stating that the results were not "conclusive." . . .

Based on Dr. Lee's letter, SEPTA removed the posters on February 16, 1996. According to the testimony of Mr. Gambaccini, SEPTA's General Manager, the "heart" of the decision to remove them was the questions about their accu-racy. . . . It is uncontested that no one at SEPTA or TDI conducted any other inquiry into the accuracy of the message on the poster, or contacted CBM for information that would support the claim made by the ad, or informed CBM of SEPTA's objections to the ad before removing the posters.

On March 13, 1996, Meara of TDI wrote to Thomas of CBM, explaining that the posters had been removed on February 16. Meara stated in his letter that the decision had been made by SEPTA as a result of "a letter from the U.S. Department of Health and Human Services in which it concluded that the ad was 'unfortunately misleading, unduly alarming and does not accurately reflect the weight of the scientific literature'." TDI included a check to CBM for $3042.60 for the "unused portion" of the contract CBM filed suit on May 10, 1996, alleg[ing] violations of CBM's rights under the First and Fourteenth Amendments and also breach of contract. . . . During the trial, three experts testified that the existing studies and research do not support the existence of a cause and effect relationship between abortion and breast cancer. These experts did, however, acknowledge that some studies show a weak "association" between induced abortions and breast cancer [a relative risk of 1.23]. One of SEPTA's experts testified that the better studies have not been consistent and that some studies show no link at all. CBM's expert, on the other hand, testified that he had analyzed 23 epidemiological studies, 12 of which, in his opinion, showed a statistically significant increase in breast cancer among women who had undergone induced abortions [a relative risk of 1.3]. He argued that this risk could not be accounted for by the presence of other variables, such as age or family. The increased risk, CBM's expert noted, was greater than the relative risk associated with oral contraceptives [1.1]. Because manufacturers of contraceptives alert the public as to the possible link between their product and breast cancer, it should not be "unduly alarming" for CBM to report a slightly greater risk purportedly associated with induced abortions.

The district court issued an opinion on August 16, 1996, holding for the defendants on all counts. The court reasoned that public transit stations do not constitute traditional public fora and that SEPTA and TDI had not created a public forum because they maintained control over the use of the advertising space. The court also found that Dr. Lee's letter was a "reasonable" basis on which to remove the advertisement. The court did not decide whether either SEPTA's or CBM's experts were "right."

## III. State Action and Commercial Speech

In this case, the parties agree that SEPTA is a state actor, as is its licensee, TDI, and that their actions are constrained by the First and Fourteenth Amendments.

[T]he posters come within the ambit of speech fully protected by the First Amendment. The defendants argue that because callers to the 1-800 number listed on the poster may receive information advertising the services of medical malpractice attorneys, CBM's message is thereby transformed into "commercial speech," and should receive substantially less constitutional protection. But the speech at issue does not advertise goods or services, nor does it refer to a specific product or service. The 1-800 number listed on the poster does not even connect callers to CBM. Any economic motive of CBM for posting the advertisement is very attenuated at best. The speech involved is accordingly not "commercial," at least in the sense that it is afforded less protection under the First Amendment.

## IV. Public Forum

The government may, as a general rule, limit speech that takes place on its own property without running afoul of the First Amendment. Where, however, the property in question is either a traditional public forum or a forum designated as public by the government, the government's ability to limit speech is impinged upon by the First Amendment. In either a traditional or a designated public forum, the government's content-based restrictions on private speech must survive strict scrutiny to pass constitutional muster. The government has, however, a far broader license to curtail speech if the forum has not been opened to the type of expression in question. In such a case, the government's restrictions need only be viewpoint neutral and "reasonable in light of the purpose served by the forum."

In order to decide whether a public forum is involved here, we must first determine the nature of the property and the extent of its use for speech.

. . . We conclude . . . that the forum at issue is SEPTA's advertising space.

SEPTA's advertising space . . . clearly does not constitute a "traditional" public forum, archetypal examples of which include streets and parks. These areas have been "held in the public trust," and dedicated to expressive activity for "time out of mind." We agree with the district court that the advertising space in the stations is not a traditional public forum.

More difficult is the question whether SEPTA has created a designated public forum by "expressly" dedicating its advertising space to "speech activity." A designated public forum is created because the government so intends. We accordingly look to the authority's intent with regard to the forum in question and ask whether SEPTA clearly and deliberately opened its advertising space to the public. . . .

## A. SEPTA's Policies

The main function of the advertising space at issue is to earn a profit for SEPTA. Although SEPTA generates approximately 99.5% of its revenues through the operation of the public transit system, it does derive about one half of one percent of its operating budget from the leasing of advertising space in its stations and in and on its vehicles. . . . TDI and SEPTA also had a secondary goal in using the space: promoting "awareness" of social issues and "providing a catalyst for change." . . . The "TDI Cares" program, in which SEPTA participates, seeks to "'give back' to the communities which TDI serves in many ways. . . ." In this program TDI picks an issue of public concern and then pays for the materials and labor involved in creating the advertisements. The purpose of the program, in TDI's words, is to assail TDI markets with "images, both poignant and creative, which are designed to elevate awareness and provide a catalyst for change." . . . SEPTA participated in TDI's annual campaign by donating unsold advertising space. . . .

[T]he nature of the forum suggests, but by no means establishes, that the government has dedicated the space to expression in the form of paid advertisements.

The contract between TDI and SEPTA provides . . . :

> All advertising displays at any time inserted or placed by the Licensee in any display devices in any vehicle and/or locations shall be of an appropriate character and quality, and the appearance of all displays shall be acceptable to SEPTA. No libelous, slanderous, or obscene advertising maybe accepted by the Licensee for display in the Authority's transit and railroad vehicles and facilities. All advertising determined by the [sic] SEPTA, in its sole discretion, as objectionable within the meaning of this subsection must not be utilized on any SEPTA vehicle or facility. SEPTA shall have the right to immediately remove any advertising material which has already been applied, in the event that the [sic] SEPTA deems material objectionable for any reason, at the expense of the Licensee.

[T]he fact that SEPTA has reserved for itself the right to reject ads for any reason at all does not signify, in and of itself alone, that no public forum has been created. If anything, we must scrutinize more closely the speech that the government bans under such a protean standard. SEPTA's purpose in operating the forum and its written policies governing access provide no conclusive answer as to whether the forum is intended to be closed or open. The goal of generating income by leasing ad space suggests that the forum may be open to those who pay the requisite fee. SEPTA has specified a few areas in which it will not freely accept advertising: alcohol and tobacco advertising beyond a specified limit and ads deemed libelous or obscene. Beyond these limitations, there are no specific restrictions on the type of advertising that SEPTA will accept. In effect, SEPTA's reservation of the right to reject any ad for any reason does not conclusively show that it intended to keep the forum closed.

## B.    SEPTA's Past Practice and the Suitability of the Forum for CBM's Ad

SEPTA has accepted a broad range of advertisements for display. These include religious messages, such as "Follow this bus to FREEDOM, Christian Bible Fellowship Church;" an ad criticizing a political candidate; and explicitly worded advertisements such as "Safe Sex Isn't" and an advertisement reminding viewers that "Virginity — It's cool to keep" and "Don't give it up to shut 'em up." Indeed, many ads address topics concerning sex, family planning, and related topics. Other examples include a controversial ad campaign on AIDS education and awareness, posters stating "The Face of Adoption" "Consider Adoption" and "Every child deserves a family," and another ad reading "Pregnant? Scared? Confused? A.R.C. Can Help Call 1-800-884-4004 or (215-844-1082.)"

On the topic of abortion, SEPTA has accepted two ads. One read "Choice Hotline, For Answers to Your Questions About: Birth Control * Pregnancy * Prenatal Care * Abortion * Adoption * HIV/AIDS * Sexually Transmitted Diseases (STDs) Abortion — Making A Decision, Call State Health Line 1-800-

692-7254 For Free Booklet on Fetal Development, Fetus is Latin for Little one — A Little Human is a Baby, Confidential * Free." The other one addressed the health benefits of legalizing abortion: "When Abortion Was Illegal, Women Died. My Mother Was One of Them. Keep Abortion Legal and Safe. Support the Clara Bell Duvall Education Fund. 471-9110."

From the broad range of ads submitted, SEPTA has requested modification of only three. One was the large wrap-around bus ad for Haynes hosiery, which would have covered the entire bus with the picture of a "scantily clad" woman; it was too "risque." The same ad was accepted as a smaller "poster" ad on the sides of buses. SEPTA also asked for modification of an ad depicting a gun with a condom stretched over it. The text of the ad, "Safe Sex Isn't," ultimately ran without the graphics. SEPTA also requested that an advertisement for a personal injury law firm delete references to rail accidents.

We conclude then, based on SEPTA's written policies, which specifically provide for the exclusion of only a very narrow category of ads, based on SEPTA's goals of generating revenues through the sale of ad space, and based on SEPTA's practice of permitting virtually unlimited access to the forum, that SEPTA created a designated public forum. Moreover, it created a forum that is suitable for the speech in question, i.e., posters which presented messages concerning abortion and health issues. CBM paid for advertising space which had previously been used for ads on those topics. We need not define the precise boundaries of the forum, particularly concerning visual images that could be considered explicit. The topic of abortion and its health effects were, however, "encompassed within the purpose of the forum."

Moreover, there is no evidence that SEPTA rejected the ad pursuant to a new or previously existing policy to close the forum to debatable or misleading speech generally, or closed it to such speech on any particular topic of health. SEPTA claims the forum is closed to all speech, and that short of viewpoint discrimination, SEPTA can make any content-based restrictions it chooses. SEPTA's prior acceptance of a broad range of advertisements cuts particularly strongly against this claim.

     . . . .

Moreover, as to the subject of abortion specifically, and family planning issues generally, permission to post advertisements has been granted as a "matter of course." There is no policy, written or unwritten, pursuant to which CBM's ads were removed.

Because we find that SEPTA has created a designated public forum, content-based restrictions on speech that come within the forum must pass strict scrutiny to comport with the First Amendment. As the Supreme Court explained in *Police Dept. of the City of Chicago v. Mosley,* "above all else, the First Amendment means that government has no power to restrict expression because of its message, its ideas, its subject matter, or its content." Thus the government "may not grant the use of a forum to people whose views it finds acceptable, but deny use to those wishing to express less favored or more controversial views. And it may not select which issues are worth discussing or debating in public facilities." The prohibited expression in this case, CBM's ad, falls within the scope of the forum created by SEPTA. Thus, SEPTA's restriction is subject to heightened review.

SEPTA has not argued that its actions survive strict scrutiny. Accordingly, we conclude that CBM's First Amendment rights were violated when SEPTA removed CBM's ads.

## V.   Reasonableness of SEPTA's Restrictions

Even if the speech in question had fallen outside the limited public forum created by SEPTA, we would nonetheless conclude that SEPTA's removal of the posters violated the First Amendment because the removal was not "reasonable."

[T]he reasonableness of the government's restriction on speech depends on the nature and purpose of the property from which it is barred. In this case, . . . [t]he subject of the speech, and the manner in which it was presented, were compatible with the purposes of the forum.

SEPTA argued that Gambaccini had testified that SEPTA "closed the debate to a situation in which there are ads or debated and dubious statements of medical fact." Consistent with this statement, SEPTA could have argued that based on Dr. Lee's letter, it viewed CBM's ad as "debated and dubious," and accordingly excluded it. A prohibition on "debated and dubious ads," put in place before, or because of the concerns about CBM's ad, might qualify as reasonable. We note, however, that SEPTA does not have a policy of protecting riders from "debated and dubious" speech generally, nor does SEPTA link this purported policy to its use of the forum.

In any event, we need not reach that question. Gambaccini did not testify to such a policy, implemented either before or after the removal of CBM's ad. Instead, when questioned if he would post an ad saying "women who choose abortion live longer and have less breast cancer," he answered "Not unless there was some credible evidence to support it." This is a different standard — a debatable advertisement may well be supported by credible evidence. And if this standard controlled, SEPTA was unreasonable because it failed to give CBM an opportunity to produce such evidence. Moreover, Gambaccini did not explain whether this standard applied generally, or just to ads on the topic of abortion and cancer. Nor did he explain SEPTA's grounds for adopting it. SEPTA has left us to guess why, in terms of the purpose of the forum, it excluded CBM's ad, and why, and to what extent, other ads will also be excluded. This makes it difficult to evaluate the extent of the governmental interest in excluding the speech from SEPTA's property.

Finally, as we have noted, SEPTA never asked CBM — the sponsor of the ad — to defend its accuracy, to explain the basis for the ad, or to clarify it. Instead, SEPTA removed the ad without contacting CBM — even though CBM had modified the poster in response to SEPTA's previous requests.

We conclude, therefore, that under the facts presented SEPTA's actions were not reasonable. SEPTA acted as a censor, limiting speech because it found it to be "misleading." SEPTA argues that it cannot investigate the accuracy of medical claims in ads. For that reason, it relied on Dr. Lee's letter. We do not hold that SEPTA must hire its own cadre of experts to evaluate medical claims made in ads. It was SEPTA, however, which accepted advertising on a permitted topic, and then decided that CBM's ad was unacceptably misleading. Having decided to exclude the posters on this basis, SEPTA did not act reasonably when it failed to ask CBM to clarify the basis on which the claim was made. This is all the more true where SEPTA has failed to explain how its content-based distinctions are related to preserving the advertising space for its intended use, and where SEPTA has in place no policy, old or new, written or unwritten, governing the display of ads making contested claims.

\* \* \*

## Aaron Wildavsky & Karl Dake, *Theories of Risk Perception*
### 119 Daedalus — J. Am. Acad. Arts & Sci. 41, 42–45, 48–51 (1990)

\* \* \*

The most widely held theory of risk perception we call the *knowledge theory*: the often implicit notion that people perceive technologies (and other things) to be dangerous because they know them to be dangerous. . . .

Another commonly held cause of risk perception follows from *personality theory*. In conversations we frequently hear personality referred to in such a way that individuals seem to be without discrimination in their risk-aversion or risk-taking propensities: some individuals love risk taking so they take many risks, while others are risk averse and seek to avoid as many risks as they can. . . .

The third set of explanations for public perceptions of danger follow two versions of *economic theory*. In one, the rich are more willing to take risks stemming from technology because they benefit more and are somehow shielded from adverse consequences. The poor presumably feel just the opposite. In "post-materialist" theory, the rationale is reversed, however: precisely because living standards have improved, the new rich are less interested in what they have (affluence) and what got them there (capitalism), than in what they think they used to have (closer social relations), and what they would like to have (better health). . . .

Other explanations for public reactions to potential hazards are based on *political theory*. These accounts view the controversies over risk as struggles over interests, such as holding office or party advantage. . . . The hope for explanatory power in such approaches to risk perception is thus placed on social and demographic characteristics such as gender, age, social class, liberal-conservative ratings, and/or adherence to political parties.

Viewing individuals as the active organizers of their own perceptions, *cultural theorists* have proposed that individuals choose what to fear (and how much to fear it), in order to support their way of life. In this perspective, selective attention to risk, and preferences among different types of risk taking (or avoiding), correspond to *cultural biases* — that is, to worldviews or ideologies entailing deeply held values and beliefs defining different patterns of social relations. Social relations are defined in cultural theory as a small number of distinctive patterns of interpersonal relationships — hierarchical, egalitarian, or individualist. . . .

. . . .

According to cultural theory, adherents of hierarchy perceive acts of social deviance to be dangerous because such behavior may disrupt their preferred (superior/subordinate) form of social relations. By contrast, advocates of great equality of conditions abhor the role differentiation characteristic of hierarchy because ranked stations signify inequality. Egalitarians reject the prescriptions associated with hierarchy (i.e., who is allowed to do what and with whom), and thus have much less concern with social deviance.

Individualists cultures support self-regulation, including the freedom to bid and bargain. The labyrinth of normative constraints and controls on behavior that are valued in hierarchies are perceived as threats to the autonomy of the individualist, who prefers to negotiate for himself. Social deviance is a threat to individualist culture only when it limits freedom, or when it is disruptive of market relationships. Our expectation is that individualists should take a stance between hierarchists, to whom social deviance is a major risk, and egalitarians, to whom it is a minor risk at most.

. . . .

People who hold an egalitarian bias (who value strong equality in the sense of diminishing distinctions among people such as wealth, race, gender, authority, etc.) would perceive the dangers associated with technology to be great, and its attendant benefits to be small. They believe that an egalitarian society is likely to insult the environment just as it exploits poor people. Those who endorse egalitarianism would also rate the risks of social deviance to be relatively low. What right has an unconscionably inegalitarian system to make demands or to set standards?

. . . .

[The authors then summarize the following findings from their research and other surveys testing how well cultural theory predicted risk perceptions among these groups.]

Our findings show that those who rate their self-knowledge of technologies highly also tend to perceive greater average benefits associated with technologies than those who are less confident about their knowledge. Those who report higher levels of education tend to perceive less threat from the risk of war. Otherwise, self-rated knowledge and education bear only weak (that is, statistically insignificant) relations to preferences for societal risk taking or to perceived risks associated with technology and the environment, social deviance, and economic troubles.

The more an individual's annual fatality estimates correspond to expert estimates, in addition, the more likely that person is to rate other risks as small — at least compared with those who are less accurate. While on the whole those who are more in accord with expert mortality estimates perceive less risk, they are also less optimistic regarding the benefits of technology. *Overall, the conclusion is compelling that self-rated knowledge and perceptual accuracy have a minimal relationship with risk perception.*

With regard to personality, we find that those who feel our society should definitely take technological risk can be described as patient, forbearing, conciliatory, and orderly (i.e., the pro-risk measure is positively correlated with the personality traits "need for order" and "deference"). Advocates of societal risk taking tend not to be aggressive, or autonomous, or exhibitionistic, but are more likely to be cautious and shy and to seek stability rather than change. *This pattern is suggestive of a technologically pro-risk personality, which emerges as that of an obedient and dutiful citizen, deferential to authority.* Such a personality structure fits extremely well with the political culture of hierarchy.

By contrast, those citizens who perceive greater risk in regard to technology and the environment tend to turn up positive on exhibitionism, autonomy, and need for change, but negative on need for order, deference, and endurance (i.e., just the opposite of those who score as favoring societal risk taking). *This technologically risk-averse pattern of personality traits also holds for those who endorse egalitarianism.*

Those who endorse egalitarianism are also more likely to be personally risk taking, but societally risk averse, while those who favor hierarchy tend to be personally risk averse, but societally pro-risk with respect to technology and the environment. Thus, *we find no evidence for a personality structure that is risk taking or risk averse across the board.* Risk taking and risk aversion are not all of a piece, but depend on how people feel about the object of attention. Cultural theory would predict, for example, that hierarchists would be risk averse when it comes to taking risks with the body politic.

Relative to conservatives, those who rate themselves as liberals tend to be technologically risk averse at the societal level, are more likely to rate the risks of technology and the environment as very great, and are comparatively unconcerned abut the risks of social deviance. As the self-rating of liberal increases, the average ratings for the risks of the 25 specific technologies increases, and the average ratings of their benefits decreases.

Political party membership is less predictive of risk perceptions and preferences than left-right ideology, especially on the Democratic side (undoubtedly because Democrats are the more heterogeneous party). When we ask what it is about thinking of oneself as a liberal or a conservative that makes such a big difference compared with thinking of oneself as a Democrat or a Republican, the findings are informative. Whether by self-rating or policy designation, *liberals have strong tendencies to endorse egalitarianism* ($r = 0.52$ and $r = 0.50$), *and to reject hierarchy* ($r = -0.55$ and $r = -0.51$) *and individualism* ($r = -0.37$ and $r = -0.31$). Likewise, membership in the Democratic party is correlated with egalitarianism ($r = 0.30$), but is not predictive of agreement or disagreement with the hierarchical or individualist point of view. *Republicans have a penchant toward individualist* ($r = 0.31$) *and hierarchical biases* ($r = 0.40$), *and an equally strong proclivity for rejecting egalitarianism* (r = −0.45). These correlations among political party membership, left-right ideology, and cultural biases are huge by the standards of survey research.

How does cultural theory compare with other approaches to perceived risk? *Cultural biases provide predictions of risk perceptions and risk-taking preferences that are more powerful than measures of knowledge and personality and at least as predictive as political orientation.* We find that egalitarianism is strongly related to the perception of technological and environmental risks as grave problems for our society (r = 0.51), and hence to strong risk aversion in this domain (r = −0.42). Egalitarianism is also related positively to the average perceived risks, and negatively to the average perceived benefits of 25 technologies. One could hardly paint a worse picture of technology — little benefit, much risk, and the risks not worth taking.

Individualist and hierarchist biases, in contrast are positively correlated to a preference for technological risk-taking (r = 0.32) and r = 0.43) and to average ratings of technological benefits (r = 0.34 and r = 0.37). Here the image is more sanguine: the benefits are great, and the risks small, so society should press on with risk taking to get more of the good that progress brings.

. . . But one should not conclude that the establishment cultures of individualism and hierarchy always favor risk taking, or that egalitarians are always risk averse. *Perception of danger is selective; it varies with the object of attention. . . .* As predicted by cultural theory, *it is not that devotees of individualism and hierarchy perceive no dangers in general, but that they disagree with those who favor egalitarianism about how dangers should be ranked. Just as technological and environmental risks are most worrisome to egalitarians, social deviance is deemed most dangerous to hierarchists, and the threat of war (which disrupts markets and subjects people to severe controls) is most feared by individualists.*

\* \* \*

## Leonard H. Glantz, Control of Personal Behavior and the Informed Consent Model
### (2006)

\* \* \*

## Control of Personal Behavior

Public health interventions have evolved over the years. The traditional public health model addressed environmental factors in order to protect the health of populations. For example, the greatest achievements in public health and those that have best protected the population produced clean water, safe milk, clean air, effective sanitation, habitable living conditions and safer workplaces. All of these interventions have one thing in common — they protect the health of the population without individuals being required to take action to protect themselves.

In recent years, in addition to these environmental interventions, there has been much more focus on changing the personal behaviors of large numbers of individuals. In 1993, an influential article was published in the Journal of the American Medical Association entitled "Actual Causes of Death in the United States," 270 JAMA 2207 (1993). The authors note that death certificates list the cause of death as the immediate medical condition that resulted in death: heart disease, cancer, cerebrovascular disease, pneumonia, influenza, diabetes, and the like. The authors claim, however, that while these are the conditions from which people die, they do not account for the underlying causes of those medical conditions. The authors propose that the actual causes of death are tobacco use, diet/activity patterns, alcohol use, fire arms, sexual behavior, motor vehicles, and illicit drug use.[2] These causes of death are seemingly all within the control of individuals. Rather than being victims of the environment people become victims of their own activity or inactivity. As this perspective became accepted one would go about preventing death and disability by getting people to cease engaging in behaviors that caused such conditions or to engage in activities that would prolong their lives and well-being. Unlike the traditional public health interventions which would make people healthier by changing their environment, these interventions are based on the notion that if each individual acts in way that makes him or her healthier, the population on the whole will be healthier — the ultimate goal of public health.

The goal of changing people's behavior, however, is not new. The seven deadly sins, which include sloth and gluttony, were seen as moral failings, not public health matters. Prohibitionists in the United States and elsewhere were opposed to the drinking of alcoholic beverages because this indulgence was perceived as unhealthy for the soul, as well as or perhaps even more than unhealthful for the body. Historically, those concerned with the moral fiber of society have tried to keep people from drinking, smoking, taking drugs, and having sex outside of marriage — all issues that are also addressed by the public health community. Is there a difference between moralistic interventions and public-health interventions? An early example of the cumulative effect of public health and moralistic concerns on social policy is found in an early United States Supreme Court case that upheld the Kansas prohibition against the manufacture of intoxicating liquors, *Mugler v. Kansas*, 123 U.S. 623 ( ). The petitioner argued that the state had no business regulating the manufacturer of liquor for his own use. The Court upheld the statute, saying that it could not ignore the fact that "Public health, public morals, and the public safety may be endangered by the general use of intoxicating drinks; nor the fact established by statistics accessible to everyone, that the idleness, disorder, pauperism, and crime existing in the country are, in some degree at least, traceable to this evil." 123 U.S. at 662.

While activities that are discouraged for either moralistic or public health reasons may be similar, the methods and goals should be different.

---

**2** Ask yourself if the authors are correct in their approach. In law, the term "causation" has a pretty distinct definition and usually refers to proximate causation. This is because there is almost no limit to how far back in time one can go to ascribe causation to a multiple of factors. For example, while describing tobacco use as the cause of death, one could ask whether the classmate in the playground who provided the first cigarette is the cause of death, or whether the tobacco farmer is the cause of death, or whether it is the economic conditions that the led the farmer to grow tobacco instead of some other crop. Ascription of causation can have a substantial political component to it.

Furthermore, public health interventions should be based on scientific knowledge about the nature of risky activities and the effectiveness of interventions designed to reduce or eliminate the risk. In the absence of a scientific and rational foundation for inducing individual behavior change, the change is being proposed for moral or aesthetic reasons rather than its implications for health.

## Does the Informed Consent Model Have a Place in Public Health Interventions?

The doctrine of informed consent for medical treatment was adopted by courts and ethicists in the late 1960s and early 1970s. Prior to its adoption, the general sense was that patients should listen to "doctor's orders." Physicians and even some family members often proposed that a patient not even be told his or her diagnosis, especially gloomy ones like cancer, so that the patient would not be come upset or "lose hope." It was not uncommon that medically proven treatments were not disclosed by physicians to their patients if those treatments were different from those the physician preferred. A stark example of this involves the treatment of breast cancer. For many years breast cancer was treated by performing a radical mastectomy, which removed all of the breast and all underlying muscle and tissue. As less radical and deforming treatments were developed, such as the removal of the cancerous tissue while saving the breast (lumpectomy), physicians who continued to believe that radical mastectomy was more likely to save lives did not discuss the availability of the less radical surgical or medical treatments. Ultimately, under pressure from organizations of women, some states adopted specific legislation requiring disclosure of alternative breast cancer therapies.

Physicians often withheld information because they feared that patients would not understand it or would act "irrationally," by which they typically meant that the patient would not choose what the physician believed to be the best chance for survival. In the breast cancer scenario, physicians who withheld information about lumpectomy often were concerned that "mere vanity" would keep women from choosing radical mastectomy. Many believed that longevity was so desirable a goal that other considerations should not be relevant.

The doctrine of informed consent to medical care created by courts in the early 1970s enables individuals to make important decisions about their health care based on their own perception of their needs, desires and fears. As the California Supreme Court noted in *Cobbs v. Grant*, 8 Cal. 3d 229, 502 P.2d 1 (1972), physicians are experts in knowing what the likely risks and benefits are of a recommended treatment, but, "the weighing of these risks against the individual subjective fears and hopes of the patient is not an expert skill. Such evaluation and decision is a nonmedical judgment reserved for the patient alone." 8 Cal. 3d at ___. This type of analysis, adopted by courts in other states, caused a reconsideration of the goals of medicine.

The goal of doctrine of informed consent is to create patients who are armed with the information they need to decide *whether or not* to accept medical care recommended by their physician. It is the fact that patients were to be well enough informed to knowledgeably *reject* a physician's recommendation that made the doctrine "radical" to physicians. It also means that a good outcome of the physician-patient interaction is not an obedient or "compliant" patient but an informed patient. Patient knowledge and autonomy became more important values than their health or longevity.

In time the medical profession came to adopt the doctrine of informed consent as a fundamental ethical underpinning of the practice of medicine:

> It is a fundamental ethical requirement that a physician should at all times deal honestly and openly with patients. . . . Only through full disclosure is a patient able to make informed decisions regarding future medical care.

AMA Opinion E-8.12 Patient Information (1994)

> The patient's right of self-decision can be effectively exercised only if the patient possesses enough information to enable an intelligent choice. The patient should make his or her own determination on treatment. The physician's obligation is to present the medical facts accurately to the patient. . . . and to make recommendations for management in accordance with good medical practice.

AMA E-8.08 Informed Consent (1981)

It is notable that the AMA acknowledged patient "self decision" as a "right." The AMA has further acknowledged that physicians must provide a patient with accurate facts but it is the patient's right to make "his or her own determination on treatment."

The question this raises is whether the philosophy behind the doctrine of informed consent plays any role in the practice of public health. Leaders in the public health profession recently adopted what is referred to as "Principles of the Ethical Practice of Public Health." Nowhere in these principles is the doctrine of informed consent mentioned. The closest to informed consent these principles comes is paragraph 6:

> 6. Public health institutions should provide communities with the information they have that is needed for decisions on policies or programs and should obtain the community's consent for their implementation.

92 American Journal of Public Health 1058 (July 2002).

It is far from clear what it means to provide communities with information and to obtain "the community's consent." Indeed the code does not require anything of a public health practitioner, unlike the AMA code of ethics that requires individual physicians to act in certain ways. Rather "public health institutions" are assigned to provide information to communities.

In the "old public health" paradigm this approach makes a certain amount of sense. If the public health goal is to create a safer water supply for a community by replacing lead water pipes, no consent of every individual who might drink that water could sensibly be required. Indeed, no particular individual in the community could "reject" the recommended water improvement project. Furthermore, community leaders such as mayors, city councilors or other elected representatives would make the decision about the water supply and should be informed about the risks and benefits of alternative approaches before making such decisions. But this is a long way from individual informed consent. It is simply a description of how policymakers arrive at decisions.

With the new public health paradigm that focuses on behavior change, there is no "community" that needs information, nor any "community" that gives consent. Behavior change is squarely focused on individuals, not communities. What might the goals of public health be in this context? Is it to have a citizenry that behaves the way public health agencies think people ought to behave or a citizenry that has enough information to make knowledgeable choices? For example, should the goal of public health be to ensure that nobody smokes cigarettes, or should the goal be to ensure that everybody knows the risks of cigarette smoking so they can make their own decision whether or not to smoke?

This raises the question of how truthful public health education campaigns need to be. If the goal is to ensure that people behave in a certain way, truth-telling could be counterproductive. For example, Viscusi argues that people in the United States tend to think that smoking is even more risky than it actually is. W. KIP VISCUSI, SMOKING: MAKING THE RISKY DECISION (1992). If the goal is to prevent people from smoking or to get smokers to stop smoking, such misinformation will help further that goal. If the goal is to have an informed populace, this goal is not met. Do public health professionals have an obligation to present accurate information even if that runs counter to their behavioral goals? If there is no obligation to tell the truth, is there some obligation not to mislead the public about risks and benefits of behavior change? If there is such an obligation, what is its source?

## Behavior Change Methods

There are many ways to change people's behavior. One way is to provide them with knowledge. This is very close to the informed consent model in which one tells the truth about risks and benefits of particular activities and leaves it up to the individual to decide whether or not to engage in those activities. For example, there can be educational advertising campaigns or even laws mandating signs in cars to inform people that they are less likely to die in an accident if they wear their seatbelts. It is well-known that education will affect some people's behaviors. Still, there will be people who will ignore or reject the information and continue to drive without seatbelts. We can try to persuade these people to use seatbelts with more appealing or effective notices or by adding a strong emotional component. For example, an advertisement might show a young family in a cemetery grieving for a family member who would be alive if only he had worn his seatbelt. This emotional manipulation will create an additional number of seatbelt users, but there will certainly still be people who do not use seatbelts. To reach this last group, the legislature might pass a law making it a crime to drive while not wearing a seatbelt. It is this last approach, state action that criminalizes otherwise innocent behaviors, that raise both legal and ethical issues.

The use of coercive measures to force people to conform their behavior in ways we think best for raises the problem of paternalism. Paternalism assumes we know what is in a person's interests better than that person does. For young children or incompetent adults, this is the case, and both law and ethics permit making decisions on their behalf. For competent adults, however, paternalism deprives them of the ability to make decisions for themselves based on what they conclude his best for them. As described above, in the pre-informed consent era physicians were endowed with paternalistic power. The movement towards informed consent was a rejection of this paternalistic way of making medical decisions. In a free and pluralistic society, Americans tend to resist paternalistic actions by the state. Indeed, one of the underpinnings of being a free adult is the ability to make poor decisions for ourselves. Because state paternalism is such a suspect doctrine in a free society, states often deny their paternalistic motives for passing legislation.

\* \* \*

## NOTES AND QUESTIONS

**1.** Wikler's article was published almost three decades ago, but the questions posed in his analysis remain quite contemporary. The general goals of health policies and laws — health itself; fair distribution of (financial) burdens; and public welfare — are widely accepted. It is the measures used to achieve those goals that generate controversy, particularly measures that compel individuals to change their personal behavior. The article examines individual policy goals in isolation, but also acknowledges that "in actuality most government programs would probably be expected to serve several purposes at once." (Wikler, *supra,* at 305.) Does the fact that a measure serves more than one goal improve its chances of justification as a matter of law, as a matter of moral theory, as a matter of political acceptability?

Does public health policy treat similar risks to health consistently? Are skiing, playing football or other recreational sports less risky than using marijuana? Risk is the result of multiplying two factors: the probability of a specific harm occurring, and the magnitude of that harm. One's perception of risk may differ, depending upon whether one focuses on the magnitude of the harm or on the probability that it may occur. (And the values of each factor may themselves be uncertain.) The probability of catching the common cold may be high during winter, but few people consider it a serious risk, because the harm it causes, while annoying, is not dreadful (unless you are immunocompromised). Moreover, as noted by Wildavsky and Dake, people may assign very different values to the same harm and to what they lose by preventing the harm. This suggests that policies may or may not be accepted depending upon whose ox is being gored. How should society decide which risks are socially acceptable and which are not? Is a simple majority vote of the legislature enough, as long as the measure serves a legitimate state purpose? Wikler's article challenges policy makers to think carefully about the accuracy of assumptions about how different measures serve legitimate public health goals. In particular, his discussion of paternalism emphasizes that measures intended to improve an individual's health for his or her own sake, rather than to prevent harm to others (as was the primary focus of Chapter Three), are both conceptually and empirically difficult to justify in a principled manner. Wilker presents an ethical analysis, not a legal one, although the arguments are relevant to legal analysis. Are the various legal doctrines applicable to criminal laws, tax laws, administrative regulation, and general civil rights and obligations sufficient to distinguish acceptable from unacceptable public health policies?

Note that Wikler mentions diabetes as an example of a disease that is beyond an individual's control. Contrast that view with current public health campaigns to reduce the incidence of diabetes by encouraging people to lose weight and take their medications consistently. (See the Mariner article on the New York City diabetes blood sugar reporting law in Chapter Four.) Is the change in how the condition is viewed the result of better scientific and epidemiological information?

**2.** A current criticism of the emphasis on personal behavioral risk factors, one recognized by Wilker (*supra,* at 305), is that it may distract attention from more important sources of risk, such as environmental and occupational factors. Contemporary serious study of the social determinants of health may have been inspired by WHY ARE SOME PEOPLE HEALTHY AND OTHERS ARE NOT? THE DETERMINANTS OF HEALTH OF POPULATIONS (Robert G. Evans, et al., eds. 2004). Some, perhaps most, environmental interventions can be less costly and more effective than laws intended to change personal behavior, primarily because they do not depend upon individual willingness to take specific actions. Moreover, they largely avoid arguments that the law violates some aspect of personal liberty. For example, building roads with safe curves, grade banking, and lighting may reduce the risk of motor vehicle crashes as much or more than enforcing speed limits. Some of these contributors to risk may be more difficult and expensive to remove. Think about what might be more appealing to you as a legislator: a bill requiring all people in motor vehicles to wear seat belts or a bill requiring the automobile industry to install air bags in all vehicles sold in the state. What constituencies might support and oppose each bill? What might each bill cost the state itself?

State laws requiring motor vehicle drivers (and more recently passengers) were encouraged as an alternative to regulatory requirements that automobile manufacturers install airbags or passive restraints in cars, which the industry had opposed since 1969. The Department of Transportation issued final standards requiring passive restraints for all cars by 1984, but reopened the rulemaking process in 1981 and ultimately rescinded the standard, when it appeared that auto makers were going to install passive seat belts instead of airbags in 99% of new cars. Some of the history of the regulatory battle between the automobile industry and the Department of Transportation is found in *Motor Vehicle Manufacturers Association of the United States v. State Farm Mutual Automobile Insurance Co.,* 463 U.S. 29 (1983). In that case, the U.S. Supreme Court overturned the agency's rescission of the standard because it was not "the product of reasoned decisionmaking." Although substantial evidence supported issuing the standard, the agency rescinded it primarily because of industry practice, which the Court found arbitrary and capricious: "If, under the statute, the agency should not defer to the industry's failure to develop safer cars, which it surely should not do, *a fortiori* it may not revoke a safety standard which can be satisfied by current technology simply because the industry has opted for an ineffective seatbelt design." 463 U.S. at 49. A presidential election resulted in a new Secretary of Transportation, however, who agreed with the industry that the airbag standard would not be issued as a final rule if two-thirds of the states enacted legislation requiring people to wear seatbelts. The effort to pass such laws was successful, although it prompted occasionally heated debates over whether such laws were unjustifiably paternalistic or a safety-conscious condition on the privilege of driving. Largely ignored in the arguments was the reason for having the debate in the first place — rejection of effective safety standards for motor vehicles.

**3.** *Christ's Bride* illustrates how different groups may view the same information and characterize similar levels of risk as negligible or significant. The decision in *Christ's Bride* turned on the reasonableness of the determination to exclude the advertising. Reasonableness in turn depended upon the degree of relative risk found in epidemiological studies, as well as the credibility of the studies' methods and statistical analysis. (Relative risk is a statistical calculation stating the risk of an outcome (*e.g.*, breast cancer) in a person with a particular risk factor (*e.g.*, having had an abortion) compared with a person without that risk factor (*e.g.*, no abortion). Relative risk is used to describe how much the risk factor increases the risk of the outcome. A relative risk of 1 means the outcome is the same with or without the risk factor. A relative risk of 2 means that a person having the risk factor has twice the risk of a person without the risk factor.) CMB's expert testified that his "metanalysis" of studies found a relative risk of breast cancer for women who had abortions of 1.3. One of SEPTA's experts had published a study finding a relative risk of 1.23. SEPTA's experts argued that a relative risk of 1.2 or 1.3 was too low to be persuasive evidence of any cause and effect relationship. They also argued that some of the breast cancer studies may have exaggerated the risk from abortion because they did not use the standard 95% confidence intervals to calculate relative risk. CMB argued that the FDA required disclosure of relative risks of 1.1 for oral contraceptives. The testimony is reviewed in the district court decision, *Christ's Bride Ministries, Inc. v. Southeastern Pennsylvania Transportation Authority*, 937 F. Supp. 425 (E.D. Pa. 1996).

What counts as a high relative risk in one case may not count as a high relative risk in another. Current estimates of the relative risk of death from heart disease among nonsmokers exposed to environmental tobacco smoke (ETS, also called secondhand smoke) are 1.3. The Environmental Protection Agency's report on environmental tobacco smoke, *Respiratory Health Effects of Passive Smoking: Lung Cancer and Other Disorders* (Dec. 1992), provided evidence for the health risks of ETS in Surgeon General's reports as well as legislative hearings on bills to ban smoking in public places. EPA produced the report as part of its statutory risk assessment determining that ETS should be classified and regulated as a Group A carcinogen, meaning that there is evidence that it causes cancer in humans. The EPA concluded that the relative risk of cancer from ETS was 1.19. (Prior to its ETS analysis, the EPA had found that higher relative risks of 2.6 and 3.0 for other chemicals were not high enough to classify the chemicals as Group A carcinogens.) The EPA's methods were challenged by the tobacco industry. In *Flue-Cured Tobacco*

*Cooperative Stabilization Corp. v. U.S. Environmental Protection Agency*, 4 F. Supp. 2d 435 (M.D. N.C. 1998), *vacated and remanded*, 313 F.3d 852 (4th Cir. 1999), the North Carolina district court found that the EPA had exceeded its statutory authority by basing its conclusion on faulty analyses that left "substantial holes in the administrative record": "EPA publicly committed to a conclusion before research had begun; excluded industry by violating the Act's procedural requirements; adjusted established procedure and scientific norms to validate the Agency's public conclusion . . . EPA disregarded information and made findings on selective information; . . . failed to disclose important findings and reasoning; and left significant questions without answers." *Id.* at 465–66. Regardless of one's views on smoking or this district court, the problems identified are unsettling: "EPA could not produce statistically significant results with its selected studies. Analysis conducted with a .05 significance level and 95% confidence level included relative risks of 1. . . In order to confirm its hypothesis, EPA maintained its standard significance level but lowered the confidence interval to 90%. This allowed EPA to confirm its hypothesis by finding a relative risk of 1.19, albeit a very weak association." *Id.* at 462. The court's rejection of the EPA's report, however, did not prevent its use as evidence of the risk of ETS among non-smokers. The Court of Appeals held that the district court lacked subject matter jurisdiction, because the EPA report was not final agency action.

Like the studies concerning abortion and breast cancer, studies of exposure to ETS have reported conflicting results, with one study reporting the implausible finding that children living with parents who smoked have a lower risk of cancer than children living with non-smokers. For our purposes, the question is to what degree can studies showing minimal risks be relied upon? Why is one set of studies believed to demonstrate no more than a negligible risk at best, while another set of studies are believed to demonstrate substantial risk? To what degree is one's attitude toward particular risks likely to affect one's willingness to believe some studies and not others?

How would you characterize the different public health responses to similar relative risks?

**4.** *AIDS Action Committee of Massachusetts, Inc. v. Massachusetts Bay Transportation Authority*, 42 F.3d 1 (1st Cir. 1994), presented a First Amendment challenge similar to that presented in Christ's Bride. The MBTA placed seven public service advertisements from AIDS Action Committee on Boston subways and trolleys. The ads showed a color picture of a packaged condom and stated that latex condoms are an effective means of preventing HIV transmission. The ad campaign provoked complaints, one-third of which included "explicit homophobic statements," 42 F.3d at 3, perhaps because the ads included text using double entendres and sexual innuendo. Shortly thereafter, the MBTA issued a new policy that required advertising to meet guidelines "with respect to good taste, decency and community standards as determined by the Authority." The policy described these standards as follows:

> [T]he average person applying contemporary community standards must find that the advertisement, as a whole, does not appeal to a prurient interest. The advertisement must not describe, in a patently offensive way, sexual conduct specifically defined by the applicable

state law. . . . Advertising containing messages or graphic representations pertaining to sexual conduct will not be accepted.

Quoted in 42 F.3d at 3-4.

The following year, the MBTA rejected six AIDS Action ads, arguing that
they violated the new policy. All the ads included text saying, "Use a latex
condom. Barring abstinence, it's the best way to prevent AIDS. For more information about HIV and AIDS, call the AIDS Action Committee Hotline at
1-800-235-2331." Introducing this text were different headlines: "Haven't you
got enough to worry about in bed?"; "Simply having one on hand won't do any
good."; "You've got to be putting me on."; "Tell him you don't know how it will
ever fit."; "One of these will make you 1/1000th of an inch larger."

The Court of Appeals found that the MBTA's rejection of the ads was content-based, in violation of the First Amendment. The Court said that the policy was not content-neutral because it did not permit sexually explicit words.
Although "the MBTA has not opposed expression of the view that the use of
condoms is effective in the fight against AIDS," *Id.* at 29. the MBTA did discriminate against the AIDS Action ads on the basis of viewpoint. The MBTA
had accepted more overtly sexual advertisements for the 1993 movie "Fatal
Instinct," which also used sexual innuendo and double entendres and which
the court found to be "at least as sexually explicit and/or patently offensive as
the AAC ads." *Id.* at 30. It added, "One might easily infer that ads tend to be
screened not because they threaten to violate the Policy but because they
appear likely to generate controversy or, even more surely, where controversy
actually results." *Id.* at 34–35. The Court did not reach the question whether
the interiors of subway cars were designated public fora. Whether or not the
MBTA could lawfully refuse to accept sexually explicit ads, it could not pick
and choose among those it did accept.

Risk behaviors involving sex and drug use are often also behaviors that
spark controversy. Public education directed at preventing or avoiding such
risks may need to be explicit — and therefore controversial — to reach the target audience. Whether the public education materials present political content
or commercial advertising, an analysis of the relevant First Amendment standards is a necessary element of deciding how to communicate. Does that analysis distinguish between advertising that states a risk and advertising that
presents a way to prevent the same risk?

The American Cancer Society's statements that the risk of breast cancer in
women is 1 in 8 generated some controversy in the 1990s. HOW MANY WOMEN
GET BREAST CANCER? www.cancer.org/docroot/CRI/content/CRI_2_2_1X_How_
many_people_get_breast_cancer_5.asp?sitearea= (last visited Jan. 2007). The
figure is derived from estimates that 13.2% (about 1 in 8) of women born today
will get breast cancer during their lifetimes. The National Cancer Institute,
part of the National Institutes of Health, statistics show that the incidence of
breast cancer in women increases with age, so that the risk reaches 1 in 8
women only among women who live past age 70. The risk among younger
women is as follows:

| Age | Risk |
|-----|------|
| 30–39 | 44% (1 in 229) |
| 40–49 | 46% (1 in 68) |
| 50–59 | 73% (1 in 37) |
| 60–69 | 82% (1 in 26) |

NATIONAL CANCER INSTITUTE, PROBABILITY OF BREAST CANCER IN AMERICAN WOMEN, www.cancer.gov/cancertopics/factsheet/Detection/probability-breast-cancer (last visited Aug. 2006).

When challenged on its use of the 1 in 8 figure, the Society responded that it was important to get women's attention to the need for prevention and screening. Is this different from Christ's Bride's use of the risk of breast cancer and abortion?

**5.** Wildavsky and Dake make clear that perceptions of risk vary from person to person. The study of risk perception continues to refine the type of analysis initiated by those authors and others. Their article offers both evidence of the presence of tendencies in attitudes toward risk and a warning against presuming that one trait can predict how a person will view a particular risk.

Fischhoff et al. attempted to identify commonalities across populations and found that people's perceptions of the magnitude of risk are influenced by factors other than numerical risk calculations. They conclude:

- Risks perceived to be voluntary are more accepted than risks perceived to be imposed.

- Risks perceived to be under an individual's control are more accepted than risks perceived to be controlled by others.

- Risks perceived to have clear benefits are more accepted than risks perceived to have little or no benefit.

- Risks perceived to be fairly distributed are more accepted than risks perceived to be unfairly distributed.

- Risks perceived to be natural are more accepted than risks perceived to be manmade.

- Risks perceived to be statistical are more accepted than risks perceived to be catastrophic.

- Risks perceived to be generated by a trusted source are more accepted than risks perceived to be generated by an untrusted source.

- Risks perceived to be familiar are more accepted than risks perceived to be exotic.

- Risks perceived to affect adults are more accepted than risk perceived to affect children.

BARUCH FISCHHOFF ET AL., FACTORS INFLUENCING RISK PERCEPTION (1981).

Although this summary may appear logical, even obvious, it is not always easy to keep in mind when analyzing something that happens to be especially frightening or especially desirable to you. How would you characterize your own perceptions of risk? If you are especially afraid of a particular risk, such as a shark attack or a drive-by shooting, do you know how many people actually die from that risk each year? For detailed statistics on causes of death, see National Center for Health Statistics, www.cdc.gov/nchs/deaths.htm.

**6.** Glantz pushes several themes raised by Wikler, most importantly in asking whether public health policies can or do accommodate the informed consent model of the physician-patient relationship. As Glantz notes, the medical profession's acceptance of patient decision making autonomy and the doctrine of informed consent was substantially nudged by ethical and judicial opinions. Jay Katz chronicled physicians' earlier paternalistic attitude toward patients in THE SILENT WORLD OF DOCTOR AND PATIENT (1984), in which he describes a conversation on breast cancer treatment he had with a surgeon-friend:

> We first discussed at some length all the uncertainties that plague the treatment of breast cancer. We readily agreed on what was known, unknown, or conjectural about the varieties of therapeutic modalities offered to patients, such as surgery, radiation, and chemotherapy. I then asked how he would speak with a patient. . . . [H]e related to me this recent experience.
>
> At the beginning of their encounter, he had briefly mentioned a number of available treatment alternatives. He added that he had done so without indicating that any of the alternatives to radical surgery deserved serious consideration. Instead, he had quickly impressed on his patient the need for submitting to this operation [complete mastectomy]. I commented that he had given short shrift to other treatment approaches even though a few minutes earlier he had agreed with me that we still are so ignorant about which treatment is best. He seemed startled by my comment but responded with little hesitation that ours had been a theoretical discussion, of little relevance to practice.

KATZ, THE SILENT WORLD OF DOCTOR AND PATIENT at 166–67.

> Dr. Katz was struck by the surgeon's confidence that patients "could neither comprehend nor tolerate an exploration of the certainties and uncertainties inherent in the treatment of breast cancer." *Id*. at 168.

Public health traditionally considered population-wide problems, not the personal health concerns of individuals. Health promotion programs, paradoxically perhaps, are intended to achieve population-wide results by having individuals stop risky behaviors for their own personal benefit. The informed consent model Glantz describes could be applied in population-based educational programs that allow individuals to make informed choices about behavioral health risks. Allowing choice respects autonomy, but it also means some people may not make the healthy choice. If the success of a public health program is judged by the extent to which rates of mortality or morbidity decrease, then the informed consent model would be judged a failure. At the same time, more coercive measures to ensure compliance confront the problem of justifying paternalism.

**7.** Many recent public health policies have wide support among people who are relatively affluent and educated. Smoking, excessive alcohol consumption, illicit drug use, and obesity, for example, are more likely to be found among people in lower socioeconomic groups than the better off and well educated classes. Morone concludes that in American history, the most coercive measures were directed most often at lower socioeconomic classes, especially people of color and immigrants, but also the working poor. *See* James Morone, HELLFIRE NATION: THE POLITICS OF SIN IN AMERICAN HISTORY (2003). Can you think of public health measures that forbid behaviors that are most prevalent among the affluent?

Great Britain has engaged in a public debate over the so-called "nanny state." One report argued for the careful use of paternalistic measures. Karen Jochelson, *Nanny or Steward: The Role of the State in Public Health* (Kings Fund, Oct. 2005). Public surveys have reported class differences in attitudes toward different public health measures, "with poorer socio-economic groups . . . more likely to feel that health is beyond an individual's control and that tackling poverty is the most effective way for a government to prevent illness." *Id.* at 7. Other surveys indicate that more educated, affluent groups support laws regulating personal behavior, while lower socioeconomic groups fear they would bear the primary burdens and instead prefer programs that improve the environment, such as bicycle paths and public parks for those who could not afford health clubs or cars.

---

## USING HEALTH INSURANCE TO IMPROVE HEALTH [OR SAVE MONEY]

Lifestyle changes may get more of a push from financial incentives than prescriptive laws. Both public and private health benefit plans are jumping on the health promotion bandwagon, offering financial incentives to reduce health risks. These plans raise many of the questions discussed in the materials in this Section: Are they unjustifiably paternalistic or a fair bargain? Do they offer rewards for staying healthy or penalties for failing to meet health standards? Do they encourage healthy social norms or discriminate against the disadvantaged? And finally, will they work? Will people live longer or better lives? Will health plans and employers save money?

In 2006, the West Virginia Medicaid Program began experimenting with a health benefit plan structure to reward personal responsibility in health care and save money. (The federal Deficit Reduction Act of 2005 allows the Centers for Medicare and Medicare to give states more flexibility in designing their Medicaid programs.) West Virginia's new standard Medicaid plan, the "Basic Benefits Plan," offers fewer benefits than in the past, but patients can qualify for an "Enhanced Benefits Plan" by agreeing in writing to the following "member responsibilities," among others, in the West Virginia Medicaid Member Agreement:

— I will do my best to stay healthy. I will go to health improvement programs as directed by my medical home. ["medical home" is defined as "where I go for check-ups or when I am sick and where my health care records will be."]

— I will read the booklets and pamphlets my medical home gives me . . .

— I will go to my medical home when I am sick.

— I will take the medicines my health care provider prescribes for me.

— I will show up on time when I have my appointments.

— I will bring my children to their appointments on time.

— I will use the hospital emergency room only for emergencies

West Virginia Medicaid Member Agreement, West Virginia State Plan Amendment, www.wvdhhr.org/bms/oAdministration/bms_admin_WV_SPA 06-02_20060503.pdf/ (last visited Aug. 2006).

The enhanced benefits (not included in the Basic Benefits package) include diabetes care, cardiac rehabilitation, nutrition education, substance abuse and mental health services, tobacco cessation programs, adult emergency dental services, and coverage for an unlimited number of medications prescribed by the Medicaid provider. *Id.* Patients can earn "rewards" for services (not yet specified) by meeting their health goals. The first year, the state Medicaid program intends to get reports from providers and Medicaid managed care organizations to track whether patient get screenings and adhere to health improvement programs, both as directed by their providers, as well as whether patients take medications and miss appointments. (See Chapter 4, Section G, for a discussion of the issues raised by this type of reporting.) The state Medicaid program can shift those who fail to perform their obligations over to the Basic Benefits Plan. *See* Comprehensive Medicaid Redesign Proposal November 2005. www.wvdhhr.org/bms/oAdministration/BMS_ RedesignDraft_20051103.pdf (last visited Jan. 2007).

The program has provoked controversy, raising the following questions: Do patients who rely on Medicaid for access to health care have a choice about which benefits plan to accept? Are there any limits on the conditions a Medicaid program can impose on its benefits? If patients do not meet their obligations, how will the Basic Benefits plan help them? Will the program reduce state Medicaid costs? West Virginia reported that in 2004, long term care and other services for 122,334 elderly, blind and disabled beneficiaries (1/3 of its Medicaid population) accounted for 65.16% of its expenditures. The Enhanced Benefit Program does not apply to this population.

The private sector is taking a similar approach in what may be a growing trend. An increasing number of employers offer health plans with reduced premiums for employees who agree to participate in "wellness," exercise or fitness programs. Others offer free screening for cholesterol, blood pressure, BMI or other health risk factors or on-site immunization or smoking cessation programs. Still others engage independent disease management companies to offer their employees advice about how to stay healthy. Such programs may serve to improve employees' health or reduce employers' health insurance costs or both. Critics worry that voluntary programs can easily become a condition of employment and that employees who do not participate could be fired or at least priced out of affordable health insurance. The Americans with Disabilities Act (ADA), 42 U.S.C. §§ 12101 *et seq.*, forbids private employers (with 15 or more employees) from discriminating in the terms and conditions of employment on the basis of disability. However, it does not prohibit charging higher insurance fees that are actuarially justified (on the basis of risk).

Whether these insurance programs achieve either of their goals, they may succeed in encouraging personal responsibility for one's health. As the materials in this section suggest, that may be a double-edged sword.

## C.   CONTROLLED SUBSTANCES

### REGINA KILMON v. MARYLAND; KELLY LYNN CRUZ v. MARYLAND
#### 2006 Md. LEXIS 479 (MD 2006)

Wilner, J.

\* \* \*

Maryland Code, § 3-204(a) (1) of the Criminal Law Article (CL) makes it a misdemeanor for a person recklessly to engage in conduct that creates a substantial risk of death or serious physical injury to another person. The question before us is whether the intentional ingestion of cocaine by a pregnant woman can form the basis for a conviction under that statute of the reckless endangerment of the later-born child. The answer is "no."

## BACKGROUND

We deal here with two prosecutions in the Circuit Court for Talbot County. In August, 2004, the State's Attorney filed a criminal information charging Regina Kilmon with second degree child abuse, contributing to conditions that render a child delinquent, reckless endangerment, and possession of a controlled dangerous substance. . . . The reckless endangerment count charged that Ms. Kilmon, "on or about the 3rd day of June through the 4th day of June, 2004, in Talbot County, Maryland, did recklessly engage in conduct, to wit: using cocaine while pregnant with Andrew Kilmon that created a substantial risk of death and serious physical harm to Andrew Kilmon."

In January, 2005, Ms. Kilmon entered a plea of guilty on the reckless endangerment count in exchange for the State's commitment to *nol pros* the other charges. [T]he State's Attorney offered . . . the following statement of facts in support of the guilty plea:

    "On June the 3rd, 2004, the Defendant . . . gave birth at the Easton Memorial Hospital to a baby boy subsequently named Andrew W. Kilmon. At the time of the birth the baby weighed 5.5 pounds. The baby was tested through a drug screen which at the hospital which showed the presence of cocaine at the level of 675 nanograms per milliliter. . . [T]he minimum sensitivity level for cocaine is 300 nanograms per milliliter. The State would have produced expert testimony that the result of using cocaine by a pregnant woman . . . is as follows: that they are more likely to experience premature separation of the placenta, spontaneous abortion and premature delivery. That cocaine may cause blood clots to develop in the brain of the fetus. May also interfere with the development of the fetus. And that low birth weight in bab[ies] born with cocaine in their system may lead to many health problems versus normal size babies. There would be further testimony that the only source of cocaine in the baby's system would have been that as derived from the blood stream of the mother prior to birth. . . ."

[T]he court accepted the plea, found Ms. Kilmon guilty of reckless endangerment, and sentenced her to four years in prison. Ms. Kilmon [appealed but the Court of Appeals granted *certiorari* before the appeal proceeded].

[In the companion case, Kelly Lynn Cruz was charged with the same crimes for using cocaine while pregnant with her child, who was born at 3 pounds 2 ounces on January 13, 2005. Cruz entered a *nol pros* to three charges, but pled not guilty to the reckless endangerment charge. The court] found her guilty and imposed a sentence of five years in prison, with two-and-a-half years suspended in favor of five years of supervised probation and drug treatment commencing on release from prison. . . .

## DISCUSSION

We pointed out in *Holbrook v. State*, 364 Md. 354, 365, 772 A.2d 1240, 1246 (2001), that "[r]eckless endangerment is purely a statutory crime" in Maryland. It exists and is defined solely by CL § 3-204. Because the issue is therefore entirely one of statutory construction, it is necessary to determine whether, in enacting § 3-204(a) (1) and its relevant antecedents, the General Assembly intended that the statute include the conduct charged. . . .

The relevant part of CL § 3-204, subsection (a) (1), makes it a misdemeanor for a person recklessly to "engage in conduct that creates a substantial risk of death or serious physical injury to another." By "another," it obviously meant another person. Aware of the Constitutional issues that may arise from regarding a fetus or embryo as a person, the State, in its briefs, makes clear its position that, for purposes of the convictions under § 3-204(a) (1), the "person" allegedly endangered by each appellant's conduct was not the fetus, but the child, after the child's live birth. The offense, in this context, according to the State, is that the prenatal ingestion of cocaine recklessly endangers the child immediately upon and after his or her live birth.

The reckless endangerment statute was first enacted in Maryland in 1989 as Art. 27, § 120. [I]t was modeled after § 211.2 of the Model Penal Code, first proposed by the American Law Institute in 1962. The later-published Commentary to § 211.2 notes that specific kinds of reckless conduct had previously been made criminal in various States — everything from reckless driving to shooting at an airplane to placing an obstruction on railway tracks — and that § 211.2 was intended to "replace the haphazard coverage of prior law with one comprehensive provision" that "reaches any kind of conduct that 'places or may place another person in danger of death or serious bodily injury.'" MODEL PENAL CODE AND COMMENTARIES, PART II (1980) at 195-96.

We have tended to construe the Maryland statute in that manner as well. In *Minor v. State*, 326 Md. 436, 443, 605 A.2d 138, 141 (1992), we held that guilt under the statute does not depend on whether the defendant actually intended that his reckless conduct create a substantial risk of death or serious injury, but whether his conduct, viewed objectively, "was so reckless as to constitute a gross departure from the standard of conduct that a law-abiding person would observe, and thereby create the substantial risk that the statute was designed to punish." In *State v. Pagotto*, 361 Md. 528, 549, 762 A.2d 97, 108 (2000), we confirmed the further point made in *Minor* that the statute was "aimed at deterring the commission of potentially harmful conduct before an injury or death occurs."

Unquestionably, the proscription against recklessly endangering conduct is, and was intended to be, a broad one. Whether it was intended to include conduct of a pregnant woman that might endanger in some way the child she is carrying is not so clear, however, as that brings into play some important policy-laden considerations not relevant with respect to acts committed by third persons.

In support of its argument that the statute should be read as including that conduct, the State observes that an injury committed while a child is still *in utero* can produce criminal liability if the child is later born alive. . . .

   . . . .

The appellants respond that acceptance of the "born alive" rule with respect to the common law relating to homicides that arise from acts committed by others does not inform whether the Legislature intended CL §3-204(a) (1) to criminalize conduct committed by a pregnant woman that might endanger the child she is carrying. The statute itself, though certainly broad in its language, does not specifically address that question. In the absence of any direct evidence of legislative intent in this regard, either clear or implicit from the language of the statute, we look for other relevant indications, and there are some very cogent ones.

Notwithstanding occasional flights of fancy that may test the proposition, the law necessarily and correctly presumes that Legislatures act reasonably, knowingly, and in pursuit of sensible public policy. When there is a legitimate issue of interpretation, therefore, courts are required, to the extent possible, to avoid construing a statute in a manner that would produce farfetched, absurd, or illogical results which would not likely have been intended by the enacting body. . . .

Keeping in mind that recklessness, not intention to injure, is the key element of the offense, if, as the State urges, the statute is read to apply to the effect of a pregnant woman's conduct on the child she is carrying, it could well be construed to include not just the ingestion of unlawful controlled substances but a whole host of intentional and conceivably reckless activity that could not possibly have been within the contemplation of the Legislature — everything from becoming (or remaining) pregnant with knowledge that the child likely will have a genetic disorder that may cause serious disability or death, to the continued use of legal drugs that are contraindicated during pregnancy, to consuming alcoholic beverages to excess, to smoking, to not maintaining a proper and sufficient diet, to avoiding proper and available pre-natal medical care, to failing to wear a seat belt while driving, to violating other traffic laws in ways that create a substantial risk of producing or exac-erbating personal injury to her child, to exercising too much or too little, indeed to engaging in virtually any injury-prone activity that, should an injury occur, might reasonably be expected to endanger the life or safety of the child. Such ordinary things as skiing or horseback riding could produce criminal lia-bility. If the State's position were to prevail, there would seem to be no clear basis for categorically excluding any of those activities from the ambit of the statute; criminal liability would depend almost entirely on how aggressive, inventive, and persuasive any particular prosecutor might be.

Confirming the strong inference that the General Assembly did not intend CL § 3-204(a) (1) to include any of this kind of self-induced activity, including the ingestion of controlled substances, is the manner in which they actually dealt with that kind of activity when they chose to deal with it.

In the same 1989 session that produced the initial enactment of the reckless endangerment law, House Bill 809 was introduced. That bill would have expanded the definition of "abuse" to include the physical dependency of a newborn infant on any controlled dangerous substance for the purposes of the Family Law Article provisions requiring reporting and investigation of sus-pected child abuse. The bill was opposed by the Secretary of Human Resources, the American Civil Liberties Union (ACLU), and the Foster Care Review Board, and it died in the House Judiciary Committee.

In 1990, a number of bills were introduced on the subject, taking differing approaches. . . .

All of those bills died in the House Judiciary Committee. . . . [T]he Department of Human Services [opposed the bills and] observed (1) that it was often difficult to establish a cause-and-effect relationship between a woman's drug use and injuries to the fetus, (2) in most cases, a woman's use of drugs during pregnancy is the result of her inability to control her addiction, the absence of adequate treatment programs, or her lack of awareness of the pos-sible effects of her drug use on the fetus, and (3) in those States where crimi-nal sanctions exist for drug use by pregnant women, the data did not indicate any decrease in the number of drug-using pregnant women. It is noteworthy that the opposition to those bills that would have established criminal liabil-ity, from both State agencies and private groups that dealt with the problem of drug-addicted pregnant women and babies, was not that the bills were unnecessary because criminal liability already existed under the reckless endangerment law, but that the approach they embraced was not good public policy.

. . . .

. . . In 1997, by 1997 Md. Laws, ch. 367 and 368, the Legislature opted to address the problem in a tri-partite civil context. It first attached to the defini-tion of a "child in need of assistance" a presumption that a child is not receiving ordinary and proper care and attention if the child was born addicted to or dependent on cocaine, heroin, or a derivative of either, or was born with a significant presence of those drugs in his or her blood. That circumstance could be taken into account by a Juvenile Court in deciding whether the child is in need of assistance. Second, the bills amended the law pertaining to the termination of parental rights to add that circumstance, plus the parent's refusal to participate in a drug treatment program, as a consideration in determining whether termination is in the child's best interest.

Finally, the Legislature required the Departments of Human Resources and Health and Mental Hygiene to develop and implement pilot drug intervention programs for the mothers of children who were born drug-exposed. As part of that intervention program, the Department of Human Resources was required to file a child in need of assistance petition on behalf of a child who was born drug-exposed if the mother failed to complete drug treatment and she and the father were unable to provide adequate care for the child. *See* Maryland Code, § 3-818 of the Cts. & Jud. Proc. Article and §§ 5-323(d) (3) (ii) and 5-706.3 of the Family Law Article.

In the 2004 session, Senate Bill 349 and House Bill 802, both captioned as the Unborn Victims of Violence Act, were introduced. Among other provisions dealing with murder, manslaughter, and assault, they would have defined the term "another," as used in CL § 3-204(a) (1), to include an unborn child, thereby making it a criminal offense recklessly to create a substantial risk of death or serious physical injury to an unborn child. There was no exemption for the conduct of the child's mother, other than in the context of a legal abortion. Neither bill passed. . . .

In 2005, the Legislature, in a more limited version of the 2004 bills, extended the law of murder and manslaughter to permit a prosecution for the murder or manslaughter of a viable fetus. *See* 2005 Md. Laws, ch. 546, enacting CL § 2-103. The statute provides that such a prosecution is warranted only if the defendant intended to cause the death of or serious physical injury to the viable fetus or wantonly or recklessly disregarded the likelihood that the defendant's action would cause death or serious physical injury to the fetus. There are at least two important differences between the 2005 enactment and the failed 2004 bills. First, the 2005 Act did *not* encompass the reckless endangerment statute but dealt only with unlawful homicides. At least equally significant, and perhaps more so, the Legislature was careful, in § 2-103(f), to make clear that "[n]othing in this section applies to an act or failure to act of a pregnant woman with regard to her own fetus."

That provision was added to the bill specifically to allay concerns expressed by the Secretary of Health and Mental Hygiene, the ACLU, and the National Organization for Women that, absent such a provision, women might be subject to prosecution for not accessing available prenatal care or causing the death of a fetus by reason of reckless behavior during pregnancy, including a drug overdose. . . .

This sixteen-year history, from 1989 to 2005, shows rather clearly that, although a pregnant woman, like anyone else, may be prosecuted for her own possession of controlled dangerous substances, the General Assembly, despite being importuned on numerous occasions to do so, has chosen not to impose additional criminal penalties for the effect that her *ingestion* of those substances might have on the child, either before or after birth. It has consistently rejected proposals that would have allowed such conduct to constitute murder, manslaughter, child abuse, or reckless endangerment. In doing so, the Legislature obviously gave credence to the evidence presented to it that criminalizing the ingestion of controlled substances — in effect criminalizing drug addiction for this one segment of the population, pregnant women — was not the proper approach to the problem and had, in fact, proved ineffective in other States in deterring either that conduct or addiction generally on the part of pregnant women. It deliberately opted, instead, to deal with the problem by providing drug treatment programs for pregnant women and using the child in need of assistance and termination of parental rights remedies if the women failed to take advantage of the treatment programs and, as a result, were unable to provide proper care for the child.

Given the exemption added to the 2005 legislation, it would be an anomaly, indeed, if the law were such that a pregnant woman who, by ingesting drugs, recklessly caused the death of a viable fetus would suffer no criminal liability for manslaughter but, if the child was born alive and did not die, could be imprisoned for five years for reckless endangerment. A *non-fatal* injury resulting from reckless conduct would be culpable; a *fatal* injury resulting from the same reckless conduct would not be.

Maryland is not the only State to address this issue. These kinds of cases — prosecutions for reckless endangerment, child abuse, or distribution of controlled substances based on a pregnant woman's ingestion of a controlled dangerous substance, or, in some cases, excessive amounts of alcohol — have arisen in other States, and the overwhelming majority of courts that have considered the issue have concluded that those crimes do not encompass that kind of activity. Indeed, only one State — South Carolina — has so far held to the contrary.

In conformance with this nearly universal view, but most particularly in light of the way in which the Maryland General Assembly has chosen to deal with the problem, we hold that it was not the legislative intent that CL § 3-204(a) (1) apply to prenatal drug ingestion by a pregnant woman. We therefore reverse the judgments entered by the Circuit Court.

\* \* \*

## NOTES AND QUESTIONS

**1.** For background information on cocaine, marijuana, and the other drugs discussed in this section, see www.drugabuse.gov/ResearchReports/ (last visited March 2006) (clearinghouse for National Institute on Drug Abuse; *see also* NATIONAL INSTITUTE ON DRUG ABUSE, COCAINE ABUSE AND ADDICTION (2004).

For references on use of cocaine and other drugs during pregnancy, see the website of the March of Dimes at http://search.marchofdimes.com/cgi-bin/MsmGo.exe?grab_id=0&page_id=994&query=pregnancy%20and%20cocai

ne&hiword=PREGNANCIES%20PREGNANCYS%20PREGNANT%20and%2
0cocaine%20pregnancy%20 (last visited August 2006).

**2.** *Kilmon v. Maryland* illustrates the issues and arguments presented in most cases concerning drug use by pregnant women, regardless of the criminal statute at issue. It collects the cases in the following footnote:

> For specific holdings, *see Johnson v. State*, 602 So. 2d 1288 (Fla. 1992) (statute prohibiting delivery of controlled substance to person under 18 not applicable to ingestion of controlled substance prior to giving birth) and *cf. State v. Ashley*, 678 So. 2d 339, 701 So. 2d 338 (Fla. 1997) (confirming *Johnson*); *State v. Gray*, 62 Ohio St. 3d 514, 584 N.E.2d 710 (Ohio 1992) (statute prohibiting creation of substantial risk to health or safety of child not applicable to abuse of drugs during pregnancy); *State v. Aiwohi*, 109 Haw. 115, 123 P.3d 1210, 1214 (Hawaii 2005) (manslaughter statute not applicable; court recognizes that "overwhelming majority of jurisdictions confronted with the prosecution of a mother for her own prenatal conduct, causing harm to the subsequently born child, refuse to permit such prosecutions"); *Com. v. Welch*, 864 S.W.2d 280 (Ky. 1993) (legislature did not intend child abuse statute to apply to prenatal self-abuse that caused drugs to be transmitted through umbilical cord to child); *Sheriff v. Encoe*, 110 Nev. 1317, 885 P.2d 596 (Nev. 1994) (child endangerment statute does not apply to transmission of illegal substances from mother to newborn through umbilical cord); *Reinesto v. Superior Court*, 182 Ariz. 190, 894 P.2d 733 (Ariz. App. 1995) (child abuse statute not applicable); *Reyes v. Superior Court*, 75 Cal. App. 3d 214, 141 Cal. Rptr. 912 (Cal. App. 1977) (child endangerment statute not applicable); *People v. Hardy*, 188 Mich. App. 305, 469 N.W.2d 50 (Mich. App. 1991) (statute prohibiting delivery of cocaine did not apply to transmission of cocaine through umbilical cord from mother to child); *People v. Morabito*, 151 Misc. 2d 259, 580 N.Y.S.2d 843 (City Ct. 1992) (child endangerment statute not applicable to that circumstance); *Collins v. State*, 890 S.W.2d 893 (Tex. App. 1994) (reckless injury statute not applicable); *State v. Deborah J.Z.*, 228 Wis. 2d 468, 596 N.W.2d 490 (Wis. App. 1999) (reckless injury statute not applicable to ingestion of excessive amount of alcohol during pregnancy causing injury to child). *Compare Whitner v. State*, 328 S.C. 1, 492 S.E.2d 777 (S.C. 1997), *cert. denied*, 523 U.S. 1145, 118 S. Ct. 1857, 140 L. Ed. 2d 1104 (1998) (holding that woman could be prosecuted for endangering fetus by prenatal substance abuse).

Like *Kilmon*, most of these cases were decided largely on public policy grounds — interpreting the statute in light of its probable effects, often bolstered by a legislative history of rejecting proposed bills that would have criminalized drug use in pregnancy in one way or another. There is little or no discussion of the woman's right to liberty or the state's power to protect the fetus or delivered child. Many state legislatures have engaged in a policy debate similar to Maryland's and described in the opinion. Would the state have the power to enact a criminal prohibition, even if it were not good policy? If so, would it have the power to impose other standards of behavior on women during pregnancy or whenever they might be pregnant? Many of the most serious risks to a fetus, particularly from cocaine, occur during the first trimester of pregnancy, perhaps even before a woman realizes she is pregnant.

**3.** Only one state — South Carolina — has interpreted its criminal statutes to include drug use during pregnancy. *Whitner v. South Carolina*, 328 S.C. 1, 492 S.E.2d 777 (1997), *cert. denied*, 523 U.S. 1145 (1998). In 1992, Cornelia Whitner was sentenced to eight years in prison after pleading guilty to criminal child neglect for taking crack cocaine during her third trimester of pregnancy. Her baby was born with cocaine metabolites in its system, but otherwise healthy. Her attorney did not advise her that the child neglect law might not apply to prenatal drug use. Whitner later petitioned for post conviction relief, claiming ineffective assistance of counsel and lack of subject matter jurisdiction. Her petition was granted on both grounds, but reversed by the state Supreme Court.

The child neglect statute at issue, S.C. CODE ANN. § 20-7-50 (1985), provided:

> Any person having the legal custody of any child or helpless person, who shall, without lawful excuse, refuse or neglect to provide, as defined in § 20-7-490, the proper care and attention for such child or helpless person, so that the life, health or comfort of such child or helpless person is endangered or is likely to be endangered, shall be guilty of a misdemeanor and shall be punished within the discretion of the circuit court.

In addition, under the Children's Code, "child" means a "person under the age of eighteen." S.C. CODE ANN. § 20-7-30(1) (1985).

The Supreme Court of South Carolina held that a viable fetus was a "person" for purposes of the Children's Code. The State argued that any maternal act that endangered or was likely to endanger "the life, comfort, or health of a viable fetus" qualified as child neglect, and the Court agreed. The Court rejected Whitner's arguments, similar to those accepted in *Kilmon* and the decisions in other states, that including viable fetuses within the definition of "child" would lead to absurd results and that the legislature had rejected bills using that approach. Instead, the Court found that the "plain meaning" of child included a viable fetus. It supported this conclusion with a discussion of developments in tort and criminal law to permit actions against a third party who injures a pregnant woman and her fetus:

> . . . In 1960, this Court decided *Hall v. Murphy,* 236 S.C. 257, 113 S.E.2d 790 (1960). That case concerned the application of South Carolina's wrongful death statute to an infant who died four hours after her birth as a result of injuries sustained prenatally during viability. The Appellants argued that a viable fetus was not a person within the purview of the wrongful death statute, because, inter alia, a fetus is thought to have no separate being apart from the mother.
>
> We found such a reason for exclusion from recovery "unsound, illogical and unjust," and concluded there was "no medical or other basis" for the "assumed identity" of mother and viable unborn child. In light of that conclusion, this Court unanimously held: "We have no difficulty in

concluding that a fetus having reached that period of prenatal maturity where it is capable of independent life apart from its mother is a person."

. . . .

Since a viable child is a person before separation from the body of its mother and since prenatal injuries tortiously inflicted on such a child are actionable, it is apparent that the complaint alleges such an "act, neglect or default" by the defendant, to the injury of the child. . . . Once the concept of the unborn, viable child as a person is accepted, we have no difficulty in holding that a cause of action for tortious injury to such a child arises immediately upon the infliction of the injury.

. . . .

Similarly, we do not see any rational basis for finding a viable fetus is not a "person" in the present [criminal] context. Indeed, it would be absurd to recognize the viable fetus as a person for purposes of homicide laws and wrongful death statutes but not for purposes of statutes proscribing child abuse. . . .

328 S.C. at 6–7.

Are there differences between allowing parents a cause of action in tort for the loss of a child at the hands of a third party and holding the mother criminally responsible for injuring her own child before birth?

Whitner argued that the statute burdened her right to privacy, specifically her right to carry her pregnancy to term. But the Court rejected the very idea of any such right:

[W]e do not think any fundamental right of Whitner's — or any right at all, for that matter — is implicated under the present scenario. It strains belief for Whitner to argue that using crack cocaine during pregnancy is encompassed within the constitutionally recognized right of privacy. Use of crack cocaine is illegal, period. No one here argues that laws criminalizing the use of crack cocaine are themselves unconstitutional. If the State wishes to impose additional criminal penalties on pregnant women who engage in this already illegal conduct because of the effect the conduct has on the viable fetus, it may do so. We do not see how the fact of pregnancy elevates the use of crack cocaine to the lofty status of a fundamental right.

328 S.C. at 18.

Ultimately, it found that the law did not affect Whitner's right to privacy, because she remained free to carry the pregnancy to term. And, pregnant or not, she never had any right to use cocaine. (This conclusion might be disputed where criminal laws prohibit only the possession, sale or distribution, and not the *use*, of a controlled substance.) Finally, the court found that the state had not only a legitimate, but a compelling interest in the potential life of the fetus, citing *Planned Parenthood of Southeastern Pennsylvania v. Casey*. But the court's treatment of the constitutional issue somewhat misses the point: This is a statute that imposes additional criminal penalties on mothers who ingest crack cocaine. The constitutional argument should focus on the status that triggers the enhanced penalty and the relationship between the mother and child. Both would appear to be the type of interest that has been regarded as "fundamental" under traditional federal constitutional analysis. Should not the state have to show a compelling interest *and* that the statute achieves that interest in the narrowest possible way? Can the state do so? Is protecting the health of the future child a compelling interest? The Attorney General of South Carolina argued publicly that the purpose of prosecuting pregnant women was to prevent harm to children, not to put women in prison. (An example of how hospitals cooperated in that endeavor is found *Ferguson v. City of Charlestown, infra.*)

Preventing harm to others has been the goal of many other criminal laws, such laws prohibiting driving while intoxicated. It is not a crime to drive, to drink alcoholic beverages, or even to be intoxicated. *See Robinson v. California*, 370 U.S. 660 (1962). Yet a person who engages in two of these lawful activities at the same time commits a crime. Are such laws analogous to laws that effectively impose more severe criminal penalties for drug possession for pregnant women than for other offenders?

4. The South Carolina court takes the view that a fetus exposed to drugs like cocaine will almost certainly suffer serious damage: "the consequences of abuse or neglect which takes place after birth often pale in comparison to those resulting from abuse suffered by the viable fetus before birth." 328 S.C. at 8. Child protection professionals in state child welfare and social service agencies might dispute this claim, since they deal with often horrifying cases of physical abuse, neglect and death of children at many ages. Nonetheless, serious injury from drug exposure *in utero* was feared when crack cocaine became widely available in the late 1980s and early 1990s. By the end of the 1990s, however, scientific evidence showed far less long term damage than originally suspected. Researchers found that even children who appeared to have some developmental delays could improve with appropriate education. A key problem is the difficulty of isolating the effect of one drug on the child of a woman who has multiple problems of her own. Pregnant women who used cocaine often used other drugs, including alcohol and tobacco, had poor nutrition, unstable housing, sometimes with abusive partners, and were often poor, all of which factors can jeopardize the physical or mental development of their children. Of course, parents who abuse or neglect their children after they are born are subject to having the children removed from their custody and even prosecution under ordinary child abuse statutes. In the absence of conditions that threaten the child, however, state child welfare agencies typically attempt to provide services to families in order to enable them to properly care for their children.

A similar approach to drug use by pregnant women would be to provide drug treatment services, as recommended by most substance abuse treatment professionals, the American Public Health Association, and other health organizations. The Maryland court notes that Maryland proposed offering treatment programs, but it was not followed up because of cost. The cost of providing drug treatment services, however, is typically less that the cost of confining someone in prison. Experts in the field argue that pregnant women who use drugs need treatment programs tailored specifically to pregnant women and that such programs almost always have long waiting lists, so that the pregnancy is likely to end before space becomes available.

# FERGUSON v. CITY OF CHARLESTON
## 532 U.S. 67 (2001)

Stevens, J.

\* \* \*

In this case, we must decide whether a state hospital's performance of a diagnostic test to obtain evidence of a patient's criminal conduct for law enforcement purposes is an unreasonable search if the patient has not consented to the procedure. More narrowly, the question is whether the interest in using the threat of criminal sanctions to deter pregnant women from using cocaine can justify a departure from the general rule that an official nonconsensual search is unconstitutional if not authorized by a valid warrant.

I

In the fall of 1988, staff members at the public hospital operated in the city of Charleston by the Medical University of South Carolina (MUSC) became concerned about an apparent increase in the use of cocaine by patients who were receiving prenatal treatment. In response to this perceived increase, as of April 1989, MUSC began to order drug screens to be performed on urine samples from maternity patients who were suspected of using cocaine. If a patient tested positive, she was then referred by MUSC staff to the county substance abuse commission for counseling and treatment. However, despite the referrals, the incidence of cocaine use among the patients at MUSC did not appear to change.

Some four months later, Nurse Shirley Brown, the case manager for the MUSC obstetrics department, heard a news broadcast reporting that the police in Greenville, South Carolina, were arresting pregnant users of cocaine on the theory that such use harmed the fetus and was therefore child abuse. Nurse Brown discussed the story with MUSC's general counsel, Joseph C. Good, Jr., who then contacted Charleston Solicitor Charles Condon in order to offer MUSC's cooperation in prosecuting mothers whose children tested positive for drugs at birth.

After receiving Good's letter, Solicitor Condon took the first steps in developing the policy at issue in this case. He organized the initial meetings, decided who would participate, and issued the invitations, in which he described his plan to prosecute women who tested positive for cocaine while pregnant. The task force that Condon formed included representatives of MUSC, the police, the County Substance Abuse Commission and the Department of Social Services. Their deliberations led to MUSC's adoption of a 12-page document entitled "POLICY M-7," dealing with the subject of "Management of Drug Abuse During Pregnancy."

The first three pages of Policy M-7 set forth the procedure to be followed by the hospital staff to "identify/assist pregnant patients suspected of drug abuse." The first section, entitled the "Identification of Drug Abusers," provided that a patient should be tested for cocaine through a urine drug screen if she met one or more of nine criteria.[3] It also stated that a chain of custody should be followed when obtaining and testing urine samples, presumably to make sure that the results could be used in subsequent criminal proceedings. The policy also provided for education and referral to a substance abuse clinic for patients who tested positive. Most important, it added the threat of law enforcement intervention that "provided the necessary 'leverage' to make the [p]olicy effective." That threat was, as respondents candidly acknowledge, essential to the program's success in getting women into treatment and keeping them there.

The threat of law enforcement involvement was set forth in two protocols, the first dealing with the identification of drug use during pregnancy, and the second with identification of drug use after labor. Under the latter protocol, the police were to be notified without delay and the patient promptly arrested. Under the former, after the initial positive drug test, the police were to be notified (and the patient arrested) only if the patient tested positive for cocaine a second time or if she missed an appointment with a substance abuse counselor. In 1990, however, the policy was modified at the behest of the solicitor's office to give the patient who tested positive during labor, like the patient who tested positive during a prenatal care visit, an opportunity to avoid arrest by consenting to substance abuse treatment.

The last six pages of the policy contained forms for the patients to sign, as well as procedures for the police to follow when a patient was arrested. The policy also prescribed in detail the precise offenses with which a woman could be charged, depending on the stage of her pregnancy. If the pregnancy was 27 weeks or less, the patient was to be charged with simple possession. If it was 28 weeks or more, she was to be charged with possession and distribution to a person under the age of 18 — in this case, the fetus. If she delivered "while testing positive for illegal drugs," she was also to be charged with unlawful neglect of a child. Under the policy, the police were instructed to interrogate the arrestee in order "to ascertain the identity of the subject who provided illegal drugs to the suspect." Other than the provisions describing the substance abuse treatment to be offered to women who tested positive, the policy made no mention of any change in the prenatal care of such patients, nor did it prescribe any special treatment for the newborns.

II

Petitioners are 10 women who received obstetrical care at MUSC and who were arrested after testing positive for cocaine. Four of them were arrested

---

[3] Those criteria were as follows:

"1. No prenatal care

"2. Late prenatal care after 24 weeks gestation

"3. Incomplete prenatal care

"4. Abruptio placentae

"5. Intrauterine fetal death

"6. Preterm labor 'of no obvious cause'

"7. IUGR [intrauterine growth retardation] 'of no obvious cause'

"8. Previously known drug or alcohol abuse

"9. Unexplained congenital anomalies."

during the initial implementation of the policy; they were not offered the opportunity to receive drug treatment as an alternative to arrest. The others were arrested after the policy was modified in 1990; they either failed to comply with the terms of the drug treatment program or tested positive for a second time. Respondents include the City of Charleston, law enforcement officials who helped develop and enforce the policy, and representatives of MUSC.

Petitioners' complaint challenged the validity of the policy under various theories, including the claim that warrantless and nonconsensual drug tests conducted for criminal investigatory purposes were unconstitutional searches. Respondents advanced two principal defenses to the constitutional claim: (1) that, as a matter of fact, petitioners had consented to the searches; and (2) that, as a matter of law, the searches were reasonable, even absent consent, because they were justified by special non-law-enforcement purposes.

. . . [The jury found for the respondents.]

. . . The Court of Appeals for the Fourth Circuit affirmed, but without reaching the question of consent. . . .

### III

Because MUSC is a state hospital, the members of its staff are government actors, subject to the strictures of the Fourth Amendment. Moreover, the urine tests conducted by those staff members were indisputably searches within the meaning of the Fourth Amendment. Neither the District Court nor the Court of Appeals concluded that any of the nine criteria used to identify the women to be searched provided either probable cause to believe that they were using cocaine, or even the basis for a reasonable suspicion of such use. Rather, the District Court and the Court of Appeals viewed the case as one involving MUSC's right to conduct searches without warrants or probable cause. Furthermore, given the posture in which the case comes to us, we must assume for purposes of our decision that the tests were performed without the informed consent of the patients.

Because the hospital seeks to justify its authority to conduct drug tests and to turn the results over to law enforcement agents without the knowledge or consent of the patients, this case differs from the four previous cases in which we have considered whether comparable drug tests "fit within the closely guarded category of constitutionally permissible suspicionless searches." In three of those cases, we sustained drug tests for railway employees involved in train accidents, for United States Customs Service employees seeking promotion to certain sensitive positions, and for high school students participating in interscholastic sports. (*See Earles, infra.*) In the fourth case, we struck down such testing for candidates for designated state offices as unreasonable.

In each of those cases, we employed a balancing test that weighed the intrusion on the individual's interest in privacy against the "special needs" that supported the program. As an initial matter, we note that the invasion of privacy in this case is far more substantial than in those cases. In the previous four cases, there was no misunderstanding about the purpose of the test or the potential use of the test results, and there were protections against the dissemination of the results to third parties. The use of an adverse test result to disqualify one from eligibility for a particular benefit, such as a promotion or an opportunity to participate in an extracurricular activity, involves a less serious intrusion on privacy than the unauthorized dissemination of such results to third parties. The reasonable expectation of privacy enjoyed by the typical patient undergoing diagnostic tests in a hospital is that the results of those tests will not be shared with non-medical personnel without her consent. In none of our prior cases was there any intrusion upon that kind of expectation.

The critical difference between those four drug-testing cases and this one, however, lies in the nature of the "special need" asserted as justification for the warrantless searches. In each of those earlier cases, the "special need" that was advanced as a justification for the absence of a warrant or individualized suspicion was one divorced from the State's general interest in law enforcement. . . . In this case, however, the central and indispensable feature of the policy from its inception was the use of law enforcement to coerce the patients into substance abuse treatment. This fact distinguishes this case from circumstances in which physicians or psychologists, in the course of ordinary medical procedures aimed at helping the patient herself, come across information that under rules of law or ethics is subject to reporting requirements, which no one has challenged here.

Respondents argue in essence that their ultimate purpose — namely, protecting the health of both mother and child — is a beneficent one. . . . In this case, a review of the M-7 policy plainly reveals that the purpose actually served by the MUSC searches "is ultimately indistinguishable from the general interest in crime control."

. . . In this case, as Judge Blake put it in her dissent below, "it . . . is clear from the record that an initial and continuing focus of the policy was on the arrest and prosecution of drug-abusing mothers. . . ." Tellingly, the document codifying the policy incorporates the police's operational guidelines. It devotes its attention to the chain of custody, the range of possible criminal charges, and the logistics of police notification and arrests. Nowhere, however, does the document discuss different courses of medical treatment for either mother or infant, aside from treatment for the mother's addiction.

Moreover, throughout the development and application of the policy, the Charleston prosecutors and police were extensively involved in the day-to-day administration of the policy. Police and prosecutors decided who would receive the reports of positive drug screens and what information would be included with those reports. Law enforcement officials also helped determine the procedures to be followed when performing the screens. In the course of the policy's administration, they had access to Nurse Brown's medical files on the women who tested positive, routinely attended the substance abuse team's meetings, and regularly received copies of team documents discussing the women's progress. Police took pains to coordinate the timing and circumstances of the arrests with MUSC staff, and, in particular, Nurse Brown.

While the ultimate goal of the program may well have been to get the women in question into substance abuse treatment and off of drugs, the immediate objective of the searches was to generate evidence *for law enforcement purposes* in order to reach that goal. The threat of law enforcement may ultimately have been intended as a means to an end, but the direct and primary purpose of MUSC's policy was to ensure the use of those means. In our opinion, this distinction is critical. Because law enforcement involvement always serves some broader social purpose or objective, under respondents' view, virtually any nonconsensual suspicionless search could be immunized under the special needs doctrine by defining the search solely in terms of its ultimate, rather than immediate, purpose. Such an approach is inconsistent with the Fourth Amendment. Given the primary purpose of the Charleston program, which was to use the threat of arrest and prosecution in order to force women into treatment, and given the extensive involvement of law enforcement officials at every stage of the policy, this case simply does not fit within the closely guarded category of "special needs."

The fact that positive test results were turned over to the police does not merely provide a basis for distinguishing our prior cases applying the "special needs" balancing approach to the determination of drug use. It also provides an affirmative reason for enforcing the strictures of the Fourth Amendment. While state hospital employees, like other citizens, may have a duty to provide the police with evidence of criminal conduct that they inadvertently acquire in the course of routine treatment, when they undertake to obtain such evidence from their patients *for the specific purpose of incriminating those patients,* they have a special obligation to make sure that the patients are fully informed about their constitutional rights, as standards of knowing waiver require.

. . . While respondents are correct that drug abuse both was and is a serious problem, "the gravity of the threat alone cannot be dispositive of questions concerning what means law enforcement officers may employ to pursue a given purpose."

Accordingly, the judgment of the Court of Appeals is reversed . . .

\* \* \*

Justice Scalia, with Justices Rehnquist and Thomas, dissenting.

There is always an unappealing aspect to the use of doctors and nurses, ministers of mercy, to obtain incriminating evidence against the supposed objects of their ministration — although here, it is correctly pointed out, the doctors and nurses were ministering not just to the mothers but also to the children whom their cooperation with the police was meant to protect. But whatever may be the correct social judgment concerning the desirability of what occurred here, that is not the issue in the present case. The Constitution does not resolve all difficult social questions, but leaves the vast majority of them to resolution by debate and the democratic process — which would produce a decision by the citizens of Charleston, through their elected representatives, to forbid or permit the police action at issue here.

The question before us is a narrower one: whether, whatever the desirability of this police conduct, it violates the Fourth Amendment's prohibition of unreasonable searches and seizures. . . .

## I

... What petitioners [and] the Court ... really object to is not the urine testing, but the hospital's reporting of positive drug-test results to police. But the latter is obviously not a search. At most it may be a "derivative use of the product of a past unlawful search," which, of course, "work[s] no new Fourth Amendment wrong" and "presents a question, not of rights, but of remedies." There is only one act that could conceivably be regarded as a search of petitioners in the present case: the *taking* of the urine sample. I suppose the *testing* of that urine for traces of unlawful drugs could be considered a search of sorts, but the Fourth Amendment protects only against searches of citizens' "persons, houses, papers, and effects"; and it is entirely unrealistic to regard urine as one of the "effects" (*i.e.,* part of the property) of the person who has passed and abandoned it.

It is rudimentary Fourth Amendment law that a search which has been consented to is not unreasonable. There is no contention in the present case that the urine samples were extracted forcibly. The only conceivable bases for saying that they were obtained without consent are the contentions (1) that the consent was coerced by the patients' need for medical treatment, (2) that the consent was uninformed because the patients were not told that the tests would include testing for drugs, and (3) that the consent was uninformed because the patients were not told that the results of the tests would be provided to the police.

. . . .

Until today, we have *never* held — or even suggested — that material which a person voluntarily entrusts to someone else cannot be given by that person to the police, and used for whatever evidence it may contain. . . . I would adhere to our established law, which says that information obtained through violation of a relationship of trust is obtained consensually, and is hence not a search.

There remains to be considered the first possible basis for invalidating this search, which is that the patients were coerced to produce their urine samples by their necessitous circumstances, to wit, their need for medical treatment of their pregnancy. If that was coercion, it was not coercion applied by the government — and if such nongovernmental coercion sufficed, the police would never be permitted to use the ballistic evidence obtained from treatment of a patient with a bullet wound. And the Fourth Amendment would invalidate those many state laws that require physicians to report gunshot wounds, evidence of spousal abuse, and like the South Carolina law relevant here, evidence of child abuse.

* * *

# BOARD OF EDUCATION OF INDEPENDENT SCHOOL DISTRICT NO. 92 OF POTTAWATOMIE COUNTY v. EARLS
### 536 U.S. 822 (2002)

Thomas, Justice.

\* \* \*

The city of Tecumseh, Oklahoma, is a rural community located approximately 40 miles southeast of Oklahoma City. The School District administers all Tecumseh public schools. In the fall of 1998, the School District adopted the Student Activities Drug Testing Policy (Policy), which requires all middle and high school students to consent to drug testing in order to participate in any extracurricular activity. In practice, the Policy has been applied only to competitive extracurricular activities sanctioned by the Oklahoma Secondary Schools Activities Association, such as the Academic Team, Future Farmers of America, Future Homemakers of America, band, choir, pom pom, cheerleading, and athletics. Under the Policy, students are required to take a drug test before participating in an extracurricular activity, must submit to random drug testing while participating in that activity, and must agree to be tested at any time upon reasonable suspicion. The urinalysis tests are designed to detect only the use of illegal drugs, including amphetamines, marijuana, cocaine, opiates, and barbiturates, not medical conditions or the presence of authorized prescription medications.

At the time of their suit, both respondents attended Tecumseh High School. Respondent Lindsay Earls was a member of the show choir, the marching band, the Academic Team, and the National Honor Society. Respondent Daniel James sought to participate in the Academic Team. Together with their parents, Earls and James brought a 42 U.S.C. § 1983 action against the School District, challenging the Policy both on its face and as applied to their participation in extracurricular activities. They alleged that the Policy violates the Fourth Amendment. . . . They also argued that the School District failed to identify a special need for testing students who participate in extracurricular activities, and that the "Drug Testing Policy neither addresses a proven problem nor promises to bring any benefit to students or the school."

Applying the principles articulated in *Vernonia School Dist. 47J v. Acton*, 515 U.S. 646 (1995), in which we upheld the suspicionless drug testing of school athletes, the United States District Court for the Western District of Oklahoma rejected respondents' claim that the Policy was unconstitutional.

The United States Court of Appeals for the Tenth Circuit reversed, holding that the Policy violated the Fourth Amendment. . . .

II

The Fourth Amendment to the United States Constitution protects "the right of the people to be secure in their persons, houses, papers, and effects, against unreasonable searches and seizures." . . .

In the criminal context, reasonableness usually requires a showing of probable cause. The probable-cause standard, however, "is peculiarly related to criminal investigations" and may be unsuited to determining the reasonableness of administrative searches where the "Government seeks to *prevent* the development of hazardous conditions." *Treasury Employees* v. *Von Raab.* . . . The Court [in *Vernonia*] also held that a warrant and finding of probable cause are unnecessary in the public school context because such requirements "'would unduly interfere with the maintenance of the swift and informal disciplinary procedures [that are] needed.'"

Given that the School District's Policy is not in any way related to the conduct of criminal investigations, respondents do not contend that the School District requires probable cause before testing students for drug use. Respondents instead argue that drug testing must be based at least on some level of individualized suspicion. It is true that we generally determine the reasonableness of a search by balancing the nature of the intrusion on the individual's privacy against the promotion of legitimate governmental interests. But we have long held that "the Fourth Amendment imposes no irreducible requirement of [individualized] suspicion." "In certain limited circumstances, the Government's need to discover such latent or hidden conditions, or to prevent their development, is sufficiently compelling to justify the intrusion on privacy entailed by conducting such searches without any measure of individualized suspicion." *Von Raab.* . . . Therefore, in the context of safety and administrative regulations, a search unsupported by probable cause may be reasonable "when 'special needs, beyond the normal need for law enforcement, make the warrant and probable-cause requirement impracticable.'"

Significantly, this Court has previously held that "special needs" inhere in the public school context. While school children do not shed their constitutional rights when they enter the schoolhouse, "Fourth Amendment rights . . . are different in public schools than elsewhere; the 'reasonableness' inquiry cannot disregard the schools' custodial and tutelary responsibility for children." In particular, a finding of individualized suspicion may not be necessary when a school conducts drug testing.

In *Vernonia*, this Court held that the suspicionless drug testing of athletes was constitutional. The Court, however, did not simply authorize all school drug testing, but rather conducted a fact-specific balancing of the intrusion on the children's Fourth Amendment rights against the promotion of legitimate governmental interests. . . .

## A

We first consider the nature of the privacy interest allegedly compromised by the drug testing. . . .

A student's privacy interest is limited in a public school environment where the State is responsible for maintaining discipline, health, and safety. School children are routinely required to submit to physical examinations and vaccinations against disease. Securing order in the school environment sometimes requires that students be subjected to greater controls than those appropriate for adults. Without first establishing discipline and maintaining order, teachers cannot begin to educate their students. And apart from education, the school has the obligation to protect pupils from mistreatment by other children, and also to protect teachers themselves from violence by the few students whose conduct in recent years has prompted national concern.

Respondents argue that because children participating in non-athletic extracurricular activities are not subject to regular physicals and communal undress, they have a stronger expectation of privacy than the athletes tested in *Vernonia*. This distinction, however, was not essential to our decision in *Vernonia*, which depended primarily upon the school's custodial responsibility and authority.

In any event, students who participate in competitive extracurricular activities voluntarily subject themselves to many of the same intrusions on their privacy as do athletes. Some of these clubs and activities require occasional off-campus travel and communal undress. All of them have their own rules and requirements for participating students that do not apply to the student body as a whole. For example, each of the competitive extracurricular activities governed by the Policy must abide by the rules of the Oklahoma Secondary Schools Activities Association, and a faculty sponsor monitors the students for compliance with the various rules dictated by the clubs and activities. This regulation of extracurricular activities further diminishes the expectation of privacy among school children.

### B

Next, we consider the character of the intrusion imposed by the Policy. Urination is "an excretory function traditionally shielded by great privacy." But the "degree of intrusion" on one's privacy caused by collecting a urine sample "depends upon the manner in which production of the urine sample is monitored."

Under the Policy, a faculty monitor waits outside the closed restroom stall for the student to produce a sample and must "listen for the normal sounds of urination in order to guard against tampered specimens and to insure an accurate chain of custody." The monitor then pours the sample into two bottles that are sealed and placed into a mailing pouch along with a consent form signed by the student. This procedure is virtually identical to that reviewed in *Vernonia*, except that it additionally protects privacy by allowing male students to produce their samples behind a closed stall. Given that we considered the method of collection in *Vernonia* a "negligible" intrusion, the method here is even less problematic.

In addition, the Policy clearly requires that the test results be kept in confidential files separate from a student's other educational records and released to school personnel only on a "need to know" basis. Respondents nonetheless contend that the intrusion on students' privacy is significant because the Policy fails to protect effectively against the disclosure of confidential information and, specifically, that the school "has been careless in protecting that information: for example, the Choir teacher looked at students' prescription drug lists and left them where other students could see them." But the choir teacher is someone with a "need to know," because during off-campus trips she needs to know what medications are taken by her students. . . . This one example of alleged carelessness hardly increases the character of the intrusion.

Moreover, the test results are not turned over to any law enforcement authority. Nor do the test results here lead to the imposition of discipline or have any academic consequences. Rather, the only consequence of a failed drug test is to limit the student's privilege of participating in extracurricular activities. Indeed, a student may test positive for drugs twice and still be allowed to participate in extracurricular activities. After the first positive test, the school contacts the student's parent or guardian for a meeting. The student may continue to participate in the activity if within five days of the meeting the student shows proof of receiving drug counseling and submits to a second drug test in two weeks. For the second positive test, the student is suspended from participation in all extracurricular activities for 14 days, must complete four hours of substance abuse counseling, and must submit to monthly drug tests. Only after a third positive test will the student be suspended from participating in any extracurricular activity for the remainder of the school year, or 88 school days, whichever is longer.

Given the minimally intrusive nature of the sample collection and the limited uses to which the test results are put, we conclude that the invasion of students' privacy is not significant.

C

Finally, this Court must consider the nature and immediacy of the government's concerns and the efficacy of the Policy in meeting them. This Court has already articulated in detail the importance of the governmental concern in preventing drug use by school children. The drug abuse problem among our Nation's youth has hardly abated since *Vernonia* was decided in 1995. In fact, evidence suggests that it has only grown worse. As in *Vernonia*, "the necessity for the State to act is magnified by the fact that this evil is being visited not just upon individuals at large, but upon children for whom it has undertaken a special responsibility of care and direction." The health and safety risks identified in *Vernonia* apply with equal force to Tecumseh's children. Indeed, the nationwide drug epidemic makes the war against drugs a pressing concern in every school.

Additionally, the School District in this case has presented specific evidence of drug use at Tecumseh schools. Teachers testified that they had seen students who appeared to be under the influence of drugs and that they had heard students speaking openly about using drugs. A drug dog found marijuana cigarettes near the school parking lot. Police officers once found drugs or drug paraphernalia in a car driven by a Future Farmers of America member. And the school board president reported that people in the community were calling the board to discuss the "drug situation." We decline to second-guess the finding of the District Court that "viewing the evidence as a whole, it cannot be reasonably disputed that the [School District] was faced with a 'drug problem' when it adopted the Policy."

Respondents consider the proffered evidence insufficient and argue that there is no "real and immediate interest" to justify a policy of drug testing non-athletes. We have recognized, however, that "[a] demonstrated problem of drug abuse . . . [is] not in all cases necessary to the validity of a testing regime," but that some showing does "shore up an assertion of special need for a suspicionless general search program." The School District has provided sufficient evidence to shore up the need for its drug testing program.

Furthermore, this Court has not required a particularized or pervasive drug problem before allowing the government to conduct suspicionless drug testing. For instance, in *Von Raab* the Court upheld the drug testing of customs officials on a purely preventive basis, without any documented history of drug use by such officials. In response to the lack of evidence relating to drug use, the Court noted generally that "drug abuse is one of the most serious problems confronting our society today," and that programs to prevent and detect drug use among customs officials could not be deemed unreasonable. Likewise, the need to prevent and deter the substantial harm of childhood drug use provides the necessary immediacy for a school testing policy. Indeed, it would make little sense to require a school district to wait for a substantial portion of its students to begin using drugs before it was allowed to institute a drug testing program designed to deter drug use.

Given the nationwide epidemic of drug use, and the evidence of increased drug use in Tecumseh schools, it was entirely reasonable for the School District to enact this particular drug testing policy. We reject the Court of Appeals' novel test that "any district seeking to impose a random suspicionless drug testing policy as a condition to participation in a school activity must demonstrate that there is some identifiable drug abuse problem among a sufficient number of those subject to the testing, such that testing that group of students will actually redress its drug problem." Among other problems, it would be difficult to administer such a test. As we cannot articulate a threshold level of drug use that would suffice to justify a drug testing program for schoolchildren, we refuse to fashion what would in effect be a constitutional quantum of drug use necessary to show a "drug problem."

Respondents also argue that the testing of non-athletes does not implicate any safety concerns, and that safety is a "crucial factor" in applying the special needs framework. They contend that there must be "surpassing safety interests," or "extraordinary safety and national security hazards," in order to override the usual protections of the Fourth Amendment. Respondents are correct that safety factors into the special needs analysis, but the safety interest furthered by drug testing is undoubtedly substantial for all children, athletes and non-athletes alike. We know all too well that drug use carries a variety of health risks for children, including death from overdose.

We also reject respondents' argument that drug testing must presumptively be based upon an individualized reasonable suspicion of wrongdoing because such a testing regime would be less intrusive. In this context, the Fourth Amendment does not require a finding of individualized suspicion, and we decline to impose such a requirement on schools attempting to prevent and detect drug use by students. Moreover, we question whether testing based on individualized suspicion in fact would be less intrusive. Such a regime would place an additional burden on public school teachers who are already tasked with the difficult job of maintaining order and discipline. A program of individualized suspicion might unfairly target members of unpopular groups. The fear of lawsuits resulting from such targeted searches may chill enforcement of the program, rendering it ineffective in combating drug use. In any case, this

Court has repeatedly stated that reasonableness under the Fourth Amendment does not require employing the least intrusive means, because "the logic of such elaborate less-restrictive-alternative arguments could raise insuperable barriers to the exercise of virtually all search-and-seizure powers."

Finally, we find that testing students who participate in extracurricular activities is a reasonably effective means of addressing the School District's legitimate concerns in preventing, deterring, and detecting drug use. While in *Vernonia* there might have been a closer fit between the testing of athletes and the trial court's finding that the drug problem was "fueled by the 'role model' effect of athletes' drug use," such a finding was not essential to the holding. *Vernonia* did not require the school to test the group of students most likely to use drugs, but rather considered the constitutionality of the program in the context of the public school's custodial responsibilities. Evaluating the Policy in this context, we conclude that the drug testing of Tecumseh students who participate in extracurricular activities effectively serves the School District's interest in protecting the safety and health of its students.

### III

Within the limits of the Fourth Amendment, local school boards must assess the desirability of drug testing school children. In upholding the constitutionality of the Policy, we express no opinion as to its wisdom. Rather, we hold only that Tecumseh's Policy is a reasonable means of furthering the School District's important interest in preventing and deterring drug use among its schoolchildren. . . .

\* \* \*

Justice Ginsberg with Stevens, O'Connor, and Souter, dissenting.

Seven years ago, in *Vernonia School Dist. 47J* v. *Acton,* 515 U.S. 646 (1995), this Court determined that a school district's policy of randomly testing the urine of its student athletes for illicit drugs did not violate the Fourth Amendment. In so ruling, the Court emphasized that drug use "increased the risk of sports-related injury" and that Vernonia's athletes were the "leaders" of an aggressive local "drug culture" that had reached "'epidemic proportions.'" Today, the Court relies upon *Vernonia* to permit a school district with a drug problem its superintendent repeatedly described as "not . . . major," to test the urine of an academic team member solely by reason of her participation in a non-athletic, competitive extracurricular activity — participation associated with neither special dangers from, nor particular predilections for, drug use.

The particular testing program upheld today is not reasonable, it is capricious, even perverse: Petitioners' policy targets for testing a student population least likely to be at risk from illicit drugs and their damaging effects. I therefore dissent.

. . . .

This case presents circumstances dispositively different from those of *Vernonia*. True, as the Court stresses, Tecumseh students participating in competitive extracurricular activities other than athletics share two relevant characteristics with the athletes of *Vernonia*. First, both groups attend public schools. . . . Concern for student health and safety is basic to the school's care-taking, and it is undeniable that "drug use carries a variety of health risks for children . . . .

Those risks, however, are present for *all* schoolchildren. *Vernonia* cannot be read to endorse invasive and suspicionless drug testing of all students upon any evidence of drug use, solely because drugs jeopardize the life and health of those who use them. Many children, like many adults, engage in dangerous activities on their own time; that the children are enrolled in school scarcely allows government to monitor all such activities. If a student has a reasonable subjective expectation of privacy in the personal items she brings to school, surely she has a similar expectation regarding the chemical composition of her urine. Had the *Vernonia* Court agreed that public school attendance, in and of itself, permitted the State to test each student's blood or urine for drugs, the opinion in *Vernonia* could have saved many words. . . .

The second commonality to which the Court points is the voluntary charac-ter of both interscholastic athletics and other competitive extracurricular activities. "By choosing to 'go out for the team,' [school athletes] voluntarily subject themselves to a degree of regulation even higher than that imposed on students generally." Comparably, the Court today observes, "students who participate in competitive extracurricular activities voluntarily subject them-selves to" additional rules not applicable to other students.

The comparison is enlightening. While extracurricular activities are "volun-tary" in the sense that they are not required for graduation, they are part of the school's educational program; for that reason, the petitioner (hereinafter School District) is justified in expending public resources to make them avail-able. Participation in such activities is a key component of school life, essen-tial in reality for students applying to college, and, for all participants, a significant contributor to the breadth and quality of the educational experi-ence. Students "volunteer" for extracurricular pursuits in the same way they might volunteer for honors classes: They subject themselves to additional requirements, but they do so in order to take full advantage of the education offered them.

Voluntary participation in athletics has a distinctly different dimension: Schools regulate student athletes discretely because competitive school sports by their nature require communal undress and, more important, expose stu-dents to physical risks that schools have a duty to mitigate. For the very rea-son that schools cannot offer a program of competitive athletics without intimately affecting the privacy of students, *Vernonia* reasonably analogized school athletes to "adults who choose to participate in a closely regulated industry." Industries fall within the closely regulated category when the nature of their activities requires substantial government oversight. Interscholastic athletics similarly require close safety and health regulation; a school's choir, band, and academic team do not.

In short, *Vernonia* applied, it did not repudiate, the principle that "the legal-ity of a search of a student should depend simply on the reasonableness, *under all the circumstances*, of the search." Enrollment in a public school, and elec-tion to participate in school activities beyond the bare minimum that the curriculum requires, are indeed factors relevant to reasonableness, but they do not on their own justify intrusive, suspicionless searches. *Vernonia,* accordingly, did not rest upon these factors; instead, the Court performed what today's majority aptly describes as a "fact-specific balancing." Balancing of that order, applied to the facts now before the Court, should yield a result other than the one the Court announces today.

*Vernonia* initially considered "the nature of the privacy interest upon which the search [there] at issue intruded." The Court emphasized that student athletes' expectations of privacy are necessarily attenuated. . . .

Competitive extracurricular activities other than athletics, however, serve students of all manner: the modest and shy along with the bold and uninhibited. Activities of the kind plaintiff-respondent Lindsay Earls pursued — choir, show choir, marching band, and academic team — afford opportunities to gain self-assurance, to "come to know faculty members in a less formal setting than the typical classroom," and to acquire "positive social supports and networks [that] play a critical role in periods of heightened stress."

On "occasional out-of-town trips," students like Lindsay Earls "must sleep together in communal settings and use communal bathrooms." But those situations are hardly equivalent to the routine communal undress associated with athletics; the School District itself admits that when such trips occur, "public-like restroom facilities," which presumably include enclosed stalls, are ordinarily available for changing, and that "more modest students" find other ways to maintain their privacy.

After describing school athletes' reduced expectation of privacy, the *Vernonia* Court turned to "the character of the intrusion . . . complained of." Observing that students produce urine samples in a bathroom stall with a coach or teacher outside, *Vernonia* typed the privacy interests compromised by the process of obtaining samples "negligible." As to the required pretest disclosure of prescription medications taken, the Court assumed that "the School District would have permitted [a student] to provide the requested information in a confidential manner — for example, in a sealed envelope delivered to the testing lab." On that assumption, the Court concluded that Vernonia's athletes faced no significant invasion of privacy.

In this case, however, Lindsay Earls and her parents allege that the School District handled personal information collected under the policy carelessly, with little regard for its confidentiality. Information about students' prescription drug use, they assert, was routinely viewed by Lindsay's choir teacher, who left files containing the information unlocked and unsealed, where others, including students, could see them; and test results were given out to all activity sponsors whether or not they had a clear "need to know."

. . . .

Finally, the "nature and immediacy of the governmental concern," faced by the Vernonia School District dwarfed that confronting Tecumseh administrators. Vernonia initiated its drug testing policy in response to an alarming situation. . . . Tecumseh, by contrast, repeatedly reported to the Federal Government during the period leading up to the adoption of the policy that "types of drugs [other than alcohol and tobacco] including controlled danger-ous substances, are present [in the schools] but have not identified themselves as major problems at this time." As the Tenth Circuit observed, "without a demonstrated drug abuse problem among the group being tested, the efficacy of the District's solution to its perceived problem is . . . greatly diminished."

The School District cites *Treasury Employees* v. *Von Raab,* 489 U.S. 656 (1989), in which this Court permitted random drug testing of customs agents absent "any perceived drug problem among Customs employees," given that "drug abuse is one of the most serious problems confronting our society today." The tests in *Von Raab* and *Railway Labor Executives,* however, were installed to avoid enormous risks to the lives and limbs of others, not dominantly in response to the health risks to users invariably present in any case of drug use.

Urging that "the safety interest furthered by drug testing is undoubtedly substantial for all children, athletes and non-athletes alike," the Court cuts out an element essential to the *Vernonia* judgment. Citing medical literature on the effects of combining illicit drug use with physical exertion, the *Vernonia* Court emphasized that "the particular drugs screened by [Vernonia's] Policy have been demonstrated to pose substantial physical risks to athletes." We have since confirmed that these special risks were necessary to our decision in *Vernonia.*

At the margins, of course, no policy of *random* drug testing is perfectly tai-lored to the harms it seeks to address. The School District cites the dangers faced by members of the band, who must "perform extremely precise routines with heavy equipment and instruments in close proximity to other students," and by Future Farmers of America, who "are required to individually control and restrain animals as large as 1500 pounds." For its part, the United States acknowledges that "the linebacker faces a greater risk of serious injury if he takes the field under the influence of drugs than the drummer in the halftime band," but parries that "the risk of injury to a student who is under the influ-ence of drugs while playing golf, cross country, or volleyball (sports covered by the policy in *Vernonia*) is scarcely any greater than the risk of injury to a stu-dent . . . handling a 1500-pound steer (as [Future Farmers of America] mem-bers do) or working with cutlery or other sharp instruments (as [Future Homemakers of America] members do)." Notwithstanding nightmarish images of out-of-control flatware, livestock run amok, and colliding tubas dis-turbing the peace and quiet of Tecumseh, the great majority of students the School District seeks to test in truth are engaged in activities that are not safety sensitive to an unusual degree. There is a difference between imperfect tailoring and no tailoring at all.

The Vernonia district, in sum, had two good reasons for testing athletes: Sports team members faced special health risks and they "were the leaders of the drug culture." No similar reason, and no other tenable justification, explains Tecumseh's decision to target for testing all participants in every competitive extracurricular activity.

Nationwide, students who participate in extracurricular activities are significantly less likely to develop substance abuse problems than are their less-involved peers. Even if students might be deterred from drug use in order to preserve their extracurricular eligibility, it is at least as likely that other students might forgo their extracurricular involvement in order to avoid detection of their drug use. Tecumseh's policy thus falls short doubly if deterrence is its aim: It invades the privacy of students who need deterrence least, and risks steering students at greatest risk for substance abuse away from extracurricular involvement that potentially may palliate drug problems.

\* \* \*

## NOTES AND QUESTIONS

**1.** As set out in the *Ferguson* decision, the Fourth Amendment generally prohibits "unreasonable searches and seizures." In most ordinary criminal investigations, this requires that a warrant be issued on the showing of probable cause; exceptions are allowed for consensual searches, searches incident to an arrest, and a few other circumstances where there is some immediate and individualized showing of probable cause. But the Supreme Court also has on a few occasions acknowledged an additional exception for certain "permissible suspicionless searches." In each of those cases, the Court has employed a balancing test that weighed the intrusion on the individual's interest in privacy against the "special needs" that supported the search. In *Skinner v. Railway Labor Executives' Ass'n*, 489 U.S. 602 (1989), the Court upheld warrantless drug testing of railway employees; in *Treasury Employees v. Von Raab*, 489 U.S. 656 (1989), the Court allowed similar testing of customs officials who were applying for promotion; in *Vernonia School Dist. 47J* v. Acton, 515 U.S. 646 (1995), the Court allowed warrantless, random drug testing of athletes participating in sports on public schools (discussed extensively in *Earles*). However, in *Chandler v. Miller,* 520 U.S. 305 (1997) the Court refused to allow for warrantless testing of candidates for political office.

These exceptional "suspicionless" search cases all derive their reasoning from a more general principle essentially distinguishing between governmental efforts to identify individual criminal conduct and government's "special need" to preemptively protect the public safety. As articulated by the *Earles* majority: "[T]he Government's need to discover such latent or hidden conditions, or to prevent their development, is sufficiently compelling to justify the intrusion on privacy entailed by conducting such searches without any measure of individualized suspicion." The Supreme Court developed this "special needs" analysis in cases involving "administrative searches" or inspections of premises, not people, in regulated industries. Examples included health and safety inspections of coal mines and warehouses, either without a warrant or with reasonable suspicion, a standard lower than probable cause. *See, e.g., Marshall v. Barlow's*, 436 U.S. 307 (1978). Other cases required that a warrant be issued prior to an administrative search (*e.g.*, a search that is part of a citywide inspection of rental property), but that the warrant could be issued based on legislative or administratively determined criteria. *See Camara v. Municipal Court of City & County of San Francisco*, 387 U.S. 523 (1967). Although the administrative search exception was initially justified primarily

on the ground that a premises search was not personal, later decisions emphasized both the government's goal in conducting the search (the "special needs")
and the fact that regulated industries — and ultimately their employees —
should have a limited expectation of privacy. In the "special needs" cases noted
above, the Court has sometimes strained to find reasons why those who are
subjected to drug testing are engaged in safety-sensitive jobs and how drug
use would result in harm to others, such as passengers on trains. Dissenting
Justices often question both the likelihood of harm and the coherence of the
"special needs" exception. For example, in *Skinner*, Justice Marshall wrote,
"There is no drug exception to the Constitution, any more than there is a
Communism exception or an exception for any other real or imagined sources
of domestic unrest." Nevertheless, as illustrated by the *Earles* case, the Court
continues to apply the special needs exception to a widening range of drug
testing policies.

**2.** In *Ferguson*, the Court rejected the government's claim that a special
needs exception comparable to that in *Skinner*, *Von Raab* and *Vernonia* justified the hospital's policy. The Court found that the invasion of privacy in this
case "is far more substantial than in those cases" and that, in any event, the
government's "special need" was little different than it was in any other criminal prosecution. Do you agree? The Court distinguished the special needs line
of cases from the general rule that searches used for law enforcement (including investigations) require a warrant or consent and found that the hospital's
policy fell within the general rule. In particular, it insisted that the determining factor was the specific — and immediate — purpose of the drug testing, not
its ultimate or long-term goal. Although both the hospital and law enforcement personnel may have intended to protect mothers and children, the policy
itself was limited to law enforcement — threatened or actual arrest and criminal prosecution for drug crimes. The Court cautioned that "Because law
enforcement always serves some broader social purpose or objective, virtually
any nonconsensual suspicionless search could be immunized under the special
needs doctrine by defining the search solely in terms of its ultimate, rather
than immediate, goal."

The Court has maintained the conceptual distinction between searches
whose immediate purpose is law enforcement and those intended to address
internal organizational safety policies. A critical factor in these cases, including *Ferguson*, is how drug test results are used. (Another factor, of rather less
conceptual weight, is how privately and sensitively the drug test itself is conducted, as a component of its reasonableness.) The Court has approved policies that require the results of drug testing to be kept confidential within the
agency and used solely for (civil) personnel decisions, such as hiring and firing
or identifying and treating employees whose drug use may pose safety risks to
others, as in *Skinner*; but has struck down policies that give test results to
police for purposes of criminal investigations.

**3.** As the dissent points out in *Ferguson*, this sort of drug testing is not the
usual sort of search or seizure. How would you respond to the Justice Scalia's
claims that there may not be a search, consensual or otherwise, that is subject
to the Fourth Amendment limitations at all — or, alternatively, that the only
search is the taking of the urine sample, a procedure to which the patients

may have consented? Compare his view of patient expectations of privacy in medical care with that expressed in the majority opinion.

Justice Scalia also argues that the special needs exception presumably upholds the validity of laws requiring physicians and other providers to report gun shot wounds, evidence of child abuse, and other data. Do you agree? If so, is this because patients have no privacy interest in controlling the use of medical information (like test results or diagnoses) that is acquired by providers as part of ordinary medical treatment? Might this view mean that public health surveillance programs could have unfettered access to anything in patients' medical records? (*See* Chapter Four.) Alternatively, might the dissent base his presumption on the idea that such reporting laws demonstrate a special need unrelated to law enforcement? The information provided by physicians under reporting laws goes to public health or social welfare agencies, not law enforcement. Does Scalia mean to suggest that law enforcement authorities can or do have the power to obtain medical records directly from providers without a warrant or probable cause?

**4.** *Earles* represents perhaps the farthest expansion of the special needs exception to date. The drug policy met some of the requirements for a special needs exception. The test results were kept confidential within the school (despite some possible laxity in keeping them secure from prying eyes) and were not delivered to law enforcement officials or used for criminal investigations. The more difficult question was whether the school had a special need for precluding participation in extracurricular programs by students who used drugs. The several opinions in *Earles* illustrate the Justices' different views of what counts as a special need. The majority opinion emphasizes the *parens patriae* role of the state — and by extension the school — as protector of children. Who is the school protecting by its policy — the students tested or other students with whom they have contact? Is this the same approach used in the cases in which a government agency's special need is to ensure the safety of its customers and passengers? The Court is obviously concerned with what it calls "the nationwide epidemic of drug use." What other risks might threaten school children? As a practical matter, how effective is the school's policy in deterring drug use among students? What other measures might a school take to protect its students from harm? (Consider school policies to offer more healthful lunches, discussed in Section D of this Chapter.)

Justice Ginsberg's dissent lays out the factual differences between the students affected in *Vernonia* and those in *Earles*. Not surprisingly, the majority minimize or ignore factual differences between the circumstances in *Earles* and *Vernonia* that are emphasized by the dissent. Do you agree with the majority that "students who participate in competitive extracurricular activities voluntarily subject themselves to many of the same intrusions in their privacy as do athletes"? Was *Vernonia* itself correctly decided? The dissent argues that the risks to students in the extracurricular programs are no different from the risks for all students and that the majority's reasoning would permit drug testing for all students. Do you agree?

**5.** As *Earles* demonstrates, the special needs exception has encouraged the adoption of drug testing policies by many government agencies, including police departments, fire departments, and schools. *See, e.g., Petersen v. City of*

*Mesa,* 207 Ariz. 35, *cert. denied,* 125 S.Ct. 51 (2004) (random, suspicionless drug testing of firemen). How effective have such policies been? Private organizations, of course, are not subject to any Fourth Amendment constraints on requiring drug testing for their employees. What, if any, differences are there between an employer's policy forbidding its employees to use unlawful controlled substances and a policy forbidding employees to smoke? Private universities and research organizations that receive federal grants and other federal funds must comply with federal policies requiring certification that staff in the funded program do not use controlled substances. Universities might also consider drug testing for enrolled students. How might a state university justify such testing?

**6.** A slightly different line of cases concerns random stops of the public at highway roadblocks or checkpoints. Such stops constitute a seizure within the meaning of the Fourth Amendment. The Supreme Court has upheld brief, suspicionless seizures at highway checkpoints to keep intoxicated drivers off the road (*See Michigan Department of State Police v. Sitz,* 496 U.S. 444 (1990), and to ask drivers if they had witnessed a hit-and-run accident (*Illinois v. Lidster,* 540 U.S. 419 (2004)). In *City of Indianapolis v. Edmond,* 531 U.S. 32 (2000), however, the Supreme Court held that a police roadblock set up to find drugs without individualized suspicion violated the Fourth Amendment. The police stopped all vehicles at six locations, checked the driver's license and registration, looked in and around the car from the outside, and walked a narcotics-detection dog around the car. About nine percent of drivers were arrested, 55% on charges of drug-related crimes. As in *Ferguson,* the Court found that "what principally distinguishes these checkpoints from those we have previously approved is their primary purpose . . . interdicting illegal narcotics." It added, "We have never approved a checkpoint program whose primary purpose was to detect evidence of ordinary criminal wrongdoing." Id. at 40–41. The safety risk posed by drivers who are impaired by drugs or alcohol may be more apparent than that presented by a customs officer, although there is little evidence that highway checkpoints have identified a significant number of impaired drivers. Are there alternative ways to keep intoxicated drivers off the road?

* * *

# GONZALES v. RAICH
## 545 U.S. 1 (2005)

Stevens, Justice.

* * *

California is one of at least nine States that authorize the use of marijuana for medicinal purposes. The question presented in this case is whether the power vested in Congress by Article I, § 8, of the Constitution "[t]o make all Laws which shall be necessary and proper for carrying into Execution" its authority to "regulate Commerce with foreign Nations, and among the several States" includes the power to prohibit the local cultivation and use of marijuana in compliance with California law.

California has been a pioneer in the regulation of marijuana. In 1913, California was one of the first States to prohibit the sale and possession of marijuana, and at the end of the century, California became the first State to authorize limited use of the drug for medicinal purposes. In 1996, California voters passed Proposition 215, now codified as the Compassionate Use Act of 1996. The proposition was designed to ensure that "seriously ill" residents of the State have access to marijuana for medical purposes, and to encourage Federal and State Governments to take steps towards ensuring the safe and affordable distribution of the drug to patients in need. The Act creates an exemption from criminal prosecution for physicians, as well as for patients and primary caregivers who possess or cultivate marijuana for medicinal purposes with the recommendation or approval of a physician. A "primary caregiver" is a person who has consistently assumed responsibility for the housing, health, or safety of the patient.

Respondents Angel Raich and Diane Monson are California residents who suffer from a variety of serious medical conditions and have sought to avail themselves of medical marijuana pursuant to the terms of the Compassionate Use Act. They are being treated by licensed, board-certified family practitioners, who have concluded, after prescribing a host of conventional medicines to treat respondents' conditions and to alleviate their associated symptoms, that marijuana is the only drug available that provides effective treatment. Both women have been using marijuana as a medication for several years pursuant to their doctors' recommendation, and both rely heavily on cannabis to function on a daily basis. Indeed, Raich's physician believes that forgoing cannabis treatments would certainly cause Raich excruciating pain and could very well prove fatal.

Respondent Monson cultivates her own marijuana, and ingests the drug in a variety of ways including smoking and using a vaporizer. Respondent Raich, by contrast, is unable to cultivate her own, and thus relies on two caregivers, litigating as "John Does," to provide her with locally grown marijuana at no charge. These caregivers also process the cannabis into hashish or keif, and Raich herself processes some of the marijuana into oils, balms, and foods for consumption.

On August 15, 2002, county deputy sheriffs and agents from the federal Drug Enforcement Administration (DEA) came to Monson's home. After a thorough investigation, the county officials concluded that her use of marijuana was entirely lawful as a matter of California law. Nevertheless, after a 3-hour standoff, the federal agents seized and destroyed all six of her cannabis plants.

Respondents thereafter brought this action against the Attorney General of the United States and the head of the DEA seeking injunctive and declaratory relief prohibiting the enforcement of the federal Controlled Substances Act (CSA), to the extent it prevents them from possessing, obtaining, or manufacturing cannabis for their personal medical use. . . . Respondents claimed that enforcing the CSA against them would violate the Commerce Clause, the Due Process Clause of the Fifth Amendment, the Ninth and Tenth Amendments of the Constitution, and the doctrine of medical necessity.

. . . The case is made difficult by respondents' strong arguments that they will suffer irreparable harm because, despite a congressional finding to the contrary, marijuana does have valid therapeutic purposes. The question before us, however, is not whether it is wise to enforce the statute in these circumstances; rather, it is whether Congress' power to regulate interstate markets for medicinal substances encompasses the portions of those markets that are supplied with drugs produced and consumed locally. . . .

## II

. . . As early as 1906 Congress enacted federal legislation imposing labeling regulations on medications and prohibiting the manufacture or shipment of any adulterated or misbranded drug traveling in interstate commerce. Aside from these labeling restrictions, most domestic drug regulations prior to 1970 generally came in the guise of revenue laws, with the Department of the Treasury serving as the Federal Government's primary enforcer. For example, the primary drug control law, before being repealed by the passage of the CSA, was the Harrison Narcotics Act of 1914, 38 Stat. 785 (repealed 1970). The Harrison Act sought to exert control over the possession and sale of narcotics, specifically cocaine and opiates, by requiring producers, distributors, and purchasers to register with the Federal Government, by assessing taxes against parties so registered, and by regulating the issuance of prescriptions.

Marijuana itself was not significantly regulated by the Federal Government until 1937 when accounts of marijuana's addictive qualities and physiological effects, paired with dissatisfaction with enforcement efforts at state and local levels, prompted Congress to pass the Marihuana Tax Act . . . Like the Harrison Act, the Marihuana Tax Act did not outlaw the possession or sale of marijuana outright. Rather, it imposed registration and reporting requirements for all individuals importing, producing, selling, or dealing in marijuana, and required the payment of annual taxes in addition to transfer taxes whenever the drug changed hands. Moreover, doctors wishing to prescribe marijuana for medical purposes were required to comply with rather burdensome administrative requirements. Noncompliance exposed traffickers to severe federal penalties, whereas compliance would often subject them to prosecution under state law. Thus, while the Marihuana Tax Act did not declare the drug illegal *per se,* the onerous administrative requirements, the prohibitively expensive taxes, and the risks attendant on compliance practically curtailed the marijuana trade.

Then in 1970, after declaration of the national "war on drugs," federal drug policy underwent a significant transformation. A number of noteworthy events precipitated this policy shift. First this Court held certain provisions of the Marihuana Tax Act and other narcotics legislation unconstitutional. Second, at the end of his term, President Johnson fundamentally reorganized the federal drug control agencies. . . . Finally, prompted by a perceived need to consolidate the growing number of piecemeal drug laws and to enhance federal drug enforcement powers, Congress enacted the Comprehensive Drug Abuse Prevention and Control Act.

Title II of that Act, the CSA, repealed most of the earlier antidrug laws in favor of a comprehensive regime to combat the international and interstate traffic in illicit drugs. The main objectives of the CSA were to conquer drug abuse and to control the legitimate and illegitimate traffic in controlled substances. Congress was particularly concerned with the need to prevent the diversion of drugs from legitimate to illicit channels. To effectuate these goals, Congress devised a closed regulatory system making it unlawful to manufacture, distribute, dispense, or possess any controlled substance except in a manner authorized by the CSA. The CSA categorizes all controlled substances into five schedules. The drugs are grouped together based on their accepted medical uses, the potential for abuse, and their psychological and physical effects on the body. Each schedule is associated with a distinct set of controls regarding the manufacture, distribution, and use of the substances listed therein. The CSA and its implementing regulations set forth strict requirements regarding registration, labeling and packaging, production quotas, drug security, and recordkeeping.

In enacting the CSA, Congress classified marijuana as a Schedule I drug. This preliminary classification was based, in part, on the recommendation of the Assistant Secretary of HEW "that marihuana be retained within schedule I at least until the completion of certain studies now underway." Schedule I drugs are categorized as such because of their high potential for abuse, lack of any accepted medical use, and absence of any accepted safety for use in medically supervised treatment. These three factors, in varying gradations, are also used to categorize drugs in the other four schedules. For example, Schedule II substances also have a high potential for abuse which may lead to severe psychological or physical dependence, but unlike Schedule I drugs, they have a currently accepted medical use. By classifying marijuana as a Schedule I drug, as opposed to listing it on a lesser schedule, the manufacture, distribution, or possession of marijuana became a criminal offense, with the sole exception being use of the drug as part of a Food and Drug Administration pre-approved research study.

The CSA provides for the periodic updating of schedules and delegates authority to the Attorney General, after consultation with the Secretary of Health and Human Services, to add, remove, or transfer substances to, from, or between schedules. Despite considerable efforts to reschedule marijuana, it remains a Schedule I drug.

III

Respondents in this case do not dispute that passage of the CSA, as part of the Comprehensive Drug Abuse Prevention and Control Act, was well within Congress' commerce power. Nor do they contend that any provision or section of the CSA amounts to an unconstitutional exercise of congressional authority. Rather, respondents' challenge is actually quite limited; they argue that the CSA's categorical prohibition of the manufacture and possession of marijuana as applied to the intrastate manufacture and possession of marijuana for medical purposes pursuant to California law exceeds Congress' authority under the Commerce Clause.

In assessing the validity of congressional regulation, none of our Commerce Clause cases can be viewed in isolation. As charted in considerable detail in *United States v. Lopez,* our understanding of the reach of the Commerce Clause, as well as Congress' assertion of authority thereunder, has evolved over time. . . .

Cases decided during that "new era," which now spans more than a century, have identified three general categories of regulation in which Congress is authorized to engage under its commerce power. First, Congress can regulate the channels of interstate commerce. Second, Congress has authority to regulate and protect the instrumentalities of interstate commerce, and persons or things in interstate commerce. Third, Congress has the power to regulate activities that substantially affect interstate commerce. Only the third category is implicated in the case at hand.

Our case law firmly establishes Congress' power to regulate purely local activities that are part of an economic "class of activities" that have a substantial effect on interstate commerce. As we stated in *Wickard*, "even if appellee's activity be local and though it may not be regarded as commerce, it may still, whatever its nature, be reached by Congress if it exerts a substantial economic effect on interstate commerce." We have never required Congress to legislate with scientific exactitude. When Congress decides that the "'total incidence'" of a practice poses a threat to a national market, it may regulate the entire class. . . . In this vein, we have reiterated that when "'a general regulatory statute bears a substantial relation to commerce, the *de minimis* character of individual instances arising under that statute is of no consequence.'"

Our decision in *Wickard* is of particular relevance. . . . *Wickard* establishes that Congress can regulate purely intrastate activity that is not itself "commercial," in that it is not produced for sale, if it concludes that failure to regulate that class of activity would undercut the regulation of the interstate market in that commodity.

. . . Like the farmer in *Wickard*, respondents are cultivating, for home consumption, a fungible commodity for which there is an established, albeit illegal, interstate market. . . . In *Wickard* we had no difficulty concluding that Congress had a rational basis for believing that, when viewed in the aggregate, leaving home-consumed wheat outside the regulatory scheme would have a substantial influence on price and market conditions. Here too, Congress had a rational basis for concluding that leaving home-consumed marijuana outside federal control would similarly affect price and market conditions.

The fact that Wickard's own impact on the market was "trivial by itself" was not a sufficient reason for removing him from the scope of federal regulation. . . . Moreover, even though Wickard was indeed a commercial farmer, the activity he was engaged in — the cultivation of wheat for home consumption- was not treated by the Court as part of his commercial farming operation. . . . [W]e have before us findings by Congress to the same effect.

In assessing the scope of Congress' authority under the Commerce Clause, we stress that the task before us is a modest one. We need not determine whether respondents' activities, taken in the aggregate, substantially affect interstate commerce in fact, but only whether a "rational basis" exists for so concluding. . . . [W]e have no difficulty concluding that Congress had a rational basis for believing that failure to regulate the intrastate manufacture and possession of marijuana would leave a gaping hole in the CSA. . . . That the regulation ensnares some purely intrastate activity is of no moment. As we have done many times before, we refuse to excise individual components of that larger scheme.

## IV

To support their contrary submission, respondents rely heavily on two of our more recent Commerce Clause cases [*Lopez* and *Morrison*]. In their myopic focus, they overlook the larger context of modern-era Commerce Clause jurisprudence preserved by those cases. Moreover, even in the narrow prism of respondents' creation, they read those cases far too broadly.

. . . .

Unlike those at issue in *Lopez* and *Morrison* the activities regulated by the CSA are quintessentially economic. "Economics" refers to "the production, distribution, and consumption of commodities." The CSA is a statute that regulates the production, distribution, and consumption of commodities for which there is an established, and lucrative, interstate market. Prohibiting the intrastate possession or manufacture of an article of commerce is a rational (and commonly utilized) means of regulating commerce in that product. Such prohibitions include specific decisions requiring that a drug be withdrawn from the market as a result of the failure to comply with regulatory requirements as well as decisions excluding Schedule I drugs entirely from the market. . . .

. . . We have no difficulty concluding that Congress acted rationally in determining that none of the characteristics making up the purported class, whether viewed individually or in the aggregate, compelled an exemption from the CSA; rather, the subdivided class of activities defined by the Court of Appeals was an essential part of the larger regulatory scheme.

First, the fact that marijuana is used "for personal medical purposes on the advice of a physician" cannot itself serve as a distinguishing factor. . . .

. . . One need not have a degree in economics to understand why a nationwide exemption for the vast quantity of marijuana (or other drugs) locally cultivated for personal use (which presumably would include use by friends, neighbors, and family members) may have a substantial impact on the interstate market for this extraordinarily popular substance. The congressional judgment that an exemption for such a significant segment of the total market would undermine the orderly enforcement of the entire regulatory scheme is entitled to a strong presumption of validity.

Second, limiting the activity to marijuana possession and cultivation "in accordance with state law" cannot serve to place respondents' activities beyond congressional reach. The Supremacy Clause unambiguously provides that if there is any conflict between federal and state law, federal law shall prevail. . . .

The exemption for cultivation by patients and caregivers can only increase the supply of marijuana in the California market. The likelihood that all such production will promptly terminate when patients recover or will precisely match the patients' medical needs during their convalescence seems remote; whereas the danger that excesses will satisfy some of the admittedly enormous demand for recreational use seems obvious. Moreover, that the national and international narcotics trade has thrived in the face of vigorous criminal enforcement efforts suggests that no small number of unscrupulous people will make use of the California exemptions to serve their commercial ends whenever it is feasible to do so. . . .

V

Respondents also raise a substantive due process claim and seek to avail themselves of the medical necessity defense. These theories of relief were set forth in their complaint but were not reached by the Court of Appeals. We therefore do not address the question whether judicial relief is available to respondents on these alternative bases. We do note, however, the presence of another avenue of relief. As the Solicitor General confirmed during oral argument, the statute authorizes procedures for the reclassification of Schedule I drugs. But perhaps even more important than these legal avenues is the democratic process, in which the voices of voters allied with these respondents may one day be heard in the halls of Congress. Under the present state of the law, however, the judgment of the Court of Appeals must be vacated. . . .

* * *

# NOTES AND QUESTIONS

**1.** Notwithstanding the constraints imposed by the Fourth Amendment, or those that may be imposed by other state or federal constitutional limitations (see discussion in Chapter Two), both the state and the federal governments have considerable discretion to regulate or prohibit the use or even the possession of narcotic or other potentially dangerous drugs. *Raich* outlines the history of the regulation of marijuana and other allegedly dangerous drugs by the federal and state governments.

*Raich* is a particularly good illustration of the distribution of power between the federal and state government and the primacy of federal laws where otherwise valid state and federal laws are in conflict. The plaintiffs in *Raich* were growing their own marijuana in conformance with California's "Compassionate Use Act," a voter-approved initiative which allowed for the individual use of marijuana for medical purposes. They sought an injunction against the enforcement of the federal Controlled Substances Act after federal agents had entered their home and destroyed their marijuana plants, claiming that the enforcement of the federal statute in this manner exceeded Congress' power to regulate interstate commerce. Despite recent decisions that had implied that the Court was inclined to narrow the scope of the commerce powers (*e.g.*, *U.S. v. Lopez*, 514 U.S. 549 (1995), and *U.S. v. Morrison*, 529 U.S. 598 (2000)), the *Raich* Court upheld the federal law on the basis of much earlier decisions — those that had allowed Congress to find that a class of regulated economic activities, taken in the aggregate, can have the necessary effect on interstate commerce, even if the particular activity subject to the regulation — in this case the individual use of marijuana — by itself would not have the requisite effect.

Justice Stevens' opinion in *Raich* was joined by four other Justices, while four Justices dissented, largely on the basis of their views of the Commerce Clause. The majority relied heavily on the case of *Wickard v. Filburn*, 317 U.S. 111 (1942), which Justice Scalia had earlier considered an unprincipled stretch of the Commerce Clause and which Justice O'Connor, dissenting, distinguishes from *Raich* on its facts. Justice O'Connor would require a factual analysis of the prohibited acts' actual effect on commerce, which she argues *Wickard* met and *Raich* did not, while the majority requires only a rational basis for Congress' assumption. Justice O'Connor writes:

> This case exemplifies the role of the States as laboratories. Today the Court sanctions an application of the federal [CSA] that extinguishes that experiment, without any proof that the personal cultivation, possession, and use of marijuana for medicinal purposes, if economic activity in the first place, has a substantial effect on interstate commerce. . . .

545 U.S. at 35.

The dissenting Justices argue the majority's interpretation of the Commerce Clause effectively grants Congress a national police power. Justice Thomas writes:

> "[T]he majority defines economic activity in the broadest possible terms. . . . If the majority is to be taken seriously, the Federal Government may now regulate quilting bees, clothes drives, and potluck suppers throughout the 50 states.
>
> . . .
>
> "If the activity is purely intrastate, then it may not be regulated under the Commerce Clause. And if the regulation of the intrastate activity is purely incidental, then it may not be regulated under the Necessary and Proper Clause."

545 U.S. at 53.

Respondents argued that California's law offered sufficiently careful state regulation to escape ties to interstate commerce, because the law carved out a local, non-economic activity distinct from criminal drug use. However, the majority considers marijuana a fungible product, one that could be used in recreation or crime as well as patient care:

> [I]f, as the principal dissent contends, the personal cultivation, possession, and use of marijuana for medicinal purposes is beyond the "'outer limits' of Congress' Commerce Clause authority," it must also be true that such personal use of marijuana (or any other homegrown drug) for recreational purposes is also beyond those "outer limits," whether or not a State elects to authorize or regulate such use.

545 U.S. at 25–26.

Having found that Congress had the power to prohibit state authorizations of marijuana use, the majority hinted that Congress might be persuaded to change marijuana's classification to permit its medical use if supporters brought supporting evidence to that body:

We do note, however, the presence of another avenue of relief. . . . the democratic process, in which the voices of voters allied with these respondents may one day be heard in the halls of Congress.

545 U.S. at 29.

Congress has rejected such attempts so far. Advocates of the use of marijuana for medical purposes complain that the FDA controls access to cannabis for use in medical research and that what is available is unsuitable for credible studies.

**2.** The Controlled Substances Act (CSA) was also at issue in *Gonzales v. Oregon*, 126 U.S. 904 (2006), which held that the United State Attorney General did not have the statutory authority to override Oregon's physician assisted suicide legislation. Oregon's law permitted physicians to prescribe drugs for patients who wished who wished to use them to commit suicide, provided that they followed a detailed procedure to ensure that the patient was terminally ill, competent, and making a fully informed decision. Attorney General John Ashcroft issued an Interpretative Rule finding that "assisting suicide is not a 'legitimate medical practice' within the meaning" of CSA regulations.

The results in *Raich* and *Oregon* can seem paradoxical, since California could not authorize patients to use marijuana to alleviate pain or even survive, while Oregon could permit physicians to prescribe drugs so that patients could end their own lives. Of course, *Raich* concerned Congress's power under the Commerce Clause to use the Controlled Substances Act to regulate intrastate marijuana use, while the issue in *Oregon* was what the CSA itself said. None of the Justices in *Oregon* challenged the conclusion that Congress had the power, if it chose, to prohibit physician-assisted suicide. The majority, however, found that Congress had not done so and had not granted the Attorney General the power to decide that prescribing medications for a patient's use to commit suicide was not legitimate medical practice. Nonetheless, the case raises policy questions about the proper locus of regulation for the practice medicine and public health. As George Annas notes:

Congress historically has been loath to legislate medical practice, preferring to see the areas in which it legislated — such as drug trafficking, recreational drug use, female genital mutilation, and even so-called partial birth abortion — not as the practice of medicine at all, but something outside it.

George J. Annas, *Congress, Controlled Substances, and Physician-Assisted Suicide — Elephants in Mouseholes*, 354 NEW ENG. J. MED. 1079, 1083–84 (2006).

Although Annas says that national medical standards have merit, he concludes: "It is one thing to decide that national standards will be set by the relevant specialty boards or other national medical organizations on the basis of evidence that supports the relevance of such standards to the health and welfare of patients; it is quite another to say that standards will be set by Congress or the attorney general on the basis of the political winds of the day." *Id.* at 1084.

**3.** For a related decision also analyzing the interplay of federal and state authority in matters relating to drug use and possession, see *State v. Mooney*, 2004 UT 49, 98 P. 3d 420 (2004) (federal law exempting use of peyote in Native American rituals incorporated into state law criminalizing the use of peyote).

# D. CASE STUDY: OBESITY

## SURGEON GENERAL, A CALL TO ACTION TO PREVENT & DECREASE OVERWEIGHT & OBESITY
### 1–17 (2001)

\* \* \*

This *Surgeon General's Call To Action* seeks to engage leaders from diverse groups in addressing a public health issue that is among the most burdensome faced by the Nation: the health consequences of overweight and obesity. This burden manifests itself in premature death and disability, in health care costs, in lost productivity, and in social stigmatization. The burden is not trivial. Studies show that the risk of death rises with increasing weight. Even moderate weight excess (10 to 20 pounds for a person of average height) increases the risk of death, particularly among adults aged 30 to 64 years.

Overweight and obesity are caused by many factors. For each individual, body weight is determined by a combination of genetic, metabolic, behavioral, environmental, cultural, and socioeconomic influences. Behavioral and environmental factors are large contributors to overweight and obesity and provide the greatest opportunity for actions and interventions designed for prevention and treatment.

For the vast majority of individuals, overweight and obesity result from excess calorie consumption and/or inadequate physical activity. Unhealthy dietary habits and sedentary behavior together account for approximately 300,000 deaths every year. Thus, a healthy diet and regular physical activity, consistent with the *Dietary Guidelines for Americans*, should be promoted as the cornerstone of any prevention or treatment effort. . . . Much work needs to be done to ensure the nutrient adequacy of our diets while at the same time avoiding excess calories. Dietary adequacy and moderation in energy consumption are both important for maintaining or achieving a healthy weight and for overall health.

Many adult Americans have not been meeting Federal physical activity recommendations to accumulate at least 30 minutes of moderate physical activity most days of the week. In 1997, less than one-third of adults engaged in the recommended amount of physical activity. Although nearly 65 percent of adolescents reported participating in vigorous activity for 20 minutes or more on 3 or more out of 7 days, national data are not available to assess whether children and adolescents meet the Federal recommendations to accumulate at least 60 minutes of moderate physical activity most days of the week. Many experts also believe that physical *inactivity* is an important part of the energy imbalance responsible for the increasing prevalence of overweight and obesity.

Our society has become very sedentary; for example, in 1999, 43 percent of students in grades 9 through 12 viewed television more than 2 hours per day.

. . . .

## MEASURING OVERWEIGHT AND OBESITY

The first challenge in addressing overweight and obesity lies in adopting a common public health measure of these conditions. An expert panel, convened by the National Institutes of Health (NIH) in 1998, has utilized Body Mass Index (BMI) for defining overweight and obesity. BMI is a practical measure that requires only two things: accurate measures of an individual's weight and height. BMI is a measure of weight in relation to height. BMI is calculated as weight in pounds divided by the square of the height in inches, multiplied by 703 [to adjust for comparisons to weights based on the metric system]. Alternatively, BMI can be calculated as weight in kilograms divided by the square of the height in meters.

Studies have shown that BMI is significantly correlated with total body fat content for the majority of individuals. BMI has some limitations, in that it can overestimate body fat in persons who are very muscular, and it can underestimate body fat in persons who have lost muscle mass, such as many elderly. Many organizations, including over 50 scientific and medical organizations . . . support the use of a BMI of 30 kg/m$^2$ . . . to identify overweight in adults. These definitions are based on evidence that suggests health risks are greater at or above a BMI of 25 kg/m$^2$ compared to those at a BMI below that level. The risk of death, although modest until a BMI of 30 kg/m$^2$ is reached, increases with an increasing Body Mass Index.

. . . .

In children and adolescents, overweight has been defined as a sex- and age-specific BMI at or above the 95th percentile, based on revised Centers for Disease Control and Prevention (CDC) growth charts. Neither a separate definition for obesity nor a definition for overweight based on health outcomes or risk factors is defined for children and adolescents.

. . . .

## HEALTH RISKS

Epidemiological studies show an increase in mortality associated with overweight and obesity. Individuals who are obese (BMI ≥ 30) have a 50 to 100 percent increase risk of premature death from all causes compared to individuals with a BMI in the range of 20 to 25. An estimated 300,000 deaths a year may be attributable to obesity.

Morbidity from obesity may be as great as from poverty, smoking, or problem drinking. Overweight and obesity are associated with an increased risk for coronary heart disease; type 2 diabetes; endometrial, colon, postmenopausal breast, and other cancers; and certain musculoskeletal disorders, such as knee osteoarthritis. Both modest and large weight gains are associated with significantly increased risk of disease. For example, a weight gain of 11 to 18 pounds increases a person's risk of developing type 2 diabetes to twice that of individuals who have not gained weight, while those who gain 44 pounds or more have four times the risk of type 2 diabetes.

A gain of approximately 10 to 20 pounds results in an increased risk of coronary heart disease (nonfatal myocardial infarction and death) of 1.25 times in women and 1.6 times in men. Higher levels of body weight gain of 22 pounds in men and 44 pounds in women result in an increased coronary heart disease risk of 1.75 and 2.65, respectively. In women with a BMI of 34 or greater, the risk of developing endometrial cancer is increased by more than six times. Overweight and obesity are also known to exacerbate many chronic conditions such as hypertension and elevated cholesterol. Overweight and obese individuals also may suffer from social stigmatization, discrimination, and poor body image.

Although obesity-associated morbidities occur most frequently in adults, important consequences of excess weight, as well as antecedents of adult disease, occur in overweight children and adolescents. Overweight children and adolescents are more likely to become overweight or obese adults; this concern is greatest among adolescents. Type 2 diabetes, high blood lipids, and hypertension, as well as early maturation and orthopedic problems also occur with increased frequency in overweight youth. A common consequence of childhood overweight is psychosocial — specifically discrimination.

These data on the morbidity and mortality associated with overweight and obesity demonstrate the importance of the prevention of weight gain, as well as the role of obesity treatment, in maintaining and improving health and quality of life.

. . . .

ECONOMIC CONSEQUENCES

Overweight and obesity and their associated health problems have substantial economic consequences for the U.S. health care system. The increasing prevalence of overweight and obesity is associated with both direct and indirect costs. . . .

In 1995, the total (direct and indirect) costs attributable to obesity amounted to an estimated $99 billion. In 2000, the total cost of obesity was estimated to be $117 billion ($61 billion direct and $56 billion indirect). Most of the cost associated with obesity is due to type 2 diabetes, coronary heart disease, and hypertension.

EPIDEMIOLOGY

The United States is experiencing substantial increases in overweight and obesity (as defined by a BMI ≥ 25 for adults) that cut across all ages, racial and ethnic groups, and both genders. According to self-reported measures of height and weight, obesity (BMI ≥ 30) has been increasing in every state in the nation. Based on clinical height and weight measurements in the 2000 National Health and Nutrition Examination Survey (NHANES), 34 percent of U.S. adults aged 20 to 74 years are overweight (BMI 25 to 29.9), and an additional 27 percent are obese (BMI ≥ 30). This contrasts with the late 1970s, when an estimated 32 percent of adults aged 20 to 74 years were overweight, and 15 percent were obese.

. . . .

The most recent data (1999) estimate that 13 percent of children aged 6 to 11 years and 14 percent of adolescents aged 12-19 years are overweight. During the past two decades, the percentage of children who are overweight has nearly doubled (from 7 to 13 percent), and the percentage of adolescents who are overweight has almost tripled (from 5 to 14 percent).

. . . .

## Disparities in Prevalence

. . . Disparities in overweight and obesity prevalence exist in many segments of the population based on race and ethnicity, gender, age, and socioeconomic status. For example, overweight and obesity are particularly common among minority groups and those with a lower family income.

. . . .

In general, the prevalence of overweight and obesity is higher in women who are members of racial and ethnic minority populations than in non-Hispanic white women. Among men, Mexican/Americans have a higher prevalence of overweight and obesity than non-Hispanic whites or non-Hispanic blacks. For non-Hispanic men, the prevalence of overweight and obesity among whites is slightly greater than among blacks.

Within racial groups, gender disparities exist, although not always in the same direction. . . .

. . . .

In addition to racial and ethnic and gender disparities, the prevalence of overweight and obesity also varies by age. Among both men and women, the prevalence of overweight and obesity increases with advancing age until the sixth decade, after which it starts to decline.

. . . .

Disparities in the prevalence of overweight and obesity also exist based on socioeconomic status. For all racial and ethnic groups combined, women of lower socioeconomic status (income ≤ 130 percent of poverty threshold) are approximately 50 percent more likely to be obese than those with higher socioeconomic status (income > 130 percent of poverty threshold). Men are about equally likely to be obese whether they are in a low or high socioeconomic group.

. . . .

HEALTH BENEFITS OF WEIGHT LOSS

The recommendations to treat overweight and obesity are based on two rationales. First, overweight and obesity are associated with an increased risk of disease and death, as previously discussed. Second, randomized controlled trials have shown that weight loss (as modest as 5 to 15 percent of excess total body weight) reduces the risk factors for at least some diseases, particularly cardiovascular disease, in the short term. Weight loss results in lower blood pressure, lower blood sugar, and improved lipid levels. While few published studies have examined the link between weight loss and reduced disease or death in the long-term, current data, as well as scientific plausibility suggest this link.

Studies have shown that reducing risk factors for heart disease, such as blood pressure and blood cholesterol levels, lowers death rates from heart disease and stroke. Therefore, it is highly probable that weight loss that reduces these risk factors will reduce the number of deaths from heart disease and stroke. Trials examining the direct effects of weight loss on disease and death are currently under way. . . . .

Families and communities lie at the foundation of the solution to the problems of overweight and obesity. Family members can share their own knowledge and habits regarding a health diet and physical activity with their children, friends and other community members. Emphasis should be placed on family and community opportunities for communication, education, and peer support surrounding the maintenance of healthy dietary choices and physical activity patterns.

. . . .

Schools are identified as a key setting for public health strategies to prevent and decrease the prevalence of overweight and obesity. Most children spend a large portion of time in school. Schools provide many opportunities to engage children in health eating and physical activity and to reinforce health diet and physical activity messages. Public health approaches in schools should extend beyond health and physical education to include school policy, the school physical and social environment, and links between schools and families and communities. Schools and communities that are interested in reducing overweight among the young people they serve can consider various options. Decisions about which options to select should be made at the local level.

. . . .

The health care system provides a powerful setting for intervention aimed at reducing the prevalence of overweight and obesity and their consequences. A majority of Americans interact with the health care system at least once during any given year. Recommendations by pediatric and adult health care providers can be influential in patient dietary choices and physical activity patterns. In collaboration with schools and worksites, health care providers and institutions can reinforce the adoption and maintenance of healthy lifestyle behaviors. Health care providers also can serve as effective public policy advocates and further catalyze intervention efforts in the family and community and in the media and communications settings.

. . . .

The media can provide essential functions in overweight and obesity prevention efforts. From a public education and social marketing standpoint, the media can disseminate health messages and display health behaviors aimed at changing dietary habits and exercise patterns. In addition, the media can provide a powerful forum for community members who are addressing the social and environmental influences on dietary and physical activity patterns.

. . . .

More than 100 million Americans spend the majority of their day at a worksite. While at work, employees are often aggregated within systems for communication, education and peer support. Thus, worksites provide many opportunities to reinforce the adoption and maintenance of healthy lifestyle behaviors. Public health approaches in worksites should extend beyond health education and awareness to include worksite policies, the physical and social environments of worksites, and their links with the family and community setting.

. . . .

[The report then discusses the separate but related roles of the individual, private organizations, and government in achieving progress against overweight and obesity.]

 . . . [T]he Surgeon General identifies the following activities as national priorities for immediate action. Individuals, families, communities, schools, worksites, health care, media, industry, organizations, and government must determine their role and take action to prevent and decrease overweight and obesity.

. . . .

The nation must take an informed, sensitive approach to communicate with and educate the American people about health issues related to overweight and obesity. Everyone must work together to:

— Change the perception of overweight and obesity at all ages. The primary concern should be one of health and not appearance.

— Educate all expectant parents about the many benefits of breastfeeding. Breastfed infants may be less likely to become overweight as they grow older. Mothers who breastfeed may return to pre-pregnancy weight more quickly.

— Educate health care providers and health profession students in the prevention and treatment of overweight and obesity across the lifespan.

— Provide culturally appropriate education in schools and communities about healthy eating habits and regular physical activity, based on the *Dietary Guidelines for Americans* [see appendix to this chapter], for people of all ages. Emphasize the consumer's role in making wise food and physical activity choices.

. . . .

The nation must take action to assist Americans in balancing healthful eating with regular physical activity. Individuals and groups across all settings must work in concert to:

— Ensure daily, quality physical education in all school grades. Such education can develop the knowledge, attitudes, skills, behaviors, and confidence needed to be physically active for life.

— Reduce time spent watching television and in other similar sedentary behaviors.

— Build physical activity into regular routines and playtime for children and their families. Ensure that adults get at least 30 minutes of moderate physical activity on most days of the week. Children should aim for at least 60 minutes.

— Create more opportunities for physical activity at worksites. Encourage all employers to make facilities and opportunities available for physical activity for all employees.

— Make community facilities available and accessible for physical activity for all people, including the elderly.

— Promote healthier food choices, including at least five servings of fruits and vegetables each day, and reasonable portion sizes at home, in schools, at worksites, and in communities.

— Ensure that schools provide healthful foods and beverages on school campuses and at school events by:

(1) Enforcing existing U.S. Department of Agriculture regulations that prohibit serving foods of minimal nutritional value during mealtimes in school food service areas, including in vending machines.

(2) Adopting policies specifying that all foods and beverages available at school contribute toward eating patterns that are consistent with the *Dietary Guidelines for Americans*.

(3) Providing more food options that are low in fat, calories, and added sugars such as fruits, vegetables, whole grains, and low-fat or nonfat dairy foods.

(4) Reducing access to foods high in fat, calories and added sugars and to excessive portion sizes.

(5) Create mechanisms for appropriate reimbursement of the prevention and treatment of overweight and obesity.

The nation must invest in research that improves our understanding of the causes, prevention, and treatment of overweight and obesity. A concerted effort should be made to:

— Increase research on behavioral and environmental causes of overweight and obesity.

— Increase research and evaluation on prevention and treatment interventions for overweight and obesity, and develop and disseminate best practice guidelines.

— Increase research on disparities in the prevalence of overweight and obesity among racial and ethnic, gender, socioeconomic, and age groups, and use this research to identify effective and culturally appropriate interventions.

\* \* \*

## UNITED NATIONS FOOD & AGRICULTURE ORGANIZATION/WORLD HEALTH ORGANIZATION, JOINT REPORT ON DIET, NUTRITION, AND THE PREVENTION OF CHRONIC DISEASES 61–71 (2003)

\* \* \*

Almost all countries (high-income and low-income alike) are experiencing an obesity epidemic, although with great variation between and within countries. In low-income countries, obesity is more common in middle-aged women, people of higher socioeconomic status and those living in urban communities. In more affluent countries, obesity is not only common in the middle-aged, but is becoming increasingly prevalent among younger adults and children. Furthermore, it tends to be associated with lower socioeconomic status, especially in women, and the urban-rural differences are diminished or even reversed.

It has been estimated that the direct costs of obesity accounted for 6.8 percent of total health care costs . . . in the United States in 1995. Although direct costs in other industrialized countries are slightly lower, they still consume a sizeable proportion of national health budgets. Indirect costs, which are far greater than direct costs, include work days lost, physician visits, disability pensions and premature mortality. Intangible costs such as impaired quality of life are also enormous. Because the risks of diabetes, cardiovascular disease and hypertension rise continuously with increasing weight, there is much overlap between the prevention of obesity and the prevention of a variety of chronic diseases, especially type 2 diabetes. . . .

The increasing industrialization, urbanization, and mechanization occurring in most countries around the world is associated with changes in diet and behavior; in particular, diets are becoming richer in high-fat, high energy foods and lifestyles more sedentary. In many developing countries undergoing economic transition, rising levels of obesity often co-exist in the same population (or even the same household) with chronic undernutrition. Increases in obesity over the past 30 years have been paralleled by a dramatic rise in the prevalence of diabetes.

Mortality rates increase with increasing degrees of overweight, as measured by BMI. As BMI increases, so too does the proportion of people with one or more comorbid conditions. . . . Eating behaviours that have been linked to overweight and obesity include snacking/eating frequency, binge-eating patterns, eating out, and (protectively) exclusive breastfeeding. Nutrient factors under investigation include fat, carbohydrate type (including refined carbohydrates such as sugar), the glycaemic index of foods, and fibre. Environmental issues are clearly important, especially as many environments become increasingly "obesogenic" (obesity-promoting).

Physical activity is an important determinant of body weight. In addition, physical activity and physical fitness (which relates to the ability to perform physical activity) are important modifiers of mortality and morbidity related to overweight and obesity. There is firm evidence that moderate to high fitness levels provide a substantially reduced risk of cardiovascular disease and all-cause mortality and that these benefits apply to all BMI levels. Furthermore, high fitness protects against mortality at all BMI levels in men with diabetes. Low cardiovascular fitness is a serious and common comorbidity of obesity, and a sizeable proportion of deaths in overweight and obese populations are probably a result of low levels of cardio-respiratory fitness rather than obesity per se. Fitness is, in turn, influenced strongly by physical activity in addition to genetic factors. These relationships emphasize the role of physical activity in the prevention of overweight and obesity, independently of the effects of physical activity on body weight.

. . . There is convincing evidence that regular physical activity is protective against unhealthy weight gain whereas sedentary lifestyles, particularly sedentary occupations and inactive recreation such as watching television, promote it. Most epidemiological studies show smaller risk of weight gain, overweight, and obesity among persons who currently engage regularly in moderate to large amounts of physical activity. Studies measuring physical activity at baseline and randomized trials of exercise programmes show more mixed results, probably because of the low adherence to long-term changes. Therefore, it is ongoing physical activity itself rather than previous physical activity or enrollment in an exercise programme that is protective against unhealthy weight gain. The recommendation for individuals to accumulate at least 30 minutes of moderate-intensity physical activity on most days is largely aimed at reducing cardiovascular diseases and overall mortality. The amount needed to prevent unhealthy weight gain is uncertain but is probably significantly greater than this. Preventing weight gain after substantial weight loss probably requires about 60-90 minutes per day. . . . Studies aimed at reducing sedentary behaviours have focused primarily on reducing television viewing in children. Reducing viewing times by about 30 minutes a day in children in the United States appears feasible and is associated with reductions in BMI.

. . . .

. . . [T]wo recent reviews of randomized trials have concluded that the majority of studies show that a high intake of NSP (dietary fibre) promotes weight loss. Pereira & Ludwig found that 12 out of 19 trials showed beneficial objective effects (including weight loss). In their review of 11 studies . . . Howarth Saltzman & Roberts reported a mean weight loss of 1.9 kg over 3.8 months. There were no differences between fibre type or between fibre consumed in food or as supplements.

There is convincing evidence that a high intake of energy-dense foods promotes weight gain. In high-income countries (and increasingly in low income countries) these energy-dense foods are not only highly processed (low NSP) but also micronutrient-poor, further diminishing their nutritional value. Energy-dense foods tend to be high in fat (*e.g.*, butter, oils, fried foods), sugars, or starch, while energy-dilute foods have a high water content (*e.g.*, fruits and vegetables). . . . While energy from fat is no more fattening than the same amount of energy from carbohydrate or protein, diets that are high in fat tend to be energy-dense. An important exception to this is diets based predominantly on energy-dilute foods (*e.g.*, vegetables, legumes, fruits) but which have a reasonably high percentage of energy as fat from added oils.

The effectiveness over the long term of most dietary strategies for weight loss, including low-fat diets, remains uncertain unless accompanied by changes in behaviour affecting physical activity and food habits. These latter changes at a public health level require an environment supportive of healthy food choices and an active life. . . . A variety of popular weight-loss diets that restrict food choices may result in reduced energy intake and short term weight loss in individuals but most do not have trial evidence of long-term effectiveness and nutritional adequacy and therefore cannot be recommended for populations.

Despite the obvious importance of the roles that parents and home environments play on children's eating and physical activity behaviours, there is very little hard evidence available to support this view. It appears that access and exposure to a range of fruits and vegetables in the home is important for the development of preferences for these foods and that parental knowledge, attitudes, and behaviours related to healthy diet and physical activity are important in creating role models. More data are available on the impact of the school environment on nutrition knowledge, on eating patterns and physical activity at school, and on sedentary behaviours at home. Some studies, but not all, have shown an effect of school-based interventions on obesity prevention. . . .

Part of the consistent, strong relationships between television viewing and obesity in children may relate to the food advertising to which they are exposed. Fast food restaurants and foods and beverages that are usually classified under the "eat least" category in dietary guidelines are among the most heavily marketed products, especially on television. Young children are often the target group for the advertising of these products because they have a significant influence on the foods bought by parents. The huge expenditure on marketing fast-foods and other "eat least" choices was considered to be a key factor in the increased consumption of food prepared outside the home in general and of energy-dense, micronutrient-poor foods in particular. Young children are unable to distinguish programme content from the persuasive intent of advertisements. The evidence that the heavy marketing of these foods and beverages to young children causes obesity is not unequivocal. . . . [T]here is sufficient indirect evidence to warrant this practice being placed in the "probable" category and thus becoming a potential target for interventions.

Diets that are proportionally low in fat will be proportionally higher in carbohydrate (including a variable amount of sugars) and are associated with protection against unhealthy weight gain, although a high intake of free sugars in beverages probably promotes weight gain. The physiological effects of energy intake on satiation and satiety appear to be quite different for energy in solid foods as opposed to energy in fluids. Possibly because of reduced gastric distension and faster transit times, the energy contained in fluids is less well "detected" by the body and subsequent food intake is poorly adjusted to account for the energy taken in through beverages. . . . The high and increasing consumption of sugars-sweetened drinks by children in many countries is of serious concern. It has been estimated that each additional can or glass of sugars-sweetened drink that they consume every day increases the risk of becoming obese by 60 percent. Most of the evidence relates to soda drinks but many fruit drinks and cordials are equally energy-dense and may promote weight gain if drunk in large quantities. Overall, the evidence implicating a high intake of sugars-sweetened drinks in promoting weight gain was considered moderately strong.

Classically the pattern of the progression of obesity through a population starts with middle-aged women in high-income groups but as the epidemic progresses, obesity becomes more common in people (especially women) in lower socioeconomic status groups. The relationship may even be bi-directional, setting up a vicious cycle (*i.e.*, lower socioeconomic status promotes obesity, and obese people are more likely to end up in groups with low socioeconomic status). The mechanisms by which socioeconomic status influences food and activity patterns are probably multiple and need elucidation. However, people living in circumstances of low socioeconomic status may be more at the mercy of the obesogenic environment because their eating and activity behaviours are more likely to be the "default choices" on offer. The evidence for an effect of low socioeconomic status on predisposing people to obesity is consistent (in higher income countries) across a number of cross-sectional and longitudinal studies, and was thus rated as a "probable" cause of increased risk of obesity.

Breastfeeding as a protective factor against weight gain has been examined in at least 20 studies involving nearly 40,000 subjects. . . . There are probably multiple effects of confounding in these studies; however, the reduction in the risk of developing obesity observed in the two largest studies was substantial. Promoting breastfeeding has many benefits, the prevention of childhood obesity probably being one of them.

. . . Large portion sizes are a possible causative factor for unhealthy weight gain. The marketing of "supersize" portions, particularly in fastfood outlets, is now common practice in many countries. There is some evidence that people poorly estimate portion sizes and that subsequent energy compensation for a large meal is incomplete and therefore is likely to lead to overconsumption.

In many countries, there has been a steady increase in the proportion of food eaten that is prepared outside the home. In the United States, the energy, total fat, saturated fat, cholesterol and sodium content of foods prepared outside the home is significantly higher than that of home prepared food. People in the United States who tend to eat in restaurants have a higher BMI than those who tend to eat at home.

Certain psychological parameters of eating patterns may influence the risk of obesity. The "flexible restraint" pattern is associated with lower risk of weight gain, whereas the "rigid restraint/periodic disinhibition" pattern is associated with a higher risk.

. . . Studies have not shown consistent associations between alcohol intake and obesity despite the high energy density of the nutrient. . . .

. . . While a high eating frequency has been shown in some studies to have a negative relationship with energy intake and weight gain, the types of foods readily available as snack foods are often high in fat and a high consumption of foods of this type might predispose people to weight gain. The evidence regarding the impact of early nutrition on subsequent obesity is also mixed, with some studies showing relationships for high and low birth weights.

The prevention of obesity in infants and young children should be considered of high priority. For infants and young children, the main preventive strategies are:

— the promotion of exclusive breastfeeding;

— avoiding the use of added sugars and starches when feeding formula;

— instructing mothers to accept their child's ability to regulate energy intake rather than feeding until the plate is empty;

— assuring the appropriate micronutrient intake needed to promote optimal linear growth.

For children and adolescents, prevention of obesity implies the need to:

— promote an active lifestyle;

— limit television viewing;

— promote the intake of fruits and vegetables;

— restrict the intake of energy-dense, micronutrient-poor foods (*e.g.* packaged snacks);

— restrict the intake of sugars-sweetened soft drinks.

Additional measures include modifying the environment to enhance physical activity in schools and communities, creating more opportunities for family interaction (*e.g.,* eating family meals), limiting the exposure of young children to heavy marketing practices of energy-dense, micronutrient-poor foods, and providing the necessary information and skills to make healthy food choices.

In developing countries, special attention should be given to avoidance of overfeeding stunted population groups. Nutrition programmes designed to control or prevent undernutrition need to assess stature in combination with weight to prevent providing excess energy to children of low weight-for-age but normal weight-for-height. In countries in economic transition, as populations become more sedentary and able to access energy-dense foods, there is a need to maintain the healthy components of traditional diets (*e.g.,* high intake of vegetables, fruits and NSP). Education provided to mothers and low socioeconomic status communities that are food insecure should stress that overweight and obesity do not represent good health.

Low-income groups globally and populations in countries in economic transition often replace traditional micronutrient-rich foods by heavily marketed, sugars-sweetened beverages (*i.e.*, soft drinks) and energy-dense, fatty, salty, and sugary foods. These trends, coupled with reduced physical activity, are associated with the rising prevalence of obesity. Strategies are needed to improve the quality of diets by increasing consumption of fruits and vegetables, in addition to increasing physical activity, in order to stem the epidemic of obesity and associated diseases.

[The report then discusses the use of BWI as a crude but useful means to measure the prevalence of obesity but notes the need to adjust the standard for different cultures and body-types.]

A total of one hour per day of moderate-intensity activity, such as walking on most days of the week, is probably needed to maintain a healthy body weight, particularly for people with sedentary occupations.

The fat and water content of foods are the main determinants of the energy density of the diet. A lower consumption of energy-dense (*i.e.*, high-fat, high-sugars, and high-starch) foods and energy-dense (*i.e.*, high free sugars) drinks contributes to a reduction in total energy intake. Conversely, a higher intake of energy-dilute foods (*i.e.*, vegetables and fruits) and foods high in NSP contributes to a reduction in total energy intake and an improvement in micronutrient intake. It should be noted, however, that very active groups who have diets high in vegetables, legumes, fruits and wholegrain cereals, may sustain a total fat intake of up to 35 percent without the risk of unhealthy weight gain.

\* \* \*

## PROBLEM: SO HOW DO WE KNOW WHAT IS GOOD TO EAT?

Everyone seems to agree that something must be done about the growing problem of obesity and, in the broader sense, what needs to be done is pretty simple: People should exercise more and eat less. In more specific terms, however, just what is and what is not healthy behavior can be harder to discern; in fact, some of things that we *think* are better for us may not be so clearly beneficial.

A good recent illustration involves the beneficial effects of a low-fat diet. For decades, physicians, dieticians, and even self-help manuals have repeated the orthodoxy that reducing the amount of fat consumed would improve health, avoid illness, and control weight gain. But a large, carefully controlled study completed in 2005 has offered a somewhat different set of conclusions. As set out in the introductory summaries to three articles in JAMA, the journal of the American Medical Association, the study found:

Among postmenopausal women, a low-fat dietary pattern did not result in a statistically significant reduction in invasive breast cancer risk over an 8.1 year average follow-up period. . . .

. . . [A] dietary intervention that reduced total fat and increased intakes of vegetables, fruits, and grains did not significantly reduce the risk of [coronary heart disease or] stroke in postmenopausal women . . . .

. . . [A] low-fat dietary pattern intervention did not reduce the risk of colorectal cancer in postmenopausal women during 8.1 years of follow-up.

[These quotes can be found in full text in the prefatory materials to the JAMA articles cited below.]

These results perplexed, perhaps even embarrassed, a number of public health experts who had long endorsed the belief that low-fat diets were better and healthier. Little could be said about the quality of the study: The researchers had followed nearly 50,000 women over the course of eight years, carefully dividing them between a group that maintained the prescribed diet and a control group that had no measurable change in their pre-study eating habits. There were some ways to qualify the results: The study only included women between the ages of 50 and 79 years. Only their diets were changed and monitored; activity levels, for examples, were not measured or controlled. Moreover, the authors of the study identified several possible sub-grouping within their study populations which appeared to have better results than the low-fat group taken as a whole, *e.g.*, women who had a higher BMI to begin with seemed to benefit more from the low-fat diets than those with lower MBI to begin with (although not in statistically measurable ways).

The surprising results were quickly picked up by the mass media, usually under headlines of the type "Fat Not As Bad As Believed" or "Low-Fat Overrated!" There also was some criticism of the presentation of the results in JAMA as the authors of the study seemed eager — almost to the point of losing their scientific discipline — to put a positive (and pro low-fat) spin on their results. The whole point, after all, of such a carefully controlled testing of a scientific hypothesis, even one that is generally accepted, is to produce quantifiable results that speak for themselves. In theory, a hypothesis that is not proven is as useful as one that is confirmed, even if that is not what the authors or anyone else had hoped the data would confirm.

This aberrational outcome is only one part of a large problem and an unusual one at that. More often the problem is interpreting the data — whether it is positive or negative or equivocal — in terms that the public can understand and put to use but not overrate. Just what a study proves or disproves involves an understanding of what a study is: an attempt to isolate one variable that may or may not have a causal connection to some outcome. Even a study with 50,000 people is just a sample. Whether it can be generalized or not is a tougher call (and depends on how representative the sample is, whether it is large enough to have statistical power, and the statistical methods used to calculate results). Even if it can be generalized, it might prove far less than most Americans and the media they rely on would like to believe. And even the best designed and controlled study can only attempt to isolate other influences well enough to assess the influence of one factor. No single study can account for all the complex influences on human behavior.

The best answer is the one most Americans are not fully prepared for: If you want to know what a study says or does not say, you should read the study in full text, apply some basic principles of statistical design, analysis, and logic, and evaluate conclusions in light of other relevant studies, just as you should do with a judicial opinion.

The text of the low-fat studies described above can be found at Ross L. Prentiss et al., *Low Fat Dietary Pattern and Risk of Invasive Breast Cancer*, 295 JAMA 629 (2005); Shirley A.A. Beresford et al., *Low-Fat Dietary Pattern and Risk of Colorectal Cancer*, 295 JAMA 643 (2005); Barbara V. Howard, *Low-Fat Dietary Pattern and Risk of Cardiovascular Disease*, 295 JAMA 655 (2005).

## KELLY BROWNELL & KATHERINE BATTLE HORGEN, FOOD FIGHT
### 3–13 (2004)

\* \* \*

It came quickly, with little fanfare, and was out of control before the nation noticed. Obesity, diabetes, and other diseases caused by poor diet and sedentary lifestyle now affect the health, happiness, and vitality of millions of men, women, and, most tragically, children and pose a major threat to the health care resources of the United States. Most alarming has been the national inaction in the face of crisis, the near-total surrender to a powerful food industry, and the lack of innovation in preventing further havoc.

The Centers for Disease Control and Prevention (CDC) labels the obesity problem an "epidemic." Within the United States, 64.5 percent of Americans are either overweight or obese, with the number growing. For many reasons, some obvious and some not, the increase in overweight children is twice that seen in adults.

Other nations are in hot pursuit. Country after country follows the American lead and grows heavier. Over consumption has replaced malnutrition as the world's top food problem. From Banff to Buenos Aires, from Siberia to the Sahara, the world need only look to America to see its future. There are now clinics for obese children in Beijing.

Similar to a new virus without natural enemies, our lifestyle of abundant food and inactivity faces little opposition. Quite the contrary, powerful forces push it forward, spreading the problem to all segments of the population. These forces are woven so tightly into our social systems (economics, health care system, even education) that change seems almost beyond imagination. Despite talk of an obesity crisis, government reports, and Presidents pushing exercise, obesity is increasing in all races, ages, income groups, and areas of the world.

. . . .

The picture with children is sad. Projecting ahead to their adult years, today's children are targeted in a relentless way by the food companies. Institutions such as schools that would like to protect children instead must sell soft drinks and snack foods to function.

. . . .

It is easy to blame parents, but they face off every day with an environment that grabs their children and won't let go. Children and the parents who raise them do not get what they deserve — conditions that support healthy eating and physical activity. The environment wins in most cases, and we have an epidemic to show for it.

By any definition, we face an emergency.

The reasons for this growing problem are simple and complex at the same time. People eat too much and exercise too little, but this easy truth masks a fascinating dance of genetics with modern lifestyle. Economics, breakthroughs in technology, how our nation thinks about food, and, of course, the powerful and sophisticated food industry, are all actors in this tragic play. Our environment is textured with risk. It intersects with genes in a way that makes an obese population a predictable consequence of modern life.

Some individuals have the biological fortune or the skills to resist this risk, leading to arguments that weight control is a matter of personal responsibility. Choices people make are important, but the nation has played the will power and restraint cards for years and finds itself trumped again and again by an environment that overwhelms the resources of most people.

The cost of inaction will multiply human suffering, place our nation at a strategic disadvantage, and have a massive impact on health care costs.

. . . .

Picture yourself a child, rather a zygote. Your father's sperm penetrates your mother's egg, unleashing a cascade of biological events. What you will eat later in life, your upper and lower limits for body weight, and how your physiology responds to being sedentary have been partially fixed.

The lives of your ancestors, dating back many thousands of years, reside in your genes. Unpredictable food supplies and looming starvation were their everyday realities. Those who adapted ate voraciously when food appeared, stored energy (as body fat) with extreme efficiency, survived later scarcity, and contributed to the gene pool from which you draw your DNA.

Married to this food biology are genes related to physical activity. Extreme exertion was once required to hunt and gather food. The body functioned optimally with bouts of heavy activity punctuated by periods of rest needed to conserve energy. Modern culture has removed strenuous exercise.

You are an exquisitely efficient calorie conservation machine. Your genes match nicely with a scarce food supply, but not with modern living conditions.

As a child, you are about to be broadsided by a "toxic" environment. Your body is unprepared for the plummeting need to be physically active and cannot anticipate the impending confrontation with Big — Big Gulp, Big Grab, Big Mac, Biggie Fries, Big everything.

If you could speak with your ancient ancestors, they would explain that people eat a lot when food is abundant, particularly foods high in fat, sugar, and calories, a fact proven by scientists thousands of years later. These foods provide quick energy but more important, are optimal for storing energy.

As you breathe for the first time outside the womb, your genes are mismatched with modern conditions. The environment is distorted beyond your body's ability to cope. It will pound you with inducements to eat, make exertion unnecessary, and do little to defend you against diseases that most threaten you.

Good fortune may bring you parents who are committed to healthy eating. They keep junk food out of the home, have healthy foods available, and teach you good nutrition. But then you go to play groups, birthday parties, and school. You see billboards, watch TV, go to movies, and travel the supermarket aisles where your favorite Disney and Nickelodeon characters are linked with sugared cereals, snack foods, and ice cream. Your parents now face Goliath.

. . . .

Biology comes undone when confronted by modern eating and exercise conditions, what we call the toxic environment. *Toxic* is a powerful word, but powerful language is needed to describe the situation. . . .

. . . .

The second half of the energy equation, physical activity, has also been affected in disastrous ways. Few children walk or bike to school; there is little physical education; computers, video games, and televisions keep children inside and inactive; and parents are reluctant to let children roam free to play.

The American landscape has been altered in profound ways. Cheeseburgers and French fries, drive-in windows and super sizes, soft drinks and candy, potato chips and cheese curls, once unusual, are as much our background as trees, grass, and clouds. We now take notice when food isn't there. Gas stations *without* a mini-market look old-fashioned and unappealing.

. . . .

The world of fast food is only one of many changing influences but may be the most dramatic. In his book *Fast Food Nation*, Eric Schlosser notes that American spending on fast food went from $6 billion to $110 billion annually in the last 30 years. . . .

. . . .

Food, not just fast food, is everywhere. Think of the modern drugstore. The items you need, like pain relievers, bandages, cough remedies, and vitamins, not to mention the pharmacy, are in the rear of the store, requiring you to pass through aisles of items you did not intend to buy. Many people gravitate naturally to the center aisles, home to a large collection of candies and foods. When you leave the pharmacy and walk back along the far aisle, notice what you encounter.

Children are valuable consumers, affecting billions of dollars in sales each year. Food marketing directed at children, almost exclusively for unhealthy foods, is as sophisticated as marketing gets. There are books, advertising journals, and conferences describing how to best market to children. It is no surprise that we have a nation of children consuming record amounts of sugar, soft drinks, fast foods, and snack foods.

. . . .

Accessibility of bad food is coupled with a key economic reality: unhealthy food is cheap. It is also convenient, fast, packaged attractively, and tasty. Healthy foods are more difficult to get, less convenient, and more expensive. If you came from Mars and knew nothing but this about a country, an epidemic of obesity is exactly what you'd predict.

This confluence of declining physical activity and in altered eating environment, both in toxic proportions, has created a human crisis.

. . . .

Food is big, but so are the companies making and selling it. Massive agribusiness companies control a surprising amount of the food chain, raising grave concerns with issues such as dwindling genetic diversity in plants and farm animals, resistant strains of bacteria resulting from the overuse of antibiotics, and undue influence on the nation's nutrition and agriculture policy.

. . . .

A consequence of this consolidation is that enormous power and influence rest in the hands of a few companies. Their presence in Washington, D.C., is visible and felt in many ways, some more obvious than others. What crops get subsidized, which commodities get shipped to schools through the National School Lunch Program, what foods get emphasized in the food guide pyramid, and whether soft drinks are permitted in schools are a few places where political influence can affect the national nutrition environment. There are many, many cases where business interests conflict with public health. People deserve to know how and when this occurs and the impact it has on them and their children.

. . . .

The word *big* applied to the food industry conjures up images of Big Oil, Big Energy, Big Tobacco, and so on. The public image of such industries is that a small number of giant companies led by ruthless executives control an entire industry and manipulate the political system, finances, and public opinion in self-serving ways that damage the public's interests. You may draw your own conclusions about whether the food industry deserves this label.

. . . .

Changing the environment is the obvious place to begin. The deteriorating environment is the clear cause of the obesity epidemic and must be the basis for its remedy. Attacking a problem by considering its causes is logical and leads squarely to a public health imperative — prevention.

Prevention is appealing for several reasons:

1. With obesity the nation's most common major chronic health problem, vast numbers of people could benefit.

2. Children are the logical focus when a disease begins early in life. Food preferences, eating habits, and, possibly, brand loyalties take shape in childhood, so the best opportunity for creating healthy habits may exist in the early years.

3. Obesity is very difficult to treat, and most people who lose weight do not keep it off. The most optimistic estimates are that 25 percent of people lose weight and maintain the loss, often requiring many tries. This lack of success combines with the very high cost of treatment to make most approaches cost-ineffective. We will never treat this problem away.

4. The nation has a long history of supporting prevention to protect its children. Child safety seats, childproof medicine bottles, warnings on toys that are choking hazards, immunization requirements, and the prohibition of tobacco sales to children are examples. Such programs show good return on investment. Improving diet and physical activity and preventing obesity rival any of these programs in importance to public health.

\* \* \*

# NOTES AND QUESTIONS

**1.** Americans have an obsession with weight. The prevalence of anorexia and bulimia has appeared to increase over time. The desire to be supermodel thin is common among teenage girls. At the same time the numbers of people who are overweight and obese also appear to have increased. Just how large that increase is and its impact on public health is less clear. The problem of obesity in the United States is qualitatively different from the problems described in previous chapters. To refer to obesity as a public health problem blurs some key distinctions and makes some causal leaps. In one sense, obesity is a public health problem because it affects the health of a large proportion of the public. On the other hand, it is not a public health threat like an epidemic of avian influenza. Obesity is neither a disease nor the result of one — at least as far as we know now. (There are some endocrine abnormalities that promote weight gain. And there is some preliminary research suggesting that mice gain weight when injected with certain viruses or microbes in the stomach and intestinal tract.) Obesity is not transmitted from person to person, or, more critically, something that directly causes harm to anyone other the individual who is labeled "obese."

And it is a label. Physicians and public health professionals use standards based on BMI to determine what counts as overweight and obese, but ultimately these are rather subjective judgments. As a result, the causes of obesity, the resulting health and economic consequences, and the possible remedial solutions are difficult even to discuss, let alone verify and assess.

Having said all that, one thing is clear: There is something happening to people in the United States and, apparently, elsewhere, that has to do with the way they live and eat and the net impact on their health. Lots of us are, to use an interesting expression, "out of shape." And while even a moment's reflection will make it clear that the body's "shape" is not a public health problem, what we all know at some level is that our "shape" is a fairly clear and visible indicator of some things that are surely problematic; moreover, if, as most observers believe, there are more and more bodies "out of shape," those problems are increasing.

**2.** According to the Surgeon General's report summarized in this section — and a host of other public health experts — lack of "shape" or, to use the term most often used in public discussions of the problem, obesity is a problem of epidemic proportions in the United States. The prevalence of obesity has increased substantially in the United States over the last two decades and appears to be increasing. In 2000, over 30 percent of American adults were described as obese (BMI index greater than 30), nearly 60 million people. As recounted by the Surgeon General, this condition is associated with higher rates of heart disease, diabetes, and a number of other medical conditions, and has resulted in nearly 300,000 premature deaths.

Obesity is a concept that is being continually redefined. In humans, the most common statistical measurement of obesity is the body mass index (BMI):

> A person with a BMI over 25.0 kg/m$^2$ is considered overweight; a BMI over 30.0 kg/m$^2$ is considered obese. A further threshold at 40.0 kg/m$^2$ is identified as urgent morbidity risk. The American Institute for Cancer Research considers a BMI between 18.5 and 25 to be an ideal target for a healthy individual (although several sources consider a person with a BMI of less than 20 to be underweight). The BMI was created in the 19th century by the Belgian statistician Adolphe Quetelet. The cut-off points between categories are occasionally redefined, and may differ from country to country. In June 1998 the NIH brought official US category definitions into line with those used by the WHO, moving the American 'overweight' threshold from BMI 27 to BMI 25. About 30,000,000 Americans moved from "ideal" weight to being 1-10 pounds "overweight" as a result.

http://encyclopedia.laborlawtalk.com/Obesity (last visited December 2006).

Some experts have even projected that the rising rates of obesity in the United States will eventually result in a reduction in *average life expectancy* in the United States. S. Jay Olshansky et al., *A Potential Decline in Life Expectancy in the United States*, 352 NEW ENG. J. MED. 1138 (2005).

Converting those human cost figures into dollar costs, the CDC has estimated that the medical costs of treating obesity-related illnesses were nearly

$100 billion in 2004, rivaling the costs associated with smoking. Nearly half of these costs were paid by Medicare and Medicaid.

For a more recent analysis of the obesity problem that reaffirms the conclusions of the Surgeon General's 2001 report, see the INSTITUTE OF MEDICINE, THE FUTURE OF THE PUBLIC'S HEALTH IN THE 21ST CENTURY (2003) at 76-83. For a more academic assessment of the data, see Ali H. Mokdad, et al., *The Spread of the Obesity Epidemic in the United States 1991-1998*, 282 JAMA 1519 (1999).

For more detailed or more recent data on the distribution of obesity among Americans, see www.cdc.gov/nccdphp/dnpa/obesity/ (last visited December 2006); www.surgeongeneral.gov/topics/obesity (last visited December 2006); www.cdc.gov/nchs/ (last visited December 2006).

For sources of information on a state-by-state basis, see www.cdc.gov/washington/overview/obesity.html (last visited December 2006); www.cdc.gov/nccdphp/dnpa/obesity/state_programs (last visited December 2006).

For an assessment of some of the efforts by each state to combat obesity, see the "Obesity Report Cards" found at www.ubalt.edu/experts/obesity (last visited December 2006).

**3.** The trends concerning obesity among American children are even more disturbing. According to a review of the literature by the IOM:

> Trends in childhood and youth obesity mirror a similar profound increase over the same approximate period in U.S. adults as well as a concurrent rise internationally, in both developed and developing countries. The obesity epidemic affects both boys and girls and has occurred in all age, race, and ethic groups throughout the United States. In addition to the increase in obesity prevalence, the heaviest group of children is getting heavier whereas the leanest group of children is staying lean. What this means is that among younger age groups of children 6 to 11 years of age and, to a lesser extent, adolescents the lowest part of the BWI distribution appears to have changed little over time.

INSTITUTE OF MEDICINE, CHILDHOOD OBESITY IN THE UNITED STATES: FACTS AND FIGURES (September 2004). For more details and a further specification of these "facts and figures," see INSTITUTE OF MEDICINE, PREVENTING CHILDHOOD OBESITY: HEALTH IN THE BALANCE (2004) (both documents can be found at www.iom.edu/ (last visited December 2006).

**4.** As reflected by the executive summary of the WHO/FAO report, the problem of obesity is hardly confined to the United States. Americans may be getting bigger and fatter, but the rest of the world is not far behind — and apparently for many of the same reasons. For the full WHO/FAO report, see www.who.int/dietphysicalactivity/publications (last visited December 2006).

For a more detailed analysis of obesity among children in other countries (and some suggestions about what should be done about it), see Cara B.

Ebbeling et al., *Childhood Obesity: Public Health Crisis, Common Sense Cure,* 360 LANCET 473 (2002).

**5.** Because of the nature of the problem — *i.e.,* obesity itself is not a disease but rather associated with many diseases and adverse effects on health — the actual costs of obesity are hard to quantify; nonetheless, the overall picture is fairly straightforward. For some good efforts to summarize and assess the effects of obesity, see, Aviva Must et al., *The Disease Burden Associated With Overweight and Obesity,* 282 JAMA 1623 (1999); David B. Allison et al., *Annual Deaths Attributable to Obesity in the United States,* 282 JAMA 1530 (1999); A.M. Wolf & Graham A. Colditz, *Current Estimates of the Economic Costs of Obesity in the United States,* 6 OBESITY RESEARCH 97 (1998); Kenneth F. Adams et al., *Overweight, Obesity, and Mortality in a Large Prospective Cohort of Persons 50 to 71 Years Old,* 355 NEW ENG. J. MED. 763–78, 773 (2006); Abel Romero-Corral et al., *Association of Bodyweight with Total Mortality and with Cardiovascular Events in Coronary Artery Disease: A Systematic Review of Cohort Studies,* 368 LANCET 666–78 (2006).

Proving how increased weight leads to bad outcomes is difficult and has produced some conflicting results. In less than a year U.S. government agencies reported that obesity caused 414,000 deaths, 280,000 deaths, and 112,000 deaths. *See* David H. Mark, *Deaths Attributable to Obesity,* 293 JAMA 1918 (2005); Edward W. Gregg et al., *Secular Trends in Cardiovascular Disease Risk Factors According to Body Mass Index in US Adults,* 293 JAMA 1868–1874 (July 14, 2005). Underweight is also associated with a higher risk of death. Katherine M. Flegal et al., *Excess Deaths Associated With Underweight, Overweight, and Obesity,* 293 JAMA 1861 (2005).

**6.** Not everyone, however, is convinced that obesity is as problematic as the data cited above seem to suggest. IN THE OBESITY MYTH: WHY AMERICA'S OBSESSION WITH WEIGHT IS HAZARDOUS TO YOUR HEALTH (2004), Paul Campos argues that the health hazards of obesity have been overstated or, at least, not convincingly proven. For example:

> . . . [H]ere are some figures from what — at the time it was compiled — was the world's largest epidemiological study to date. This study, conducted in Norway in the mid-1980s, followed 118 million people for ten years. Consider the following data in light of the government's and the medical establishment's claims that a BMI of 18.5 to 24.9 is optimal and that people with BMI figures of 25 and above are running major health risks. The highest life expectancy (79.7 years) was found among people with BMI figures between 26 and 28. . . . The lowest life expectancy (74.2 years) was found among those with BMI figures below 18 (A woman of average height who is 5 pounds below what the government claims to be her "optimal" BMI will fall into that category). Those with BMI figures between 18 and 20 . . . had a lower life expectancy than those with BMI figures between 34 and 36. . . .

Campos at 10.

Whether Campos' assessment is correct, it is clear that we know far less about the health effects of obesity than we do about most disease-related health problems or even about the health effects of tobacco use. There is a growing body of empirical research finding an association between obesity and a number of medical conditions, but determining whether there is a direct causal relationship between obesity and illness — or vice versa — is a more complicated epidemiological problem. We also don't know very much about some important practical questions, questions that will have to be answered in order to shape effective, remedial solutions. In this regard, consider the following:

a. The data concerning morbidity and mortality are most convincing for people who are "very obese". The data assessing a connection between "slightly obese" people and risk of death or illness is practically nonexistent. (There are even some studies, as Campos points out, that suggest that slightly "obese people" live longer, healthier lives.) Contrast smoking: There seems to be a direct one-to-one correlation between each increment of increased exposure to tobacco smoke and an incremental increase in risk of death or illness. Perhaps obesity is only a health risk beyond some threshold (*e.g.*, BMI 30).

b. Smokers who quit can actually improve their health and lower their risk of illness and death. They may not be as healthy as non-smokers, but the sooner a smoker stops smoking, the better. Is the same true for obesity? Is a former obese person healthier than a current one — but less healthy than someone who has avoided the problem throughout their lifetime? What about people who gain and lose weight cyclically? Is it "worth it" to lose weight? Again, are the answers different for "very obese" or "slightly obese" people?

c. What is the relationship between obesity and good nutrition? Is it more important to eat the right foods or to maintain caloric intake/exercise levels in proper balance? For that matter, what are the right foods and what happens if you only eat healthy foods some of the time — or some healthy foods all of the time?

Note how the answers to these questions may bear on the questions of food labeling, advertising limits, and potential liability for fast food and other, allegedly hazardous food products.

**7.** The discussion of possible remedial solutions in the Surgeon General's report and, to a lesser extent, the WHO/FAO report follows the same pattern later adopted in the IOM report discussed in Chapter One: They envision a grand, cooperative partnership of everyone involved — government, business, food producers, schools, etc. — that would work together to solve the problem. There is little realistic discussion of the role that some of these actors play in producing the problem in the first place. Nor is there any realistic game plan for what should happen if this fanciful coalition does not join hands in cooperation.

The excerpt from Brownell and Horgen, on the other hand, focuses on these more controversial aspects of the problem. As Brownell and Horgen argue, Americans don't just eat too much and exercise too little because many of them are stupid. They do so, in part, because of the social and economic environment in which they live. And at least part of that environment has been structured by the entities that directly profit from Americans' bad eating habits. Moreover, since these entities profit from that environment, they will resist any changes in that environment, whatever the merits of the public health-based justifications for doing so. Thus advocacy of "grand cooperative effort" to fight obesity is at least naïve — if not politically disingenuous.

Brownell and Horgen are hardly alone in their more realistic analysis of the problem. For other interesting works with similar political messages, see ERIC SCHLOSSER, FAST FOOD NATION (2002) (particularly the chapter on the safety of meat generally and, in particular, that used to prepare fast food); DAVID G. HOGAN, SELLING 'EM BY THE SACK (1998) (the history of White Castle hamburgers and their pioneering of various means for increasing consumption of fast food); MARION NESTLE, FOOD POLITICS: HOW THE FOOD INDUSTRY INFLUENCES NUTRITION AND HEALTH (2002).

For a useful source of current information on nutrition politics and related matters, see www.cspinet.org/ (the website of the Nutrition Action Newsletter) (last visited December 2006). *See also* www.phaionline.org/ (the website of the Public Health Advocacy Institute) (last visited December 2006).

## PELMAN v. McDONALD'S
### 237 F. Supp. 2d 512 (S.D.N.Y. 2003) ("Pelman I")

Sweet, Judge.

\* \* \*

This action presents unique and challenging issues. The plaintiffs have alleged that the practices of McDonalds in making and selling their products are deceptive and that this deception has caused the minors who have consumed McDonalds' products to injure their health by becoming obese. Questions of personal responsibility, common knowledge, and public health are presented, and the role of society and the courts in addressing such issues.

The issue of determining the breadth of personal responsibility underlies much of the law: Where should the line be drawn between an individual's own responsibility to take care of herself, and society's responsibility to ensure that others shield her? Laws are created in those situations where individuals are somehow unable to protect themselves and where society needs to provide a buffer between the individual and some other entity — whether herself, another individual, or a behemoth corporation that spans the globe. Thus Congress provided that essentially all packaged foods sold at retail shall be appropriately labeled and their contents described [in the Nutrition Labeling and Education Act of 1990]. Also, as a matter of federal regulation, all alcoholic beverages must warn pregnant women against their use. Congress has gone further and made the possession and consumption of certain products criminal because of their presumed effect on the health of consumers. Other products have created health hazards and resulted in extensive and expensive class action litigation. . . . Public health is one, if not the, critical issue in society.

This opinion is guided by the principle that legal consequences should not attach to the consumption of hamburgers and other fast food fare unless consumers are unaware of the dangers of eating such food. . . . If consumers know (or reasonably should know) the potential ill health effects of eating at

McDonalds, they cannot blame McDonalds if they, nonetheless, choose to satiate their appetite with a surfeit of super-sized McDonalds products. On the other hand, consumers cannot be expected to protect against a danger that was solely within McDonalds' knowledge. Thus, one necessary element of any potentially viable claim must be that McDonalds' products involve a danger that is not within the common knowledge of consumers. As discussed later, plaintiffs have failed to allege with any specificity that such a danger exists.

McDonalds has also, rightfully, pointed out that this case, the first of its kind to progress far enough along to reach the stage of a dispositive motion, could spawn thousands of similar "McLawsuits" against restaurants. Even if limited to that ilk of fare dubbed "fast food," the potential for lawsuits is great: Americans now spend more than $110 billion on fast food each year, and on any given day in the United States, almost one in four adults visits a fast food restaurant. (citation to Fast Food Nation) The potential for lawsuits is even greater given the numbers of persons who eat food prepared at other restaurants in addition to those serving fast food. . . .

The interplay of these issues and forces has created public interest in this action, ranging from reports and letters to the Court to television satire. Obesity, personal liberty, and public accountability affect virtually every American consumer.

. . .

### Facts

Ashley Pelman, a minor, and her mother and natural guardian Roberta Pelman are residents of the Bronx, New York. . . . The [class of] infant plaintiffs are consumers who have purchased and consumed the defendants' products and, as a result thereof, have become overweight and have developed diabetes, coronary heart disease, high blood pressure, elevated cholesterol intake, and/or other detrimental and adverse health effects as a result of the defendants' conduct and business practices. Defendant McDonald's Corp. is a Delaware corporation with its principal place of business at One McDonald's Plaza, Oak Brook, Illinois. It does substantial business with outlets in the State of New York, as well as throughout the fifty states and the world. Defendant McDonalds of New York is a New York State corporation. . . . It does substantial business with outlets and/or franchises in the State of New York.

McDonalds is the owner, manager, franchisee, and operator of defendants the Bruckner Boulevard and Jerome Avenue outlets. . . .

### Obesity in Young Persons and Its Effects

Today there are nearly twice as many overweight children and almost three times as many overweight adolescents as there were in 1980. In 1999, an estimated 61 percent of U.S. adults were overweight or obese and 13 percent of children aged 6 to 11 years and 14 percent of adolescents aged 12 to 19 years were overweight. In 1980, those figures for children were 7 percent for children aged 6 to 11 years and 5 percent for adolescents aged 12 to 19 years. Obese individuals have a 50 to 100 percent increased risk of premature death from all causes. Approximately 300,000 deaths a year in the United States are currently associated with overweight and obesity. . . . Obesity and overweight classification are associated with increased risk for coronary heart disease; type 2 diabetes; endometrial, colon, postmenopausal breast, and other cancers; and certain musculoskeletal disorders, such as knee osteoarthritis.

Studies have shown that both modest and large weight gains are associated with significantly increased risk of diseases. . . .

## Claims

The plaintiffs allege five causes of action as members of a putative class action of minors residing in New York State who have purchased and consumed McDonalds products. Counts I and II are based on deceptive acts and practices in violation of the Consumer Protection Act, New York General Business Law §§ 349 and 350. . . . Count I alleges that McDonalds failed to adequately disclose the ingredients and/or health effects of ingesting certain of their food products with high levels of cholesterol, fat, salt, and sugar; described their food as nutritious; and engaged in marketing to entice consumers to purchase "value meals" without disclosing the detrimental health effects thereof. Count II focuses on marketing techniques geared toward inducing children to purchase and ingest McDonalds' food products. Count III sounds in negligence, alleging that McDonalds acted at least negligently in selling food products that are high in cholesterol, fat, salt, and sugar when studies show that such foods cause obesity and detrimental health effects. Count IV alleges that McDonalds failed to warn the consumers of McDonalds' products of the ingredients, quantity, qualities, and levels of cholesterol, fat, salt and sugar content and other ingredients in those products, and that a diet high in fat, salt, sugar and cholesterol could lead to obesity and health problems. Finally, Count V also sounds in negligence, alleging that McDonalds acted negligently in marketing food products that were physically and psychologically addictive.

## Discussion

[The court then considers whether it should remand the case to state court.]

This lawsuit is not the typical products liability case because, as referred to above, the issue is over-consumption of products created, manufactured, and advertised at a national level. A McDonalds' Big Mac is the same at every outlet in the Bronx, New York; the same at every outlet in the State of New York; and the same at every outlet throughout the United States. Clearly what is at issue in this lawsuit is the national menu and national policy of McDonalds Corp., and the plaintiffs' real beef is with McDonalds Corp.

As a result, the motion to remand is denied.

[The court then discusses the defendants' motion to dismiss the case.]

Counts I and II allege that McDonalds violated the New York Consumer Protection Act, §§ 349 and 350 by (1) deceptively advertising their food as not unhealthful and failing to provide consumers with nutritional information (Count I) and (2) inducing minors to eat at McDonalds through deceptive marketing ploys (Count II).

Section 349 makes unlawful "[d]eceptive acts or practices in the conduct of any business, trade, or commerce or in the furnishing of any service in this state." Section 350 prohibits "[f]alse advertising in the conduct of any business." To state a claim for deceptive practices under either section, a plaintiff must show: (1) that the act, practice, or advertisement was consumer-oriented; (2) that the act, practice, or advertisement was misleading in a material respect, and (3) that the plaintiff was injured as a result of the deceptive practice, act, or advertisement.

[The court then rejects the defendants argument that the federal nutritional labeling laws which exempts restaurants from the laws applicable to retail products preempts any state law which relating to the labeling of food.]

In Count I, plaintiffs allege that McDonalds violated the act both by commission (*e.g.,* stating that its products were nutritious, encouraging consumers to "supersize" their meals without disclosing the negative health effects) and by omission (*e.g.,* failing to provide nutritional information for products). Because the Complaint does not identify a single instance of deceptive acts, Count I shall be dismissed to the extent it alleges deceptive practices. . . .

. . . .

. . . [I]t is worth noting that, even in their opposition papers, the plaintiffs only cite to two advertising campaigns ("McChicken Everyday!" and "Big N' Tasty Everyday") and to a statement on the McDonalds' website that "McDonalds can be part of any balanced diet and lifestyle." These are specific examples of practices, act, or advertisements and would survive a motion to dismiss based on lack of specificity. Whether they would survive a motion to dismiss on the substantive issue of whether such practices, act, and advertisements are deceptive is less clear. The two campaigns encouraging daily forays to McDonalds and the statement regarding making McDonalds a part of a balanced diet, if read together, may be seen as contradictory — a balanced diet likely does not permit eating at McDonalds everyday. However, the advertisements encouraging persons to eat at McDonalds "everyday!" do not include any indication that doing so is part of a well-balanced diet, and the plaintiffs fail to cite any advertisement where McDonalds asserts that its products may be eaten for every meal of every day without any ill consequences. Merely encouraging consumers to eat its products "everyday" is mere puffery, at most, in the absence of a claim that to do so will result in a specific effect on health. As a result, the claims likely would not be actionable if alleged.

On December 11, 2002, the Court accepted from plaintiffs a number of documents concerning actions taken against McDonalds' advertising practices in the late 1980's by the state attorneys general from several states, including New York State. While any claim based on the advertisements at issue likely would be time barred, a review of those advertisements and the state attorney generals' analysis of them may assist plaintiffs in shaping a claim under the

Consumer Protection Act. For instance, by letter dated April 24, 1987 (the "Abrams Letter"), Robert Abrams, the then-Attorney General of the State of New York, addressed several specific allegedly deceptive claims in McDonalds advertisements: 1. The advertisement discussing salt (sodium) content in foods says, "Our sodium is down *across the menu*." (emphasis added) This is not true. That same advertisement lists four products (regular fries, regular cheeseburger, 6-piece McNuggets, and vanilla milkshake), none of which have had their sodium content lowered in the past year.

2. The advertisement touting the "real" milk in McDonald's shakes says that they contain "Wholesome milk, natural sweeteners, a fluid ounce of flavoring, and stabilizers for consistency. And that's all." In fact, that's not really all. McDonald's own ingredient booklet shows that a typical shake, such as vanilla or strawberry, actually contains artificial flavor and sodium benzoate and sodium hexametaphosphate, two chemical preservatives. This advertisement tells only part of the story. . . .

The second subset of Claim I focuses on McDonalds' failure to label its foods with their nutritional content. Unlike above, the plaintiffs clearly have out-lined the allegedly deceptive practice: The fact that McDonalds failed to post nutritional labeling on the products and at points of purchase. However, because this is a purportedly deceptive act based on an omission, it is not suf-ficient for the plaintiffs to point to the omission alone. They must also show why the omission was deceptive — a duty they have shunned.

. . . .

The plaintiffs fail to allege that the information with regard to the nutri-tional content of McDonalds' products was solely within McDonalds' posses-sion or that a consumer could not reasonably obtain such information. It cannot be assumed that the nutritional content of McDonalds' products and their usage was solely within the possession of McDonalds. (Although the plaintiffs do not allege it as part of Count I or II, the allegations contained in Count V — that McDonalds serves addictive products — would present a closer question as to a deceptive omission in violation of the Act, as such infor-mation is not available to the public.)

Count II, which focuses on representations targeting children, fails for the same reasons discussed above. The Complaint does not identify a single spe-cific advertisement, promotion, or statement directed at infant consumers, and Count II must be dismissed in the absence of such specificity.

The plaintiffs' common law claims against McDonalds sound in negligence, alleging that McDonalds was negligent in manufacturing and selling its prod-ucts and negligent in failing to warn consumers of the potential hazards of eating its products. . . .

Count III essentially alleges that McDonalds' products are inherently dan-gerous because of the inclusion of high levels of cholesterol, fat, salt, and sugar. McDonalds argues that because the public is well aware that hamburgers, fries, and other fast food fare have such attributes, McDonalds cannot be held liable.

. . . .

When asked at oral argument to distinguish this case from those cases involving injuries purportedly caused by asbestos exposure, counsel for the defendants stated that in this case, the dangers complained of have been well-known for some time, while the dangers of asbestos did not became apparent until years after exposure. The Restatement [of Torts] confirms this analysis, recognizing that the dangers of over-consumption of items such as alcoholic beverages, or typically high-in-fat foods such as butter, are well-known. Thus any liability based on over-consumption is doomed if the consequences of such over-consumption are common knowledge.

It is worth noting, however, that the Restatement provision cited above included tobacco as an example of products such as whiskey and butter, the unhealthy over-consumption of which could not lead to liability. As the successful tobacco class action litigation and settlements have shown, however, the fact that excessive smoking was known to lead to health problems did not vitiate liability when, for instance, tobacco companies had intentionally altered the nicotine levels of cigarettes to induce addiction. . . .

Thus, in order to state a claim, the Complaint must allege either that the attributes of McDonalds products are so extraordinarily unhealthy that they are outside the reasonable contemplation of the consuming public or that the products are so extraordinarily unhealthy as to be dangerous in their intended use. The Complaint — which merely alleges that the foods contain high levels of cholesterol, fat, salt and sugar, and that the foods are therefore unhealthy — fails to reach this bar. It is well-known that fast food in general, and McDonalds' products in particular, contain high levels of cholesterol, fat, salt, and sugar, and that such attributes are bad for one.

This rule makes sense in light of the policy issues discussed at the outset of this opinion. If a person knows or should know that eating copious orders of super-sized McDonalds' products is unhealthy and may result in weight gain (and its concomitant problems) because of the high levels of cholesterol, fat, salt, and sugar, it is not the place of the law to protect them from their own excesses. Nobody is forced to eat at McDonalds (except, perhaps, parents of small children who desire McDonalds' food, toy promotions, or playgrounds and demand their parents' accompaniment).

. . . .

For the first time in their opposition papers, the plaintiffs attempt to show that over-consumption of McDonalds is different in kind from, for instance, over-consumption of alcoholic beverages or butter because the processing of McDonalds' food has created an entirely different — and more dangerous — food than one would expect from a hamburger, chicken finger, or French fry cooked at home or at any restaurant other than McDonalds. They thus argue that McDonalds' food is "dangerous to an extent beyond that which would be contemplated by the ordinary consumer who purchases it, with the ordinary knowledge common to the community as to its characteristics." . . .

Similarly, plaintiffs argue that McDonalds' products have been so altered that their unhealthy attributes are now outside the ken of the average reasonable consumer. They point to McDonalds' ingredient lists to show that

McDonalds' customers worldwide are getting much more than what is commonly considered to be a chicken finger, a hamburger, or a French fry. . . .

For instance, Chicken McNuggets, rather than being merely chicken fried in a pan, are a McFrankenstein creation of various elements not utilized by the home cook. . . .

In addition, Chicken McNuggets, while seemingly a healthier option than McDonalds hamburgers because they have "chicken" in their names, actually contain twice the fat per ounce as a hamburger. It is at least a question of fact as to whether a reasonable consumer would know — without recourse to the McDonalds' website — that a Chicken McNugget contained so many ingredients other than chicken and provided twice the fat of a hamburger.

Similarly, it is hardly common knowledge that McDonalds' French fries are comprised, in addition to potatoes, of partially hydrogenated soybean oil, natural flavor (beef source), dextrose, and sodium acid pyrophosphate (to preserve natural color); they are cooked in partially hydrogenated vegetable oils, ("may contain partially hydrogenated soybean oil and/or partially hydrogenated corn oil and/or partially hydrogenated canola oil and/or cottonseed oil and/or corn oil"); TBHQ and citric acid are added to preserve freshness; Dimethylpolysiloxane is added as an anti-foaming agent.

This argument comes closest to overcoming the hurdle presented to plaintiffs. If plaintiffs were able to flesh out this argument in an amended complaint, it may establish that the dangers of McDonalds' products were not commonly well known and thus that McDonalds had a duty toward its customers. The argument also addresses McDonalds' list of horribles, *i.e.*, that a successful lawsuit would mean that "pizza parlors, neighborhood diners, bakeries, grocery stores, and literally anyone else in the food business (including mothers cooking at home)," could potentially face liability. Most of the above entities do not serve food that is processed to the extent that McDonalds' products are processed, nor food that is uniform to the extent that McDonalds' products are throughout the world. Rather, they serve plain-jane hamburgers, fries and shakes — meals that are high in cholesterol, fat, salt and sugar, but about which there are no additional processes that could be alleged to make the products even more dangerous. In addition, there is the problem of causation; hardly any of the entities listed above other than a parent cooking at home serves as many people regularly as McDonalds and its ilk.

. . .

Plaintiffs also argue in their papers, less successfully, that McDonalds has a duty to plaintiffs because they have an "allergic sensitivity" to McDonalds fare. . . .

Plaintiffs also attempt to ground a duty in a claim that eating McDonalds with high frequency is a "misuse" of the product of which McDonalds is aware. Again, such allegation was not in the Complaint, and, in any case, plaintiffs fail to allege even in their papers that what is at issue is a misuse "in the sense that it was outside the scope of the apparent purpose for which the [products] were manufactured." . . .

A better argument based on over-consumption would involve a claim that McDonalds' products are unreasonably dangerous for their intended use. The intended use of McDonalds' food is to be eaten, at some frequency that presents a question of fact. If plaintiffs can allege that McDonalds products' intended use is to be eaten for every meal of every day, and that McDonalds is or should be aware that eating McDonalds' products for every meal of every day is unreasonably dangerous, they may be able to state a claim.

. . . .

Because Count III has failed to state a claim, it is dismissed.

McDonalds also argues that Count III should be dismissed because the plaintiffs may not as a matter of law allege that the unhealthy attributes of McDonalds' products were the proximate cause of their obesity and other health problems.

In order to show proximate cause, a plaintiff must establish that the defendant's conduct was a substantial cause in bringing about the harm. . . .

Several factors are considered, including "the aggregate number of actors involved which contribute towards the harm and the effect which each has in producing it," and "whether the situation was acted upon by other forces for which the defendant is not responsible." . . .

No reasonable person could find probable cause based on the facts in the Complaint without resorting to "wild speculation." . . .

First, the Complaint does not specify how often the plaintiffs ate at McDonalds. The class action proposed by plaintiffs could consist entirely of persons who ate at McDonalds on one occasion. As a result, any number of other factors then potentially could have affected the plaintiffs' weight and health. In order to survive a motion to dismiss, the Complaint at a minimum must establish that the plaintiffs ate at McDonalds on a sufficient number of occasions such that a question of fact is raised as to whether McDonalds' products played a significant role in the plaintiffs' health problems. While the assignment of such a frequency is beyond the competency of this Court at this time, it seems like the frequency must be more than once per week — a figure cited by plaintiffs' counsel in oral argument as a potentially not unhealthy figure. Naturally, the more often a plaintiff had eaten at McDonalds, the stronger the likelihood that it was the McDonalds' food (as opposed to other foods) that affected the plaintiffs' health.

Second, McDonalds points out that articles on which plaintiffs rely in their Complaint suggest that a number of factors other than diet may come into play in obesity and the health problems of which plaintiffs complain. As a result, in order to allege that McDonalds' products were a significant factor in the plaintiffs' obesity and health problems, the Complaint must address these other variables and, if possible, eliminate them or show that a McDiet is a substantial factor despite these other variables. Similarly, with regard to the plaintiffs' health problems that they claim resulted from their obesity (which they allege resulted from their McDonalds habits) it would be necessary to allege that such diseases were not merely hereditary or caused by environmental or other factors.

Because the Complaint fails to allege that the danger of the McDonalds' products were not well-known and fails to allege with sufficient specificity that the McDonalds' products were a proximate cause of the plaintiffs' obesity and health problems, Count III shall be dismissed.

Count IV alleges a failure to warn of the unhealthy attributes of McDonalds' products. While the cause of action differs from Count III, McDonalds' arguments that this claim fails because the dangers of its fare were well-known and that plaintiffs have failed to show proximate cause are nonetheless applicable.

. . . .

As discussed above, the Complaint fails to allege that the McDonalds' products consumed by the plaintiffs were dangerous in any way other than that which was open and obvious to a reasonable consumer. While the plaintiffs have presented the outline of a substantial argument to the contrary in their papers, as discussed *supra,* their theory is not supported in their Complaint, and thus cannot save Count IV from dismissal. In addition, as also discussed above, the Complaint does not allege with sufficient specificity that the plaintiffs' consumption of McDonalds' products was a significant factor in their obesity and related health problems. As a result, Count IV must be dismissed.

The exact basis of Count V is unclear. It appears to be a products liability claim, *i.e.,* McDonalds' products are inherently dangerous in that they are addictive. The claim may also be read to allege that McDonalds failed to warn its customers that its products were addictive. This claim, unlike the one above based on unhealthy attributes, does not involve a danger that is so open and obvious, or so commonly well-known, that McDonalds' customers would be expected to know about it. In fact, such a hypothesis is even now the subject of current investigations. . . . Such a finding would go far in explaining why fast-food sales have climbed to more than $100 billion a year . . . despite years of warnings to limit fats. Therefore, it does not run into the same difficulties discussed above with regard to clarifying that the unhealthy attributes are above and beyond what is normally known about fast food.

While it is necessary to accept as true the allegation in the Complaint that McDonalds' products are addictive for the purposes of this motion, such allegation standing alone is, nonetheless, insufficient as overly vague. The Complaint does not specify whether it is the combination of fats and sugars in McDonalds products that is addictive, or whether there is some other additive, that works in the same manner as nicotine in cigarettes, to induce addiction. Further, there is no allegation as to whether McDonalds purposefully manufactured products that have these addictive qualities. In addition, the Complaint fails to specify whether a person can become addicted to McDonalds' products after eating there one time or whether it requires a steady diet of McDonalds in order to result in addiction. There is also no allegation as to whether plaintiffs, as infants, are more susceptible to the addiction than adults.

While some of these questions necessarily may not be answered until discovery (should this claim be re-plead and survive a motion to dismiss), and likely then only with the aid of expert witnesses, to allow a complaint to survive merely because it alleges product liability on the basis of addiction would be to allow any complaint that alleges product liability based on the addictive nature of the products to survive dismissal, even where such addiction is likely never to be proven. As a result, a complaint must contain some specificity in order to survive a motion to dismiss.

A claim that a product causes addiction and that reasonable consumers are unaware of that danger must at the very least (1) allege that the plaintiffs are addicted, with allegations revealing ways in which their addiction may be observed, and (2) specify the basis of the plaintiffs' belief that they and others became addicted to the product. Further allegations addressing questions raised above would further strengthen the claim. In the absence of any such specific allegations, Count V must be dismissed.

In any case, as discussed above, the Complaint fails to allege sufficiently that the addictive nature of McDonalds' food and the plaintiffs' resulting ingestion thereof is a proximate cause of the plaintiff's health problems. As a result, Count V is dismissed.

. . . [T]he plaintiffs may amend their complaint to address the deficiencies listed above.

\* \* \*

## PELMAN v. McDONALD'S
### 2003 WL 2205277 (S.D.N.Y.) ("Pelman II")

Sweet, Judge.

\* \* \*

[Following the decision in *Pelman I*, the plaintiffs amended their complaint. The defendants again moved to have lawsuit dismissed. The court began its decision by summarizing the earlier proceeding and repeated much of the background information discussed in *Pelman I*, as the following:]

## McDonald's Advertising Campaigns

In one survey of the frequency of purchases by visitors to McDonald's restaurants, McDonald's found that 72% of its customers were "Heavy Users," meaning they visit McDonald's at least once a week, and that approximately 22% of its customers are "Super Heavy Users," or "SHUs," meaning that they eat "at McDonald's ten times or more a month." Super Heavy Users make up approximately 75% of McDonald's sales. Many of McDonald's advertisements, therefore, are designed to increase the consumption of Heavy Users or Super Heavy Users. The plaintiffs allege that to achieve that goal, McDonald's engaged in advertising campaigns which represented that McDonald's foods are nutritious and can easily be part of a healthy lifestyle.

Advertising campaigns run by McDonald's from 1987 onward claimed that it sold: "Good basic nutritious food." "Food that's been the foundation of well-balanced diets for generations. And will be for generations to come." McDonald's also represented that it would be "easy" to follow USDA and

Health and Human Services guidelines for a healthful diet "and still enjoy your meal at McDonald's." McDonald's has described its beef as "nutritious" and "leaner than you think." And it has described its French fries as "well within the established guidelines for good nutrition." While making these broad claims about its nutritious value, McDonald's has declined to make its nutrition information readily available at its restaurants. In 1987, McDonald's entered into a settlement agreement with the New York State Attorney General in which it agreed to "provide [nutritional] information in easily understood pamphlets or brochures which will be free to all customers so they could take them with them for further study [and] to place signs, including in-store advertising to inform customers who walk in, and drive-through information and notices would be placed where drive-through customers could see them." Despite this agreement, the plaintiffs have alleged that nutritional information was not adequately available to them for inspection upon request.

In the amended complaint, the plaintiffs alleged four causes of action as members of a putative class action of minors residing in New York State who have purchased and consumed McDonald's products. Shortly before oral argument, however, the plaintiffs informed the Court that they are dropping their fourth cause of action, which alleged negligence by McDonald's because of its failure to warn plaintiffs of the dangers and adverse health effects of eating processed foods from McDonald's. The three remaining causes of action are based on deceptive acts in practices in violation of the Consumer Protection Act . . . .

Count I alleges that McDonald's misled the plaintiffs, through advertising campaigns and other publicity, that its food products were nutritious, of a beneficial nutritional nature or effect, and/or were easily part of a healthy lifestyle if consumed on a daily basis. Count II alleges that McDonald's failed adequately to disclose the fact that certain of its foods were substantially less healthier, as a result of processing and ingredient additives, than represented by McDonald's in its advertising campaigns and other publicity. Count III alleges that McDonald's engaged in unfair and deceptive acts and practices by representing to the New York Attorney General and to New York consumers that it provides nutritional brochures and information at all of its stores when in fact such information was and is not adequately available to the plaintiffs at a significant number of McDonald's outlets.

The plaintiffs allege that as a result of the deceptive acts and practices enumerated in all three counts, they have suffered damages including, but not limited to, an increased likelihood of the development of obesity, diabetes, coronary heart disease, high blood pressure, elevated cholesterol intake, related cancers, and/or detrimental and adverse health effects and/or diseases.

. . . .

[The court then describes § 349 and § 350. It goes on to conclude that any violation of the act cannot be claimed for actions before 1987 because of the statute of limitations.]

McDonald's argues that the consumer protection claims must be dismissed because the plaintiffs do not "allege that any of them ever saw even one of the McDonald's statements and advertisements described in the Amended Complaint." The plaintiffs counter that they have alleged that their misconceptions about the healthiness of McDonald's food resulted from "a long-term deceptive campaign by Defendant of misrepresenting the nutritional benefits of their foods over the last approximate [sic] fifteen (15) years." Plaintiffs are correct that it is not necessary to allege reliance on defendant's deceptive practices in the context of a § 349 claim. . . . To state a claim under § 350 for false advertising, however, it is necessary to allege reliance on the allegedly false advertisement.

While plaintiffs have alleged that McDonald's has made it difficult to obtain nutritional information about its products, they have not alleged that McDonald's controlled all relevant information. Indeed, the complaint cites the complete ingredients of several McDonald's products. Plaintiffs are therefore required to allege reliance in order to survive a motion to dismiss. The plaintiffs' vague allegations of reliance on a "long-term deceptive campaign" are insufficient to fulfill the reliance requirement. . . . Even assuming that the specific advertisements cited by the plaintiffs would be considered deceptive, it cannot be determined that the other advertisements upon which the plaintiffs are alleged to have relied are also deceptive without citing at least one instance of such advertisements. Absent an example of an alleged false advertisement on which plaintiffs relied, the amended complaint states only a legal conclusion — that the campaign in its entirety is deceptive — without making a factual allegation. Such conclusory allegations are not entitled to a presumption of truthfulness. . . .

          . . . .

Making all reasonable inferences in favor of the plaintiffs, the complaint implicitly alleges only one instance in which the infant plaintiffs were aware of allegedly false advertisements. The plaintiffs implicitly allege that they were aware of McDonald's national advertising campaign announcing that it was switching to "100 percent vegetable oil" in its French fries and hash browns, and that McDonald's fries contained zero milligrams of cholesterol, when they claim that they "would not have purchased or consumed said French fries or hash browns, or purchased and consumed in such quantities," had McDonald's disclosed the fact that these products "contain beef or extracts and trans fatty acids." . . .

The most formidable hurdle for plaintiffs is to demonstrate that they "suffered injury as a result of the deceptive act." . . .

          . . . .

Even if plaintiffs were able sufficiently to allege that their injuries were causally related to McDonald's representations about its French fries and hash browns, that claim must still be dismissed because the plaintiffs have not alleged that those advertisements were objectively misleading.

The essence of the plaintiffs' claim of deception with regard to McDonald's French fries and hash browns is that McDonald's represented that its fries are cooked in "100 percent vegetable oil" and that they contain zero milligrams of cholesterol whereas in reality they "contain beef or extracts and trans fatty acids." However, the citations in the amended complaint to McDonald's advertisements, and the appended copies of the advertisements, do not bear out the plaintiffs' claims of deception. The first citation is to an advertisement titled "How we're getting a handle on cholesterol," alleged to have commenced in 1987 and to have continued for several years thereafter. The text cited by the plaintiffs states: "a regular order of French fries is surprising low in cholesterol *and saturated fat: only 9 mg of cholesterol* and 4.6 grams of saturated fat. Well within established guidelines for good nutrition." The advertisement also states that McDonald's uses "a specially blended beef and vegetable shortening to cook our world famous French fries and hash browns."

The plaintiffs next allege that beginning on or around July 23, 1990, McDonald's announced that it would change its French fry recipe and cook its fries in "100 percent vegetable oil," a change that rendered its fries cholesterol-free. They allege that from the time of the change until May 21, 2001, McDonald's never acknowledged "that it has continued the use of beef tallow in the French fries and hash browns cooking process." On its website, however, McDonald's is alleged to have "admitted the truth about its French fries and hash browns": "A small amount of beef flavoring is added during potato processing — at the plant. After the potatoes are washed and steam peeled, they are cut, dried, par-fried and frozen. It is during the par-frying process at the plant that the natural flavoring is used. These fries are then shipped to our U.S. restaurants. Our French fries are cooked in vegetable oil at our restaurants."

. . . .

Plaintiffs further allege that McDonald's claims that its French fries and hash browns are cholesterol-free is also misleading because the oils in which those foods are cooked contain "trans fatty acids responsible for raising detrimental blood cholesterol levels (LDL) in individuals, leading to coronary heart disease." However, plaintiffs have made no allegations that McDonald's made any representations about the *effect* of its French fries on blood cholesterol levels.

Because the plaintiffs have failed to allege both that McDonald's caused the plaintiffs' injuries or that McDonald's representations to the public were deceptive, the motion to dismiss the complaint is granted. . . .

\* \* \*

# PELMAN v. McDONALD'S CORP.
### 396 F.3d 508 (2d Cir. 2005) ("Pelman III")

Rakoff, Judge.

\* \* \*

In this diversity action, plaintiffs . . . by their respective parents . . . appeal from the dismissal of Counts I-III of their amended complaint. Each of the these counts purports to allege, on behalf of a putative class of consumers, that defendant McDonald's Corporation violated both § 349 and § 350 of the New York General Business Law, commonly known as the New York Consumer Protection Act, during the years 1987 through 2002.

Specifically, Count I alleges that the combined effect of McDonald's various promotional representations during this period was to create the false impression that its food products were nutritionally beneficial and part of a healthy lifestyle if consumed daily. Count II alleges that McDonald's failed adequately to disclose that its use of certain additives and the manner of its food processing rendered certain of its foods substantially less healthy than represented. Count III alleges that McDonald's deceptively represented that it would provide nutritional information to its New York customers when in reality such information was not readily available at a significant number of McDonald's outlets in New York visited by the plaintiffs and others. The amended complaint further alleges that as a result of these deceptive practices, plaintiffs, who ate at McDonald's three to five times a week throughout the years in question, were "led to believe that [McDonald's] foods were healthy and wholesome, not as detrimental to their health as medical and scientific studies have shown . . . [and] of a beneficial nutritional value," and that they "would not have purchased and/or consumed the Defendant's aforementioned products, in their entire[t]y, or on such frequency but for the aforementioned alleged representations and campaigns." Finally, the amended complaint alleges that, as a result, plaintiffs have developed "obesity, diabetes, coronary heart disease, high blood pressure, elevated cholesterol intake, related cancers, and/or other detrimental and adverse health effects. . . ." What is missing from the amended complaint, however, is any express allegation that any plaintiff specifically relied to his/her detriment on any particular representation made in any particular McDonald's advertisement or promotional material. The district court concluded that, with one exception, the absence of such a particularized allegation of reliance warranted dismissal of the claims under § 350 which prohibits false advertising. As to the exception — involving McDonald's representations that its French fries and hash browns are made with 100% vegetable oil and/or are cholesterol-free — the district court found that, while the amended complaint might be read to allege implicit reliance by plaintiffs on such representations, the representations themselves were objectively non-misleading.

Although plaintiffs' notice of appeal states that they challenge the judgment "dismissing the Plaintiffs' Amended Complaint," their brief on appeal contains no argument as to why the district court's dismissal of the claims asserted under § 350 was incorrect. Accordingly, we regard any challenge to the dismissal of the § 350 claims as abandoned.

Plaintiffs' appellate brief does, however, challenge the district court's dismissal of the claims under § 349 which makes unlawful "[d]eceptive acts or practices in the conduct of any business, trade, or commerce, or in the furnishing of any service in this state." Unlike a private action brought under § 350, a private action brought under § 349 does not require proof of actual reliance. Additionally, § 349 extends well beyond common-law fraud to cover a broad range of deceptive practices . . . and because a private action under § 349 does not require proof of the same essential elements (such as reliance) as common-law fraud, an action under § 349 is not subject to the pleading-with-particularity requirements . . . but need only meet the bare-bones notice-pleading requirements. . . .

Although the district court recognized that § 349 does not require proof of reliance, the district court nonetheless dismissed the claims because it concluded that "[p]laintiffs have failed, however, to draw an adequate causal connection between their consumption of McDonald's food and their alleged injuries." Thus, the district court found it fatal that the complaint did not answer such questions as:

> What else did the plaintiffs eat? How much did they exercise? Is there a family history of the diseases which are alleged to have been caused by McDonald's products? Without this additional information, McDonald's does not have sufficient information to determine if its foods are the cause of plaintiffs' obesity, or if instead McDonald's foods are only a contributing factor.

This, however, is the sort of information that is appropriately the subject of discovery, rather than what is required to satisfy the limited pleading requirements. . . .

So far as the § 349 claims are concerned, the amended complaint more than meets the [minimum pleading] requirements . . . .

Accordingly, the district court's dismissal of those portions of Counts I-III of the amended complaint as alleged violations of § 349 [is vacated].

\* \* \*

# PELMAN v. McDONALD'S
### 452 F. Supp. 2d 320 (2006) ("Pelman V")

Sweet, Judge.

\* \* \*

## Facts

In this diversity action, Plaintiffs allege that McDonald's engaged in a scheme of deceptive advertising . . . during the years 1987 to 2002. The facts underlying the Plaintiffs' complaint have been outlined extensively by this Court and by the Second Circuit in *Pelman I, Pelman II,* and *Pelman III,* familiarity with which is assumed.

Count I [of the Second Amended Complaint (SAC)] alleges that the combined effect of McDonald's various promotional representations was to create the false impression that its food products were nutritionally beneficial and part of a healthy lifestyle if consumed daily. Count II alleges that McDonald's failed to adequately disclose that its use of certain additives and the manner of its food processing rendered certain of its foods substantially less healthy than represented. Count III alleges that McDonald's deceptively represented that it would provide nutritional information to its New York customers when in reality such information was not readily available at a significant number of McDonald's outlets in New York. The Second Circuit held that Counts I-III alleges claims under New York General Business law § 349 sufficient for Rule 8(a). . . .

In *Pelman IV*, this Court ordered the Plaintiffs to provide a more definite statement of their claims, including:

(1) identification of the advertisements about which the plaintiffs are complaining; (2) a brief explanation of why the advertisements are materially deceptive to an objective consumer; (3) a brief explanation of how the plaintiffs were aware of the acts alleged to be misleading; and (4) a brief description of the injuries suffered by each plaintiff by reason of defendant's conduct.

. . . In accordance with the first directive above, the SAC identifies a number of advertisements being claimed as part of the Defendant's deceptive practices. Additionally, the SAC outlines why the advertisements are objectively deceptive. In response to the third requirement, the SAC alleges that Plaintiffs were aware of McDonald's deceptive practices through their exposure to the advertisements and statements annexed to their pleading and that such statements were disseminated in the specified fora of: television, radio, internet, magazine, periodical, in-store poster advertisements, and press releases issued in New York State from 1985 and continuing through filing in 2002. The SAC also alleges that the Plaintiffs' beliefs were affected through their contact and interaction with third-parties, i.e., parents, friends, and relatives, who were influenced by McDonald's allegedly misleading nutritional advertisements.

With respect to a more definite statement of the injuries suffered by Plaintiffs, the SAC alleges that each named Plaintiff was injured as a result of Defendant's practices, in the following respects:

> obesity, elevated levels of Low-Density Lipoprotein, or LDL, more commonly known as "bad" cholesterol, significant or substantial increased factors in the development of coronary heart disease, pediatric diabetes, high blood pressure, and/or other detrimental and adverse health effects and/or diseases as medically determined to have been causally connected to the prolonged use of Defendants products. . . .

## Applicable Standards

. . . [A] pleading to which a responsive pleading is permitted is so vague or ambiguous that a party cannot reasonably be required to frame a responsive pleading, the party may move for a more definite statement before interposing a responsive pleading.". . .

## Discussion

. . . First, McDonald's contends that the SAC fails to provide a brief explanation of how each Plaintiff became aware of the alleged deceptive advertisements . . . . Second, McDonald's contends that the Plaintiffs have failed to comply with the Court's order in that the SAC fails to describe briefly the injuries each Plaintiff allegedly suffered. Third, McDonald's seeks to limit this case to the allegedly deceptive advertisements specifically identified in the SAC. Finally, McDonald's seeks to limit Plaintiffs' case to only those advertisements identified that McDonald's contends have been properly alleged as objectively unreasonable.

## A. *Plaintiffs Have Sufficiently Described How They Were Aware of the Nutritional Schemes Alleged to be Deceptive*

. . . According to Defendant, the allegations that the Plaintiffs "were aware" of the alleged acts "through recent exposure . . . disseminated in various . . . forms of media" and through "contact and communication with . . . third parties" do not comply with the Court's order because they do not address each Plaintiff separately or outline the specific facts surrounding the Plaintiff(s)' exposure to each advertisement. In essence, McDonald's argues — as it did in its motion for a more definite statement — that Plaintiffs have not alleged that they heard or saw the allegedly deceptive advertisements.

As noted above, the Second Circuit held that Plaintiffs adequately alleged a cause of action under § 349, including the causation element . . . . Accordingly, as this Court explained in *Pelman IV*, Plaintiffs need not have seen or heard each advertisement, but rather only to have been exposed to them in some manner. Specifically, this Court explained:

. . . [R]eliance is not a necessary element of a § 349 claim. (noting that "New York courts . . . show only that the practice complained of was objectively misleading or deceptive and that he had suffered injury " 'as a result' of the practice." . . . Defendant's argument for this more particular information rests on its contention that "New York decisions have repeatedly held that a court must dismiss a claim based on an advertisement or statement never seen by the plaintiffs.". . . [T]he amended complaint has already been upheld . . . as having adequately alleged the elements of a § 349 claim. Defendant has failed to show, and this Court fails to see, that the absence of this information makes the complaint vague and conclusory such that defendant cannot interpose a response in good faith. Accordingly, plaintiffs need not confirm that each plaintiff saw or heard each advertisement.

As such, in *Pelman IV*, this Court did not order the specificity requested by McDonald's, but rather simply ordered Plaintiffs to provide a brief explanation of how they "were aware of the nutritional schemes they allege to have been deceptive." . . . .

It is concluded that Plaintiffs' SAC complies with this directive. First, Plaintiffs have alleged that they were aware of the advertisements and statements comprising McDonald's allegedly deceptive nutritional scheme through their exposure to certain advertisements and statements annexed to their pleading and that such statements were disseminated in the specified forums of television, radio, internet, magazine, periodical, in-store poster advertisements, and press releases issued in New York State from 1985 through 2002. Additionally, the Plaintiffs alleged that their beliefs were affected through their contact and interaction with third-parties who were exposed to and influenced by McDonald's allegedly misleading advertisements. This information is sufficient to allow Defendant to interpose a response, and Defendant's motion to strike is denied.

### B. *Plaintiffs Have Sufficiently Described the Injuries Each of Them Allegedly Suffered*

Defendant also argues that Plaintiffs have not complied with the portion of *Pelman IV* that ordered Plaintiffs to provide "a brief description of the injuries suffered by each plaintiff by reason of defendant's conduct." According to McDonald's, the SAC fails to comply with the Court's directive because it provides only a list of potential injuries from overeating, but fails to link particular injuries with a particular plaintiff.

As set forth above, the SAC alleges that Plaintiff Ashley *Pelman* was injured as a result of McDonald's conduct in the following respects:

> obesity, elevated levels of Low-Density Lipoprotein, or LDL, more commonly known as "bad" cholesterol, significant or substantial increased factors in the development of coronary heart disease, pediatric diabetes, high blood pressure, and/or other detrimental and adverse health effects and/or diseases as medically determined to have been causally connected to the prolonged use of Defendant's products . . . .

This language appears identically for every Plaintiff in Counts I and II of the SAC. Defendant contends that this language does not comply with the Court's directive as it does not name specific injuries suffered by each Plaintiff and that the boilerplate allegation renders McDonald's incapable of answering the SAC.

Contrary to McDonald's contentions, it is concluded that the SAC outlines the injuries sustained by each Plaintiff in a manner sufficient for McDonald's to answer. Allegations less specific than those outlined above were held adequate to state a cause of action by the Second Circuit. Moreover, while McDonald's conclusorily claims that it does not have information relating to Plaintiffs' injuries sufficient to interpose an answer, they fail to offer specific arguments in support of this contention.

Each of the Plaintiffs has separately alleged that, as a direct result of Defendant's actions, he or she sustained: (1) physical injuries of weight gain, obesity, hypertension, and elevated levels of LDL cholesterol; (2) false beliefs as to the nutritional contents and effects of Defendant's foods; and (3) economic losses in the form of the costs of the Defendant's products that they would not have purchased but for Defendant's misconduct.

The SAC also outlines the McDonald's menu items and food portions consumed, the frequency of consumption of the menu items, and the time period of consumption with respect to each Plaintiff. Additionally, each Plaintiff separately alleges that they exceed the Body Mass Index as established by the U.S. Surgeon General, National Institute of Health, Centers for Disease Control, U.S. Food and Drug Administration, and all acceptable scientific medical guidelines for the classification of clinical obesity. Finally, the SAC details the injuries and costs associated with each Plaintiff's physical injuries.

These allegations are deemed in compliance with the Court's October 24, 2005 directive and sufficient for McDonald's to answer Plaintiffs' complaint.

## C.  *Plaintiffs' Case Shall Be Limited to the Advertisements Identified in the SAC*

Defendant further contends that Plaintiffs should be limited to the forty advertisements specifically identified in the SAC.

In *Pelman IV*, the Court noted that "the absence of information as to the specific advertisements at issue renders plaintiffs' complaint vague and conclusory." The Court further concluded that "[w]ithout information as to which of McDonald's representations comprised the nutritional schemes alleged to have injured plaintiffs, McDonald's can neither admit, nor in good faith deny, the Consumer Protection Act violations." Accordingly, the Court ordered Plaintiffs to "identify the advertisements that collectively amount to the alleged deceptive nutritional schemes."

In addition to identifying forty specific allegedly deceptive advertisements, Plaintiffs also openly signal their intention to add "other" advertisements to their case at some later date. McDonald's contends that the Court's October 24, 2005 directive forecloses Plaintiffs from later identifying additional advertisements and that the SAC's reference to unidentified "other" advertisements leaves McDonald's unable to answer the SAC in full.

It is concluded that Plaintiffs shall be limited to the advertisements identified in the SAC, with leave granted to permit Plaintiffs to amend the SAC with additional advertisements for good cause shown.

## D.  *The Court Will Not Address the Sufficiency of Plaintiffs' Allegations Under § 349*

Finally, Defendant argues that Plaintiffs have identified only seven advertisements that conceivably could be read as objectively misleading and urges the Court to limit Plaintiffs' case to these advertisements. With respect to the remaining allegations, Defendant urges the Court to strike portions of the SAC that refer to claims that have already been dismissed by the Court, including references to parents as individual Plaintiffs and McDonald's representation that its French fries are "cholesterol-free," which this Court previously held to be objectively non-deceptive as a matter of law. Second, McDonald's argues that Plaintiffs' allegations that certain advertisements are misleading because they mention just one ingredient are as a matter of law not objective misleading. Third, McDonald's challenges Plaintiffs' allegation that McDonald's advertisements contain a hidden message that its products are "healthier-than-in-fact" or that consumers should disregard other aspects of their diets. Fourth, McDonald's contends that its statements that its food is "nutritious" are objectively non-misleading. Finally, McDonald's challenges the legal sufficiency of the portions of the SAC that allege that Plaintiffs were misled due to McDonald's alleged failure to abide by the terms of a 1986 settlement with the Attorneys General of three states, including New York, which allegedly required McDonald's to post certain nutritional and ingredient information about its products.

.  .  .  .

With respect to Defendant's first contention, this Court previously dismissed all claims brought directly by parent co-plaintiffs, finding that the statute of limitations barred their claims. The Plaintiffs did not appeal that holding. . . . Plaintiffs have conceded this point. Therefore, the portions of the SAC that refer to the parents individually as Plaintiffs and that state that two parents "purchased and/or consumed the Defendant's products for herself," . . . are hereby stricken.

With respect to references in the SAC to Plaintiffs' French fry allegations, this Court previously concluded that "McDonald's representation that its fries are 'cholesterol-free' or contain zero milligrams of cholesterol is . . . objectively non-deceptive." Similarly, this Court held that Plaintiffs' allegation with respect to McDonald's Mighty Kids Meal "is mere puffery rather than any claim that children who eat a 'Might[y] Kids Meal' will become mightier." On appeal, the Second Circuit did not disturb these rulings. As such, these rulings constitute the law of the case, and Plaintiffs are precluded from revisiting these allegations. Accordingly, the portions of the SAC that refer to McDonald's representation that its fries are "cholesterol-free" is hereby stricken.

With respect to Defendant's remaining contentions, McDonald's has not asserted that the challenged allegations render it incapable to interpose an answer, but rather challenges the legal sufficiency of the allegations as not objectively misleading . . . .

### Conclusion

As set forth above, McDonald's motion to strike and dismiss the SAC in its entirety is denied. Those portions of the SAC that refer to parents as individual co-plaintiffs shall be stricken, as shall the Plaintiffs' allegations concerning McDonald's "cholesterol-free" French fry representation and McDonald's Mighty Kids Meals. McDonald's is hereby ordered to answer the SAC within thirty days.

It is so ordered.

* * *

## Richard A. Daynard, P. Tim Howard & Cara L. Wilking, *Private Enforcement: Litigation as a Tool to Prevent Obesity*
### 25 J. Pub. Health Pol'y 408–14 (2004)

* * *

Unlike tobacco, which is harmful when consumed in any quantity, food is necessary for life. But successful tobacco litigation was based not on the dangers of the products but on the misdeeds of the manufacturers. Similarly, cases against food manufacturers are likely to be based on evidence that manufacturers misrepresented nutritional properties of products, took advantage of the credulity of children to sell them high calorie density products that helped launch them on a career of unhealthy eating, marketed addictive high calorie sodas to teenagers in their own school buildings, or otherwise violated consumer protection laws that prohibit "unfair or deceptive acts or practices in commerce.

. . . .

One of litigation's first benefits is access to industry documents through the discovery process. Evidence essential to proving cases of unfair trade practices, negligence, or product liability, will undoubtedly flow from discovery requests made of food manufacturers and retailers, and information obtained through depositions and interrogatories answered under oath. . . .

An increase in industry self-policing is another benefit of litigation. Some food manufacturers and retailers already are responding to public concerns about obesity and their own concerns about litigation, and have chosen to modify certain business practices. . . . This self-regulation is not merely an incidental effect of litigation: consumer protection laws and product liability principles, like almost all law, are primarily designed to discourage the proscribed conduct, with the application of legal sanctions and compensatory damage awards reserved for the occasional instance where the legal standard was violated nonetheless.

## APPLICABLE LEGAL PRINCIPLES

### Unfair and Deceptive Trade Practices

State and federal consumer protection laws prohibit manufacturers and retailers of food and other products from inducing consumers to purchase products through unfair, deceptive, and misleading trade practices. The Federal Trade Commission Act (FTCA) proscribes unfair and deceptive trade practices, but it can only be invoked by the Federal Trade Commission.

State consumer protection laws are largely modeled after the FTCA but, with the exception of one state, provide consumers with a private right of legal action. State consumer protection statutes are broadly drafted and deem unlawful such unfair and deceptive trade practices as direct misrepresentation and failure to disclose material information. State consumer protection jurisprudence, however, reflects disparities in the willingness of state courts to enforce consumer protection laws. State statutes, moreover, vary considerably with respect to the requirement that a plaintiff prove intent to deceive and/or induce reliance by consumers on false or misleading statements made. . . .

An early example of use of consumer protection laws to counter practices that encourage childhood obesity is the 1983 California Supreme Court decision *Committee on Children's Television v. General Food*. The plaintiff NGO alleged that advertisements on children's television programs for high-sugar breakfast cereals made by General Foods and other manufacturers were unfair and deceptive because they were designed to make children believe these products would help make them strong and healthy, whereas they were minimally nutritious and tended to cause tooth decay. . . .

The strength of claims brought under *unfair and deceptive acts and practices statutes* is that while plaintiffs must show that the representations and/or omissions made by the defendant in the marketing of the food product was unfair and deceptive, they do not have to show that the consumption of the product caused obesity and its medical consequences. However, finding private counsel willing to take on a consumer protection case may be difficult. The financial losses to each consumer, measured by the money spent on unfairly or deceptively marketed products, are likely small. While consumer protection laws generally allow successful plaintiffs to recover their attorneys' fees, courts are not always sufficiently generous in awarding such fees to provide economic incentives commensurate with the enormous resources necessary to successfully litigate such a claim. Class action claims, which could combine the small financial losses suffered by each of tens or hundreds of thousands of consumers, may prove to be the most effective vehicle to make a case "large" enough to justify a large award in the minds of most judges.

### Personal Injury Claims

Personal injury claims may also provide relief to consumers harmed by food products and can be brought either on the theory that there was something wrong with the product or the manufacturer improperly marketed the product. In general, for a *product liability* action to be successful, a plaintiff must prove that: (1) the danger from the food was not apparent to the average consumer; (2) the food was unreasonably dangerous for its intended use; and (3) the harm would not have occurred had an adequate warning about the food been given.

Defining the "average consumer" depends on the age and sophistication of the consumer. Courts may be more receptive to claims brought on behalf of children because they lack the ability to analyze critically advertising claims and promotions directly targeted at them. . . .

The *improper marketing theory*, which can be based either on consumer protection laws or on traditional common law negligence or fraud, requires that the seller deceived the consumer in a material way about the health effects of eating the food, and that this deception caused the consumer to consume the food. If a seller explicitly or implicitly represented, for example, that one could eat a typical McDonald's meal every day without putting on weight, and a customer reasonably relied on this representation, such a case could be brought. The consumer, however, would have to prove that his reliance on these misrepresentations continued to be reasonable even as he put on weight and his waistline expanded.

Under either a product liability or improper marketing theory, the plaintiff must prove that his obesity and its sequelae were caused by consuming the food in question. This requires the plaintiff to show, at a minimum, that the defendant's food was a "substantial factor" in causing the obesity, and that the obesity was a "substantial factor" in causing the subsequent medical condition. The latter link can frequently be proven through ordinary etiological evidence — studies in the public health or medical literature. Establishing a causal link between a particular food product and an individual's weight gain, while more difficult, may not be impossible. . . .

. . . .

*Personal Responsibility of the Plaintiff*

Resistance to obesity-related litigation is consistently couched in personal responsibility terms — responsibility for the injury should lie entirely on the afflicted consumer. This argument was frequently used to discredit attempts to hold the tobacco industry responsible for harms to consumers, and, while an initially attractive argument, does not withstand analysis. Various factors mitigate consumers' blameworthiness. Predictable over-consumption on the part of a consumer does not excuse decisions by food marketers to exploit this consumer behavior for their own benefit and to the detriment of consumers' health.

Attributing primary causal responsibility to the individual consumer denies the power of the new food environment — ubiquitous and inexpensive food with little nutritional value. . . .

## DIRECT RESPONSES TO THE THREAT OF LITIGATION: PROPOSED IMMUNITY FOR THE FOOD INDUSTRY

In the United States, widespread media attention to the threat of obesity-related litigation has inspired federal and state *tort reform* legislation that would grant the food industry blanket immunity from obesity-related lawsuits. In the spring of 2004, proposed federal legislation, entitled the "Personal Responsibility in Food Consumption Act," seeking to grant the food industry immunity from "claims of injury relating to a person's weight gain or obesity" passed the House of Representatives. And at least nineteen states have considered or are considering similar legislation. Dubbed "cheeseburger bills" by the popular media, state-level legislation would bar lawsuits by consumers alleging harm in the form of obesity and obesity-related illness. . . .

## CONCLUSION

Food producers and restaurants argue that obesity-related litigation is inherently frivolous, and that they will be bankrupted from the legal costs of defending against such litigation. Defendants, they certainly know, can quickly get genuinely frivolous litigation dismissed, and may even obtain their attorneys' fees from the plaintiffs if the lawsuit is found to be frivolous. Plaintiffs' lawyers in the United States, on the other hand, receive compensation only if the cases are settled or won: they have no incentive to bring frivolous cases. There has not been, and there will not be, a flood of frivolous obesity-related lawsuits. The industry's real fear, rather, is of well-founded lawsuits, amply supported by compromising memos, obtained in discovery from company files that would demonstrate how many food companies engage in unfair or deceptive acts and practices that substantially contribute to the obesity epidemic.

\* \* \*

# Cheryl L. Hayne, Patricia A. Moran & Mary M. Ford, *Regulating Environments to Reduce Obesity*
### 25 J. PUB. HEALTH POL'Y 391–99 (2005)

\* \* \*

. . . [R]egulatory interventions can help create a food environment more conducive to healthy dietary practices. Regulatory interventions may come in many forms. In order to illustrate two potential regulatory fulcra for legal levers, we will focus here on product labeling and advertising restrictions, and two federal agencies.

. . . .

## Restaurant Food Labeling

The Food and Drug Administration has authority to regulate nutritional labeling of processed foods in the United States. The Federal Food, Drug and Cosmetic Act, however, exempts restaurants. They are not required to disclose nutrition information. This exemption seems out-of-date, as Americans now spend about half of their food budget purchasing meals and drinks outside of the home. Exempting the restaurant and fast-food industry from disclosing the content and nutritional value makes it difficult for consumers to estimate the energy content of the food they consume away from home. And food eaten outside of the home is generally higher in fat and lower in other nutrients than food prepared at home. Many popular table-service restaurants serve 1000–2000 calories per meal, or 35% to 100% of a full day's energy required for most adults. . . . Mandating point-of-sale nutritional information for customers could combat increased portion sizes and decreased nutritional value of fast-food and restaurant meals as eating out becomes a larger part of U.S. food consumption. This information might enable consumers to make informed dietary decisions. It could also encourage restaurants to modify their ingredients and menus to provide greater healthy and nutritious food and beverage options to their customers.

## Advertising

Food manufacturers' and restaurant chains' advertising encourages consumers to purchase unhealthy foods and make poor dietary decisions. Children are a particularly attractive marketing target. Their increasing buying power and influence on goods purchased for the wider household have encouraged the food industry to target children. In many countries, advertising for energy-dense food targeting children has increased relative to other age group targets. Considerable effort goes into planning the seeds of brand loyalty with this vulnerable group.

High exposure of children to advertisements for foods high in fat and sugar is believed to be a major contributor to obesity. [A study found that] eight in ten adults agree that business marketing and advertising exploit children by convincing them to buy things that are bad for them or that they don't need.

The study found these concerns highest in relation to food and nutrition issues. Most foods advertised to children — fast food, sweets, ice creams, and carbonated drinks — are highly processed, high in fat and/or sugar and low in nutrients; providing "empty calories." Food marketing has not only undermined parents' dietary preferences, but these highly marketed foods in children's diets contribute to early increasing weight and associated health problems. Eighty percent of obese adolescents remain obese as adults, primarily because dietary habits developed when young persist for a lifetime. That advertising of these products is a direct cause of children's weight and health problems appears to be widely accepted by critics and by some policy makers. Advertising must be effective or why else would the food industry spend so much on it?

In the United States alone, the U.S. food industry spends about $11 billion annually on advertising in addition to another $22 billion on other consumer promotions. Such expenditures dwarf the National Cancer Institute's $1 million annual investment in its educational "5-A-Day" campaign to increase fruit and vegetable consumption or the $1.5 million budget of the National Heart, Lung and Blood Institute's National Cholesterol Education Campaign. . . .

Governments both here and elsewhere might intervene with regulatory actions restricting food marketing practices to overcome this market failure. No one has suggested that governments are likely to spend enough on informational efforts to overcome current industry advertising practices. Provided with balanced information and no longer bombarded pervasively by advertisements for high-calorie, high-fat and high-sugar products, perhaps consumers will have the ability to make healthier food purchasing decisions.

Unlike the FDA, which would need legislative changes before regulating restaurants, the Federal Communications Commission already regulates radio and television broadcasting. Might it consider requiring broadcasters to provide equal time for messages promoting healthy eating and physical activity? Perhaps a greater opportunity comes from restricting advertising of high-calorie, low-nutrient foods on television programming commonly watched by children. If the FCC prohibited "junk food" advertisers from targeting children under a specific age, would children be less likely to purchase, or ask their parents to purchase, unhealthy foods?

The United States could make substantial contributions to the international obesity epidemic, were it to step up efforts to regulate the industry and the food environment to promote healthier and more informed consumer choice. Regulatory actions are already gaining acceptance abroad. . . .

. . . .

The nutritional labeling of foods consumed away from home and health-conscious advertising limitations are two areas that are worthy of regulatory consideration. As discussed above, children have become targets for aggressive advertising of unhealthy foods. Advertising, however, is only one factor fueling the overweight epidemic; certain aspects of the school environment also encourage weight gain and inactivity among children. The school environment offers some promising opportunities for regulators.

# THE SCHOOL ENVIRONMENT

Schools offer an opportunity to address the increasing incidence and prevalence of overweight among children and adolescents. Because children spend a high percentage of their formative years at school, a healthy school environment could influence a child's eating and fitness habits for years to come. . . .

## The National School Lunch Program

The National School Lunch Program (NSLP), administered by the United States Department of Agriculture (USDA), serves lunch to approximately 2.5 million American children each school day. Schools choosing to participate receive donated commodities and cash subsidies. They are obliged to provide free or reduced-price lunches to eligible low-income children. All lunches and snacks served under the NSLP must meet federal nutritional guidelines: no more than 30% of calories may be from total fat and no more than 10% from saturated fat; and the lunch must contain one-third of Recommended Daily Allowances for calories, protein, iron, calcium, and vitamins A and C.

Many school cafeterias also offer foods not currently regulated by the USDA. Products sold á la carte or in vending machines, in competition with the NSLP, generally lack comparable nutritional value. Researchers studying 20 Minnesota secondary schools found that high-fat foods such as chips, crackers and ice cream constituted 21.5% of the available á la carte items; while a mere 4.5% of the á la carte items were fruits and vegetables. Two-thirds of the schools examined had soft drink contracts for vending machines. Adolescents have increased their consumption of high-sugar soft drinks by 100% in the last 20 years. Not surprisingly, this energy intake has been linked to weight gain.

Improvements to the NSLP could help combat the obesity epidemic. Expanding NSLP authority to regulate á la carte items and vending may be an avenue to control the types of foods offered to students. With greater authority, it would be possible to replace high-fat and high-sugar food with more nutritious choices.

## Physical and Nutrition Education

One key regulatory opportunity at the state level lies in improvements to physical and nutrition education programs. A recent survey shows that state physical education mandates are usually general and include only minimum recommendations leaving interpretations up to local school districts. Resulting physical education programs often fail to meet the recommendations of the Surgeon General and CDC for daily physical education. A report published by the National Center for Education Statistics shows similar deficits in nutrition education: In grades kindergarten to eight only 50% of schools were required by state or district mandates to provide nutrition education. This figure drops to 40% for grades 9 and 10 and to 20% for grades 11 and 12. Failure to fund nutrition and physical education ultimately results in increased state and federal healthcare spending. State mandates to require daily physical education and quality nutrition education in all primary and secondary schools might reduce obesity, but could prove costly to school districts.

*Vending Contracts*

Local schools have the power to make the greatest and most immediate impact to combat overweight children and adolescents by eliminating soft drink vending machines. Soft drink vending machines have become a ubiquitous fixture in schools in the United States. In Minnesota, 98% of secondary schools and 44% of elementary schools . . . have vending machines. Researchers have found that each daily serving of a sugar-sweetened beverage increases the odds of becoming obese by 1.6.

If vending machine contracts can be modified or eliminated so that machines are either removed or promote healthy beverages, students would have less access to sugary beverages and consumption would decline. This is not unprecedented: The Los Angeles Board of Education has taken action to eliminate the availability of soft drinks in all elementary, middle and high schools and Texas has recently started controlling soft drinks, as well.

But special consideration must be given to school budget constraints and dependence on revenues from vending machines and other food marketing. When Texas took a first step to regulate food choices in the Texas Public School System by issuing new nutrition policies and restricting the availability of soft drinks and high-fat foods, it tried to offset any disruption to school fundraising with a program from the Texas Department of Agriculture to help school districts learn to raise funds without using food.

*Limitations of Regulations in the School Environment*

Students spend about 7 hours a day for 180 days a year in the school environment and most consume at least one of three meals per day in school. From 35% to 40% of adolescents' total energy intake is being consumed in secondary school. Schools influence a child's eating, drinking and fitness behavior. At home, many children live (and consume most of their calories) in the company of family members who eat poorly. Schools can temper this problem by involving parents in the school's nutrition initiatives. Intense academic requirements and limited budgets often leave little time for physical and nutrition education. Children must be healthy and ready to learn, thus, curriculum reform to improve academic results might well be approached holistically, taking into account not only intellectual growth but physical health and fitness.

. . . .

# THE BUILT ENVIRONMENT

[The authors then discuss their views on the "built environment," the various aspects of a community's physical layout, which creates opportunities for exercise and physical activity.]

\* \* \*

## THE CALIFORNIA CHILDHOOD OBESITY PREVENTION ACT OF 2005

The Legislature finds and declares as follows:

In the past two decades obesity has doubled in children, and tripled in adolescents. On average, 30 percent of California's children are overweight, and in some school districts, anywhere from 40 to 50 percent of California's pupils are overweight. Only 2 percent of California's adolescents, between the ages of 12 and 17 years, inclusive, have eating habits that meet national dietary recommendations. Only 23 percent of pupils in grades 5, 7, and 9 are physically fit. Almost half of the children and adolescents diagnosed with diabetes have the Type 2 form of the disease, which is strongly linked to obesity and lack of exercise. One in four obese children have early signs of Type 2 diabetes.

Overweight and physical inactivity costs California an estimated 24.6 billion dollars annually, approximately seven hundred fifty dollars ($750) per person — a cost that is expected to rise by another 32 percent by the year 2005. Poor nutrition and physical inactivity account for more preventable deaths (28 percent) than anything other than tobacco — more than AIDS, violence, car crashes, alcohol, and drugs combined. The long-term impact of childhood obesity on California's economy, and on our children's increased risk of death from heart disease, cancer, stroke, and diabetes will be staggering. Approximately 300,000 deaths in the United States per year are currently associated with obesity and overweight; the total direct and indirect costs attributed to overweight and obesity amounted to 117 billion dollars in the year 2000. Obesity is linked to a larger increase of chronic health conditions and accounts for a significantly higher amount of health expenditures than those associated with smoking, heavy drinking, or poverty.

Each additional daily serving of sugar-sweetened soda increases a child's risk for obesity by 60 percent. Twenty years ago, boys consumed more than twice as much milk as soft drinks, and girls consumed 50 percent more milk than soft drinks. By 1996, both boys and girls consumed twice as many soft drinks as milk. Soft drinks now comprise the leading source of added sugar in a child's diet. Teenage boys consume twice the recommended amount of sugar each day, almost one-half of which (44 percent) comes from soft drinks. Teenage girls consume almost three times the recommended amount of sugar, 40 percent of which comes from soft drinks.

A study of 9th and 10th grade girls found that those who drank colas were five times more likely to develop bone fractures, and girls who drank other carbonated beverages were three times more likely to suffer bone fractures than non-consumers of carbonated beverages. Decreased milk consumption means that children are no longer getting required amounts of calcium in their diets. The average teenage girl now consumes 40 percent less calcium than she needs, putting her at high risk of osteoporosis in her later years.

[The legislation then amended the pre-existing law concerning sale of beverages to pupils at elementary, middle, or junior high schools, California Education Code § 49931.5 to read in part:]

(a) (1) Regardless of the time of day, only the following beverages may be sold to a pupil at an elementary school:

(A) Fruit-based drinks that are composed of no less than 50 percent fruit juice and have no added sweetener.

(B) Vegetable-based drinks that are composed of no less than 50 percent vegetable juices and have no added sweetener.

(C) Drinking water with no added sweetener.

(D) Two-percent-fat milk, one-percent-fat milk, nonfat milk, soy milk, rice milk, and other similar nondairy milk.

(a) (2) An elementary school may permit the sale of beverages that do not comply with paragraph (1) as part of a school fundraising event in any of the following circumstances:

(A) The items are sold by pupils of the school and the sale of those items takes place off and away from the premises of the school.

(B) The items are sold by pupils of the school and the sale of those items takes place one-half hour or more after the end of the school day.

(a) (3) From one-half hour before the start of the school day to one-half hour after the end of the school day, only the following beverages may be sold to a pupil at a middle or junior high school:

(A) Fruit-based drinks that are composed of no less than 50 percent fruit juice and have no added sweetener.

(B) Vegetable-based drinks that are composed of no less than 50 percent vegetable juice and have no added sweetener.

(C) Drinking water with no added sweetener.

(D) Two-percent-fat milk, one-percent-fat milk, nonfat milk, soy milk, rice milk, and other similar nondairy milk.

(E) An electrolyte replacement beverage that contains no more than 42 grams of added sweetener per 20-ounce serving.

(a) (4) A middle or junior high school may permit the sale of beverages that do not comply with paragraph (3) as part of a school event if the sale of those items meets all of the following criteria:

(A) The sale occurs during a school-sponsored event and takes place at the location of that event at least one-half hour after the end of the school day.

(B) Vending machines, pupil stores, and cafeterias are used later than one-half hour after the end of the school day.

(a) (5) This subdivision does not prohibit an elementary, or middle or junior high school from making available through a vending machine any beverage allowed under paragraph (1) or (3) at any time of day, or, in middle and junior high schools, any beverage that does not comply with paragraph (3) if the beverage only is available not later than one-half hour before the start of the school day and not sooner than one-half hour after the end of the school day.

(b) (1) Commencing July 1, 2007, no less than 50 percent of all beverages sold to a pupil from one-half hour before the start of the school day until one-half hour after the end of the school day shall be those enumerated by paragraph (3).

(b) (2) Commencing July 1, 2009, all beverages sold to a pupil from one-half hour before the start of the school day until one-half hour after the end of the school day shall be those enumerated by paragraph (3).

(b) (3) Beverages allowed under this subdivision are all of the following:

(A) Fruit-based drinks that are composed of no less than 50 percent fruit juice and have no added sweetener.

(B) Vegetable-based drinks that are composed of no less than 50 percent vegetable juice and have no added sweetener.

(C) Drinking water with no added sweetener.

(D) Two-percent-fat milk, one-percent-fat milk, nonfat milk, soy milk, rice milk, and other similar nondairy milk.

(E) An electrolyte replacement beverage that contains no more than 42 grams of added sweetener per 20-ounce serving.

\* \* \*

## Rogan Kersh & James A. Morone, *Obesity, Courts, & The New Politics of Public Health*
### 30 J. HEALTH POL., POL'Y & L. 839 (2005)

\* \* \*

The image is among the most memorable in recent political history. Seven tobacco company executives stood before a House subcommittee in April 1994, affirming under oath that nicotine is not addictive and that cigarette smoking does not cause cancer. Both claims were quickly exposed as fraudulent, inspiring public outrage, official inquiries, legislative proposals, and denunciations from every quarter including the Oval Office. Government action eventually followed, but it took a distinctive form — one that does not fit neatly into our usual models of health care policy making.

Congress debated bold changes but failed to enact any significant legislation affecting the tobacco industry. Parts of the executive branch also attempted strong action and fell short; the U.S. Food and Drug Administration (FDA) moved to regulate tobacco as a drug but the industry blocked the effort in the courts. State and local governments wrestled with the issue and came up with limited restrictions, most notably smoking bans in some public places. Decisive government actions — a whopping $246 billion financial settlement, dramatic limits on marketing, restrictions on advertising, and selective smoking bans — all took place in the judicial branch. In a relatively speedy and creative burst, the courts broke a legislative logjam, dramatically reshaped a vast public health domain, and changed the public policy calculus for activists, policy makers, medical professionals, the tobacco industry, and millions of smokers.

The tobacco case marked an important change in American health policy. In particular, it introduced two features that are, we argue, increasingly typical of the political process.

First, tobacco turned the political focus onto what had once been seen as purely private behavior. . . . Today, however, the political urge to regulate private behavior extends to a growing array of issues: tobacco, obesity, abortion, the right to die, drug abuse, and even a patient's relationship with his or her managed care organization. The list goes on. Traditional health policy debates turned on avowedly public matters such as building a health care infrastructure (through programs like Hill-Burton), increasing access to health care (national health insurance), or organizing research (Centers for Disease Control). . . .

Second, regulating private behavior prompts a distinctive political process. To place an issue on the political agenda, advocates must persuade others that private behavior holds important public ramifications. [T]hat threshold puts a particular premium on demonizing either users or providers. Although regulating private behavior . . . often bogs down in legislative stalemate, the focus on individuals makes it especially well suited for judicial action. The emphasis on regulating private behavior leads to an increasing reliance on the courts. . . .

. . . .

Understanding the new health policy frame is crucial for analyzing the politics of obesity, and obesity, in turn, offers a clear illustration of the emerging political pattern. . . .

## Making the Problem Political

. . . .

Obesity's rise to political prominence — to a "crisis demanding action" — has been astonishingly swift. Fewer than a dozen stories on obesity-related public policy appeared in major U.S. media outlets during the final quarter of 1999. The surgeon general issued an alarm, in the form of the first official report on obesity, in 2001. By the final quarter of 2002, the stack of obesity articles topped 1200 — a thousand-fold increase. Over 1400 stories appeared during the second quarter (April-June) of 2003, and the total has remained well over 1000 stories per quarter since. Most national publicity offers variations on the same theme: Americans face a crisis. The obesity epidemic reaches beyond adults and increasingly endangers children. An estimated one in three U.S. adolescents are overweight (15 percent are clinically obese), a figure that has tripled in the past twenty years; some 80 percent of this group will become obese adults.

Two institutional forces propel the problem onto the public agenda: the medical establishment and the financial incentives in our high-cost health care system. Both are longstanding features of the American policy scene. They helped drive the tobacco wars, and they are likely to turn other risky private behaviors into policy problems in the future.

. . . When the health care establishment converges on a message, especially a warning of danger, it becomes front-page news. Obesity had been a medical concern since the 1950s, but it was much more recently — and very suddenly — that medical leaders such as the Surgeon General, prominent physicians, and health researchers began targeting fat as the nation's greatest public health danger.

Physicians urge the government to combat obesity on two broad grounds. First, reducing obesity clearly has life-saving and life-prolonging effects. Second, reduced obesity can significantly enhance the quality of life, especially among adolescents and young adults. Health specialists have powerfully documented these claims. . . .

. . . .

America's high — and rising — health care costs mean that people's risky private behavior raises taxes (for government health care) and increases premiums (for private insurance). There is a direct economic logic to arresting bad health behavior. In an era when no policy assessment is complete without cost-benefit analysis, the fight against obesity gets plenty of attention.

. . . .

Many policy makers who dismiss the health alarms find themselves moved by budgetary arguments, especially when they are made by business leaders. Prominent business periodicals showcased a 1998 study analyzing the economic burden of obesity on American businesses; the increased costs of health insurance, sick leave, and disability insurance came to an estimated $12.7 billion. . . .

Identifying a national health problem does not, in itself, guide policy makers to a solution. A comprehensive public-opinion survey undertaken by political scientists . . . suggests a distinct lack of public consensus about the topic; however, media attention to the politics of fat has spiraled since their survey was conducted in spring 2001. As public health warnings mount, pressure for some kind of government action increases. In fact, the spotlight on obesity has drawn attention from the White House, Congress, and all fifty states. A nation that is extremely chary of explicit limits on health care — we dread rationing health care — is always eager to identify a culprit behind inexorably rising costs. But what might policy makers do about eating?

Framing a response requires explaining the root of the problem. Why are people overweight and obese? Two overarching explanations define two very different kinds of solutions, involving dramatically different policy recommendations. The responses are not mutually exclusive. Indeed, in the past, both worked together to prompt government action. However, in our highly partisan political environment, political activists often seize on one and dismiss the other.

An explanation dating to the early twentieth century blames individuals for getting fat. They lack willpower; they make foolish food choices; they live unhealthy lifestyles. A century of diets is built on this logic. So are endless late-night advertisements touting (rather dangerous-looking) devices that promise to restore American abs to their prelapsarian condition. Fat people, the argument goes — like smokers or heavy drinkers — make their own personal choices. . . .

. . . .

An alternative definition of the problem targets an "unhealthy food environment." Suddenly, a dizzying variety of health snares snap into focus. For starters, American portion sizes have undergone an extraordinary expansion. The typical hamburger in 1957, for example, weighed in at one ounce (and 210 calories). Today, that burger is up to six ounces (618 calories) — and that is before you add bacon, cheese, super-sized fries (another 610 calories all by themselves), and a double gulp (sixty-four-ounce) soft drink. . . .

A subtler version of the same problem lies in hidden ingredients. Food specialists, such as Brownell and Horgen, point out that even relatively healthy products come loaded with sugar, which is "a cheap way to make food taste good.". . .

Obesity as a policy problem is redefined, in this perspective, and focuses on a powerful food industry organized to push ever more calories into the American public. The problem includes hidden content, portion size, relentless advertising, and the ubiquity of high-fat junk food. (Your airport terminal gate is never far from a donut).

Some critics take the next step and identify corporate villains. Food merchants cynically manipulate children. They put soda machines in schools and fast-food outlets in the lunchrooms. Nothing moves the political system like tales of greed and profit — especially when they menace kids. . . .

When policy makers trace the problem partially to the industry (or, less pointedly, the "food environment") rather than obese people themselves, an entirely different set of solutions comes into view. These include more detailed food labels, controlling the advertising directed at children, rethinking school nutrition, regulating the fat content of foods, imposing higher taxes on unhealthy ingredients, punishing false or misleading nutritional claims, and subsidizing healthy alternatives. This roster of strong action — echoing tobacco policy outcomes — represents a series of strategies for shifting the incentives that face the food industry today.

Of course, redefining the problem also redefines the politics. At first, most industries resist government regulation and this one has done so extremely effectively. The food industry — well organized, well financed, and politically savvy — does not deny the obesity crisis or epidemic. Rather, it shifts attention to the first definition of the problem, focusing on individual diet and lifestyle.

Still, as long as public attention remains focused on obesity, the definition of the problem — personal or environmental or both — will remain contested. Policy makers typically begin by following the path of least political resistance.

Public policy focuses on individuals and unexceptional efforts (strong on exhortation and symbols) to help them stay healthy. If the problem (or, rather, the publicity) persists, the prospect of more complex and intrusive public action emerges. Actual decisions — concrete policy choices — turn our attention to the political arenas themselves.

## Traditional Health Policy Institutions Respond

Issues often move through the policy stream fueled more by rhetoric than action. Obesity has been no exception. A drumbeat of messages from the Bush administration and congressional leaders primarily encourages self-help activities such as exercise and sensible eating. Congress's highest profile activity concerning obesity has involved efforts to ban lawsuits against the food industry. Will government action grow bolder?

. . . .

[S]tudents of recent health policy know that change — especially at the national level — has been either halting or nonexistent. Health care reform, a patient's bill of rights, the tobacco settlement, medical privacy regulations, malpractice reform, and a host of other policies have all failed to pass Congress. The most significant health care measure enacted in recent years, a prescription drug benefit, has encountered massive criticism (including from former backers such as the American Association of Retired Persons [AARP]) and is likely to be revamped considerably. . . .

Congress's principal response to obesity has been a wealth of rhetoric deploring the crisis, along with occasional expressions of concern about consumption habits and (from the Democratic minority) industry practices. Scant legislation has resulted. . . .

Why such congressional inaction in the face of what observers on both the left and the right define as a policy crisis? Political scientists have perhaps over-explained the stalemate. The checks and balances of the American political system make any ambitious change difficult, and barriers have multiplied in recent years. Congress is evenly divided and fiercely partisan. Recent trends in political campaigning exacerbate this partisanship, thanks to a revolution in political information technology that permits the majority party in each state to craft safe congressional districts. . . .

Obesity politics is further complicated by the dizzying array of foods and the complicated claims and counterclaims about nutrition. Naturally, food companies and their lobbyists play a major political role. . . . However, food producers are different from tobacco companies. Once regulations begin to take hold, different sectors of the industry — health foods, organic producers, fruit companies — might abandon the united front and seek market advantage in a new anti-fat regulatory regime. Still, these are speculations for the distant future. . . .

The Department of Health and Human Services (DHHS) has also been rhetorically active. In May 2003 alone, for example, Secretary Tommy Thompson issued major statements on Americans' physical activity and on the

costs of obesity, sponsored a national town meeting on obesity-related diabetes, and called for society to "pressure the food industry, the fast food industry, [and] the soft-drink industry . . . to offer healthier foods" (while rejecting
lawsuits as an option for doing so). In the early Fall [of 2004] Thompson publicly challenged overweight employees of the Department of Health and
Human Services to improve their health and launched a weight-loss regimen
himself. . . .

But no concrete policy recommendations, much less integrated programs for
combating obesity, have been issued from the DHHS secretary's office. . . .

The FDA has also moved slowly with respect to obesity politics. . . .

. . . [T]he executive branch is subject to multiple and overlapping jurisdictions over personal health behaviors such as smoking and obesity. The DHHS,
the Agriculture Department, the FDA, and even the Office of Management
and Budget (through its central clearance authority) all have important
responsibilities for various aspects of the food and obesity issue. As with
Congress, the executive branch's institutional framework blunts policy action.
And where national executive and legislative officials tread cautiously (or not
at all), other actors move to fill the void.

The obesity epidemic has set off a flurry of activity in the states. . . . A patchwork quilt of state laws now seeks to reduce obesity rates by getting tough
with food industry (through policies like junk food taxes) on the one hand and
protecting the industry (by banning lawsuits) on the other. Inconsistent programs across different states — and the vulnerability of state regulatory
regimes to industry lobbying efforts — push anti-obesity advocates and stakeholders such as school officials to seek coherent national policies. And the
judiciary may be the easiest venue in which to pursue such a systematic policy.
The emerging politics of public health — with its emphasis on regulating private behavior — makes the courts an increasingly important locus of decision.

## The New Litigation and Public Health

The judiciary remains the most active venue for social change in health politics, especially on the federal level. In part this is by simple default — the
other branches are not inclined (or not able) to act. Moreover, issues of private
behavior fit easily into the judicial process. . . .

. . . .

Litigious approaches to public policy take several different forms. The most
prominent has traditionally been class-action lawsuits and a subset of these,
mass torts. Each has entered a new phase in recent years. During their initial
surge in the 1960s, class-action suits primarily concerned civil rights, securities, or consumer issues; lawyers aimed to recover compensation for injured
parties or to encourage regulatory enforcement. These goals are present in the
recent public health court cases, but are supplemented by a novel twist. [There
is] a shift to a "new litigation" characterized by an emerging form of social policy torts: "In addition to seeking monetary compensation for individuals and
public entities, the new litigation seeks the kind of industry-wide changes in

corporate products and practices that advocates have pursued, without much success, in state and federal legislatures. . . ."

The most prominent social policy torts have directly addressed public health issues blocked in Congress. Many of these cases involve private behavior, including tobacco, obesity, dietary supplements, patients' rights, and gun safety. Efforts to regulate private behavior have traditionally landed in the courts, perhaps because such issues require governments to negotiate the tension between public needs and private rights. Now, however, a much broader range of public health matters — managed care, asbestos, pharmaceutical costs and imports, diesel emissions, and so forth — have also moved from Congress to the courts.

Why does this new litigation have such a distinctly public health tint? Perhaps the answer lies in common denominators running across the cases: a large collection of affected individuals (smokers, health-plan members, pharmaceutical users, etc.); an easily identifiable corporate target ("Big Tobacco," gun manufacturers, managed care bureaucracies, fast food companies); widespread demands for action; and stalemate on Capitol Hill, in the White House, or both. In each case a coalition of advocates has formed, often led by state attorneys general and private class-action attorneys — a novel public-private combination in American politics.

The first obesity cases are now just reaching the courts, accompanied by angry complaints from politicians seeking to block intrusive action in the legislatures and administrative agencies. What does the future hold for this new spate of suits? A closer look at the tobacco example may provide a rough guide. It also offers cautions for every political side. Tobacco illustrates both the promises and the pitfalls of the new litigation.

[The authors then review the history of the tobacco litigation discussed in Chapter Five of these materials.]

This wave of new litigation featured three principal elements. First, a broad coalition of state and federal actors, including attorneys general and tort lawyers, formed around the tobacco issue. . . . Second, this coalition sought not merely punitive or civil damages, but sweeping changes in the tobacco industry's products and practices — in short, they pursued policy goals more normally associated with legislatures. Enormous media attention marked the tobacco case, as it does other social-policy torts. Third, the anti-smoking coalition adopted a multi-district litigation strategy, collecting lawsuits arising from similar circumstances and bringing them before a single court or judge. . . .

This description of the new litigation helps explain how courts became the key locus of action in the tobacco wars, a development that increasingly characterizes health politics more generally. First, inaction in national elective branches led an aroused public (spurred by interest-group advocates and expansive media coverage) to demand other means of redress. Second, a set of entrepreneurial actors, some relatively new to national politics, actively promoted their cause in the courts. Foremost among these were state attorneys general, who since the 1970s had become far more active, expanding their caseloads and filing more amicus briefs in Supreme Court cases. Initially their heightened workload was primarily in antitrust, civil rights, and consumer protection; with tobacco they turned to public health on a national scale. Similarly, tort lawyers have increased their presence in various realms of national policy making, including health care, during and after the 1980s. These plaintiffs' attorneys also adopted a much more coordinated strategy during the tobacco fight, a practice that has continued in other public health suits.

. . . .

Anti-smoking activists' jurisprudential strategy was not an unmitigated success. The courts blocked the FDA's effort to expand its authority and regulate tobacco as a drug; that move would have permitted extensive government intervention in the tobacco business. In effect, multiple court rulings add up to a kind of judicially imposed compromise between public health advocates and the tobacco industry. As the courts begin to dominate public health politics, the limits of judicial capacity become more important.

The tobacco case as well as class actions affecting managed care, gun manufacturers, asbestos producers, diesel engine emissions, and other industries — all pursued in the name of protecting public health — suggests that courts can be the locus for sweeping policy change. But should they perform this role? . . .

. . . [C]ritics argue that the constitutionality of court decision making is ambiguous. The Constitution plainly emphasizes policy making through elected — and therefore more accountable — officials in Congress, the executive branch, and state legislatures. Critics of judicial policy making caution further that the rights approach favored by courts is inappropriate for addressing complex social issues; the stare decisis requirement binds judges in ways that limit their inclination or ability to create policy innovations. . . .

Moreover, continue the critics, courts are usually inadequately equipped to deal with the technical, specialized nature of most policy concerns. Judges and litigators are trained as generalists, leaving them poorly situated to resolve complex questions concerning health effects, medical technologies, and the like. On another critical front, a glut of cases can result from mass-tort action in a public health arena, overwhelming the judiciary's capacity to address the issue. . . .

Beyond these principled reasons to oppose court involvement in public policy making, some critics question the effectiveness of judicial activity. In the tobacco case, the aftermath of the 1998 settlement has witnessed only a slight decline in smoking rates across the United States. . . . Alongside these evolving empirical judgments, a related matter colors the tobacco case — and, by extension, the broader implications of new social policy litigation: the politics of implementation. Courts are rarely able to devote sustained attention or significant resources to implement their policy directives; the tobacco settlement provides a prominent example of this difficulty with regulation by litigation.

A related source of controversy is the distribution of settlement funds. The 1998 Master Settlement Agreement includes no restrictions on how states spend their share of the $246 billion — monies that will be provided in perpetuity and that may well be replenished by additional judgments against tobacco companies. Thus, a new set of distributional political issues arises in the wake of regulatory controversies. Some states, including Montana and Michigan, opted for state constitutional amendments governing their settlement allocations; others, including Pennsylvania and North Carolina, fought the matter out in their legislatures and in state courts. Thus one result of the new litigation approach to tobacco, again mirrored in other public health debates, is a fresh round of legal battles in the implementation stage — further cause for lament to critics of judicial policy making.

The limited-capacity view of judicial involvement has won wide currency in contemporary political science scholarship on law and courts. But as a few legal scholars counter, we are constantly thrown back to the legislative stalemate. As demands for action — even cries of crisis — meet a divided legislature, political action flows willy-nilly to the courts. . . .

Other responses to judicial incapacity question the empirical evidence of courts' inability to act. . . . Courts have always been the final arbiters when private behaviors turn political. Now they have turned to a broad range of public health matters. Initial evidence confirms the judgment that the courts possess adequate institutional capacity. For better or worse, U.S. courts are remaking health policy related to tobacco, guns, asbestos, and HMOs. The food industry is now shaping up as the new litigators' next target.

* * *

# NOTES AND QUESTIONS

**1.** Are lawsuits such as *Pelman* viable? If they are, will they help reduce obesity and its consequent results?

The answer to the first question is yet to be determined. *Pelman V* left the plaintiff with a viable cause of action, at least sufficient to survive summary judgment, but the plaintiffs face substantial problems of proof if they take their case to trial. Moreover, the courts seem to have rejected most of the causes of action except for those under the New York trade laws; there may not be analogous legislation in other jurisdictions. On the other hand, both the trial judge and the appellate judges imply that they had some sympathy for the plaintiffs and some animus for the behavior of the defendants.

The barriers faced by future plaintiffs may even be greater than those faced by the *Pelman* plaintiffs. Louisiana and at least 12 other states have enacted laws since 1992 attempting to immunize the fast food industry from these sorts of lawsuits. For a review of pending lawsuits, legislation intended to immunize potential defendants, and references to other sources, see http://www.banzhaf.net/obesity/links/ (last visited December 2006).

The legal literature has been sparse but not particularly enthusiastic about these "chesseburger lawsuits." *See, e.g.,* Amy Vroom, *Fast Food or Fat Food: Food Manufacturer Liability for Obesity*, 72 DEF. COUNS. J. 56 (2005).

The public reaction to these lawsuits has paralleled the apparent view of the state legislatures in Louisiana and other states; Many if not most people think it is silly to claim that fast food purveyors have caused, in the legal sense of the term, people to become obese. But are these lawsuits as specious as they may appear at first glance? Are their parallels to the tobacco litigation discussed in Chapter Five — which many people thought were silly until all of the facts came out? Can you imagine some set of facts that may be discovered, comparable to the revelations about the nicotine cover-up and other fraudulent practices of the tobacco companies that might make these lawsuits more factually plausible or legally viable?

For a good history of food-related litigation, see Ellen J. Fried, *The Potential for Policy Initiatives to Address the Obesity Epidemic: A Legal Perspective From the United States* 270–80 in DAVID CRAWFORD & ROBERT W. JEFFERY, OBESITY PREVENTION AND PUBLIC HEALTH (2005).

**2.** Assume for the moment that "cheeseburger lawsuits" are not completely mooted by immunization legislation or rejected outright by the courts. What *should be* the standard for liability, even if causation and other related issues can be satisfied? Consider the following options:

     a. sellers or manufacturers of food should be liable if they fail to disclose a substantial health risk of which the average consumer would otherwise be unaware (a negligence standard)

     b. sellers or manufacturers of food should be liable if it is found that any product they sell is unreasonably dangerous (a strict liability standard)

     c. sellers or manufacturers of food should be liable if it is found that they have affirmatively concealed a substantial health risk associated with their product (a requirement of intentional malfeasance)

**3.** If privately initiated lawsuits are either not viable or not effective in combating the problems of obesity, are there market-based strategies that may resolve the problem? If Americans consumers started demanding more healthy foods, surely the retail food and restaurant industries would start selling more of them. But part of the problem is that many people don't know what is and is not healthy and lack the information to make those decisions.

Would better nutritional labeling help resolve this problem? The Food and Drug Administration has the authority to regulate the nutritional labeling of processed foods, although food served in restaurants is exempted from their authority. Should that exemption be removed? Are the current efforts of the FDA appropriate or sufficient? For a discussion, see Rebecca Fribush, *Putting Calories and Fat Counts on the Table: Should Mandatory Nutritional Disclosure laws Apply to Restaurant Foods?* 73 GEO. WASH. L. REV. 377 (2005).

Or is the problem more a matter of the *misinformation* and the other demand-inducing effects of food advertising? Should the government regulate food advertising more closely? Alternatively, should the government engage in more counter-advertising and consumer education? Any effort to regulate food advertising, of course, would have to overcome the same First Amendment concerns as discussed with respect to the regulation of tobacco advertising in

Chapter Five: It would have to be carefully tailored to meet the demands of the so-called *Central Hudson* test. For a good discussion, see Rachel Weiss & Jason Smith, *Legislative Approaches to the Obesity Epidemic*, 25 J. PUB. HEALTH POL'Y 379, 383–385 (2005).

**4.** There is a larger question here: whether public health policy should be made by the legislature — state or federal — or whether it should be made by the judiciary as part of resolving lawsuits initiated by individuals or other representatives of the public. As Kersh and Morone describe, plaintiffs brought litigation against the tobacco industry and the food industry after failing to persuade the legislature to take action. Are litigants more representative of the public than the legislature? If legislators are so secure in their seats that they do not need to respond to voters' concerns, is there any alternative? Kersh and Morone may view the courts as more influential than they are, but courts can at least respond to specific controversies. Whether or not litigation is a realistic tool, both the public and policy makers are increasingly considering legislation and liability rules to improve public health. These authors also note that issues that in past might have been characterized simply as public policy concerns, are increasingly considered public health issues: obesity, smoking, firearms, domestic violence, and even managed care. As with tobacco, public acceptance of social policies to address obesity increased dramatically when obesity was characterized as a serious health problem, rather than a cosmetic concern.

**5.** A few local communities and states have experimented with "fat taxes," taxes on soft drinks, fast foods, or other less-than-healthy food. Apparently such taxes can be a good source of revenue and, as "sin taxes," are somewhat less controversial than other forms of taxation. Whether they can have any effect on the consumption of these foods is harder to assess. For an extended review of "fat taxes," their effects, and related matters, see JEFF STRNAD, CONCEPTUALIZING THE "FAT TAX": THE ROLE OF FOOD TAXES IN DEVELOPED ECONOMIES (Working Paper July 2004) (*available at* http://ssrn.com/abstract_id=561321) (last visited March 2005). According to Strnad,

> As of the middle of 2000, 17 states and two major cities imposed junk food taxes. Eight other states have imposed junk food taxes in the past, but repealed them prior to 2000. . . .

> . . . Advocates now propose extending these taxes as a way to fund public health initiatives with respect to diet and exercise. The envisioned initiatives would counter what the advocates see as a "toxic environment" that provides access to and encourages consumption of a diet high in fat, high in calories, delicious, widely available, and low in cost. . . . The advocates emphasize that the taxes would not have to be very heavy, *e.g.*, on the order of a penny per can of soda, in order to raise substantial revenues, and they note that surveys indicates substantial support for small taxes conditional on the revenues being spent to fund health education programs.

> Tying junk food taxes to health initiative expenditures may create public appeal, but from a normative standpoint the justification for connecting the tax and the expenditure is not clear. . . .

A second set of tax proposals is much more ambitious. These proposals often fall under the moniker of the "fat taxes" because many of the proposed taxes would apply to fatty foods or to the fat content of foods. Some of the proposals are not limited to fat content. The most general simply call for taxing unhealthy foods and subsidizing healthy foods. In contrast to junk food taxes, fat taxes explicitly attempt to influence behavior to meet public health goals. [S]uch taxes are concerned about the impact of food taxes on consumption [not raising revenue].

. . . Focusing on this goal raises the question of why the government should interfere with individual choice with respect to diet. . . .

STRNAD at 5–6.

**6.** In Adam Benforado et al., *Broken Scales: Obesity and Justice in America,* 53 EMORY L. J. 1645 (2004) the authors attempt to assess the linkage between the availability of food, the efforts by corporate entities to encourage its consumption, and the apparent epidemic of obesity. They come to some interesting conclusions. As reflected in the following paragraph, they too challenge the assumption that obese people simply make bad decisions about what they choose to eat:

The point of this excursion into the realities of human eating has been to enable a critical, realistic analysis of the obesity crisis. The experience of eating is driven in powerful ways by the unseen realities of our interior situation and because these realities are hidden, our conceptions of the obese and overweight end up being tragically distorted. When we see fat people eating, we assume that hunger has nothing to do with it because we "know" that we feel hungry and eat when our bodies need more food, and their bodies clearly do not need more food. Eating by the obese and the overweight, we therefore mistakenly conclude, must be driven not by legitimate hunger and food needs, but by something less legitimate — something like gluttony, or at the very least, something arising from personal, dispositional choice.

Benforado at 1687–88.

**7.** As discussed in the Hayne article, the federal government has been involved in underwriting better nutrition in the nation's schools since 1946 when the first national school lunch program (NSLP) was enacted. Since that time, the program has been expanded to include federal aid for pre-school meals and "snacks," and grown to become a multi-billion undertaking serving tens of millions of children. While the program has been publicized as an attempt to ensure that the nation's children get enough to eat, the program's efforts to ensure that the meals that are provided are, in fact, healthy have been limited and enforcement of the program's dietary standards has been questionable.

According to amendments to the NSLP enacted in 2004, all participating schools must establish "local wellness policies" including goals for improving nutrition, physical activity, and nutrition education by July 2006. *See* Pub.

Law. No. 108-265, § 204, codified at 42 U.S.C. § 1751. Whether this will be still another unenforceable federal requirement remains to be seen.

For additional description of the NSLP, related legislation, and references to other sources, see www.schoolnutrition.org/Index (last visited December 2006).

**8.** One issue that has drawn considerable public attention and some political action is the extent to which soft drink and other fast-food retailers have been allowed to advertise in schools, either as part of the "Channel One" in-school television programming or through logos or other advertisements on school facilities, athletic score boards, or vending machines. During the last decade many schools — as many as 75 percent nationwide — have entered some sort of contractual arrangement with one or another soft drink company, allowing advertising privileges in return for cash or in-kind contributions. Should schools be able to do this? Should this be considered as part of the education of students or simply as a matter of revenue raising?

For a relevant and provocative study that seems to indicate that consumption of soda pop is an important and direct cause of obesity in children, see David Ludwig et al., *Relation Between Consumption of Sugar-Sweetened Drinks and Childhood Obesity: A Prospective, Observational Analysis,* 357 LANCET 505 (2001). Among other things, the authors concluded that "the odds of becoming obese among children increased 1.6 times for each additional can or glass of sugar-sweetened drink that they consumed every day." Ludwig at 507.

In what may be regarded as one hopeful sign, Coca-Cola, Pepsico, and other soft drink companies announced in August of 2005 that they had agreed to limit — voluntarily — the sale of soft drinks in elementary, middle, and high schools. According to a statement published August 17, 2005, and distributed through the media, no carbonated soft drinks, diet or regular, will be sold in vending machines in elementary schools; in middle schools regular carbonated soft drinks will not be sold in vending machines, although diet soft drinks, and "alternative drinks" such as bottled water, sports drinks, and juice may be. In high schools, no more than half the vending machines can be filled with carbonated soft drinks. Whether this policy will be followed or not, remains to be seen. More importantly, whether it will have any measurable impact on the amount of soft drinks consumed or, more importantly, the health status of school children, also is yet to be determined.

**9.** As set out in the text, in 2005 California passed legislation that may have mooted the voluntary efforts of the soft drink industry and gone several steps further in efforts to improve the nutrition available in its public schools.

Arkansas has undertaken a more active program aimed at the obesity problem among the state's children. In 2005, the state made an assessment of the BWI of virtually all (98 percent) of the children in the state's schools. The results were sobering: 21 percent of the state's public school students were rated as overweight and an additional 17 percent were considered "at risk for overweight." (Less than 2 percent were considered "underweight.") The results were not uniform through the state. In some school districts nearly 50 percent of the children were considered overweight. The rates also were somewhat higher for males and for members of racial minority groups. As a result of these findings, each school district was required to implement a school nutrition and physical activity program. For a description and assessment, see http://www.achi.net (last visited December 2006).

**10.** Is obesity a public health problem in the sense that public health agencies should be undertaking efforts comparable to those described in earlier chapters? Beyond school-based programs targeting children, what other public health measures are currently under consideration? For one interesting effort to devise a comprehensive attack on obesity, see WALTER C. WILLETT & SERENA DOMOLKY, STRATEGIC PLAN FOR THE PREVENTION AND CONTROL OF OVERWEIGHT AND OBESITY IN NEW ENGLAND found at www.neconinfo. org/docs/StrategicPlan (last visited December 2006).

For a related academic review, see Marion Nestle & Michael F. Jacobson, *Halting the Obesity Epidemic: A Public Health Policy Approach,* 115 PUB. HEALTH REP. 12 (2000).

**11.** Everyone seems to agree that American eat too much of the wrong foods — and get too little exercise to burn their excess calories. But what should Americans eat? For one attempt to outline what are healthy eating habits, see U.S. DEPT. OF AGRICULTURE AND DEPT. OF HEALTH AND HUMAN SERVICES, DIETARY GUIDELINES OF AMERICANS (5th ed. 2005) (found at www.health.gov/dietaryguidelines/ (last visited December 2006). See also the newly revised "food pyramid," *available at* www.mypyramid.gov (last visited December 2006).

# Chapter 7

# FIREARMS AND GUN CONTROL

## A. INTRODUCTION

At first encounter, any suggestion that firearms and gun control should be considered as public health issues may seem somewhat overreaching. After all, as gun enthusiasts are fond of saying, guns don't kill people; people kill people. If anything needs to be viewed as a public health problem, it is the individual who misbehaves, not the instrument that is used in that misbehavior. Moreover, to the extent that guns and the people that use them should be controlled, most of the gun-related conduct that leads to death and injury involves activities that are already governed by the criminal law. What value is there in viewing guns and their use through the same lens that we used to examine such things as unhealthy behavior, exposure to disease, and other traditional public health matters?

To begin with, guns are not really that qualitatively different than many of the other matters already discussed in these materials. Tobacco, as we have seen, appears to provide pleasure notwithstanding its well-established dangers to its users; junk food is not all that bad for your health unless and until it is ingested excessively; cars without seat belts and air-bags (and motorcyclists without helmets) are not unsafe to their occupants until there is an accident. Yet in these cases, government policymakers may regulate the products themselves, not just the individuals who use (or abuse) them. (Airbags are mandatory in cars; helmets much meet manufacturing requirements. Indeed, countless products must meet health and safety requirements in order to be sold at all). For that matter, civil and/or criminal law enforcement and public health remedies are not mutually exclusive, either as a matter of efficiency or political choice.

More importantly, viewing firearms and gun control in the same manner as other public health topics allows us to shift away from identifying individual "culprits" and affixing individual blame for death and harm — or at least from doing so exclusively — and towards the identification of causation in the broader sense of the term: What are the causal factors that lead to gun-related harm in various populations? How can those causal links be altered to reduce the frequency of death and injury? What is the most cost-effective way to produce the maximum beneficial impact — given the range of interventions public health analysis invites us to consider?

As the material in the first part of this chapter is intended to demonstrate, the number of people injured or killed with guns is a real and growing problem, whether or not it is properly labeled as a public health problem. If current estimates are correct, 30,000 or more Americans die each year from gunshots; tens of thousands more are wounded or injured. The direct and indirect costs, in dollars and social well-being, are enormous. And while there are some legitimate uses of guns — hunting, self-defense, policing and maintaining public security — guns are used in many criminal activities that are themselves a risk to the health and safety of the public.

What can be done to eliminate or reduce all this is not as clear. As the first several articles in this chapter document, few of the various gun control measures that have been adopted by various states, some localities, and, on occasion, the federal government have been measurably successful. For some critics, this means more and more restrictive measures will be needed. Others argue that what is needed is a more objective assessment of what works and what does not. One critic even argues that limiting gun ownership not only will *not* reduce gun violence, it may cause it to increase.

Most critically, at least from a legal perspective, the options for gun control must be considered in light of the possible limits on government action created by the Second Amendment to the federal Constitution as well as by the comparable language included in most state constitutions. The language securing the "right to bear arms" is ambiguous and it has been infrequently interpreted by the courts; notwithstanding, it is clear is that gun ownership and use has a unique constitutional status and one that may drastically limit some options for gun control, regardless of their merits. As the cases in the second section of this chapter are intended to illustrate, there is a lively and passionate debate over the meaning and implications of the federal and state protections of the right to bear arms and the principles that define the federal and state government's discretion to regulate gun use and possession.

At the same time that gun control and regulatory measures are being debated in legislative bodies and evaluated in light of the Second Amendment limitations by the courts, a second judicial debate has concerned the extent to which private parties and, in some cases, state and local governments can bring lawsuits against gun owners, distributors, and manufacturers seeking injunctive relief or damages for the harm caused by their guns.

## B.  THE IMPACT OF GUNS ON HEALTH AND SAFETY

### DAVID HEMENWAY, PRIVATE GUNS/PUBLIC HEALTH
#### 1–7 (2004)

* * *

On an average day during the 1990s in the United States, firearms were used to kill more than 90 people and to wound three hundred more. Each day guns were also used in the commission of about three thousand crimes. The U.S. rates of death and injury due to firearms and the rates of crimes committed with firearms are far higher than those of any other industrialized country, yet our rates of crime and non-lethal violence are not exceptional. For example, the U.S. rates of rape, robbery, non-lethal assault, burglary, and larceny resemble those of other high-income countries; however our homicide rate is far higher. . . .

. . . Australia, Canada, and New Zealand . . . have roughly similar per capita incomes, cultures, and histories. . . . In 1992, the rates of property crimes and violent crime were comparable across these four countries; with the decline in U.S. crime, by the end of the century, U.S. crime rates were actually lower than in these other countries. What distinguishes the United States is the high rate of lethal violence. In 1992, our murder rate was five times higher than the average of these three other countries. In 1999–2000 it was three times higher. In contrast to these other nations, most of our murderers used guns. . . .

Canada, Australia, and New Zealand all have many guns, though not nearly as many hand guns as the United States. The key difference is that these other countries do a much better job of regulating their guns. Their experience and that of all high-income nations shows that when there are reasonable restrictions on guns, gun injuries need not be such a large public health problem. Their experience shows that it is possible to live in a society with many guns yet one in which relatively few crimes are committed with guns.

. . . [A] comparison of violent deaths of five- to fourteen-year-olds in the United States and in the other 25 high-income countries during the 1990s shows that the United States has much higher suicide and homicide rates, almost entirely because of the higher gun death rates. The United States has ten times the firearm suicide rate and the same non-firearm suicide rate as these other countries, and the United States has 17 times the firearm homicide rate and only a slightly higher non-firearm homicide rate. Our unintentional firearm death rate is 9 times higher.

. . . [B]etween 1950 and 1993, the overall death rate for U.S. children under 15 years declined substantially because of decreases in deaths from both illness and unintentional injury. However, during the same period, childhood homicide rates tripled and suicide rates quadrupled; these increases resulted almost entirely from gun violence.

Though gunshot wounds often result in death, even nonfatal wounds can be devastating, leading to permanent disability. . . . [N]onfatal gunshot injuries are currently the second leading cause of spinal cord injury in the United States. . . .

The psychological ravages of firearm trauma can be especially long-lasting. . . .

The direct medical costs of gunshot wounds were estimated at $6 million a day in the 1990s. The mean medical cost of a gunshot injury is about $17,000 and would be higher except that the medical costs for deaths at the scene are low. Half of these costs are borne directly by U.S. taxpayers; gun injuries are the leading cause of uninsured hospital stays in the United States. . . .

. . . .

The total number of firearms in civilian hands has increased rapidly in the past 40 years, 70 percent of all new guns purchased in American during the 20th century were bought after 1960. The type of gun purchased has also changed. In 1960, only 27 percent of the yearly additions to the gunstock were handguns; by 1994, that number had doubled to 54 percent.

While the number of guns has increased, the percentage of American households reporting that they own guns has declined markedly in recent years from about 48 percent to about 35 percent. This decline appears in part to result from the decreasing number of adults in each household and, since 1997, from a decline in the proportion of adults who personally own firearms. . . .

Currently, one in four adults owns a gun of some kind, but owners of four or more guns are in possession of 77 percent of the total. . . . Approximately 40 percent of adult males and 10 percent of adult females are gun owners. . . .

The percentage of households with long guns (rifles) fell from 40 percent in 1973 to 32 percent in 1994, but household handgun ownership rose from 20 percent to 25 percent. Since the mid-1990s, even household handgun ownership has been declining. Perhaps 16 percent of U.S. adults currently own handguns.

. . . .

One of the most important predictors of gun ownership is whether one's parents had a gun in the home. Gun ownership is highest among those over 40 years old and is more prevalent among those with higher incomes. While gun owners come from the entire spectrum of American society, people who admit to having been arrested for a non-traffic offense are more likely to own guns; owners of semiautomatics are more likely than other gun owners to report that they binge drink; and combat veterans with PTSD appear more likely than other veterans to own firearms (and to engage in such potentially harmful behavior as aiming guns at family members, patrolling their property with loaded guns, and killing animals in fits of rage).

. . . .

Between 1965 and 2000, more than 60,000 Americans died from unintentional firearms shootings. . . . Young people are the primary victims. More than half of all unintentional firearm fatalities are individuals under 25 years of age. Although relatively few adolescents own guns, the 15 to 19 year old age group has by far the highest rate of unintentional firearm fatalities; second is the 20 to 24 age group.

. . . One study examined data from 1979 to 1997 and found that for every age group, for men and women, for blacks and whites, people living in states with more guns were for more likely to die in gun accidents. Even after accounting for poverty, urbanization, and region, the differences were enormous.

There are currently 2 to 3 accidental firearm deaths each day, but this is, of course, only the tip of the iceberg. For every unintentional firearm fatality, it is estimated that approximately 13 victims are injured seriously enough to be treated in hospital emergency departments. In other words, more than 30 people a day are shot unintentionally but do not die. . . .

. . . .

. . . Since 1965, more than half a millions Americans have committed suicide with a firearm, nearly ten times as many as have died from gun-related accidents. In the United States, more people kill themselves with guns than by all other methods combined. . . .

. . . .

Since 1960, approximately 500,000 Americans have been murdered with guns. Gun murders account for more than two-thirds of all murders, and our murder rate for this period was five times higher than the average rate for other developed nations.

. . . .

Youth have been disproportionately not only the victims but also the perpetrators of homicide. In the early 1990s, the rate of murder arrest was highest among 18–20 year olds, followed by 17 year olds and 16 year olds. . . . Adolescents were killing adolescents and firearms were used in 80 percent of teenage homicides.

. . . .

Overall, the literature on the link between gun availability and homicide is compelling. Most studies . . . show the higher levels of gun prevalence are linked not only with higher levels of gun homicide but also with a higher overall homicide rate.

Focusing exclusively on incidents that result in injury or death would severely underestimate the extent of the gun violence problem in the United States. Guns are often used in crime with no bullets being fired and no one being shot. Many such crimes, including cases of assault, rape, and robbery, are not reported to police. . . .

On an average day in 2001, there were 1700 robberies in the United States, including holdups, muggings, purse snatching, and other violent confrontations motivated by theft. Guns were uses in more than 500 of these robberies. Higher levels of gun ownership appear to be associated with higher rates of robbery with guns but not with overall robberies levels. Victims of gun robberies are less likely to resist and less likely to be non-fatally injured than victims of robberies without guns. . . .

Victims of gun robberies, however, are far more likely to be murdered. . . .

\* \* \*

## Jon S. Vernick & Julie Samia Mair, *How the Law Affects Gun Policy in the United States: Law as Intervention or Obstacle to Prevention*
### 30 J. L. MED. & ETHICS 692, 693–95 (2002)

\* \* \*

The public health approach inherent in the science of injury prevention suggests that interventions focusing as far "upstream" as possible — for example, on the manufacturer of a potentially dangerous product like firearms — may be preferable to those focusing on the end user. Ultimately, it may be easier to change the practices of a small group of manufacturers than those of a much larger group of end users. For firearms, however, relatively few of the legal interventions in the United States have focused on manufacturers. But there are some notable exceptions that may represent the beginnings of a future trend.

Banning the manufacture or sale of certain firearms deemed to be especially dangerous directly targets the companies that make them. At the federal level, the Gun Control Act of 1968 prohibits the importation of handguns deemed not "particularly suitable for or readily adaptable to sporting purposes." This has had the effect of preventing the importation of so-called Saturday night special handguns. Sometimes also called "junk guns," these handguns have been described as small, poorly made, inexpensive, inaccurate, and unreliable. As a result, they have much less utility for lawful users and may be favored by some, particularly price-sensitive, criminals. Several states have also banned the *domestic* manufacture or sale of Saturday night specials, including Massachusetts and California within the past three years.

Federal law also bans the manufacture of assault weapons, defined as semi-automatic firearms that possess a combination of military-style features, such as a folding stock, bayonet mount, or flash suppressor. Several states and localities also ban assault weapons under a variety of similar definitions. Some localities even ban all handguns. Washington, D.C., and Chicago, Illinois have banned most handgun ownership for many years. . . .

. . . .

Finally, the design of the gun itself can be changed through legislation or regulation to make it safer. Unlike virtually all other consumer products, however, there is no federal agency with the authority to regulate the safe design of guns. [T]he federal Consumer Product Safety Commission (CPSC) has been expressly forbidden to regulate the safety of firearms or ammunition. Recently, though, two states — Massachusetts and Maryland — have required manufacturers to incorporate safety features into handguns sold within the states.

In 1997, the Attorney General of Massachusetts, using his existing consumer protection authority, promulgated regulations to require, in part, that all new handguns sold in Massachusetts contain: (1) a device to prevent a young child from firing the gun; (2) a tamper-resistant serial number to assist in the tracing of guns used in crime; and (3) a loaded chamber indicator or magazine safety to reduce the risk of unintended shootings where the shooter believed the gun was unloaded. . . .

In 2000, Maryland also enacted a law that will change how guns are designed. Under the Responsible Gun Safety Act of 2000, handguns manufactured after December 31, 2002 may not be sold in Maryland unless they have a device built into the gun itself "designed to prevent the handgun from being discharged unless the device is deactivated." The purpose of the law is to prevent shootings caused by unauthorized users of the gun. A built-in key or combination lock, but not a separately applied trigger lock, would probably satisfy the requirements of the law. Bills have also been introduced, but not yet enacted, in other states to require even more high-tech solutions to the problem of shootings caused by unauthorized users. Some of these bills would require that new handguns be "personalized," to automatically permit the gun to fire only for authorized users. For example, a high-tech personalized gun might incorporate a fingerprint reader or other device for recognizing its authorized user, without relying on a key or combination.

## Laws targeting dealers or distributors

Like many other consumer products, most firearms are not sold directly by manufacturers to consumers. Instead, manufacturers supply firearms to a large number of independent dealers and distributors, who then make direct sales to the public. This distribution system creates the opportunity for another set of legal interventions focused on those dealers.

At the federal level, persons who are "engaged in the business" of selling firearms must obtain a federal firearms license. To obtain this license, persons must undergo a background check and pay a fee. Although a recent analysis suggests that approximately one percent of all firearms dealers are responsible for selling more than half of all traced crime guns, federal law currently provides little opportunity to investigate potential scofflaw dealers. Most states also require a state dealer's license for those selling firearms. Just two states (Massachusetts and Rhode Island), however, require periodic inspection of dealers.

Recently, some California localities began considering various ways to use local law as an intervention to prevent gun violence. Several chose to enact ordinances restricting the location or other business practices of gun dealers, such as requiring certain anti-theft measures. Other municipalities have used the law to target those selling firearms at gun shows. At gun shows, both dealers and non-dealers congregate to buy and sell firearms, among other activities. Montgomery County, Maryland, for example, recently forbade gun shows from operating in county-owned facilities. There is evidence to suggest that some criminals use gun shows as a ready source of firearms.

## Laws targeting buyers or users

Despite the potential benefits of concentrating more prevention efforts on manufacturers and distributors, the majority of legal interventions regarding firearms in the United States focus "downstream" on the gun buyers and users. Many of these, though, are criminal laws simply forbidding certain dangerous acts with guns. . . .

Under the Gun Control Act of 1968, as amended by the Brady Handgun Violence Prevention Act in 1994, certain categories of persons are prohibited from purchasing firearms. These include convicted felons, minors, fugitives, those who have been "adjudicated as a mental defective," and illegal aliens. Persons buying guns from licensed dealers (those with a federal firearm license) are required to undergo a background check to determine if they fit one of the prohibited categories. Sales between private individuals rather than from dealers, however, do not require a background check under federal law, though a few states do require checks for *all* gun sales.

Some states implement their own background check laws through a system that requires the prospective buyer to first obtain a license or permit to purchase the firearm. These licensing systems often require a long waiting period to conduct an extensive background check. Some states also require the firearm itself to be registered, much as a car is registered, to assist law enforcement officials in tracing guns used in crimes and holding sellers criminally accountable for unlawful sales. There is evidence to suggest that states with both a licensing and registration system make it harder for criminals to obtain firearms from in-state sources.

Because gun laws vary so greatly from state to state, interstate trafficking of weapons is a common source of guns for criminals. One legal intervention adopted in just four states limits the number of handguns that may be purchased by one person to one handgun per month. The goal of these one-gun-per-month laws is to make it more difficult for gun traffickers to stock up on firearms for resale to criminals. The second such law in the nation, enacted in Virginia in 1993, appears to have greatly reduced the proportion of guns from Virginia used in crimes in other states.

Once the gun has been acquired, seventeen states mandate that the gun be stored safely. Child access prevention (CAP) laws make it a crime to store a firearm so that a child can gain ready access. Florida enacted its CAP law in 1989 in response to a number of high profile accidental shootings involving children. Public health practitioners in other states saw the opportunity to use the law as an intervention, and by 1999, sixteen additional states had their own CAP law. There is mixed evidence regarding the effectiveness of CAP laws in preventing accidental deaths among children. CAP laws are most likely to be effective if the law mandates felony prosecution and is well publicized.

* * *

## John R. Lott, Jr., More Guns, Less Crime: Understanding Crime and Gun-Control Laws
### 160–66 (2d ed. 2000)

* * *

Many factors influence crime, with arrest and conviction rates being the most important. However, nondiscretionary concealed-handgun laws are also important, and they are the most cost-effective means of reducing crime. The cost of hiring more police in order to change arrest and conviction rates is much higher, and the net benefits per dollar spent are only at most a quarter as large as the benefits from concealed-handgun laws. Even private, medium-security prisons cost state governments about $34 a day per prisoner ($12,267 per year). For concealed handguns, the permit fees are usually the largest costs [and are] borne by private citizens. The durability of guns allows owners to recoup their investments over many years. Using my yearly cost estimate of $43 per concealed handgun for Pennsylvanians, concealed handguns pay for themselves if they have only 1/285 of the deterrent impact of an additional year in prison. This calculation even ignores the other costs of the legal system, such as prosecution and defense costs — criminals will expend greater effort to fight longer prison sentences in court. No other government policy appears to have anywhere near the same cost-benefit ratio as concealed-handgun laws.

Allowing citizens without criminal records or histories of significant mental illness to carry concealed handguns deters violent crimes and appears to produce an extremely small and statistically insignificant change in accidental deaths. If the rest of the country had adopted right-to-carry concealed-handgun provisions in 1992, about 1500 murders and 4000 rapes would have been avoided. On the other hand, consistent with the notion that criminals respond to incentives, county-level data provide some evidence that concealed-handgun laws are associated with increases in property crimes involving stealth and in crimes that involve minimal probability of contact between the criminal and the victim. Even though both the state-level data and the estimates that attempt to explain why the law and the arrest rates change indicate that crime in all the categories declines, the deterrent effect of nondiscretionary handgun laws is largest for violent crimes. Counties with the largest populations, where the deterrence of violent crimes is the greatest, are also the counties where the substitution of property crimes for violent crimes by criminals is the highest. The estimated annual gain in 1992 from allowing concealed handguns was over $5.74 billion.

Many commonly accepted notions are challenged by these findings. Urban areas tend to have the most restrictive gun-control rules and have fought the hardest against nondiscretionary concealed handgun laws, yet they are the very places that benefit the most from nondiscretionary concealed handgun laws. Not only do urban areas tend to gain in their fight against crime, but reductions in crime rates are greatest precisely in those urban areas that have the highest crime rates, largest and most dense populations, and greatest concentrations of minorities. To some this might not be too surprising. After all, law-abiding citizens in these areas must depend on themselves to a great extent for protection. Even if self-protection were accepted, concerns would still arise over whether these law-abiding citizens would use guns properly. This study provides a very strong answer: a few people do and will use permitted concealed handguns improperly, but the gains completely overwhelm these concerns.

Another surprise involves women and blacks. Both tend to be the strongest supporters of gun control, yet both obtain the largest benefits from nondiscretionary concealed-handgun laws in terms of reduced rates of murder and other crimes. Concealed handguns also appear to be the great equalizer among the sexes. Murder rates decline when either more women or more men carry concealed handguns, but the effect is especially pronounced for women. An additional woman carrying a concealed handgun reduces the murder rate for women by about three to four times more than an additional man carrying a concealed handgun reduces the murder rate for men. Providing a woman with a concealed handgun, represents a much larger change in her ability to defend herself than it does for a man.

The benefits of concealed handguns are not limited to those who use them in self-defense. Because the guns may be concealed, criminals are unable to tell whether potential victims are carrying guns until they attack, thus making it less attractive for criminals to commit crimes that involve direct contact with victims. Citizens who have no intention of ever carrying concealed handguns in a sense get a "free ride" from the crime-fighting efforts of their fellow citizens. However, the "halo" effect created by these laws is apparently not limited to people who share the characteristics of those who carry the guns. The most obvious example is the drop in murders of children following the adoption of nondiscretionary laws. Arming older people not only may provide direct protection to these children, but also causes criminals to leave the area. Nor is the "halo" effect limited to those who live in areas where people are allowed to carry guns. The violent-crime reduction from one's own state's adopting the law is in fact greatest when neighboring states also allow law-abiding citizens to carry concealed handguns. The evidence also indicates that the states with the most guns have the lowest crime rates. Urban areas may experience the most violent crime, but they also have the smallest number of guns. Blacks may be the racial group most vulnerable to violent crime, but they are also much less likely than whites to own guns.

These estimates make one wonder about all the attention given to other types of gun legislation. My estimates indicate that waiting periods and background checks appear to produce little if any crime deterrence. Yet President Clinton credits the Brady law with lowering crime because it has, according to him, been "taking guns out of the hands of criminals." During the 1996 Democratic National Convention, Sarah Brady, after whose husband the bill was named, boasted that it "has helped keep more than 100,000 felons and other prohibited purchasers from buying handguns. . . ." From 1994 until the Supreme Court's decision in 1997, backers of the Brady law focused almost exclusively on the value of background checks, the one part of the law that the Supreme Court specifically struck down.

Actually, the downward crime trend started in 1991, well before the Brady law became effective in March 1994. . . .

Others estimate a much smaller effect of the Brady law on gun sales. In 1996 the General Accounting Office reported that initial rejections based on background checks numbered about 60,000, of which over half were for purely technical reasons, mostly paperwork errors that were eventually corrected! A much smaller number of rejections, 3000, was due to convictions for violent crimes, and undoubtedly many of the people rejected proceeded to buy guns on the street. By the time the background-check provision was found unconstitutional, in June 1997, only four people had gone to jail for violations.

Presumably, no one would argue that rejected permits are meaningful by themselves. They merely proxy for what might happen to crime rates, provided that the law really stops criminals from getting guns. Do criminals simply get them from other sources? Or do the restrictions primarily inconvenience law-abiding citizens who want guns for self-defense? The results presented in this book are the first systematic national look at such gun laws, and if the national Uniform Crime Report data through 1994 or state waiting periods and background checks are any indication, the empirical evidence does not bode well for the Brady law. No statistically significant evidence has appeared that the Brady law has reduced crime, and there is some statistically significant evidence that rates for rape and-aggravated assault have actually risen by about 4 percent relative to what they would have been without the law.

Yet research does not convince everybody. Perhaps the Supreme Court's June 1997 decision on the constitutionality of the Brady law's national background checks will shed light on how effective the Brady law was. The point of making the scope of the background check national was that without it, criminals would buy guns from jurisdictions without the checks and use them to commit crimes in the rest of the country. As these national standards are eliminated, and states and local jurisdictions discontinue their background checks, will crime rates rise as quickly without this provision of the law as gun-control advocates claimed they fell because of it? My bet is no, they will not. . . .

Since 1994, aside from required waiting periods, many new rules making gun ownership by law-abiding citizens more difficult have come into existence. There were 279,401 active, federal gun-dealer licenses in the nation when the new licensing regulations went fully into effect in April 1994. By the beginning of 1997 there were 124,286, a decline of 56 percent, and their number continues to fall. This has undoubtedly made purchasing guns less convenient. Besides increasing licensing fees from $30 to $200 for first-time licenses and imposing renewal fees of $90, the 1994 Violent Crime Control and Law Enforcement Act imposed significant new regulatory requirements that were probably much more important in reducing the number of licensees.

The Bureau of Alcohol, Tobacco, and Firearms (BATF) supports this decrease largely because it believes that it affects federal license holders who are illegally selling guns. The BATT's own (undoubtedly high) estimate is that about 1 percent of federal license holders illegally sell guns, and that this percentage has remained constant with the decline in licensed dealers. If so, 155,115 licensees have lost their licenses in order to eliminate 1,551 illegal traffickers. Whether this lopsided trade-off justifies stiffer federal regulation is unclear, but other than simply pointing to the fact that crime continued on its downward course nationally during this period, no evidence has been offered. No attempt has been made to isolate this effect from many other changes that occurred over the same period of time.

Changes in the law will also continue to have an impact. Proposals are being made by the U.S. Department of justice to require owners of "firearms arsenals" to provide notice to law enforcement, where the definition of what constitutes an "arsenal" seems to be fairly subjective, and to require gun owners to record the make, model, and serial number of their firearms as a condition of obtaining gun insurance. Other proposals would essentially make it impossible for private individuals to transfer firearms among themselves.

It is too early to conclude what overall impact these federal rules have had on gun ownership. Surely the adoption of the Brady law dramatically increased gun ownership as people rushed out to buy guns before the law went into effect. . . . But without annual gun-ownership data, we cannot separate all the different factors that have altered the costs and benefits of gun ownership.

Other changes are in store during the next couple of years that could affect some of the discussion in this book. The Clinton administration has been encouraging the development of devices for determining at a distance what items a person is carrying. Such devices will enable police to see whether individuals are carrying guns and can help disarm criminals, but criminals who managed to acquire them could also use them to determine whether a potential victim would offer armed resistance. The ability to target unarmed citizens would lower the risks of committing crime and reduce the external benefits produced by concealed handguns. Since both police and criminals might use them, the net effect on crime rates of their use is not immediately clear.

. . . Before granting the government the right to use such long-range devices, we must answer some novel questions regarding constitutional rights. For example, would the ability to take a picture of all the objects that a person is carrying amount to an invasion of privacy? Would it constitute an illegal search?

What implications does this study have for banning guns altogether? This book has not examined evidence on what the crime rate would be if all guns could be eliminated from society — no data were present in the data set for areas where guns were completely absent for any period of time, but the findings do suggest how costly the transition to that gun-free goal would be. If outlawing guns would primarily affect their ownership by law-abiding citizens, this research indicates that at least in the short run, we would expect crime rates to rise. The discussion is very similar to the debate over nuclear disarmament. A world without nuclear weapons might be better off, but unilateral disarmament may not be the best way to accomplish that goal. The large stock of guns in the United States, as well as the ease with which illegal items such as drugs find their way across borders implies that not only might the transition to a gunfree world be costly (if not impossible), but the transition might also take a long time.

Further, not everyone will benefit equally from the abolition of guns. For example, criminals will still maintain a large strength advantage over many of their victims (such as women and the elderly). To the extent that guns are an equalizer, their elimination will strengthen criminals relative to physically weak victims. As we have seen in discussing international crime data, eliminating guns alters criminals' behavior in other ways, such as reducing their fear of breaking into homes while the residents are there.

All these discussions, of course, ignore the issues that led the founding fathers to put the Second Amendment in the Constitution in the first place — important issues that are beyond the scope of this book. They believed that an armed citizenry is the ultimate bulwark against tyrannical government. Possibly our trust in government has risen so much that we no longer fear what future governments might do. Having just fought a war for their independence against a government that had tried to confiscate their guns, the founding fathers felt very strongly about this issue.

## WHAT CAN WE CONCLUDE?

How much confidence do I have in these results? The largest previous study on gun control produced findings similar to those reported here but examined only 170 cities within a single year. This book has examined over 54,000 observations across 3,000 counties for eighteen years and has controlled for a range of other factors never accounted for in previous crime studies. I have attempted to answer numerous questions. For example, do higher arrest or conviction rates reduce crime? What about changes in other handgun laws, such as penalizing the use of a gun in the commission of a crime, or the well-known waiting periods? Do income, poverty, unemployment, drug prices, or demographic changes matter? All these factors were found to influence crime rates, but no previous gun study had accounted for changing criminal penalties, and this study is the first to look at more than a few of any of these other considerations. Preventing law-abiding citizens from carrying handguns does not end violence; it merely makes victims more vulnerable to attack. While people have strong views on either side of this debate, and one study is unlikely to end this discussion, the size and strength of my deterrence results and the lack of evidence that holders of permits for concealed handguns commit crimes should at least give pause to those who oppose concealed handguns. In the final analysis, one concern unites us all: Will allowing law-abiding citizens to carry concealed handguns save lives? The answer is yes, it will.

* * *

# NOTES AND QUESTIONS

**1.** How many guns are there (in private hands) in the United States? No one really knows; there is no national reporting system for sale or ownership. Hemenway's estimates of private gun ownership are just that, estimates. The Bureau of Alcohol, Tobacco, and Firearms (ATF) (a source cited in several of the excerpts in this chapter) has estimated that 192 million guns were privately owned in the United States in 1999, 65 million of which were handguns. For additional sources, an attempt to assess the accuracy of the data, and interesting comparisons between gun ownership in Canada and that in the United States, see Philip J. Cook & Jens Ludwig, *Principles for Effective Gun Policy,* 73 FORDHAM L. REV. 589, 590-92 (2004).

Data about how much harm these guns cause is also surprisingly sparse. All sources seem to agree that there is some good news: Gun-related injuries declined in the 1990s. Nonetheless, they remain the second leading cause of injury mortality in the United States. In the year 2002, the CDC reports that over 30,000 people died from gun-related injuries, about 20 percent of all injury deaths. (This is comparable to the rates reported by Hemenway for the 1990s.) Over half of these were suicides (representing about 50 percent of all suicides); about 40 percent were homicides. Males were six times more likely to die of a gunshot wound; blacks were twice as likely as whites. By way of comparison, there were roughly 26,000 deaths form poisoning and 44,000 deaths from traffic accidents in 2002. *See* National Center for Health Statistics, *Deaths: Final Data for 2002,* 53 NAT'L VITAL STAT. REP. No. 5, 1-15 (2004). *See also* www.cdc.nchs/fastats/injury.htm (last visited December 2006); www.ojp.usdoj.gov/bjs/guns.html (last visited December 2006).

According to Hemenway, an average of more than 80,000 Americans per year suffered nonfatal gunshot wounds from 1993 to 1997. Similar estimates are made by Vernick & Mair, *infra* at 692. Vernick & Mair also estimate that gun deaths and injuries are associated with substantial costs to both individual Americans and society at large — including $2.3 billion in lifetime medical costs for gunshot wounds occurring in 1994; about half of these costs were paid from public sources (mostly Medicaid and Medicare expenditures).

These estimates notwithstanding, there does not appear to be a good, regularly updatable source of information on either fatal or non-fatal injuries or their associated costs that can be attributable to guns. Indeed, many observers have claimed that the government should improve the surveillance of gun deaths and injuries to make it comparable to the surveillance efforts that are made for infectious diseases and other sources of injuries.

There are, of course, no good sources of quantifiable data on the many other "costs" associated with gun ownership and use, *e.g.*, the number of people intimidated or harassed with guns, the loss of property values in neighborhoods associated with gun use, the increased insecurity or loss of "peace of mind" of people who live near gun use areas, and so on.

**2.** As should be clear from Vernick & Mair, gun control is a collective term. There are a number of ways in which ownership and possession of guns can be regulated or prohibited or even encouraged. (One city in Colorado has enacted a law requiring all adult males to own a firearm.) Most gun control laws, however, are intended to limit their distribution and use, either by regulating their manufacture, sale, or possession.

For a good source of gun control laws on a state-by-state basis, see www.stategunlaws.org (last visited December 2006). For an additional source with a somewhat different orientation, see www.keepandbeararms.com (last visited December 2006).

Do any of these gun control laws really save lives or prevent injury? Most people assume the answers to such questions are obvious: Fewer, safer guns means lower rates of morbidity and mortality from gunshots. As Lott argues, however, the reality of gun control may differ from the dictates of common sense, at least with regard to concealed weapon laws. According to Lott, states that adopt "shall issue" concealed weapons laws may reduce their rates of murder and other violent crimes, presumably because criminals are afraid that their potential victims may be carrying concealed weapons. As a result, more armed, law-abiding citizens means fewer crimes, a counters intuitive and provocative claim.

Lott backs up his claims with impressive empirical evidence. Nonetheless, not everyone has accepted either the reliability or validity of the data he has amassed or the conclusions that he has drawn from that data. Indeed, his critics have challenged the sources of his data, some of the ways in which he has analyzed it, and even his motives. None, however, have been completely successful in discounting his work. For one example, see JOHN DONOHUE, DOES MORE GUN CARRYING REDUCE CRIME? (Brookings Institute 2005) (*available at* www.brookings.edu/es/urban) (last visited April 2005). See also Lott's point-by-point rebuttal of his critics efforts in the epilogue to the second edition of his book.

For another work that attempts to develop a thesis similar to that of Lott with regard to gun ownership and crime rates in Great Britian, see JOYCE LEE MALCOM, GUNS AND VIOLENCE: THE ENGLISH EXPERIENCE (2002) (comparing the experience with and without gun control laws in England and the United States, making the case that gun control laws do not reduce gun-related violence).

A recent review of the literature sponsored by the CDC concerning the impact of various types of gun-control laws, declines to endorse either Lott's view or that of his critics:

> The substantial number of studies of shall-issue laws largely derives from and responds to one landmark study [The Lott study]. Many of these studies were considered to be non-independent because they assessed the same intervention in the same population during similar time periods. A review of these revealed critical problems, including misclassification of laws, unreliable county-level crime data, and failure to use appropriate denominators for the available numerator crime data. Methodological problems, such as failure to adjust for auto-correction in time series data, were also evident. Results across studies were inconsistent or conceptually implausible. Therefore, the evidence is insufficient to determine the effect of shall issue laws on violent outcomes.

CDC, FIRST REPORTS EVALUATING THE EFFECTIVENESS OF STRATEGIES FOR PREVENTING VIOLENCE: FIREARMS LAWS 6 (2005) (written by the independent Task Force on Community Prevention Services).

For other works attempting to assess the effectiveness of various gun control measures, see Arthur L. Kellerman et al., *Gun Ownership as a Risk Factor for Homicide in the Home*, 329 NEW ENG. J. MED. 1084 (2005) (arguing that a gun in the home raises the risk of homicide and claiming that most in-home deaths from guns are a result of a homicide by a family member or friend); Daniel W. Webster & Marc Starnes, *Reexamining the Association Between Child Access Prevention Gun Laws and Unintentional Shooting Deaths of Children*, 106 PEDIATRICS 1466 (2000); Peter Cummings et al., *State Gun Safe Storage Laws and Child Mortality Due to Firearms*, 278 JAMA 1084 (1997); PHILLIP COOK & JENS LUDWIG, EVALUATING GUN POLICY (2003); Phillip Cook & Anthony Braga, *Comprehensive Firearms Tracing: Strategic and Investigative Uses of New Data on Firearms Markets*, 43 ARIZ. L. REV. 277 (2001).

Perhaps most importantly, the same CDC-sponsored review of the literature quoted *supra* declines to endorse either the effectiveness or ineffectiveness of *any* gun control measure. In short, the empirical data concerning the efficacy of gun control measures are rather inconclusive — across the board. *See also* NATIONAL RESEARCH COUNCIL, NATIONAL ACADEMIES, FIREARMS AND VIOLENCE: A CRITICAL REVIEW (2005) *available at* www.national-academies.org (last visited December 2006).

**3.** From a legal or policymaking point of view, what difference does it make if, in fact, the empirical data does not clearly document that one or another legal strategy will be effective? Obviously it would be nice to know what works and what doesn't, especially in such a highly controversial area of public policy, but how often do policymakers really know, in advance, that a particular legal or political strategy will be effective? What happens in other contexts such as proposals to improve automobile safety or to increase limits on alcohol availability? Do we typically wait until the available data is overwhelming? Is "fairly convincing" evidence enough? How about "more likely than not to be accurate" data? In other situations, the opinions of experts — and even non-experts — are sufficient to uphold legislation. Is there something about gun control legislation that leads political decision makers to be especially cautious before acting?

There is one good, legal reason to be cautious: the potential application of the Second Amendment. Good data to support various options for gun control may be relevant to the constitutional analysis of these measures under the various levels of judicial review required by the Second Amendment or other constitutional principles, as outlined in the section that follows.

## C.  THE CONSTITUTIONAL AUTHORITY OF THE STATE AND FEDERAL GOVERNMENTS TO REGULATE GUN USE AND OWNERSHIP

"A well-regulated Militia being necessary to the security of a free State, the right of the people to keep and Arms, shall not be infringed."

— Second Amendment to the Constitution of the United States

### UNITED STATES v. WRIGHT
### 117 F.3d 1265 (11th Cir. 1997)

Kravitch, Judge.

* * *

The Second Amendment to the United States Constitution provides: "A well regulated Militia, being necessary to the security of a free State, the right of the people to keep and bear Arms, shall not be infringed." In this case, we must decide whether this amendment grants constitutional protection to an individual whose possession or use of machineguns and pipe bombs is not reasonably related to an organized state militia. . . .

### I. Background

In June 1994, the Bureau of Alcohol Tobacco and Firearms received information that Donald Wright was looking for someone to reassemble a .50 caliber machinegun. Subsequently, two undercover local law enforcement agents were introduced to Wright as individuals capable of reassembling this gun. At this meeting, Wright produced the disassembled machinegun and told the agents that, once it was reassembled, he planned to shoot the gun, grease it, and then bury it. Agents arrested Wright in possession of the disassembled machinegun as he drove away from the meeting. Upon arrest, Wright consented to a search of his residence during which agents discovered a .223 caliber Olympic Arms model Car-AR automatic assault machinegun and three pipe bombs in a shed outside his home. Agents also found several other unregistered assault weapons, ammunition, and assorted documents and videotapes describing threats to United States sovereignty posed by the "New World Order."

Wright was charged with one count of possessing machineguns in violation of 18 U.S.C. § 922(o) and with one count of possessing unregistered destructive devices in violation of 26 U.S.C. § 5861(d). He filed a motion to dismiss the indictment on the grounds that the charging statutes violated, among other constitutional provisions, the Commerce Clause and the Second Amendment. In support of his motion, Wright submitted the seized documents and videotapes to demonstrate that his weapons possession was motivated by what he perceived to be the danger of the "New World Order." He also offered the testimony of a firearms expert to establish that the machineguns and pipe bombs were the type of weapons used by contemporary militias. The district court, adopting the magistrate judge's report and recommendation, denied his motion.

. . . .

## II. Discussion

. . . .

## B.   Second Amendment

Wright . . . contends that §§ 922(o) and 5861(d) violate his right to bear arms under the Second Amendment. As a member of Georgia's unorganized militia, Wright claims that he has a constitutional right to possess machineguns and pipe bombs because these weapons are used by contemporary militia fighting forces. . . .

. . . [T]he Supreme Court has provided us with important guidance in interpreting this constitutional provision. In United States v. Miller, 307 U.S. 174 (1939), the Court considered whether the National Firearms Act of 1934, 26 U.S.C. § 1132, which required the registration of certain firearms, violated the Second Amendment rights of two individuals indicted for transporting unregistered sawed-off shotguns in interstate commerce. In reversing the district court's order . . . the Court stated:

> In the absence of any evidence tending to show that possession or use of a "shotgun having a barrel of less than eighteen inches in length" at this time has some reasonable relationship to the preservation or efficiency of a well regulated militia, we cannot say that the Second Amendment guarantees the right to keep and bear such an instrument.

Because the Court concluded that there was no evidence that the sawed-off shotgun was "any part of the ordinary military equipment or that its use could contribute to the common defense," the Court held that the statute did not violate the Second Amendment rights of the defendants.

The fact that the *Miller* Court did not examine the possession or use of the sawed-off shotguns in that case in no way suggests, as appellant contends, that individual possession of a military-type weapon is protected by the Constitution irrespective of whether the possession or use of that weapon is reasonably related to a "well regulated militia." Without any evidence that the sawed-off shotgun at issue in that case could have been used as a weapon by a well regulated militia group to provide for the common defense, there was no need for the Court to determine if the actual possession or use of the weapons bore a reasonable relationship to a well regulated militia.

Therefore, in order to claim Second Amendment protection, Wright must demonstrate a reasonable relationship between his possession of the machine-guns and pipe bombs and "the preservation or efficiency of a well regulated militia." Wright claims that he has satisfied this test because his weapons possession is reasonably related to his membership in Georgia's unorganized militia, which he asserts is "well regulated" within the meaning of the Second Amendment.

Because the sawed-off shotguns in *Miller* were not susceptible to use in any militia, the Court did not need to determine explicitly what constituted a "well regulated militia." A careful reading of *Miller,* however, strongly suggests that only militias actively maintained and trained by the states can satisfy the "well regulated militia" requirement of the Second Amendment. As the *Miller* Court emphasized, the "obvious purpose" of the Second Amendment was to "render possible the effectiveness of" the governmental militia described in the Militia Clauses of the Constitution.

At the time of ratification, and as remains the case today, the militia was defined broadly and was understood to include "all males physically capable of acting in concert for the common defense." But because the Constitution protects only the possession or use of guns reasonably related to a "well regulated militia," membership in this broad segment of the population is constitutionally insignificant. In determining the scope of Second Amendment protection, the *Miller* Court did not rely on the commonly understood and wide-reaching definition of the militia, but rather turned to early militia laws of New York, Massachusetts, and Virginia, which provided for the training, maintenance, and equipping of these states' respective militias. We find the *Miller* Court's reliance on these statutory provisions regulating "the organization and government of the Militia," to be significant. In our view, it indicates that the *Miller* Court understood the Second Amendment to protect only the possession or use of weapons that is reasonably related to a militia actively maintained and trained by the states.

Moreover, after examining the text and history of the Second Amendment, we conclude that this reading of *Miller* is consistent with the motivating purposes of the drafters of the Second Amendment. The amendment describes a "well regulated militia" as "being necessary to the security of a free State." The fact that the drafters qualified "well regulated militia" by reference to state security suggests to us that they intended this term to refer only to governmental militias that are actively maintained and used for the common defense. We find substantial support for this textual reading in the history of the drafting and ratification of the Constitution and the Bill of Rights.

The Militia Clauses in Article I authorized Congress to organize, arm, and discipline the militia, but reserved to the states the authority to train the militia and appoint its officers. This dual grant of authority reflected the tension between two competing concerns at the Constitutional Convention: the widespread distrust of a national standing army versus the danger of relying on inadequately trained soldiers as the primary means of providing for the common defense. . . . The Second Amendment was inserted into the Bill of Rights to protect the role of the states in maintaining and arming the militia. It was designed to protect the state militias from federal legislation enacted to undermine the role of state militias. . . .

The concerns motivating the creation of the Second Amendment convince us that the amendment was intended to protect only the use or possession of weapons that is reasonably related to a militia actively maintained and trained by the states. With this conclusion, we join every other federal court that has been called on to consider the "well regulated militia" requirement of the Second Amendment, several of which have considered and rejected the claim made by Wright in this case that membership in a state's unorganized militia is sufficient to bring gun possession within the protection of the Second Amendment.

Faced with this overwhelming body of contrary authority, Wright nevertheless maintains that Georgia's unorganized militia is sufficiently well regulated to trigger constitutional protection. He notes that under Georgia law the Governor has the authority to prescribe and to establish regulations governing the unorganized militia. Wright also refers to statutes that allow, under certain circumstances, "the Governor [to] call for and accept from the unorganized militia as many volunteers as are required for service in the organized militia." (citation omitted)

In our view, these statutes fall far short of rendering the Georgia unorganized militia "well regulated" for the purposes of the Second Amendment. The possibility that in responding to a future crisis state authorities might seek the aid of members of the unorganized militia does not speak to the militia's current state of regulation. Wright has not directed us to any Georgia statutes governing the actual, as opposed to potential, organization, training, and equipping of the members of the unorganized militia. . . .

Because Wright has presented no evidence to demonstrate any connection, let alone a "reasonable relationship," between his possession of the machineguns and pipe bombs and the preservation or efficiency of a militia actively trained and maintained by the State of Georgia, his weapons possession is entitled to no constitutional protection. Therefore, we conclude in this case that neither § 922(o)'s blanket ban of machinegun possession nor the registration requirements of § 5861(d) infringe on any constitutionally protected liberties.

* * *

# SILVEIRA v. LOCKYER
## 312 F.3d 1052 (9th Cir. 2002)

Reinhardt, Judge.

\* \* \*

In 1999, the State of California enacted amendments to its gun control laws that significantly strengthened the state's restrictions on the possession, use, and transfer of the semi-automatic weapons popularly known as "assault weapons." Plaintiffs, California residents who either own assault weapons, seek to acquire such weapons, or both, brought this challenge to the gun control statute, asserting that the law, as amended, violates the Second Amendment, the Equal Protection Clause, and a host of other constitutional provisions. . . .

## I. INTRODUCTION

In response to a proliferation of shootings involving semi-automatic weapons, the California Legislature passed the Roberti-Roos Assault Weapons Control Act ("the AWCA") in 1989. The immediate cause of the AWCA's enactment was a random shooting earlier that year at the Cleveland Elementary School in Stockton, California. An individual armed with an AK-47 semi-automatic weapon opened fire on the schoolyard, where three hundred pupils were enjoying their morning recess. Five children aged 6 to 9 were killed, and one teacher and 29 children were wounded.

. . . [T]he AWCA, was the first legislative restriction on assault weapons in the nation, and was the model for a similar federal statute enacted in 1994. The AWCA renders it a felony offense to manufacture in California any of the semi-automatic weapons specified in the statute, or to possess, sell, transfer, or import into the state such weapons without a permit. The statute contains a grandfather clause that permits the ownership of assault weapons by individuals who lawfully purchased them before the statute's enactment, so long as the owners register the weapons with the state Department of Justice. The grandfather clause, however, imposes significant restrictions on the use of weapons that are registered pursuant to its provisions. Approximately forty models of firearms are listed in the statute as subject to its restrictions. The specified weapons include "civilian" models of military weapons that feature slightly less firepower than the military-issue versions, such as the Uzi, an Israeli-made military rifle; the AR-15, a semi-automatic version of the United States military's standard-issue machine gun, the M-16; and the AK-47, a Russian-designed and Chinese-produced military rifle. The AWCA also includes a mechanism for the Attorney General to seek a judicial declaration in certain California Superior Courts that weapons identical to the listed firearms are also subject to the statutory restrictions.

. . . .

In 1999, the legislature amended the AWCA in order to broaden its coverage and to render it more flexible in response to technological developments in the manufacture of semi-automatic weapons. The amended AWCA retains both the original list of models of restricted weapons, and the judicial declaration procedure by which models may be added to the list. The 1999 amendments to the AWCA statute add a third method of defining the class of restricted weapons: The amendments provide that a weapon constitutes a restricted assault weapon if it possesses certain generic characteristics listed in the statute. . . .

Plaintiffs in this case are nine individuals, some of whom lawfully acquired weapons that were subsequently classified as assault weapons under the amended AWCA. They filed this action in February, 2000, one month after the 1999 AWCA amendments took effect. Plaintiffs who own assault weapons challenge the AWCA requirements that they either register, relinquish, or render inoperable their assault weapons as violative of their Second Amendment rights. Plaintiffs who seek to purchase weapons that may no longer lawfully be purchased in California also attack the ban on assault weapon sales as being contrary to their rights under that Amendment. Additionally, plaintiffs who are not active or retired California peace officers challenge on Fourteenth Amendment Equal Protection grounds two provisions of the AWCA: one that allows active peace officers to possess assault weapons while off-duty, and one that permits retired peace officers to possess assault weapons they acquire from their department at the time of their retirement. . . .

## II. DISCUSSION

### A. *Background and Precedent.*

A robust constitutional debate is currently taking place in this nation regarding the scope of the Second Amendment, a debate that has gained intensity over the last several years. . . . There are three principal schools of thought that form the basis for the debate. The first, which we will refer to as the "traditional individual rights" model, holds that the Second Amendment guarantees to individual private citizens a fundamental right to possess and use firearms for any purpose at all, subject only to limited government regulation. This view, urged by the NRA and other firearms enthusiasts, as well as by a prolific cadre of fervent supporters in the legal academy, had never been adopted by any court until the recent Fifth Circuit decision in United States v. Emerson, 270 F.3d 203 (5th Cir. 2001). The second view, a variant of the first, we will refer to as the "limited individual rights" model. Under that view, individuals maintain a constitutional right to possess firearms insofar as such possession bears a reasonable relationship to militia service. The third, a wholly contrary view, commonly called the "collective rights" model, asserts that the Second Amendment right to "bear arms" guarantees the right of the people to maintain effective state militias, but does not provide any type of individual right to own or possess weapons. Under this theory of the amendment, the federal and state governments have the full authority to enact prohibitions and restrictions on the use and possession of firearms, subject only to generally applicable constitutional constraints, such as due process, equal protection, and the like. Long the dominant view of the Second Amendment, and widely accepted by the federal courts, the collective rights model has recently come under strong criticism from individual rights advocates. After conducting a full analysis of the amendment, its history, and its purpose, we reaffirm our conclusion in Hickman v. Block, 81 F.3d 98 (9th Cir. 1996), that it is this collective rights model which provides the best interpretation of the Second Amendment.

[The court then discussed the limited relevance of the Supreme Court's decision in *United States v. Miller*.]

. . . .

In light of the United States government's recent change in position on the meaning of the amendment, the resultant flood of Second Amendment challenges in the district courts, the Fifth Circuit's extensive study and analysis of the amendment and its conclusion that *Miller* does not mean what we and other courts have assumed it to mean, the proliferation of gun control statutes both state and federal, and the active scholarly debate that is being waged across this nation, we believe it prudent to explore Appellants' Second Amendment arguments in some depth, and to address the merits of the issue, even though this circuit's position on the scope and effect of the amendment was established in *Hickman*.

## B.   *Appellants Lack Standing to Challenge the Assault Weapons Control Act on Second Amendment Grounds*

Appellants contend that the California Assault Weapons Control Act and its 1999 revisions violate their Second Amendment rights. We unequivocally reject this contention. We conclude that although the text and structure of the amendment, standing alone, do not conclusively resolve the question of its meaning, when we give the text its most plausible reading and consider the amendment in light of the historical context and circumstances surrounding its enactment we are compelled to reaffirm the collective rights view we adopted in *Hickman:* The amendment protects the people's right to maintain an effective state militia, and does not establish an individual right to own or possess firearms for personal or other use. . . . Because we hold that the Second Amendment does not provide an individual right to own or possess guns or other firearms, plaintiffs lack standing to challenge the AWCA.

The Second Amendment states in its entirety: "A well regulated Militia being necessary to the security of a free State, the right of the people to keep and bear Arms, shall not be infringed." As commentators on all sides of the debate regarding the amendment's meaning have acknowledged, the language of the amendment alone does not conclusively resolve the question of its scope. . . . What renders the language and structure of the amendment particularly striking is the existence of a prefatory clause, a syntactical device that is absent from all other provisions of the Constitution, including the nine other provisions of the Bill of Rights. Our analysis thus must address not only the meaning of each of the two clauses of the amendment but the unique relationship that exists between them.

### a. The Meaning of the Amendment's First Clause: "A Well Regulated Militia Being Necessary to the Security of A Free State."

The first or prefatory clause of the Second Amendment sets forth the amendment's purpose and intent. An important aspect of ascertaining that purpose and intent is determining the import of the term "militia." Many advocates of the traditional individual rights model, including the Fifth Circuit, have taken the position that the term "militia" was meant to refer to all citizens, and, therefore, that the first clause simply restates the second in more specific terms. . . . Relying on their definition of "militia," they conclude that the prefatory clause was intended simply to reinforce the grant of an individual right that they assert is made by the second clause. . . .

We agree that the interpretation of the first clause and the extent to which that clause shapes the content of the second depends in large part on the meaning of the term "militia." If militia refers, as the Fifth Circuit suggests, to all persons in a state, rather than to the state military entity, the first clause would have one meaning — a meaning that would support the concept of traditional individual rights. If the term refers instead, as we believe, to the entity ordinarily identified by that designation, the state-created and organized military force, it would likely be necessary to attribute a considerably different meaning to the first clause of the Second Amendment and ultimately to the amendment as a whole.

We believe the answer to the definitional question is the one that most persons would expect: "militia" refers to a state military force. We reach our conclusion not only because that is the ordinary meaning of the word, but because contemporaneously enacted provisions of the Constitution that contain the word "militia" consistently use the term to refer to a state military entity, not to the people of the state as a whole. We look to such contemporaneously enacted provisions for an understanding of words used in the Second Amendment in part because this is an interpretive principle recently explicated by the Supreme Court in a case involving another word that appears in that amendment — the word "people." That same interpretive principle is unquestionably applicable when we construe the word "militia."

"Militia" appears repeatedly in the first and second Articles of the Constitution. . . . Nevertheless, the contexts in which the term is used demonstrate that even without the prefatory word, "militia" refers to state military organizations and not to their members or potential members throughout these two Articles. . . .

. . . .

Finally, our definition of "militia" is supported by the inclusion of the modifier "well regulated.". . .

### b. The Meaning of the Amendment's Second Clause: "The Right of the People to Keep and Bear Arms Shall Not Be Infringed."

. . . We consider it highly significant . . . that the second clause does not purport to protect the right to "possess" or "own" arms, but rather to "keep and bear" arms. This choice of words is important because the phrase "bear arms" is a phrase that customarily relates to a military function.

Historical research shows that the use of the term "bear arms" generally referred to the carrying of arms in military service — not the private use of arms for personal purposes. . . .

We also believe it to be significant that the first version of the amendment proposed by Madison to the House of Representatives concluded with an exemption from "bearing arms" for the "religiously scrupulous." . . . Accordingly, the exemption from bearing arms for the religiously scrupulous can only be understood as an exemption from carrying arms in the service of a state militia, and not from possessing arms in a private capacity. . . .

Finally, we address the use of the term "keep" in the second clause. The reason why that term was included in the amendment is not clear. . . . Arms can be "kept" for various purposes — military, social, or criminal. The question with respect to the Second Amendment is not whether arms may be kept, but by whom and for what purpose. If they may be kept so that the possessor is enabled to "bear arms" that are required for military service, the words would connote something entirely different than if they may be kept for any individual purpose whatsoever. In this connection, some scholars have suggested that "keep and bear" must be construed together (like "necessary and proper") as a unitary phrase that relates to the maintenance of arms for military service. . . . In the end, however, the use of the term "keep" does not appear to assist either side in the present controversy to any measurable extent.

### c. The Relationship Between the Two Clauses

. . . As we have noted, and as is evident from the structure of the Second Amendment, the first clause explains the purpose of the more substantive clause that follows, or, to put it differently, it explains the reason necessitating or warranting the enactment of the substantive provision. Moreover, in this case, the first clause does more than simply state the amendment's purpose or justification: it also helps shape and define the meaning of the substantive provision contained in the second clause, and thus of the amendment itself. . . .

When the second clause is read in light of the first . . . we believe that the most plausible construction of the Second Amendment is that it seeks to ensure the existence of effective state militias in which the people may exercise their right to bear arms, and forbids the federal government to interfere with such exercise. This conclusion is based in part on the premise, explicitly set forth in the text of the amendment, that the maintenance of effective state militias is essential to the preservation of a free State, and in part on the historical meaning of the right that the operative clause protects — the right to bear arms. . . .

In the end, however, given the history and vigor of the dispute over the meaning of the Second Amendment's language, we would be reluctant to say that the text and structure alone establish with certainty which of the various views is correct. Fortunately, we have available a number of other important sources that can help us determine whether ours is the proper understanding. These include records that reflect the historical context in which the amendment was adopted, and documents that contain significant portions of the contemporary debates relating to the adoption and ratification of the Constitution and the Bill of Rights. . . .

[The court then engages in an extended review of the historical context in which the Second Amendment was debated and adopted.]

What our historical inquiry reveals is that the Second Amendment was enacted in order to assuage the fears of Anti-Federalists that the new federal government would cause the state militias to atrophy by refusing to exercise its prerogative of arming the state fighting forces, and that the states would, in the absence of the amendment, be without the authority to provide them with the necessary arms. Thus, they feared, the people would be stripped of their ability to defend themselves against a powerful, over-reaching federal government. The debates of the founding era demonstrate that the second of the first ten amendments to the Constitution was included in order to preserve the efficacy of the state militias for the people's defense — not to ensure an individual right to possess weapons. Specifically, the amendment was enacted to guarantee that the people would be able to maintain an effective state fighting force — that they would have the right to bear arms in the service of the state.

   . . . .

. . . Our review of the debates during the Constitutional Convention, the state ratifying conventions, and the First Congress, as well as the other historical materials we have discussed, confirmed what the text strongly suggested: that the amendment was adopted in order to protect the people from the threat of federal tyranny by preserving the right of the states to arm their militias. The proponents of the Second Amendment believed that only if the states retained that power could the existence of effective state militias — in which the people could exercise their right to "bear arms" — be ensured. The historical record makes it equally plain that the amendment was not adopted in order to afford rights to individuals with respect to private gun ownership or possession. Accordingly, we are persuaded that we were correct in *Hickman* that the collective rights view, rather than the individual rights models, reflects the proper interpretation of the Second Amendment. Thus, we hold that the Second Amendment imposes no limitation on California's ability to enact legislation regulating or prohibiting the possession or use of firearms, including dangerous weapons such as assault weapons. Plaintiffs lack standing to assert a Second Amendment claim, and their challenge to the Assault Weapons Control Act fails.

[The court then held that the exceptions allowed for off-duty law enforcement officers did not violate principles of equal protection, but that there was no rational basis for an exception to allow for possession of prohibited weapons by retired police officers.]

* * *

## NORDYKE v. KING
### 364 F.3d. 1025 (9th Cir. 2004)

\* \* \*

[Introductory note: In an earlier phase of this litigation, a three-judge panel of the Ninth Circuit refused to hear a Second Amendment challenge to an ordinance of Alameda County, California, which prohibited the possession of firearms on county property and thus barred the plaintiffs' participation in a gun show held at the county's fairgrounds. *Nordyke v. King,* 319 F.3d 1185 (9th Cir. 1185 (2000). That three-judge panel viewed itself as bound by a prior *en banc* ruling of the 9th Circuit, *Hickman v. Block,* which essentially read the Second Amendment as protecting a collective, and not an individual, right. The panel took note of the 9th Circuit's post-*Hickman* decision in *Lockyer, supra,* but criticized the *Lockyer* court (also a three-judge panel) for not likewise considering itself bound by *Hickman,* which would have precluded its engaging in its own lengthy analysis of the Second Amendment.

That history brings us to the proceedings of which the opinion below is a part. The opinion is a dissent to the decision by a majority of the justices on the Ninth Circuit denying the *Nordyke* plaintiffs' petition for a rehearing, before the circuit court *en banc,* of the three-judge panel's refusal to hear the Second Amendment challenge. In substance, the dissent is a rejection of *Hickman, Lockyer,* and the three-judge decision in *Nordyke.*]

Gould, Judge, dissenting.

I respectfully dissent from our denial of rehearing en banc. This case presents an important issue of the scope of the constitutional guarantee of the Second Amendment, arising in the context of state restriction of gun shows. The panel decision in this case was compelled by our circuit's prior holding . . . in which we embraced a "collective rights" reading of the Second Amendment. . . . An "individual rights" interpretation, as was recently adopted by the Fifth Circuit [in *United States v. Emerson*] . . . is more consistent with the text, structure, purposes, and history of the Second Amendment, as well as colonial experience and pre-adoption history. It also reflects what I consider to be the scholarly consensus that has recently developed on the question of how to best interpret the Second Amendment. We should recognize that individual citizens have a constitutional right to keep and bear arms, subject — in the same manner as all other core constitutional rights — to certain limits. Thereafter, the chips will fall where they may, and decisions in due course will clarify what is and is not constitutionally permissible regulation, and the further standards for addressing it.

. . . .

I

The Second Amendment . . . contains a substantive guarantee and a prefatory clause. The collective rights view of the Second Amendment places undue weight on a confused interpretation of the prefatory clause to reach the conclusion that the Second Amendment grants only a collective right. . . . [E]ven if it were assumed that the Second Amendment's prefatory clause did limit the scope of the substantive guarantee to those in the "militia," the militia should be defined to encompass the people as a whole. The plain meaning of the language of the Second Amendment mandates an individual rights interpretation.

As with all of the first eight amendments of the Bill of Rights, the Second Amendment makes clear that its purpose is to grant a right to the people. As used throughout the text of the Constitution, "rights" and "powers" are granted to the people, whereas government only has "power" or "authority.". . . The Second Amendment states that the right it provides for is one "of the people." Apart from the Second Amendment, the phrase "the people" appears in four other places in the Bill of Rights. There is no question that "the people," as used in the First, Fourth, Ninth, and Tenth Amendments refers to individuals. . . .

The right granted to the people by the Second Amendment is one to "keep and bear arms." Those who support the collective rights view maintain that "keep and bear" should be read as a unitary phrase . . . or that the word "keep," as used in the Second Amendment, has no independent content because the Second Amendment does not protect a right to "own" or to "possess" arms. . . . Collective rights supporters argue further that the term "bear arms" refers only to members of an organized militia during actual service. . . . These interpretations of "keep and bear arms" are inconsistent with basic principles of constitutional interpretation, and conflict with the historical use and meaning of the words "keep" and "bear."

. . . .

I also disagree with the conclusion of collective rights proponents that the term "bear arms" has only military connotations. In *Emerson,* the Fifth Circuit conducted an extensive analysis of the use of "bear arms" in early state constitutions and declarations of rights. From this analysis, the *Emerson* court concluded that early nineteenth century constitutions and declarations of rights in at least ten different states gave "people" or "citizens" the right to "bear arms" in their own personal defense. Such widespread use of the phrase "bear arms" in state grants of individual rights undercuts the argument that the drafters of the Second Amendment chose this phrase as a manner of indicating a collective right.

However, even if "bear" is presumed to have a military definition, the Second Amendment's further use of the word "keep" takes the scope of the Second Amendment beyond the right to bear arms in military defense. Had the drafters of the Second Amendment intended only to grant the people a right to carry arms while serving in the organized militia, the use of "bear" alone would have been sufficient. The most common definition of "keep," both today as well as at the time the Second Amendment was drafted, is to have custody or possession of. . . .

. . . .

The Second Amendment's prefatory clause states: "A well regulated Militia, being necessary to the security of a free State." As the Second Amendment's substantive guarantee confers an individual right to keep and bear arms, the question is whether the language of the Amendment's preamble modifies the right conferred by the substantive guarantee to limit it to a "collective" right. I am convinced that it does not.

Supporters of a collective rights interpretation read the term "militia" as used in the Second Amendment to mean "essentially a state military entity," and "not some amorphous body of the people as a whole." However, the Second Amendment's language indicates that the "Militia" rests upon the shoulders of the people. And protecting the right of an individual to keep and bear arms certainly serves the Second Amendment's prefatory goal. Allowing citizens to keep arms furthers the effectiveness of a well-regulated militia, which is in turn necessary to the security of a free state. . . .

This interpretation is also consistent with the purposes and structure of the Second Amendment. The Second Amendment serves two purposes: (1) to protect against external threats of invasion; and (2) to guard against internal threats to our republic. . . . As I wrote in [a related case]:

> Those who debated and framed the Bill of Rights were educated in practical political concepts and doubtless recognized that an opening gambit for tyrants is to disarm the public. If the Second Amendment is held to protect only a state-regulated militia, then there would be no constitutional bar to a federal government outlawing possession of all arms by hunters and those with legitimate needs for protection. A general confiscation of guns could become the order of the day. I believe that result is foreclosed by the salient purpose of the Second Amendment to guard against tyranny, and that an individual right to keep and bear arms must be recognized.

However, even if I were to assume that the prefatory clause did modify the Second Amendment's substantive guarantee, I would still reach the conclusion that the Second Amendment guarantees an individual right. The First Militia Act of 1792, 1 Stat. 271 (1792), passed only a few years after ratification of the Constitution, provides a contemporaneous window on the accepted meaning of the term "militia" at the time the Constitution was drafted. . . . The Militia Act of 1792 defined the "militia" as: "each and every free able-bodied white male citizen of the respective states, resident therein, who is or shall be of the age of eighteen years, and under the age of forty-five years." Thus, contrary to the "collective rights" notion . . . the militia was precisely *not* "a state entity, a state fighting force," limited to those who are active members of such a collective organization. It was *all* the able-bodied white male citizens from 18 to 45, whether they were organized into a state fighting force or not.". . .

Furthermore, the Supreme Court has also had opportunity to expound on the historical meaning of the word "militia." In *Miller* the most recent Supreme Court precedent interpreting the Second Amendment, the Court devoted a substantial portion of its opinion to a discussion of the scope of the "militia." Looking to "the debates in the [constitutional] Convention, the history and legislation of the Colonies and States, and the writings of approved commentators," the Supreme Court concluded that the militia referred to by the Second Amendment was neither an organized fighting force nor a formal state military entity . . . In the words of the Court: "the Militia comprised all males physically capable of acting in concert for the common defense. A body of citizens enrolled for military discipline."

I do not read the prefatory clause of the Second Amendment to limit the scope of the substantive guarantee of the right to keep and bear arms. Even if a limiting purpose is attributed to the prefatory clause's reference to "militia," the First Militia Act, the current federal statutory definition of "militia" and the Supreme Court's review of the historical meaning and purpose of the militia at the time of the framers are in accord that a "militia" is not restricted to the organized state military. Instead, these authorities support the conclusion that the militia consists of everyday civilians from a broad swath of the population. It is by granting these ordinary civilians the right to keep and bear arms that the Second Amendment aims to further the effectiveness of a "well-regulated militia," which in turn is "necessary to the security of a free State."

## II

Historical analysis also supports the conclusion that the framers of the Bill of Rights intended for the Second Amendment to create an individual right to keep and bear arms. The Fifth Circuit devoted a substantial portion of the *Emerson* opinion to a detailed review of the debate between the Federalists, those in favor of a strong federal government, and Anti-Federalists, those skeptical of a powerful government, over the strength of the federal government established by the Constitution. A summary of the history of the Bill of Rights shows that contemporaneous concern over the strength of the federal government led to the creation of an individual right to keep and bear arms in the Second Amendment.

Although the government contemplated by the Constitution was one of limited, enumerated powers, the Anti-Federalists feared that the federal government would use its power to infringe on the fundamental rights of the people. One concern was the federal government's broad military power under the Constitution, including the power to call forth and organize the militia, and the power to raise and support a standing army. . . . The Anti-Federalists worried that this power could be used to control or destroy the militia, and that a tyrannical federal government could further use this power to leave the states and their citizens defenseless against the federal government's transgressions.

The concerns of the Anti-Federalists did not stop adoption of the Constitution, which was soon ratified by the required nine states. However, these concerns did persuade the first Congress to consider the need to amend the Constitution to include a Bill of Rights. During consideration of what eventually became the Second Amendment, the Senate rejected a proposed amendment that would have granted states the power to arm and train their own militias. In other words, the Senate expressly rejected an amendment proposing language that would support a collective rights view of the Second Amendment. . . .

Contemporaneous legal commentary further shows that persons living in the late eighteenth and nineteenth centuries viewed the Second Amendment as conferring an individual right. . . .

## III

The individual rights view of the Second Amendment has also "enjoyed recent widespread academic endorsement." Scholars with such wide-ranging views as Laurence Tribe, Akhil Reed Amar, William Van Alstyne, and Eugene Volokh have come to a consensus that the Second Amendment protects an individual right to keep and bear arms. . . .

. . . .

### IV

The Second Amendment protects the right "of the people." It protects the people's right not only to "bear arms," which may be read as having a military connotation, but also to "keep arms," which can only be interpreted as having an individual one. By rejecting the individual right to keep arms, *Hickman* fails to do justice to the language of the Second Amendment. *Hickman* also disregards the important lesson of history that an armed citizenry can both repel external aggression and check the danger of an internal government degenerating to tyranny.

. . . The Second Amendment was designed to provide national security not only when our country is strong but also if it were to become weakened or otherwise subject to attack. As the people bear the risk of loss of their freedom and the pain of any attack, our Constitution provides that the people have a right to participate in defense of the Nation. The Second Amendment protects that fundamental right.

\* \* \*

## BACH v. PATAKI
### 408 F.3d 75 (2d Cir. 2005)

Wesley, Judge.

\* \* \*

David Bach, a Virginia resident and domiciliary, wants to carry his Ruger P-85 9 mm pistol while visiting his parents in New York. He has a permit from the Commonwealth of Virginia to carry a concealed weapon. Bach is a model citizen — he holds a Department of Defense top secret security clearance, is a commissioned officer in the United States Naval Reserve, a veteran Navy SEAL, a lawyer employed by the Navy's Office of the General Counsel, a father of three, and, perhaps most laudably, a son who regularly visits his parents in upstate New York. "During the ten-hour drive between Virginia and Upstate New York, [his] family and [he] travel on dimly lit rural roads and busy streets and highways[,] some of which are in densely populated areas that have extremely high violent crimes rates." Bach has read "about unarmed, law-abiding citizens being slain by sadistic predators despite the exceptional efforts of law enforcement" and believes that carrying a pistol will help him protect his family.

However, as a nonresident without New York State employment, Bach is not eligible for a New York firearms license. The State Police informed Bach that "no exemption exists which would enable [him] to possess a handgun in New York State" and that "[t]here are no provisions for the issuance of a carry permit, temporary or otherwise, to anyone not a permanent resident of New York State nor does New York State recognize pistol permits issued by other states." The State Police further explained that persons "who maintain seasonal residen[ce] in New York State likewise are not eligible for a New York State Pistol Permit" and warned Bach that if he were found in possession of his pistol in New York he "would be subject to automatic forfeiture of the firearm in question and criminal prosecution."

Bach filed this action against State and local officials to contest his exclusion from New York's licensing scheme. His complaint requests that the district court declare New York's licensing laws unconstitutional, facially and as applied, in violation of both the "right to keep and bear arms" set out in the Second Amendment and the Privileges and Immunities Clause of Article IV of the United States Constitution. [which states that "[t]he Citizens of each State shall be entitled to all Privileges and Immunities of Citizens in the several States."].

. . . .

## II

New York State has regulated the possession of weapons since 1849. That year, the State criminalized possession of the "slung [sling] shot." Thirty-five years later, New York instituted a statewide licensing requirement for minors carrying weapons in public, and soon after the turn of the century, the State expanded its licensing requirements to include all persons carrying concealed pistols. With the passage of the Sullivan Act in the spring of 1911, New York's licensing requirement applied to all persons possessing pistols or any other firearm small enough to be carried concealed.

The State's earliest firearms-licensing statutes delegated licensing to municipalities. When the State first established statewide application requirements, it limited licenses to "have and carry concealed" to those "citizen[s] of and usually a resident in the state of New York," but permitted the licensing official — judges in most parts of the State, but the police commissioner in New York City — to make an exception, so long as the officer received certificates of good moral character regarding the applicant and the official "state[d] in such license the particular reason for the issuance thereof."

In 1963, New York altered its statewide licensing procedures, making two significant and related changes. First, it granted licensing officers the authority to revoke licenses "at any time." Second, it limited carry licensees to New York residents and in-state employees. As explained below, the licensing officers' revocation authority and the residency requirement remain features of the current statutory regime.

Today, New York regulates handguns primarily though Articles 265 and 400 of the Penal Law. Article 265 creates a general ban on handgun possession, with specific exemptions thereto. . . . The exemption at issue here is a licensed use exemption defined in Article 400: "[the p]ossession of a pistol or revolver by a person to whom a license therefor has been issued."

Article 400 of the Penal Law "is the exclusive statutory mechanism for the licensing of firearms in New York State." Licenses are limited to persons over twenty-one, of good moral character, without a history of crime or mental illness, and "concerning whom no good cause exists for the denial of the license."

There are several types of pistol and revolver licenses, including licenses for household possession, for workplace possession, and to "have and carry concealed." The last, a carry license, may issue only for "proper cause."

Licensing is a rigorous and principally local process that begins with the submission of a signed and verified application to a local licensing officer. Applicants must demonstrate compliance with certain statutory eligibility requirements as well as any facts "as may be required to show the good character, competency and integrity of each person or individual signing the application." Every application triggers a local investigation. "[T]he police authority of the city or county where the application is made is responsible for investigating the statements in the application." Local police, therefore, investigate applicants' mental health history, criminal history, moral character, and, in the case of a carry license, representations of proper cause. Police officers also take applicants' fingerprints and check them against the records of the State Division of Criminal Justice Services and the FBI. Upon completion of the investigation, the police authority reports its results to the licensing officer.

Local licensing officers, often local judges, have considerable discretion in deciding whether to grant a license application. . . .

A licensing officer is also "statutorily invested with the power to *sua sponte* revoke or cancel a license.". . .

An officer's revocation decision may be triggered by local incidents; in light of the highly destructive potential of a firearm, local officials may revoke a license if a licensee engages in behavior that portends of future problems. . . . Local incidents may also lead a licensing officer to conclude that a licensee lacks the mental fitness to continue to possess a firearm and to revoke the license on that basis.

Licensing is thus a locally controlled process. . . .

The only nonresidents eligible for a license are local workers, who may apply to the licensing officer in the city or county of their principal employment or principal place of business. The statute does not provide a mechanism for any other nonresident applications. One New York appellate court has explained that nonresident applications would be inconsistent with "the purposes underlying the pistol permit procedures, namely, to insure that only persons of acceptable background and character are permitted to carry handguns and to provide a method for reporting information on the identity of persons possessing weapons and the weapons themselves. . . ."

Some classes of nonresidents may nonetheless possess or carry handguns in New York. Although New York generally "does not recognize or give effect to licenses to carry firearms issued by . . . other state[s]," federal law grants a limited right to transport unloaded firearms through the State. Additionally, Article 265 sets forth a number of provisions permitting nonresidents to possess or carry firearms. For instance, police officers of other States may possess pistols while conducting official business in New York, and nonresidents licensed within their own States may use pistols in competitive shooting matches in New York . . .

### III

[The court then decides that Bach has standing to bring his constitutional claims even though he did not apply for a license.]

### IV

Bach argues that New York's licensing scheme unreasonably infringes upon his "right to keep and bear arms" under the Second Amendment. . . . He contends that the Second Amendment's right to keep and bear arms is a right of individual citizens, that it limits the States in regulating firearms, and that New York's statutory scheme cannot withstand the resultant heightened scrutiny.

Bach focuses primarily on the question of whether the right to keep and bear arms is an individual right. Applying textualist and originalist approaches to interpreting the Amendment, proffering historical and contemporary scholarship, and buttressed by the recent conclusions of both the Fifth Circuit and the Department of Justice, Bach asks this Court to declare the "right to keep and bear arms" an individual, rather than collective, right. Defendants, by contrast, construe the Amendment as merely a "guarantee . . . to the states [of] the collective right to arm or fortify their respective 'well regulated' militias" and insist that the Amendment "does not establish an individual right to 'bear arms' for any purpose." . . .

Although the sweep of the Second Amendment has become the focus of a national legal dialogue, we see no need to enter into that debate. Instead, we hold that the Second Amendment's "right to keep and bear arms" imposes a limitation on only federal, not state, legislative efforts. We thus join five of our sister circuits.

Our holding is compelled by the Supreme Court's opinion in Presser v. Illinois, 116 U.S. 252 (1886). In 1879, Herman Presser led four hundred armed members of a society called the *Lehr und Wehr Verein* through the streets of Chicago. Illinois's Military Code required that any "parade with arms" be licensed by the Governor. Presser lacked a license, and was charged and convicted under the Code. Presser argued to the Supreme Court that Illinois had exercised a power "forbidden to the States by the Constitution of the United States." He relied on both the Second and Fourteenth Amendments.

The Supreme Court rejected Presser's argument. Justice Woods explained, "[A] conclusive answer to the contention that [the Second Amendment] prohibits the legislation in question lies in the fact that the amendment is a limitation only upon the power of Congress and the National government, and not upon that of the States." . . .

*Presser* stands for the proposition that the right of the people to keep and bear arms, whatever else its nature, is a right only against the federal government, not against the States. . . .

Bach does not distinguish *Presser*. Rather, he contends that *Presser* is "outdated" and "do[es] not reflect the Court's modern view." He relies on two footnotes for support — the Fifth Circuit's comment in *Emerson* that *Presser* "came well before the Supreme Court began the process of incorporating certain provisions of the first eight amendments into the Due Process Clause of the Fourteenth Amendment," and the Ninth Circuit's similar note in *Silveira*. . . .

We must follow *Presser*. Where, as here, a Supreme Court precedent "has direct application in a case, yet appears to rest on reasons rejected in some other line of decisions, the Court of Appeals should follow the case which directly controls, leaving to th[e Supreme] Court the prerogative of overruling its own decisions." . . . We cannot overrule the Supreme Court.

Accordingly, we hold that the "right to keep and bear arms" does not apply against the States and affirm the district court's dismissal of Bach's Second Amendment claim.

V

Bach also challenges New York's licensing regime under the Privileges and Immunities Clause of Article IV, section two of the Constitution. He contends that "New York's prohibition on allowing nonresidents such as Bach to obtain a firearms license violates the Privileges and Immunities Clause."

Bach suggests that New York's licensing scheme unconstitutionally discriminates against both his protected rights under the Privileges and Immunities Clause and the "right to travel" secured therein. But the "right to travel," at least in this context, is simply a shorthand for the protections of the Privileges and Immunities Clause of Article IV, as travel — movement from one State to another — is at the core of every Privileges and Immunities Clause challenge. As the Supreme Court has explained, the "right to travel," in the constitutional context, "embraces at least three different components." Two of those components, "'the right of free ingress and regress to and from' neighboring states," and "the right of the newly arrived citizen to the same privileges and immunities enjoyed by other citizens of the same State," are inapplicable here. The third and only relevant component is merely a restatement of rights arising under Article IV — "the right to be treated as a welcome visitor rather than an unfriendly alien when temporarily present in [a] second State." Bach's appeal depends on only this last guarantee that, "by virtue of a person's state citizenship, a citizen of one State who travels in other States, intending to return home at the end of his journey, is entitled to enjoy the 'Privileges and Immunities of Citizens in the several States' that he visits." His appeal thus condenses to the challenge that New York's handgun licensing scheme unconstitutionally discriminates against nonresidents with regard to a protected privilege under the Clause.

The Privileges and Immunities Clause provides that "[t]he Citizens of each State shall be entitled to all Privileges and Immunities of Citizens in the several States." This clause, like the Commerce Clause of Article I, section 8, derives from the fourth of the Articles of Confederation, and had the primary purpose of "fus[ing] into one Nation a collection of independent, sovereign States," . . . It operates to "place the citizens of each State upon the same footing with citizens of other States, so far as the advantages resulting from citizenship in those States are concerned." Indeed, "[t]he Privileges and Immunities Clause, by making noncitizenship or nonresidence an improper basis for locating a special burden, implicates not only the individual's right to nondiscriminatory treatment but also, perhaps more so, the structural balance essential to the concept of federalism."

In order to prevail on a Privileges and Immunities challenge, a plaintiff must demonstrate that the "State has, in fact, discriminated against out-of-staters with regard to the privileges and immunities it accords its own citizens." The challenged "privilege" must come within the scope of the Clause. "The Clause '. . . establishes a norm of comity without specifying the particular subjects as to which citizens of one State coming within the jurisdiction of another are guaranteed equality of treatment.' "Only those activities " 'sufficiently basic to the livelihood of the Nation'" are protected. Other "distinctions between residents and nonresidents merely reflect the fact that this is a Nation composed of individual States."

Where a protected privilege or immunity is implicated, the State may defeat the challenge by showing sufficient justification for the discrimination, *i.e.,* "'something to indicate that non-citizens constitute a peculiar source of the evil at which the statute is aimed.'"A state may defend its position by demonstrating: "(a) a substantial reason for the discrimination, and (b) a reasonable relationship between the degree of discrimination exacted and the danger sought to be averted by enactment of the discriminatory statute." "The availability of less restrictive means is considered when evaluating the measure and degree of the relationship between the discrimination and state interest." This evaluation must "be conducted with due regard for the principle that States should have considerable leeway in analyzing local evils and prescribing appropriate cures."

Insofar as a plaintiff challenges a State's discrimination against him with regard to privileges and immunities — an "as-applied" challenge — he need only demonstrate that his own "nonresidency presents [no] special threat to any of the State's interests that is not shared" by residents. "A facial challenge to a legislative Act is, of course, the most difficult challenge to mount successfully, since the challenger must establish that no set of circumstances exist under which the Act would be valid." . . .

Bach argues that New York's licensing regime discriminates against nonresidents with regard to a protected right under Article IV's Privileges and Immunities Clause without sufficient justification. Defendants do not dispute that New York's laws discriminate against nonresidents, who, unlike residents, may only apply for a license if they work principally within the State. Instead, they respond, first, that possession of a firearm is not within the ambit of the Privileges and Immunities Clause and, second, that, even if the Clause did apply, New York's pistol permit scheme would remain valid because it "is closely related to a substantial state interest in restricting firearms possession to persons of acceptable temperament and character."

Bach can prevail only if New York's grant of an Article 400 license should be considered a "privilege" under Article IV. Neither the Supreme Court, this Court, nor any other Court of Appeals has considered whether the Privileges and Immunities Clause protects what Bach calls "the right to self-defense through the use of a firearm.". . .

. . . .

. . . Because we agree with defendants and the district court that New York's licensing scheme is sufficiently justified, we will assume, without deciding, that entitlement to a New York carry license is a privilege under Article IV.

There is no question that New York discriminates against nonresidents in providing handgun licenses under Article 400. Defendants do not contest this fact. Instead, they argue that the discrimination is sufficiently justified by New York's public safety interest in monitoring handgun licensees. We do not doubt, and Bach does not dispute, that "[t]he State has a substantial and legitimate interest . . . in insuring the safety of the general public from individuals who, by their conduct, have shown themselves to be lacking the essential temperament or character which should be present in one entrusted with a dangerous instrument."

New York's monitoring interest is, in essence, an interest in continually obtaining relevant behavioral information. The State's licensing scheme vests broad revocation discretion in a local licensing officer, permitting that officer to revoke a license on the basis of a wide variety of behavioral data, including information reported from local incidents. The operative information available to licensing officers is not restricted to the legal formalities of an arrest warrant, an accusatory instrument, or a judgment of conviction. Licensing officers have the discretion to revoke licenses upon displays of "poor judgment. . . .

But the degree of discrimination exacted must be substantially related to the threatened danger. This is the more difficult inquiry: With regard to New York's monitoring interest, is there any "particularized evil presented uniquely by nonresident[s] . . . that warrants the degree of outright discrimination imposed"? Defendants argue:

> The ongoing flow of information to a licensing officer as a result of the licensee's tie to a particular residence or community is an important element of the State's regulatory scheme. It substantially increases the likelihood that a licensing officer will be alerted to facts that cast doubt on a licensee's fitness to possess a firearm.

Bach challenges the substantiality of this relationship. He contends: (1) nonresidents within the State are no more difficult to monitor than residents, and (2) New York has not shown that it could not obtain the same quality of information from other States. Thus, Bach concludes, defendants have not shown any "palpable and unique risks" posed by out-of-state residents. . . .

First, although it may be true that New York can monitor nonresidents as easily as residents while either are in the State, New York has an interest in the entirety of a licensee's relevant behavior. Information regarding a licensee's adherence to license conditions is information that may only exist when the gun owner is in-state, but information regarding the licensee's character and fitness for a continued license is not so limited. New York has just as much of an interest, for example, in discovering signs of mental instability demonstrated in New Jersey as in discovering that instability in New York. The State can only monitor those activities that actually take place in New York. Thus, New York can best monitor the behavior of those licensees who spend significant amounts of time in the State. By limiting applications to residents and in-state workers, New York captures this pool of persons. It would be much more difficult for New York to monitor the behavior of mere visitors like Bach, whose lives are spent elsewhere.

Second, we think it self-evident that, at least in Bach's case, other States, like Virginia, cannot adequately play the part of monitor for the State of New York or provide it with a stream of behavioral information approximating what New York would gather. They do not have the incentives to do so. First, other States are not bound to impose a discretionary revocation system like New York's. Therefore, they need not engage in monitoring of licensees similar to New York's monitoring. Second, because a New York license operates only in New York, other States, like Virginia, have very little to gain from a revocation of a New York license — a revocation would affect the safety of New Yorkers, not Virginians. Obviously, New Yorkers have a much greater interest in reporting misbehavior to New York local licensing officers than do out-of-state persons and their government officers. Monitoring is incentive-driven; without these incentives, there is little reason to expect effective monitoring, if any.

Moreover, Bach does not point to any adequate alternative method for New York to collect this information. Bach argues that New York can and does rely on out-of-state reporting. . . . But New York's system permits license revocations for a range of misbehavior of which serious offenses and felonies form only a small part, and Bach does not point to any reason to expect Virginia or any other State to report such behavior to New York. Bach also suggests that New York could require nonresidents to submit to more frequent renewals or periodic interviews with local officials. However, New York's proffered interest is in monitoring the relevant day-to-day behavior of license-holders; it is unclear how an accelerated renewal schedule or a round of interviews with local officials would supply this information.

Bach also suggests that reference letters or certifications from a nonresident's local authorities could fill New York's informational gap. Perhaps in other contexts references or similar informational requests might provide an adequate substitute source of information. For instance, when a State has an interest in monitoring the fitness of a licensed professional, references from persons involved in professional relationships with the licensee might be an adequate source of information. Or, where a State has an interest in monitoring the fitness of a licensed user of some universally-insured activity — driving an automobile, for instance — submission of updated insurance reports might prove adequate. In both examples, there may be strong arguments that another party has an equally strong incentive to monitor the licensee's relevant behavior — the professional's clients will often have a personal stake in the professional's work; the insurer will have a financial stake in the insured's risk profile. Here, however, Bach has not pointed to any monitor with a similar interest in assessing a nonresident's fitness to carry a handgun. Other States are not bound by New York's monitoring system. Thus, Bach has not shown how New York could "protect its interests through less restrictive means."

New York's monitoring rationale is distinct from rationales rejected in other Privileges and Immunities Clause cases. Most importantly, the monitoring rationale is not an interest of merely "general concern," to which a resident/nonresident distinction would not be tailored, but, rather, actually turns on where a person spends his or her time. The exception for nonresidents working in-state is consistent with this criterion. . . . New York's exception is relevant because the location of a licensee's principal employment correlates with the State's monitoring interest in a manner similar to the place of the licensee's residence — both present opportunities for the State to monitor the licensee. New York's nonresident distinction, with the in-state worker exception, is thus tailored to the State's monitoring interest.

Defendants have demonstrated that "'non-citizens constitute a peculiar source of the evil at which the statute is aimed.'" Bach's failure to prevail on his as-applied challenge renders his facial challenge likewise invalid. Accordingly, we affirm the district court's rejection of Bach's Privileges and Immunities Clause claim.

\* \* \*

## NOTES AND QUESTIONS

**1.** Unlike so many other public health measures considered in this textbook, the activity that gun control legislation seeks to regulate or prohibit is specifically protected by the federal and state constitutions — at least to some extent. That alone counsels some caution in designing and implementing gun control measures. But the protection of the Second Amendment to the federal Constitution and the protections of the "right to bear arms" that appear in most state constitutions are not easily defined and do not parallel the substantive protections of other protected activities such as speech, religion, or privacy.

Somewhat oddly, there has been virtually no guidance from the U.S. Supreme Court as to the meaning and application of the Second Amendment. The only Supreme Court decision directly addressing the Second Amendment is *United States v. Miller*, 307 U.S. 174 (1939), which upheld a prosecution under the 1934 federal gun control law of individuals who were trafficking in "sawed-off shotguns" across state lines. As discussed in *Wright,* the Court held that since there was no possible linkage between a "well-regulated militia" and the activities of the defendants, the Second Amendment was no bar to the prosecution. Subsequent courts have debated the implications of that holding, but, in fact, the *Miller* decision does little more than recognize that the Second Amendment can, in some circumstances (other than those before the Court), limit the scope of otherwise constitutional federal government activities.

Subsequent to *Miller*, most courts, as reflected in the *Wright* and *Silveira* decisions, have adopted the narrower view that the Second Amendment is a *collective right*, essentially imposing limits on the extent to which the federal government can restrict the states in matters relating to their maintenance of the state's militia. In its narrowest form, this would mean that the Second Amendment does not apply to state government limitations on guns at all.

This narrow view of the reach of the Second Amendment was adopted in *Quilici v. Village of Morton Grove*, 695 F.2d 261 (7th Cir. 1982), which observed that the Supreme Court has never held that the Second Amendment should be viewed as "incorporated" into the substantive requirements of the Fourteenth Amendment; as a consequence, *Quilici* held that the Second Amendment was inapplicable to a local ordinance (or to any other local or state law).

The *Bach* decision comes to the same conclusion as *Quilici*, although somewhat indirectly. Most other courts reviewing local or state gun control laws, even those adopting a collective rights approach to the Second Amendment, as demonstrated by *Silveira*, have at least considered the Second Amendment as potentially applicable to state laws, even while denying that the limits of the Second Amendment invalidate the laws they were evaluating.

As noted in each of the Second Amendment cases excerpted in this chapter, there has been a recent trend towards reexamining the meaning and application of the Second Amendment. In *United States v. Emerson*, 270 F.3d 203 (5th Cir. 2001, the Fifth Circuit, after a lengthy review of the deliberations leading to the adoption of the Second Amendment, the political and historical record of that time, and the ever-growing literature concerning the "right to bear arms," held that the Second Amendment does protect an individual's ability to "bear arms" (although the *Emerson* court went on to uphold the conviction under state law of the defendant who had possession of a handgun in violation of a court order).

Since *Emerson*, a number of justices and a few other courts have indicated that they may prefer the individual rights approach of *Emerson* to the collective rights approach of *Wright, Silveira,* and most other courts. In 2004, the Bush Administration also took the position (under the urging of Attorney General Ashcroft) that the Second Amendment should be viewed as an individual right. *See* www.usdoj.gov/olc/ (last visited December 2006).

**2.** The *Nordyke* decisions provide a good illustration of the unsettled status of the law in the last few years and of the issues that are the focus of this highly emotional debate. As noted in *Silveira*, the Ninth Circuit, sitting en banc, adopted a collective rights approach to the Second Amendment in *Hickman v. Block*, 81 F.3d 98 (9th Cir. 1996). *Silveira*, a three-judge panel decision, affirmed that view. In the first *Nordyke* decision, another panel came to the same conclusion: The Second Amendment confers a collective right and, as a result, individuals cannot claim that the Second Amendment protects them from state or federal gun control laws. The second *Nordyke* decision was a refusal by the whole Circuit to rehear the first *Nordyke* decision en banc. The dissent to that decision, excerpted *supra*, outlines the arguments in support of the individual right perspective (and makes reference to the other decisions that also have taken a "new look" at these issues.).

**3.** One related issue that has not been addressed at length in any of these cases is the applicable level of judicial scrutiny, if and when the Second Amendment is applied to a state or federal law. As reviewed in earlier chapters, when the government acts in a manner that affects constitutionally protected rights such as privacy, speech, or religion, that fact does not establish an absolute bar to government action, but instead leads the courts to more closely examine the government's purposes or objectives and the means by which they are sought to be achieved. Even speech, perhaps the most closely protected constitutional right, can be subject to regulation or even prohibited altogether if the government's purpose is "compelling" and the means for achieving that purpose are "sufficiently tailored." Assuming the Second Amendment does apply to a state or federal gun control law, that is only the beginning of the inquiry; the courts must still apply some enhanced level of judicial review to that legislation. In this regard, *Emerson* is a good illustration: Even while recognizing that the "right to bear arms" is implicated by a state law, it still upheld the enforcement of that law (with, unfortunately, little discussion of the applicable standard of judicial review).

What governmental purposes might be sufficiently important to justify a regulation or denial of "the right to bear arms"? How narrow or "tailored" does that legislation have to be? Is a general objection to some types of guns, *e.g.*, assault rifles, enough of a justification for a categorical ban? If misuse of a gun is a crime, is a prohibition on the possession of guns to avoid that misuse an overbroad effort to prevent the crime? Perhaps most important from a public health perspective, will the courts require advocates of gun control to show empirical support for their claims that one or another gun control law is constitutionally justified?

**4.** A second relatively-overlooked issue arises from the fact that some, though not all, states have a "right to bear arms" in their state constitutions. Often these state constitutional provisions are worded differently than the Second Amendment. As such, they may provide a wholly separate basis for opposing a state or local gun control law, one that may be of special relevance in those jurisdictions that view the Second Amendment as inapplicable to the states. More broadly, the state right could be interpreted as an individual one, even by a court or justice inclined to read the Second Amendment as protecting only collective rights.

Interestingly, this was a non-issue in the Ninth Circuit decisions in *Lockyer* and *Nordyke* since there is not an explicit "right to bear arms" in the California state constitution. In other states with state constitutional rights to bear or keep arms, the issue could be much more important if not wholly determinative.

The State of Washington provides an interesting example. Washington State Constitution article 1, § 24 provides:

> The right of the individual citizen to bear arms in defense of himself, or the state, shall not be impaired, but nothing in this section shall be construed as authorizing individuals or corporations to organize, maintain, or employ an armed body of men.

This provision clearly enough contemplates an individual right, which would limit the state's ability to regulate or prohibit various forms of use or possession of arms. But as applied by the state's supreme court, this individual right is subject to "reasonable regulation under the state's police powers." What this means varies from context to context but does not appear to be the kind of stringent protection of the individual's right typically seen in privacy, speech, or religion cases. *See, e.g., Seattle v. Montana*, 129 Wash. 2d 583, 919 P.2d 1218 (1996) (local ordinance banning the possession of dangerous knives upheld); *State v. Schelin*, 147 Wash. 2d 562, 55 P.3d 632 (2002) (evidence of gun collection admissible where constructive possession of firearms is an element of the crime); *cf. State v. Rupe*, 101 Wash. 2d 664, 683 P.2d 571 (1984) (admission into evidence of defendant's gun collection in penalty phase of homicide prosecution reversible error).

Other states also have recognized a state constitutional individual right to bear arms, but also have allowed the state some discretion in designing and implementing gun control legislation. Again, the critical issue may be the state courts' formulation of the applicable level of judicial scrutiny. For example, in *Mosby v. Devine*, 851 A.2d 1031 (R.I. 2004), the Rhode Island Supreme Court held that the state constitution creates an individual (not collective) right to bear arms, but that the state's gun permit law was a reasonable exercise of the police power (implying a minimal level of judicial review). For a similar decision upholding a state law banning assault weapons, see *Benjamin v. Bailey*, 662 A.2d 1226 (Conn. 1995).

Kentucky's constitution protects an individual right to bear arms, subject only to legislative regulation of carrying concealed weapons. Nonetheless, the Kentucky Supreme Court recently recognized a broader zone of permissible legislative restriction of the right. In *Posey v. Commonwealth*, 185 S.W.3d 170, (Ky. 2006), the defendant, a felon, was convicted under a state law that made it a crime for a felon to possess a firearm. Posey claimed that the state law violated the state's constitution. Section 1(7) of the Kentucky Constitution reads:

> All men are, by nature, free and equal, and have certain inherent and inalienable rights, among which may be reckoned . . . [t]he right to bear arms in defense of themselves and of the State, subject to the power of the General Assembly to enact laws to prevent persons from carrying concealed weapons.

The Kentucky Supreme Court interpreted that language broadly:

> While we agree that it may be reasonable to infer from this language . . . that the 1890 constitutional convention desired to expand the lot of persons entitled to possess firearms, we disagree that this expansion reasonably or necessarily included convicted felons. It is generally accepted that certain classes of persons are thought to lack the ability or the natural attributes to possess many of the rights which are recognized under our constitution. For example, none of the parties dispute the premise that children and insane or incompetent persons are likely not endowed with the natural right to bear arms. . . . Historically, convicted felons were similarly accorded diminished status when it came to being endowed with certain natural rights.
>
> Indeed, the view prevailing at the time our modern constitution was formulated was that felons were not endowed with the natural right to possess firearms. . . . Thus, without further evidence to suggest that convicted felons were somehow accorded more status by the 1890 constitutional convention than was historically attributed to them, we

cannot say that the use of the word "men" within our modern constitution was intended to necessarily encompass those men who were
convicted felons.

. . . .

In fact, the concept of an individual right to bear arms sprung from
classical republican ideology which required the individual holding
that right to maintain a certain degree of civic virtue. . . . This concept
of civic virtue is similarly reflected in other provisions contained in
[the state constitution], such as the rights of all persons to life, liberty,
and the pursuit of happiness. Yet, neither party would claim that
these rights are absolute or somehow immune from reasonable limitations in the interest of public safety and welfare.

. . . .

. . . In balance, we defer to the reasonable interpretation of our legislature, finding that the constitution permits some reasonable regulation of the people's right to bear arms, but only to the extent that such
regulation is enacted to ensure the liberties of all persons by maintaining the proper and responsible exercise of the general right contained
in Section 1(7).

185 S.W.3d at 177-78.

**5.** Note that the *Bach* decision also considered a separate constitutional
problem. Bach was claiming that the state's requirement that handgun
licenses only be issued to residents violated his privileges and immunities as
secured by Article IV, § 2 of the Constitution (as opposed to the privileges and
immunities referenced in § 1 of the Fourteenth Amendment). Essentially
Article IV prohibits states from discriminating between residents and nonresidents with regard to unspecified "privileges and immunities." The courts have
had few opportunities to interpret which activities are regarded as "privileges
and immunities" or the discretion allowed to the states. The *Bach* court avoids
the first problem by assuming for purposes of argument that a hand gun
license would fall within the category of "privileges and immunities," but holding that the state had a sufficient justification for denying licenses to nonresidents notwithstanding the prohibition of Article IV, § 2. For background, see
*United Building & Construction Trades Council of Camden County & Vicinity
v. Mayor and Council of City of Camden*, 465 U.S. 208 (1984).

**6.** As mentioned in several of the excerpts in this chapter, a separate constitutional debate was sparked by the enactment of the "Brady Act" in 1993,
amending the Gun Control Act of 1968, 18 U.S.C. § 921 *et seq.*, and requiring
dealers to be licensed and requiring dealers to make background checks to
determine whether purchasers of handguns were eligible under state and federal law to own handguns. The 1993 amendments included a requirement that
gun dealers submit background information to state and local law enforcement agencies who were required to make "reasonable efforts" to verify the
accuracy of the information obtained by the dealers. The legislation anticipated that eventually an "instant" verification system would be developed.

In *Printz v. United States*, 521 U.S. 898 (1997), the Supreme Court held that the requirements relating to state and local law enforcement were unconstitutional. According to the Court, Tenth Amendment principles prohibit the Congress from imposing mandatory obligations on state officials (and their local counterparts). The Court did not, however, invalidate the entire "Brady Act" (as suggested by one of the authors above ) nor did the Court in any way rely on the Second Amendment or give any significance to the facts that this was a federal law regulating the ownership or sale of guns. The focus of the decision was federalism, specifically the impermissibility of the federal government's directly imposing regulatory responsibilities on state and local officials.

## D.  THE ROLE OF LITIGATION IN DETERMINING PUBLIC POLICY ON GUN USE AND OWNERSHIP

### 1.   The Government as Plaintiff

### CITY OF CINCINNATI v. BERETTA U.S.A. CORP.
95 Ohio St. 3d 416, 768 N.E.2d 1136 (2002)

Sweeney, Justice.

\* \* \*

On April 28, 1999, plaintiff-appellant, the city of Cincinnati, filed a complaint against fifteen handgun manufacturers, three trade associations, and one handgun distributor, seeking to hold them responsible under nuisance, negligence, and product liability theories of recovery, for the harm caused by the firearms they manufacture, sell, or distribute. The gist of the complaint is that appellees have manufactured, marketed, and distributed their firearms in ways that ensure the widespread accessibility of the firearms to prohibited users, including children and criminals.

. . . .

This case represents one of a growing number of lawsuits brought by municipalities against gun manufacturers and their trade associations to recover damages associated with the costs of firearm violence incurred by the municipalities. . . .

. . . .

### A.   Public Nuisance

Appellant alleged in its complaint that appellees have created and maintained a public nuisance by manufacturing, marketing, distributing, and selling firearms in ways that unreasonably interfere with the public health, welfare, and safety in Cincinnati and that the residents of Cincinnati have a common right to be free from such conduct. Appellant further alleged that appellees know, or reasonably should know, that their conduct will cause handguns to be used and possessed illegally and that such conduct produces an ongoing nuisance that has a detrimental effect upon the public health, safety, and welfare of the residents of Cincinnati.

. . . [A]ppellees maintain that Ohio's nuisance law does not encompass injuries caused by product design and construction, but instead is limited to actions involving real property or to statutory or regulatory violations involving public health or safety. We disagree. . . . "Unreasonable interference" includes those acts that significantly interfere with public health, safety, peace, comfort, or convenience, conduct that is contrary to a statute, ordinance, or regulation, or conduct that is of a continuing nature or one which has produced a permanent or long-lasting effect upon the public right, an effect of which the actor is aware or should be aware. . . . Contrary to appellees' position, there need not be injury to real property in order for there to be a public nuisance.

. . . .

Appellees further argue that they cannot be held liable for the harm alleged because they did not have control over the alleged nuisance at the time of injury. Contrary to appellees' position, it is not fatal to appellant's public nuisance claim that appellees did not control the actual firearms at the moment that harm occurred.

Appellant's complaint alleged that appellees created a nuisance through their ongoing conduct of marketing, distributing, and selling firearms in a manner that facilitated their flow into the illegal market. Thus, appellant alleged that appellees control the creation and supply of this illegal, secondary market for firearms, not the actual use of the firearms that cause injury. Just as the individuals who fire the guns are held accountable for the injuries sustained, appellees can be held liable for creating the alleged nuisance.

Appellees also contend that appellant's nuisance claim cannot go forward because the distribution of firearms is highly regulated and covers "legislatively authorized conduct.". . . Even though there exists a comprehensive regulatory scheme involving the manufacturing, sales, and distribution of firearms . . . the law does not regulate the distribution practices alleged in the complaint.

Finally, appellees argue that the public nuisance claim fails because appellant has failed to plead an underlying tort to support either an absolute public nuisance claim based on intentional or ultra-hazardous activity or a negligence-based claim of qualified public nuisance. However, the complaint clearly alleged both intentional and negligent misconduct on appellees' part. . . .

## B.   Negligence

Appellant further alleged in its complaint that appellees were negligent in failing to exercise reasonable care in designing, manufacturing, marketing, advertising, promoting, distributing, supplying, and selling their firearms without ensuring that the firearms were safe for their intended and foreseeable use by consumers. In addition, the complaint alleged that appellees failed to exercise reasonable care to provide a full warning to consumers of the risks associated with firearms.

In order to maintain a negligence action, the plaintiff must show the existence of a duty, a breach of that duty, and that the breach of that duty proximately caused the plaintiff's injury.

. . . [T]he negligence issue before us is not whether appellees owe appellant a duty to control the conduct of third parties. Instead, the issue is whether appellees are themselves negligent by manufacturing, marketing, and distributing firearms in a way that creates an illegal firearms market that results in foreseeable injury. Consequently, the "special relationship" rule is not determinative of the issue presented here. . . .

        . . . .

## C.   Product Liability

Appellant also seeks recovery under two products liability theories, for defective design and failure to warn. In its complaint, appellant alleged that the guns manufactured or supplied by appellees were defective because they do not incorporate feasible safety devices that would prevent unauthorized use and foreseeable injuries. As to the cause of action for failure to warn, appellant alleged that appellees manufactured or supplied guns without adequate warning of their dangerousness or instruction as to their use.

The court of appeals upheld the dismissal of these claims, finding that the complaint was deficient because it did not allege with specificity "a single defective condition in a particular model of gun at the time it left its particular manufacturer.". . .

. . . [S]ince Ohio is a notice-pleading state, Ohio law does not ordinarily require a plaintiff to plead operative facts with particularity. . . . [A] complaint need only contain "a short and plain statement of the claim showing that the party is entitled to relief." Consequently, as long as there is a set of facts, consistent with the plaintiff's complaint, which would allow the plaintiff to recover, the court may not grant a defendant's motion to dismiss. Appellant's complaint withstands this test of notice pleading, since it alleged that appellees had manufactured or supplied defective guns without appropriate safety features.

Nevertheless, appellant is precluded from bringing its statutory product liability claims. Under the Product Liability Act, a claimant (including a governmental entity) cannot recover economic damages alone. Instead, in order to fall within the purview of the Act, and to be considered a "product liability claim". . . the complaint must allege damages other than economic ones. . . . However, the failure to allege other than economic damages does not necessarily destroy the right to pursue common-law product liability claims.

We likewise find that appellant can bring a common-law failure-to-warn claim. . . . To recover under a failure-to-warn theory at common law, the plaintiff must prove that the manufacturer knew or should have known, in the exercise of reasonable care, of the risk or hazard about which it failed to warn and that the manufacturer failed to take precautions that a reasonable person would take in presenting the product to the public. . . .

The court of appeals reasoned that the failure-to-warn claim could not go forward because the defendants owe no duty to warn of the dangers associated with firearms, which are open and obvious dangers. Although, in general, the dangers associated with firearms are open and obvious, appellant has alleged sufficient facts in its complaint to overcome a motion to dismiss. . . . [S]ome of the allegations involve risks that are not open and obvious, such as the fact that a semiautomatic gun can hold a bullet even when the ammunition magazine is empty or removed. . . .

## II. Remoteness

Appellees maintain that even if appellant could establish any of the elements of the individual torts it alleged, the injuries to the city are still too remote to create liability on the part of the gun manufacturers and trade associations. In essence, appellees argue that remoteness bars recovery, since the causal connection between the alleged wrongdoing and the alleged harm is too tenuous and remote and because the claims asserted are indirect and wholly derivative of the claims of others.

Remoteness is not an independent legal doctrine but is instead related to the issues of proximate causation or standing. Thus, a complaint will fail on remoteness grounds if the harm alleged is the remote consequence of the defendant's misconduct (causation) or is wholly derivative of the harm suffered by a third party (standing).

. . . [In] handgun litigation, the courts have taken divergent positions. While some courts have found that remoteness bars recovery [others] have rejected the remoteness argument. . . .

The complaint in this case alleged that as a direct result of the misconduct of appellees, appellant has suffered "actual injury and damages including, but not limited to, significant expenses for police, emergency, health, prosecution, corrections and other services.". . . [I]n taking the allegations in the complaint as true, we find that the alleged harms are direct injuries to appellant, and that such harms are not so remote or indirect as to preclude recovery by appellant as a matter of law.

With regard to whether causation is too remote in this case, we turn to the three factors. . . . The first concern, difficulty of proof, is minimal in this case, since appellant is seeking recovery, in part, for police expenditures and property repairs, which can be easily computed. Under the second factor, there is little risk of double recovery, since appellant is seeking recovery for injuries to itself only. . . . Finally, no other person is available to bring suit against appellees for these damages. Under the third factor, [we consider] whether "the general interest in deterring injurious conduct" will be better served by requiring that suit be brought by more directly injured victims. Although appellant is indirectly attempting to protect its citizens from the alleged misconduct by the gun manufacturers and trade associations, appellant is seeking recovery for its own harm. Under these circumstances, the general interest will be best served by having this plaintiff bring this lawsuit. . . .

## III.   Recoupment of Cost of Governmental Services

Appellant alleged in its complaint that due to the misconduct of appellees, it has sustained damages, including "significant expenses for police, emergency, health, corrections, prosecution and other services." Appellees contend that the cost of these public services is non-recoverable, since these are services the city is under a duty to provide.

Although a municipality cannot reasonably expect to recover the costs of city services whenever a tortfeasor causes harm to the public, it should be allowed to argue that it may recover such damages in this type of case. . . . [T]he misconduct alleged in this case is ongoing and persistent. The continuing nature of the misconduct may justify the recoupment of such governmental costs. Therefore, if appellant can prove all the elements of the alleged torts, it should be able to recover the damages flowing from appellees' misconduct. . . .

## IV.   Constitutional Arguments

Appellees further argue that appellant is attempting to regulate a national firearms industry and, therefore, its claims are barred under the Commerce Clause and the Due Process Clause of the United States Constitution.

. . . .

We find no impediment in the Due Process or Commerce Clause that requires dismissal of this lawsuit.

## V.   Conclusion

In conclusion, we find that the court of appeals erred in upholding the dismissal of the complaint, since sufficient facts have been alleged to withstand scrutiny under Civ. R. 12(b) (6). Reversal of the judgment, however, does not mean that appellant will prevail upon remand. What it does mean is that appellant has alleged the facts necessary to withstand a motion to dismiss and will now have the opportunity to pursue its claims. While we do not predict the outcome of this case, we would be remiss if we did not recognize the importance of allowing this type of litigation to go past the pleading stages. As two commentators so aptly noted: "If as a result of both private and municipal lawsuits, firearms are designed to be safer and new marketing practices make it more difficult for criminals to obtain guns, some firearm-related deaths and injuries may be prevented. While no one should believe that lawsuits against gun manufacturers and dealers will solve the multifaceted problem of firearm violence, such litigation may have an important role to play, complementing other interventions available to cities and states."

. . . .

Moyer, Chief Justice, dissenting.

I respectfully dissent from the majority's decision. Appellant alleges an "epidemic of handguns in the hands of persons who cannot lawfully possess them, which has brought terror to the streets, schoolyards, playgrounds, and homes of Cincinnati and has resulted in thousands of preventable shootings of innocent citizens, especially children and police officers." These are serious allegations, and portray a city under siege virtually overrun with criminals bearing illegally obtained handguns. However, the issue before us is not whether the city could prove that appellees fail to take reasonable measures that would prevent handguns they sell from being possessed by criminals and minors. Nor is the issue whether this alleged failure "unreasonably interferes with the public's health, safety, welfare, and peace," as alleged by appellant. The issue is not whether we agree with appellant that there exists in Cincinnati an epidemic of violence due to handguns illegally obtained.

This appeal simply involves a question of law: Does the city have standing to assert its claims? The majority holds that appellant has standing. I disagree with this conclusion, and would find the city's alleged injuries to be too remote from the conduct of appellees and too derivative of the harms suffered by victims of handgun violence to establish proper standing to sue the appellees.

As the majority's discussion regarding remoteness and proximate causation aptly demonstrates, the harm alleged by the city must not be a remote or tenuous consequence of the appellees' alleged misconduct. . . . The limitation of proximate causation rests in a very large part on the nature and degree of the connection between the defendant's acts and the events of which the plaintiff complains.

. . . .

In the instant case, the city characterizes appellees as corporations that design, manufacture, advertise, import and/or sell firearms that can be fired by unauthorized or unintended users in Cincinnati. Therefore, the links in the factual chain between appellees' conduct and harms [are from] manufacturer to distributor or wholesaler, distributor or wholesaler to retailer, retailer to authorized or unauthorized buyers, and ultimately accidental misuse by authorized buyers or criminal misuse by unauthorized buyers. Accidental and criminal misuse of handguns then results in increased expenses for the city for "additional police protection, overtime, emergency services, pension benefits, health care, social services and other necessary facilities and services." In addition, the city alleges that it has sustained "a loss of investment, economic development and tax revenue due to lost productivity — all associated with the defective design, and negligent manufacture, assembly, marketing, distribution, promotion and sale of guns."

. . . The very fact that there are multiple links between the conduct of the manufacturers and the harms suffered by the city demonstrates the difficulty in determining damages. For example, where a criminal wrongdoer harms another with an illegally obtained handgun, that criminal offender is responsible for injuries caused to the victim. Depending upon how the wrongdoer obtained the handgun, there may be a number of persons linking the offender to the retailer or distributor, who may also be liable. Additionally, there will be enormous difficulties in determining exactly how much of municipal expenses such as police, emergency services, pension benefits, health care, social services and other necessary facilities and services, as well as loss of revenue and investment and economic development, are a result of *only* the manufacturers' actions and *not the actions of the criminal wrongdoer, the retailer, distributor, or persons who possess guns legally.*

Finally, factors other than the manufacture, advertisement, distribution, and retail sales of handguns may contribute to the various harms claimed by the plaintiffs. . . . [T]hese may include "illegal drugs, poverty, illiteracy, inadequacies in the public educational system, the birth rates of unmarried teenagers, the disintegration of family relationships, the decades-long trend of the middle class moving from city to suburb, the upward track of health costs generally, and unemployment.

. . . [I]n addition to remoteness, the harms suffered by the plaintiffs were derivative of those suffered by the victims and their families. In other words, the city would not suffer the harm of increased costs for municipal services but for the fact that certain residents of the city had been the primary victims of handgun violence. . . .

The majority characterizes this first factor as one of "difficulty of proof," and believes the difficulty to be minimal, as the city "is seeking recovery, in part, for police expenditures and property repairs, which can be easily computed." However, in order to prove damages, the city must first identify which incidents involved the use of illegal handguns or legal handguns in the hands of unauthorized users, and then link that portion of the city's costs to that incident. In many instances the weapon used in a crime is never recovered. How, under these circumstances, can the city prove that the weapon involved was either illegal or in the hands of an unauthorized user?

. . . .

The question is not whether the city can prove that it has suffered damages, but whether the city can prove that those damages are attributable to the wrongdoing of the gun manufacturers as opposed to other, independent factors. Given the multiple links in the factual chain between the gun manufacturers' conduct and harms suffered by the city, the derivative nature of the harms when viewed in conjunction with harms suffered by the primary victims of handgun violence, as well as the multiple societal factors that contribute to the misuse of handguns, I would find a very high degree of difficulty in determining the amount of the city's damages attributable to the conduct of the gun manufacturers.

. . . .

In its complaint, the city paints a horrific picture of murder, assault, suicides, and accidental killings involving either illegal handguns or legal handguns in the hands of unauthorized users. As a result of these violent acts, the city, "in its role of providing protection and care for its citizens, . . . provide[s] or pay[s] for additional police protection, emergency services, pension benefits, health care and other necessary services due to the threat posed by the use of defendants' products." In addition, the city alleges harm as a result of "injuries to certain of its residents and police officers caused by the defendants' products, as well as by the loss of substantial tax revenue."

Taking, as we must, these pleadings as true, it follows that for practically every harm the city has suffered, there is at least one injured victim standing between the city and the gun manufacturers. In its complaint, the city states that it is seeking reimbursement for police, emergency, health, corrections, prosecution, and other services. Support for the conclusion that this is a derivative action is found in the complaint itself, which expressly connects the city's damages to death and injuries by individual citizens allegedly resulting from illegal handguns or the use of legal handguns by unauthorized users. This would suggest that many of the city's expenses would not have been incurred but for injuries to the primary victim. For example, the city may incur expenses for police, emergency services, and health care when someone has been injured because of the use of an unauthorized or illegal handgun. The injured person may also have a claim against the gun manufacturers.

. . . [Our prior case law] requires courts to analyze not whether these damages are capable of being proven, but whether the difficulties inherent in fashioning complicated rules apportioning damages among multiple plaintiffs is justified. Thus . . . because directly injured victims can generally be expected to vindicate the law "as private attorneys general" without the problems described by factors one and two, the need for courts to grapple with these problems is simply unjustified by the general interest in deterring injurious conduct. . . .

. . . .

Cook, Justice, dissenting.

Like the Chief Justice, I would find that Cincinnati's negligence-based claims are barred by remoteness principles. I write separately, however, because our views on remoteness ultimately diverge in one subtle respect. I also write separately to illustrate why the city has failed to state cognizable claims for products liability and public nuisance.

. . . I would find that the remoteness of the alleged harm precludes the city from establishing *proximate cause* as a matter of law. . . .

. . . .

. . . [R]emoteness principles also support dismissal of the city's causes of action sounding in products liability. Remoteness aside, however, the city's claims also fail for their failure to plead a compensable injury.

The majority correctly determines that the city has failed to state a valid statutory claim for relief insofar as an action for purely economic harm is not maintainable under the Ohio Products Liability Act. I disagree, however, with the majority's holding that the city may maintain its common-law products-liability claims alleging defective design and failure to warn. Even assuming that the Act does not preempt these claims . . . the city has not pleaded valid common-law causes of action. As the majority acknowledges, the city pleaded facts suggesting that it has suffered purely economic damages (*i.e.*, increased municipal costs allegedly attributable to the actions of the various defendants). The majority cites no case, however, in which we have allowed products liability to be a viable theory of recovery for a plaintiff situated similarly to the city in this case — namely, a plaintiff whose economic harm is *not* attributed to having been a user, consumer, or foreseeable person present at the time of product failure. . . .

As to the public-nuisance cause of action, it is true that principles of remoteness do not necessarily prevent the city from stating a valid claim. . . . Nevertheless, even this cause of action fails because the reach of public-nuisance law does not go as far as the city would have us extend it.

First, the city's allegations of harm cut against holding the named defendants responsible under a public-nuisance theory. The defendants' allegedly wrongful conduct would never ripen into a public nuisance without the conduct of various unnamed third parties, such as criminals and persons who negligently allow minors to obtain guns. . . . Where acts of independent third parties cause the alleged harm, it cannot be said that the defendants — here, gun manufacturers, trade associations, and a gun distributor — have the requisite degree of control over the source of the nuisance to allow liability.

Second, to allow the public-nuisance doctrine to reach the defendants in this case amounts to an unwarranted legislative judgment by this court. By its decision today, the majority subjects the defendants to potential nuisance liability for the way they design, distribute, and market lawful products. In extending the doctrine of public nuisance in this manner, this court takes the ill-advised first step toward transforming nuisance into "a monster that would devour in one gulp the entire law of tort."

* * *

# IN RE FIREARMS
## 126 Cal. App. 4th 959, 24 Cal Rptr. 3d 657 (2005)

Marchiano, Judge.

* * *

In 1999, the city attorneys of several jurisdictions, including the cities of San Francisco, Berkeley, Sacramento, and the counties of San Mateo and Alameda, filed an unfair business practices and nuisance action on behalf of the general public in San Francisco Superior Court against a large number of manufacturers and distributors of handguns and three trade associations, alleging that the defendants marketed and distributed handguns in violation of the UCL [the state's unfair competition law].

. . . .

The complaints in the three coordinated actions generally alleged that the defendants market, distribute, promote and design handguns in a manner that facilitates the use of the weapons to commit violent crime, fails to incorporate safety features, deceives the public about the dangers of firearms, circumvents federal, state and local laws and creates a public nuisance. Plaintiffs characterized their case as one that sought civil penalties and injunctive relief for the selling of guns to retail dealers that supplied the illegal black market with firearms. Plaintiffs contended that they possessed evidence showing that each defendant repeatedly sold its guns to "high-risk" retail dealers who were associated with large quantities of guns that were traced by law enforcement authorities as having been used in crimes.

In early 2001, defendants moved for an order compelling the plaintiffs to disclose facts supporting their claims. On March 26, 2001, the court granted the request and ordered plaintiffs to disclose evidence reflecting how criminals and others acquired the firearms manufactured and/or sold by defendants and whether the manner of acquisition had a factual nexus to defendants' alleged conduct.

Following multiple disagreements over discovery matters, certain defendants, including Beretta U.S.A. Corp. and Sturm, Ruger & Company, Inc., moved for an order precluding evidence that defendants' conduct caused the acquisition of firearms by criminals. The preclusion request was based on plaintiffs' failure to produce documents to support its sales and distribution theories of liability. Plaintiffs responded that they were not required to link a specific instance to a particular defendant and proposed to prove their case with expert testimony based on statistical studies of illegal gun purchases. The court denied the motion, but noted that without access to the evidentiary foundation for expert testimony, the expert opinions would be nothing more than policy arguments.

Manufacturer, distributor and retailer defendants renewed their arguments in a summary judgment motion. The motion was based on the arguments that plaintiffs could not establish a causal connection between defendants' business practices and the acquisition of firearms by criminals, and that expert opinion could not be substituted for evidence. Specifically, defendants' statement of undisputed facts consisted of 10 numbered statements contending that there was no evidence of any incident connecting a defendant with a shooting or a criminal's acquisition of a weapon through an improper purchase from a retail source.

Plaintiffs' responded with a separate statement of 478 numbered items in 104 pages, and what the trial court characterized as "a mountain of argument" and "120 pounds of paper." The court noted that most of the purported evidence submitted by plaintiffs consisted of inadmissible hearsay studies, monographs and reports, but did not make specific evidentiary rulings.

On April 10, 2003, the trial court filed a carefully reasoned and thorough 45-page opinion granting the omnibus motion of the manufacturer and distributor defendants. The court examined plaintiffs' evidence and recognized that it showed only that there are some bad retailers whose actions facilitate the transfer of guns to criminals. . . . The court also noted the definition of "unfair competition" . . . and reasoned that under any test, there must be some causal connection between the harm and the conduct of the defendants.

The court deduced that the only connection between the high-risk gun sales practices and the gun manufacturers was their failure to police the entire gun industry. Absent some connection between any practice of the gun manufacturer defendants and the harm caused by illegal guns, the trial court found no unfairness could be shown. The court also stated that defendants' mere failure to implement changes in their business practices does not establish a UCL violation or a public nuisance.

In addition, the court also granted summary judgment for the trade association defendants, finding no authority for the argument that a trade association had a duty to adopt firearms safety standards or that the failure to do so was connected to harm to the public.

The court denied summary judgment to distributor defendants Ellett Brothers, Inc., MKS Supply, Inc., and Southern Ohio Gun Distributors, stating that they failed to negate plaintiffs' evidence that they violated state law by distributing firearms to purchasers without receiving documentation of the purchasers' possession of state and local firearms dealer licenses. The court also denied summary judgment to retailer defendants Andrew's Sporting Goods, Inc. (Andrew's), and Trader's Sports, Inc. (Trader's), because the evidence, in the form of gun trace data, raised questions of fact concerning involvement in high-risk business practices.

Judgment was entered dismissing manufacturer, distributor and trade association defendants according to the summary judgment orders. . . .

## DISCUSSION

We are aware of the toll taken on society by firearm violence and the improper acquisition and use of firearms. . . .

Plaintiffs in this case seek to hold the gun manufacturer and distributor defendants liable, not for any wrongful or illegal action taken by them, but for failing to take proactive steps to control the practices of a small percentage of the federal firearms licensees (FFL) that they ultimately supply. These few FFL's to whom the gun distributors supply firearms have allegedly engaged in various business practices that experts state are associated with a high risk that guns will be diverted to criminals. After considering the voluminous expert studies and declarations submitted in opposition to the defendants' motion for summary judgment, the trial court found that the evidence did not support the basic theory of the plaintiffs' case.

Plaintiffs' legal theory of expanding UCL liability to those who profit from downstream dealer sale of guns that end up in criminal hands is creative and thought provoking. But based on the evidence presented, we conclude that endorsing the theory in this case would stretch the already expansive boundaries of the UCL beyond any principled reading of the statute. In addition, supervision of the sweeping measures sought would be a Herculean task for court oversight.

. . . .

The complaints allege that the defendants have marketed handguns using practices that encourage sales to unauthorized users without adequately monitoring their distributors and dealers or setting standards for distributors and dealers regarding how to legally and responsibly sell handguns.

Specific unfair policies include: failing to place controls on the actions of retail dealers; distribution policies that make sales to straw men likely; sales of large numbers of handguns in a single transaction; allowing sales to "kitchen table" dealers who do not maintain retail places of business; failing to prevent sales by private citizens at gun shows; distributing guns to dealers without ensuring that the dealers adequately check purchasers' identification for accuracy; distributing more guns than defendants reasonably expect to sell to legal purchasers; and failing to monitor gun sales in jurisdictions outside California with weak gun control laws.

In addition, the complaints alleged that defendants design guns without making serial numbers tamper proof, and that they design handguns to appeal to criminals without incorporating safety features to prevent unintentional shootings and unauthorized use. The complaints also alleged that defendants engaged in a "campaign of deception and misrepresentation concerning the dangers of their firearms" by implying that gun ownership will increase home safety. The parties have not addressed issues regarding gun design or false advertising on appeal.

Each of the three complaints also alleged creation of a public nuisance. Specifically, the complaints alleged that California residents are injured and killed by firearms supplied to criminals. The complaints alleged that defendants' conduct results in supplying thousands of handguns to the illegitimate secondary market that are illegally possessed and remain in the hands of criminals for years.

### Moving Party's Showing to Negate Plaintiffs' Claims

The theory of defendants' motion for summary judgment was that plaintiffs had no evidence that any defendants' act or omission caused any criminal to acquire a firearm. In addition, they argued that there was no evidence that any design feature of a firearm caused a shooting. Defendants also emphasized the existing extensive array of federal, state and local laws regulating firearms and urged the court to reject what defendants characterized as plaintiffs' mere policy arguments.

Defendants argued that plaintiffs did not produce evidence of a factual nexus between any defendant and incidents of firearm purchases by straw men, criminal acts by retailers, sales at gun shows or swap meets, sales to "kitchen table" vendors, firearms acquired by theft, multiple sales, acquisition of guns by criminals, accidental shootings, or intentional shootings.

Defendants relied on the deposition testimony of several of plaintiffs' experts, including Gerald Nunziato, a former official of the United States Department of Treasury, Bureau of Alcohol, Tobacco and Firearms (ATF) and Joseph Vince, a former chief of the ATF and president of Crime Gun Solutions, a company that assists police in the collection and analysis of crime gun data. Excerpts from depositions were offered to show the absence of any link between defendants' conduct and the alleged harm. . . .

*Plaintiffs' Attempted Showing of a Triable Issue of Fact*

Plaintiffs argued that an action brought under [the UCL] assesses only the extent to which a defendant has created an unreasonable risk to the public, and does not concern concepts of negligence law such as duty and causation. They presented studies showing the methods used by criminals to obtain guns from irresponsible gun retailers, including straw man purchases, thefts, and multiple sales.

Plaintiffs offered declarations from firearm experts stating their opinions that retailers linked to a significant number of such sales were more likely than not engaged in sales to gun traffickers or high-risk business practices that facilitate diversion of guns to the criminal market. . . .

The evidence presented by plaintiffs was predominately information pertaining to the gun industry as a whole. Plaintiffs presented several gun tracing profiles . . . concluding that firearms recovered in crimes in California were sold through FFL's that exhibited many of the ATF's gun trafficking indicators. The ATF's information was available to any defendant who requested it.

One tracing profile showed FFL's associated with each defendant distributor, the number of guns sold by the FFL and included in the crime gun trace database from 1995 to 2001 (with dealer identities redacted after 1996) and showed percentages of guns with high-risk factors. Plaintiffs also offered a California dealer profile that associated high-risk gun trafficking indicators with each FFL.

Plaintiffs' expert Gerald Nunziato concluded that the profiles and data he reviewed indicated that all defendants sold firearms that were recovered in crimes and traced. He also concluded that the traced guns were sold through numerous dealers that showed significant high-risk indicators of gun trafficking. He also opined that the defendants could have gathered and analyzed the same data plus additional data from their own files to help identify the high-risk dealers and utilize this information to "self-police their distribution partners. . . ."

Plaintiffs also offered the declaration of Carole Bridgewater, former gun shop owner and secretary/treasurer of the National Alliance of Stocking Gun Dealers stating that the gun industry has known "for a long time that there are serious problems in the way it distributes its products." . . .

Attorney Robert Ricker, a former gun lobbyist, stated in his declaration that gun manufacturers and distributors know of illegal practices by some retailers, but adopt a "see-no-evil, hear-no-evil, speak-no-evil" approach rather than requiring retailers to stop making questionable gun sales. He stated that industry leaders stifled discussions about the gun industry taking voluntary action to control the distribution of guns. In Ricker's opinion, if manufacturers investigated retailers whose records reflect a disproportionate number of crime gun traces, high-risk retail gun transfers would decrease.

Plaintiffs listed a number of proposed business practices that manufacturers and distributors could require of all their dealers that they claimed would cut down on black market sales of guns. . . .

. . . .

*UCL Definition of "Unfair" — Need for a Showing of Causation*

[The UCL] defines unfair competition to "mean and include any unlawful, unfair or fraudulent business act or practice and unfair, deceptive, untrue or misleading advertising and any act prohibited by [the Business and Professions Code]. The statute does not define the term "unfair," but . . . our Supreme Court signaled the need to put restrictions on its potentially limitless application.

Plaintiffs argue that *Cel-Tech* does not apply in this case and urge use of the pre-*Cel-Tech* definitions of an unfair practice. Plaintiffs contend that the trial court applied the wrong standard in deciding whether there was an issue of fact as to whether defendants' actions were "unfair" under the UCL.

    . . . .

Plaintiffs argue that a finding of unfairness . . . requires only a showing that defendants engaged in a business practice that offended the public policy of keeping guns out of the hands of criminals. Under the balancing test, plaintiffs argue that distributing guns to retailers who engage in high-risk practices is so dangerous to the public as to outweigh any benefit of defendants' business practice. . . .

According to plaintiffs, the trial court improperly injected the tort element of legal causation into the analysis. . . . We do not read the court's comment so strictly. In context, the court was referring, not to concepts of legal causation, but to the need to show some connection between conduct by defendants and the alleged harm to the public. Even in a UCL unfairness case, there must be such a connection. Without evidence of a causative link between the unfair act and the injuries or damages, unfairness by itself merely exists as a will-o'-the-wisp legal principle.

    . . . .

In [*Cel-Tech*] our Supreme Court rejected prior definitions of unfairness as "too amorphous." "Although the unfair competition law's scope is sweeping, it is not unlimited. Courts may not simply impose their own notions of the day as to what is fair or unfair." For that reason, the court took care to ensure that the definition of unfairness to competitors was "tethered to some legislatively declared policy or proof of some actual or threatened impact on competition." . . .

Accordingly, the court defined "unfair" in the context of an action by a plaintiff claiming injury from a competitor's act as conduct "that threatens an incipient violation of an antitrust law, or violates the policy or spirit of one of those laws because its effects are comparable to or the same as a violation of the law, or otherwise significantly threatens or harms competition." The court expressly stated that its definition is not applicable to actions brought by consumers, but its disapproval of the older unstructured definitions of unfairness cannot be ignored.

As this court noted in [a subsequent decision] "*Cel-Tech,* however, may signal a narrower interpretation of the prohibition of unfair acts or practices in all unfair competition actions and provides reason for caution in relying on the broad language in earlier decisions that the court found to be too amorphous. Moreover, where a claim of an unfair act or practice is predicated on public policy, we read *Cel-Tech* to require that the public policy which is a predicate to the action must be tethered to specific constitutional, statutory or regulatory provisions.

. . . .

We follow the lead of the *Cel-Tech* court in consulting parallel federal authority to assist in determining the appropriate reach of the UCL. Federal authorities clearly require a causative link between the defendant's actions and the resulting harm. . . . In determining whether an act or practice is unfair, the Commission may consider established public policies as evidence to be considered with all other evidence. Such public policy considerations may not serve as a primary basis for such determination."

To satisfy the federal definition of unfairness, the practice must cause or be likely to cause substantial injury, must not be outweighed by countervailing benefits, and the injury must be one that consumers themselves could not reasonably avoid. . . . The latter element was not supported by the plaintiffs' showing in this case.

In light of the Supreme Court's caution that businesses must be able to "know, to a reasonable certainty, what conduct California law prohibits and what it permits," we do not believe a UCL violation may be established without a link between a defendant's business practice and the alleged harm. . . .

. . . .

No evidence in this case hints that any of the manufacturer defendants provided weapons to criminals or failed to properly record sales or did any of the other acts that plaintiffs characterize as high-risk business practices. They did not control the wrongful acts or encourage others to engage in questionable acts. Neither did they change their business practices to avoid proposed regulations or advise retailers on ways to circumvent the law. The record in this case shows that the only business practice that these defendants engage in is the manufacture and sale of firearms to dealers that are licensed as such by the federal government. Plaintiffs have cited no cases finding a manufacturer has engaged in an unfair practice solely by legally selling a non-defective product based on actions taken by entities further along the chain of distribution. Even plaintiffs' experts could not present an evidentiary link between the manufacturer of a firearm and a retail gun dealer who sold guns that ended up in criminal circumstances.

It is important to emphasize that the evidence presented did not show that any defendant had actual knowledge that specific retailers were illegally supplying guns to the crime gun market or took any action to aid or encourage such activity. At best, defendants had access to inconclusive statistics concerning the actions of a minority of retailers. [The] data indicating a retailer sold numerous crime guns, without more, would not support a conclusion of wrongdoing. Plaintiffs' evidence raises only a suspicion regarding the acts of a small number of retailers that may justify additional investigation and fact finding.

While that evidence may be sufficient to justify a trial of the retailers, it does not implicate any act by the manufacturers.

Furthermore, the crime gun trace data and expert declarations did not, without more specific evidence, establish wrongdoing on the part of a specific retailer such that viewing the data alone would justify imposition of sanctions for gun trafficking. . . . Where the evidence in this case did support the inference that some retailers engaged in high-risk sales, the trial court denied summary judgment as to those entities.

While plaintiffs' attempt to add another layer of oversight to a highly regulated industry may represent a desirable goal, the record in this case does not present sufficient evidence to impose unannounced and uncodified requirements on business enterprises based on an expert's opinion of what constitutes good public policy. . . .

### The Trial Court Properly Rejected Plaintiffs' Nuisance Theory

Plaintiffs' complaints alleged that defendants' conduct constitutes a public nuisance because it results in supplying handguns to the criminal market that remain in the hands of criminals for years and causes death and injury to the public. Plaintiffs contend that the trial court ignored the public nuisance cause of action, which, if supported, could also establish a violation of [the UCL]. But the court did discuss the issue of public nuisance in its opinion and concluded that plaintiffs' evidence failed to show causation, a necessary element of a public nuisance claim.

A nuisance is: "anything that is injurious to health . . . or is indecent or offensive to the senses, or an obstruction to the free use of property, [that] interfere[s] with the comfortable enjoyment of life or property, or unlawfully obstructs the free passage or use, in the customary manner, of any navigable lake, or river, bay, stream, canal, or basin, or any public park, square, street, or highway. . . . [California statutory law divides] the types of nuisance into public and private. A public nuisance is one which affects at the same time an entire community or neighborhood, or any considerable number of persons.

Plaintiffs assert that the Restatement Second of Torts (Restatement) § 821(b) provides that no showing of causation is necessary when only an injunction is sought. They contend that they need only show that defendants created a risk of some threatened harm. The Restatement is not so loosely worded. Section 821(b) subdivision (2) explains: "Circumstances that may sustain a holding that an interference with a public right is unreasonable include the following: (a) Whether the conduct involves a significant interference with the public health, the public safety, the public peace, the public comfort or the public convenience, or (b) whether the conduct is proscribed by a statute, ordinance or administrative regulation, or (c) whether the conduct is of a continuing nature or has produced a permanent or long-lasting effect, and, as the actor knows or has reason to know, has a significant effect upon the public right." This listing of examples of public nuisance illustrates the need for a relationship between the conduct and the impending harm. Thus, a defendant's action must not only create a risk of some harm, it must also be likely to lead to invasion of the public right at issue.

The language of the Restatement presumes that the necessary elements for proof of a cause of action for public nuisance include the existence of a duty and causation. "The conduct necessary to make the actor liable for either a public or a private nuisance may consist of (a) an act; or (b) a failure to act under circumstances in which the actor is under a duty to take positive action to prevent or abate the interference with the public interest or the invasion of the private interest." If a plaintiff could obtain an injunction absent a showing of causation of an interference with a public right, the plaintiff could enjoin the manufacturing of a firearm solely because the mere existence of the firearm creates a risk of harm. A connecting element to the prohibited harm must be shown.

Cases cited by plaintiffs as examples of public nuisance in other contexts are distinguishable because the acts of defendants in those cases were illegal or violated regulatory provisions and did more than create a risk of harm. The actions of the defendants in the cited cases were highly likely to cause imminent harm to the public. . . .

Although it is not necessary to show that harm actually occurred, plaintiffs must show that a defendants acts are likely to cause a significant invasion of a public right. . . .

   . . . .

In this case, there is no causal connection between any conduct of the defendants and any incident of illegal acquisition of firearms or criminal acts or accidental injury by a firearm. Defendants manufacture guns according to federal law and guidelines.

Plaintiffs list cases from other jurisdictions that have upheld public nuisance claims against gun manufacturers and distributors, arguing that the trial court erred by not following those cases. No California state case is cited that analyzes the issue. . . .

The out-of-state cases allowing a nuisance action to go forward are distinguishable. . . . In *Ileto v. Glock, Inc.*, 349 F.3d 1191 (9th Cir. 2003) a Ninth Circuit panel majority reinstated claims of negligence and nuisance against gun manufacturers and distributors brought by individual victims and survivors of an assault by a gunman. It is significant that the court declined to reinstate the action against manufacturers and distributors whose guns were not actually fired during the shooting because the claims for nuisance and negligence could not stand without a showing that those guns caused the alleged injury. . . .

. . . Even if we were to accept the *Ileto* court's interpretation of what our Supreme Court may decide when faced with this issue, the conclusions in that case (aside from the need to show causation) are not applicable here, where there is no evidence of either of the contentions underlying the causes of action. . . .

We find the views expressed by the dissenters to the denial of rehearing en banc in *Ileto* instructive. Circuit Judge Callahan explained the potential reach of the *Ileto* decision allowing the nuisance claim against defendant Glock, Inc., to go forward. "The potential impact of the panel's decision is staggering: Any manufacturer of an arguably dangerous product that finds its way into California can be hauled into court in California to defend against a civil action brought by a victim of the criminal use of that product. The manufacturers' liability will turn not on whether the product was defective, but whether its legal marketing and distribution system somehow promoted the use of its product by criminals and underage end users. Thus, General Motors could be sued by someone who was hit by a Corvette that had been stolen by a juvenile. The plaintiff would allege that General Motors knew that cars that can greatly exceed the legal speed limit are dangerous, and through advertising and by offering discounts, it increased the attractiveness of the car and the number of Corvettes on the road and thus increased the likelihood that a juvenile would steal a Corvette and operate it in a injurious manner. . . .

. . . [As set out by a concurring opinion in *Ileto*]: "*In* effect, it is a form of regulation administered through the courts rather than the states regulatory agencies. It is, moreover, a peculiarly blunt and capricious method of regulation, depending as it does on the vicissitudes of the legal system, which make results highly unpredictable in probability and magnitude. Courts should therefore be chary of adopting broad new theories of liability, lest they undermine the democratic process through which the people normally decide whether, and to what degree, activities should be fostered or discouraged within the state. . . ."

Plaintiffs public nuisance claim fails for lack of any evidence of causation. Their complaint attempts to reach too far back in the chain of distribution when it targets the manufacturer of a legal, non-defective product that lawfully distributes its product only to those buyers licensed by the federal government.

We do not hold that the theories asserted would never be tenable under different evidence. We merely find, based on the evidence presented here, that the evidence does not sufficiently establish the alleged acts of the defendants caused the diversion of firearms to the criminal market.

\* \* \*

## 2.    Private Litigation

## SMITH v. BRYCO ARMS
### 131 N.M. 87, 33 P.3d 638 (2001)

Bustamante, Justice.

\* \* \*

In this case we consider, under theories of strict products liability and negligence, the liability of the manufacturer and distributor of a .22 caliber handgun, referred to as the J-22, for the accidental shooting of an Albuquerque boy, 14-year-old Sean Smith (Sean), by his 15-year-old friend D.J. Valencia (D.J.). The trial court granted summary judgment to the gun manufacturer, Defendant Bryco Arms (Bryco), and to the gun distributor, Defendant Jennings Firearms, Inc. . . .

Plaintiff raises strict products liability and negligence theories of recovery against Bryco and Jennings. Both theories are predicated upon the fact that the J-22 handgun does not incorporate a "magazine-out safety," a "chamber load indicator," or a written warning on the gun itself alerting users that the J-22 can fire even though the magazine has been removed. The issues on appeal are (1) whether the court erred in ruling that, as a matter of law, Bryco and Jennings were not negligent because they had no duty to incorporate the safety features described above; (2) whether the trial court erred in ruling that, as a matter of law, the J-22 does not present an unreasonable risk of injury for purposes of strict product liability; and (3) whether Plaintiff came forward with evidence sufficient to raise a genuine issue of material fact that the failure to incorporate the above safety features was a proximate cause of Sean's injury. . . .

## FACTUAL AND PROCEDURAL BACKGROUND

The shooting occurred on January 29, 1993, at Sean's house. No parents were home at the time. Sean, Michael Brummett (Michael) age 15, and Brian Romero (Brian) age 16, were at Sean's house. The three boys decided to go out to get some food. While they were out, Michael legally purchased the J-22 handgun and ammunition for $40 from an individual identified only as Bernard. The sale occurred in a parking lot in Albuquerque. While purchasing the gun, Michael examined the chamber and saw it was empty and asked to see the ammunition magazine. Michael inserted the magazine into the gun and purchased it. The three boys examined the gun in the car. When they got back to Sean's house, the boys again examined the gun. Michael put the gun and magazine clip in his jacket, brought it into the house, and took the gun with him into the bathroom. At some point, Sean also called D.J. to come over. Michael removed the magazine and kept it with him in the bathroom while the other boys passed the gun around in the living room. Sean, D.J., and Brian testified that they thought the gun was unloaded and would not fire with the magazine out. The boys testified that they did not realize that a bullet might remain in the chamber even though the magazine had been removed. When the gun was passed to D.J., he "stupidly" pulled the trigger and unintentionally shot Sean as Sean was talking on the telephone, hitting him in the mouth and seriously injuring him.

Sean and his parents, Patrick and Jeanne Smith (Plaintiffs), initially filed a complaint to recover damages for personal injury, alleging that the parents of D.J., Michael, and Brian were negligent for failing to supervise the boys properly. The complaint was then amended to name the three boys and their parents, alleging negligence of minors, negligence as a matter of law, vicarious parental liability, and parental negligence. The complaint was amended a second time to add Bryco, the manufacturer of the J-22, and Jennings, the distributor of the J-22. [The parents and the other boys settled out of court with plaintiffs.]

. . . .

. . . .

. . . [T]he trial court applied a restrictive definition of defect. In the trial court's view, a defect consisted of a flaw in the fabrication of the particular J-22 involved in this case. . . .

The trial court's unwillingness to consider possible design and warning defects sidestepped the true gravamen of the Plaintiffs' case: that the gun as designed was defective because it did not incorporate available and economically reasonable design features and warnings which would have prevented the shooting. . . . Apparently viewing the application of normal products liability and negligence concepts to handguns as a significant change in the law, the trial court deferred to our Supreme Court for action. . . .

. . . .

The trial court was perhaps concerned that applying our tort law to handguns could have the effect of infringing on the constitutional right to bear arms. N.M. Const. art. XI, § 6. We recognize that firearms are different than other products in the sense that they are the subject of a constitutional right. However, as the following discussion will demonstrate, we do not perceive anything so unique about handguns that they cannot or should not be subject to normal tort law concepts, norms, and methods of analysis. . . .

## A. The Strict Products Liability Theory

. . . The purpose behind the strict products liability doctrine is to allow an injured user or consumer to recover against a supplier or manufacturer without the requirement of proving negligence. The policy underpinnings supporting imposition of strict liability on product manufacturers and suppliers include (1) ensuring that the risk of loss for injury resulting from defective products is borne by the suppliers, principally because they are in a position to absorb the loss by distributing it as a cost of doing business; (2) encouraging suppliers to select reputable and responsible manufacturers who generally design and construct safe products and who generally accept financial responsibility for injuries caused by their defective products; and (3) promoting fairness by ensuring that plaintiffs injured by an unreasonably dangerous product are compensated for their injuries.

Under the strict products liability theory, a supplier of products is liable for harm proximately caused by an unreasonable risk of injury resulting from a condition of the product or from a manner of its use. This rule applies even though all possible care has been used by the supplier in putting the product on the market. . . .

Whether a product is unreasonably dangerous, and therefore defective, is ordinarily a question for the jury. New Mexico's "unreasonable-risk-of-injury" test allows for proof and argument under any rational theory of defect. The jury instructions covering strict products liability are designed to encourage a risk-benefit calculation by defining "unreasonable risk of injury" in a way which requires the jury to balance meritorious choices for safety made by the manufacturer while minimizing the risk that the public will be deprived needlessly of beneficial products. . . .

Plaintiffs allege that the J-22 handgun was in an unreasonably dangerous and defective condition because it (1) "[i]nadequately lacked a proper safety mechanism which would prevent the handgun from firing when the ammunition magazine was removed," (2) "was not designed so as to sufficiently warn foreseeable users when a round of ammunition has been loaded," and (3) lacked "a warning adequate to apprise all foreseeable users, especially minor users, of the fact that the handgun could fire a projectile even if the ammunition magazine were removed."

We perceive nothing new or unusual in these theories of defect. . . .

## B.   The Negligence Theory

In support of their negligence claims, Plaintiffs allege that Defendants had a duty to Plaintiffs (1) "to use reasonable care in the design, manufacture and [marketing] of the J-22 handgun to ensure that it would be reasonably safe for its foreseeable uses" and (2) to warn Plaintiffs "of all inherent dangers to the J-22 handgun including the fact the weapon could fire a projectile even if the ammunition magazine was removed." Plaintiffs further allege that Defendants failed to fulfill this duty because they did not design the J-22 with a magazine-out safety, or a chamber load indicator, or a printed warning on the J-22.

It is well-established in New Mexico negligence law that manufacturers and distributors of products have a duty to use ordinary care in producing products so as to avoid a foreseeable risk of injury caused by a condition of the product or manner in which it is used. . . . These are bedrock propositions of New Mexico products liability and negligence law. It can thus be stated without risk of contradiction that the duty of a product supplier to use ordinary care to avoid foreseeable risks of injury caused by a condition of the product or manner in which it is used exists as a matter of law. . . .

Stated positively, the general duty imposed on manufacturers and suppliers of products to use ordinary care includes a duty to consider risks of injury created by foreseeable misuse of the product. . . .

Defendants argue that they had no duty of care to Sean because they had no "special relationship" with him. Defendants base this contention on the theory that the injury was caused by D.J.'s criminal act in pointing and firing the handgun at Sean. Because the trigger was pulled by a third party, Defendants contend, they cannot be held liable unless it can be found that they had a special relationship with Sean which imposed a duty to control the conduct of the third person. . . .

The basic inquiry in all of these cases is whether the defendant has the ability to exercise control over a premise or an activity such that it is reasonable to impose a duty of ordinary care on it as to the management of the premises or activities. At times a duty is found based on the existence of a "special relationship" between plaintiff and defendant. A special relationship can arise as part of a commercial connection between parties, or it can be more or less voluntarily undertaken. . . .

These difficulties are not present in a products liability context. The basic policy decision has been made that the duty of a product distributor extends to persons who can be foreseeably injured by a defective product — including injuries caused by foreseeable misuse of the product if the defect proximately contributes to the injury. Thus, contrary to Defendants' contentions, a "special relationship" between manufacturer/distributor and user is not required to establish a product supplier's duty to make or distribute safe products.

Further, the presence or absence of a special relationship between Defendants and Sean is immaterial because Plaintiffs are clearly not attempting to hold Defendants responsible for failing to control D.J. Plaintiffs are attempting to hold Defendants liable in negligence or strict liability for harm proximately caused by Defendants' affirmative acts of designing and distributing a defective product which combined with D.J.'s subsequent misconduct to injure Sean. . . . It is sufficient if it occurs with some other cause acting at the same time, which in combination with it, causes the injury.". . . .

Once it has been determined that a duty exists, the limits on that duty under a specific set of facts are ordinarily questions for the jury. . . .

## C.  Material Issues of Fact Were Raised by Plaintiffs in Response to Defendants' Motions for Summary Judgment

[On a motion for summary judgment, once the moving party makes a] prima facie showing, the burden shifts to the party opposing the motion to demonstrate the existence of specific evidentiary facts which would require trial on the merits." Defendants contend that as a matter of law, the J-22 was not a defectively designed product and Defendants were not negligent in the manufacture and design of it. Defendants contend they are entitled summary judgment as to the design and warning defects issues because the J-22 has the following safety features which they argue are sufficient as a matter of law: (1) the J-22 Operator's Parts and Instructions Sheet, which accompanies the newly manufactured gun in its display box, explains all safety concerns, including the safe loading and unloading of the gun; and (2) the word "Fire" is visible when the handgun is in a firing position, and there is a manual safety, which when applied makes the word "Safe" visible and keeps the gun from firing.

Defendants also assert the J-22 handgun was not defectively manufactured because it operated as intended when D.J. intentionally pulled the trigger while pointing it at Sean, even if he did not intend to injure him. Bryco and Jennings representatives testified that had the boys put the existing safety on and not pointed the gun at anyone, as they had been taught by their parents and guardians not to do, the shooting could not have occurred. Defendants also contend they are entitled to summary judgment because the safety devices and warnings Plaintiffs advocate are not feasible for the J-22, and that, in general, there are pros and cons to the desirability . . . of magazine safeties.

Defendants also contend they are entitled to summary judgment because as a matter of law, Bryco and Jennings had no duty to protect these minors against their intentional, reckless, and criminal use of the product. The President of Jennings, Janice Jennings, testified that in her opinion, the boys' reckless conduct made the accident inevitable. The boys' actions were so reckless, willful, and criminal, Defendants contend, that as a matter of law, this misuse of the gun could not reasonably be foreseen by Bryco and Jennings. Finally, Defendants argue that the boys' actions interrupt the chain of proximate causation. Defendants point to the boys' depositions where they each admitted their actions were "stupid." In addition, the boys admitted that they acted contrary to what they had been taught by their parents or guardians about not handling guns, not pointing them at anyone, and assuming a gun is loaded at all times. The boys admitted that they initially lied to the police about how they got the gun and how the shooting occurred. They also admitted to initially hiding the gun from their parents and the police.

To counter Defendants' criminal and per se negligence theories, Plaintiffs provided evidence that the boys purchased the gun legally at the time. . . . To counter Defendants' assertions that the gun is sufficiently safe, Plaintiffs provided evidence that when purchased, there was no Parts and Instruction Sheet that came with the gun, and that this was a common occurrence in gun sales. In addition, Plaintiffs provided evidence that without the instruction sheet and in the absence of a magazine-out safety, chamber load indicator, or suitable warning (e.g., "check the chamber for a bullet at all times"), that loading and unloading the gun is confusing depending on whether the chamber is checked while the magazine is in or out. If the chamber is viewed while the magazine is in the gun, the chamber will appear empty, but a bullet will then be loaded into the chamber. Removing the magazine, therefore, does not necessarily unload the gun.

While D.J. testified that he "stupidly" pulled the trigger, each of the boys testified that he thought the gun was unloaded because the magazine was out. There was some evidence that Sean or Brian actually, though inadvertently, may have loaded the gun while the magazine was in the gun and before returning it to Michael who thought that, by removing the magazine and keeping it with him while the other boys examined the gun in another room after D.J. showed up, he had made it safe. Michael testified that the chamber was empty when he examined the gun while purchasing it. Then, when Michael removed the magazine and kept it with him in the bathroom while the other boys examined it in another room, Michael testified that he thought the gun was safe and unloaded.

In response to Defendants' contentions that the J-22 had sufficient safety devices and warnings as designed, Plaintiffs provided evidence that patents for magazine-out safeties have been filed in 1912, 1914, 1916, 1921, 1922, 1927, 1945, 1949, 1951, 1977, 1980, 1981, 1984, and 1986. These patent applications specifically articulate the known danger that people will remove the gun magazine and think they have unloaded the gun and then fire it, unintentionally injuring someone. The United States Patent Office granted the first patent for a magazine-out safety device on April 30, 1912. The Patent Abstract for this patent, No. 1,024,932, describes a device with the purpose and effect of preventing accidents such as the one in which Sean was injured:

A number of accidents occur in connection with automatic fire arms owing to the fact that if the fire arm is loaded and the magazine withdrawn, persons little acquainted with the operation of these fire arms often believe it to be unloaded while in reality a cartridge remains in the barrel. The present invention has for its object to obviate such accidents by providing means for setting the weapon automatically at a position of safety immediately the magazine is withdrawn.

In response to Defendants' contentions that the boys' misuse of the gun was unforeseeable or interrupted proximate causation, Plaintiffs provided government studies that show that the kind of unintentional shooting that occurred in this case is relatively common and might have been prevented if the person handling the gun had known it was loaded. For example, a nationally published study by the United States General Accounting Office reported in 1991 that 23% of unintentional shootings in America might have been prevented if the person handling the gun had known it was loaded. Another study showed that in New Mexico, 25 children aged 0-14 years old were killed in unintentional shootings between 1984 and 1988. During depositions, Defendants admitted they could foresee that children and teenagers would be able to access the J-22, and could be injured from handling a gun they believed to be unloaded. Plaintiffs' evidence would permit a reasonable jury to find that at the time the J-22 handgun was manufactured, Defendants were on notice, knew, or should have known of the risks posed by bullets in the chamber through the numerous patents filed about this issue, existing designs by other gun manufacturers, and through lawsuits against gun manufacturers and distributors.

Documents and advertisement flyers showed that recent handguns manufactured and distributed by Defendants have incorporated a magazine-out safety that blocks the trigger bar and disables the handgun so that it cannot fire when the magazine is removed, and a chamber load indicator device to guard against the risks posed by a bullet hidden in the chamber. Plaintiffs quoted Defendants' testimony that, notwithstanding, Defendants did not consider additional safety devices for the J-22; that no product analyses were conducted on the J-22; that no one reviews Bryco products to see if they can be made safer; and that Bryco did not investigate what other manufacturers were doing to make their firearms safer.

Defendants admitted that had a magazine-out safety been in the J-22 at the time D.J. fired, the gun would not have fired and Sean would not have been shot.

This is not a case where the use to which the product was put is so unforeseeable as a matter of law that the case should be taken from the jury under either a strict products liability or negligence theory. . . .

In addition, Plaintiffs' feasibility evidence conflicted with Defendants' contentions on that point. Plaintiffs provided evidence indicating that installing the safety devices and warnings were both feasible and inexpensive. The cost of the magazine out safety parts is about 22 cents and the cost of the chamber load indicator parts about 8 cents, adding about 30 cents to the manufacturing price of the J-22. Finally, Plaintiffs presented the affidavits of three experts on the issues of feasibility, foreseeability, and causation. Vaughn P. Adams, Jr., Ph.D., P.E., is a registered industrial and safety engineer who has qualified as an expert in numerous cases and has testified on safety devices and firearms. In his opinion, Bryco and Jennings failed to provide reasonable safeguarding means which were available and widely known at the time the J-22 handgun was designed, manufactured, and distributed, to control the recognized hazard of unintentional discharge of their handgun under foreseeable conditions, including the occurrence of a cartridge unknowingly remaining in the chamber when the magazine was removed. He also opined that it was foreseeable that severe injury and death will be caused when individuals handle a loaded handgun which they believe is unloaded. David P. Sklar, M.D., Chairman of the Department of Emergency Medicine, Professor of Internal Medicine, and Medical Director of the Center for Injury Prevention, Research, and Education at the University of New Mexico School of Medicine, also opined about the foreseeability of accidental shootings like the one that injured Sean. Robert L. Hillberg, a firearms manufacturer and designer, opined about the feasibility of installing additional safeties and warnings on the J-22.

## CONCLUSION

. . . In this case, we are applying existing principles of products liability under New Mexico law to another type of product supplier: the manufacturer and distributor of the J-22 handgun. We are not changing the law.

Plaintiffs' claims pose the question whether the gun could function as intended and yet be made safer. Plaintiffs contend that the J-22 is defective because it did not incorporate safety devices and warnings designed to prevent foreseeable unintentional shooting accidents, a claim well within existing New Mexico products liability and negligence law. We note that the open and obvious danger rule has been abolished in New Mexico and a risk is not made reasonable simply because it is made open and obvious to persons exercising ordinary care. . . .

Whether the type of misuse evident in this case was foreseeable, whether the existing features of the J-22 are sufficiently safe, and whether it was feasible without impairing the utility of the gun or being unduly expensive for Bryco and Jennings to incorporate the advocated safety devices and/or warnings into the design of the J-22, are all issues for the jury to decide. To determine whether Bryco and Jennings are strictly liable for Sean's injuries, the jury will assess whether the product as designed posed an unreasonable risk of injury to these minors. To determine whether Bryco and Jennings are liable under a negligence theory, the jury will assess whether they were negligent in adopting the particular design of the J-22.

Because there remain material issues of fact for resolution by the jury, Defendants are not entitled to judgment as a matter of law.

* * *

## PROTECTION OF LAWFUL COMMERCE IN ARMS ACT
### Pub. L. No. 109-92 (2005)

FINDINGS; PURPOSES.

(a) FINDINGS. Congress finds the following:

(1) The Second Amendment to the United States Constitution provides that the right of the people to keep and bear arms shall not be infringed.

(2) The Second Amendment to the United States Constitution protects the rights of individuals, including those who are not members of a militia or engaged in military service or training, to keep and bear arms.

(3) Lawsuits have been commenced against manufacturers, distributors, dealers, and importers of firearms that operate as designed and intended, which seek money damages and other relief for the harm caused by the misuse of firearms by third parties, including criminals.

(4) The manufacture, importation, possession, sale, and use of firearms and ammunition in the United States are heavily regulated by Federal, State, and local laws. Such Federal laws include the Gun Control Act of 1968, the National Firearms Act, and the Arms Export Control Act.

(5) Businesses in the United States that are engaged in interstate and foreign commerce through the lawful design, manufacture, marketing, distribution, importation, or sale to the public of firearms or ammunition products that have been shipped or transported in interstate or foreign commerce are not, and should not, be liable for the harm caused by those who criminally or unlawfully misuse firearm products or ammunition products that function as designed and intended.

(6) The possibility of imposing liability on an entire industry for harm that is solely caused by others is an abuse of the legal system, erodes public confidence in our Nation's laws, threatens the diminution of a basic constitutional right and civil liberty, invites the disassembly and destabilization of other industries and economic sectors lawfully competing in the free enterprise system of the United States, and constitutes an unreasonable burden on interstate and foreign commerce of the United States.

(7) The liability actions commenced or contemplated by the Federal Government, States, municipalities, and private interest groups and others are based on theories without foundation in hundreds of years of the common law and jurisprudence of the United States and do not represent a bona fide expansion of the common law. The possible sustaining of these actions by a maverick judicial officer or petit jury would expand civil liability in a manner never contemplated by the framers of the Constitution, by Congress, or by the legislatures of the several States. Such an expansion of liability would constitute

a deprivation of the rights, privileges, and immunities guaranteed to a citizen of the United States under the Fourteenth Amendment to the United States Constitution.

(8) The liability actions commenced or contemplated by the Federal Government, States, municipalities, private interest groups and others attempt to use the judicial branch to circumvent the Legislative branch of government to regulate interstate and foreign commerce through judgments and judicial decrees thereby threatening the Separation of Powers doctrine and weakening and undermining important principles of federalism, State sovereignty and comity between the sister States.

(b) PURPOSES. The purposes of this Act are as follows:

(1) To prohibit causes of action against manufacturers, distributors, dealers, and importers of firearms or ammunition products, and their trade associations, for the harm solely caused by the criminal or unlawful misuse of firearm products or ammunition products by others when the product functioned as designed and intended.

(2) To preserve a citizen's access to a supply of firearms and ammunition for all lawful purposes, including hunting, self-defense, collecting, and competitive or recreational shooting.

(3) To guarantee a citizen's rights, privileges, and immunities, as applied to the States, under the Fourteenth Amendment to the United States Constitution, pursuant to section 5 of that Amendment.

(4) To prevent the use of such lawsuits to impose unreasonable burdens on interstate and foreign commerce.

(5) To protect the right, under the First Amendment to the Constitution, of manufacturers, distributors, dealers, and importers of firearms or ammunition products, and trade associations, to speak freely, to assemble peaceably, and to petition the Government for a redress of their grievances.

(6) To preserve and protect the Separation of Powers doctrine and important principles of federalism, State sovereignty and comity between sister States.

(7) To exercise congressional power under article IV, section 1 (the Full Faith and Credit Clause) of the United States Constitution.

## PROHIBITION ON BRINGING OF QUALIFIED CIVIL LIABILITY ACTIONS IN FEDERAL OR STATE COURT.

(a) IN GENERAL. A qualified civil liability action may not be brought in any Federal or State court.

(b) DISMISSAL OF PENDING ACTIONS. A qualified civil liability action that is pending on the date of enactment of this Act shall be immediately dismissed by the court in which the action was brought or is currently pending.

(c) DEFINITIONS.

In this Act:

(1) ENGAGED IN THE BUSINESS. The term "engaged in the business" has the meaning . . . as applied to a seller of ammunition, means a person who devotes time, attention, and labor to the sale of ammunition as a regular course of trade or business with the principal objective of livelihood and profit through the sale or distribution of ammunition.

(2) Manufacturer. The term "manufacturer" means, with respect to a qualified product, a person who is engaged in the business of manufacturing the product in interstate or foreign commerce and who is licensed to engage in business as such a manufacturer. . . .

(3) PERSON. The term "person" means any individual, corporation, company, association, firm, partnership, society, joint stock company, or any other entity, including any governmental entity.

(4) QUALIFIED PRODUCT. The term "qualified product" means a firearm . . . , including any antique firearm . . . , or ammunition (as defined in section 921(a) (17) (A) of such title), or a component part of a firearm or ammunition, that has been shipped or transported in interstate or foreign commerce.

(5) QUALIFIED CIVIL LIABILITY ACTION.

(A) IN GENERAL. The term "qualified civil liability action" means a civil action or proceeding or an administrative proceeding brought by any person against a manufacturer or seller of a qualified product, or a trade association, for damages, punitive damages, injunctive or declaratory relief, abatement, restitution, fines, or penalties, or other relief, resulting from the criminal or unlawful misuse of a qualified product by the person or a third party, but shall not include —

(i) an action brought against a transferor convicted under (the federal law requiring the licensing of gun dealers), or a comparable or identical State felony law, by a party directly harmed by the conduct of which the transferee is so convicted;

(ii) an action brought against a seller for negligent entrustment or negligence per se;

(iii) an action in which a manufacturer or seller of a qualified product knowingly violated a State or Federal statute applicable to the sale or marketing of the product, and the violation was a proximate cause of the harm for which relief is sought, including —

(I) any case in which the manufacturer or seller knowingly made any false entry in, or failed to make appropriate entry in, any record required to be kept under Federal or State law with respect to the qualified product, or aided, abetted, or conspired with any person in making any false or fictitious oral or written statement with respect to any fact material to the lawfulness of the sale or other disposition of a qualified product; or

(II) any case in which the manufacturer or seller aided, abetted, or conspired with any other person to sell or otherwise dispose of a qualified product, knowing, or having reasonable cause to believe, that the actual buyer of the qualified product was prohibited from possessing or receiving a firearm or ammunition under (federal law).

(iv) an action for breach of contract or warranty in connection with the purchase of the product;

(v) an action for death, physical injuries or property damage resulting directly from a defect in design or manufacture of the product, when used as intended or in a reasonably foreseeable manner, except that where the discharge of the product was caused by a volitional act that constituted a criminal offense, then such act shall be considered the sole proximate cause of any resulting death, personal injuries or property damage; or

(vi) an action or proceeding commenced by the Attorney General to enforce (federal laws relating to licensing of gun dealers or other related federal laws).

(B) NEGLIGENT ENTRUSTMENT. As used in subparagraph (A) (ii), the term "negligent entrustment" means the supplying of a qualified product by a seller for use by another person when the seller knows, or reasonably should know, the person to whom the product is supplied is likely to, and does, use the product in a manner involving unreasonable risk of physical injury to the person or others.

(C) RULE OF CONSTRUCTION. The exceptions enumerated under clauses (i) through (v) of subparagraph (A) shall be construed so as not to be in conflict, and no provision of this Act shall be construed to create a public or private cause of action or remedy.

(D) MINOR CHILD EXCEPTION. Nothing in this Act shall be construed to limit the right of a person under 17 years of age to recover damages authorized under Federal or State law in a civil action that meets one of the requirements under clauses (i) through (v) of subparagraph (A).

. . . .

(9) UNLAWFUL MISUSE. — The term "unlawful misuse" means conduct that violates a statute, ordinance, or regulation as it relates to the use of a qualified product.

CHILD SAFETY LOCKS.

(a) SHORT TITLE. This section may be cited as the "Child Safety Lock Act of 2005".

(b) PURPOSES. The purposes of this section are —

(1) to promote the safe storage and use of handguns by consumers;

(2) to prevent unauthorized persons from gaining access to or use of a handgun, including children who may not be in possession of a handgun; and

(3) to avoid hindering industry from supplying firearms to law abiding citizens for all lawful purposes, including hunting, self-defense, collecting, and competitive or recreational shooting.

(c) FIREARMS SAFETY.

(1) MANDATORY TRANSFER OF SECURE GUN STORAGE OR SAFETY DEVICE. Section 922 of title 18, United States Code, is amended by inserting at the end the following:

"(z) SECURE GUN STORAGE OR SAFETY DEVICE.

"(1) IN GENERAL. Except as provided under paragraph (2), it shall be unlawful for any licensed importer, licensed manufacturer, or licensed dealer to sell, deliver, or transfer any handgun to any person other than any person licensed under this chapter, unless the transferee is provided with a secure gun storage or safety device . . . for that handgun.

"(2) EXCEPTIONS. Paragraph (1) shall not apply to

"(A) (i) the manufacture for, transfer to, or possession by, the United States, a department or agency of the United States, a State, or a department, agency, or political subdivision of a State, of a handgun; or

"(ii) the transfer to, or possession by, a law enforcement officer employed by an entity referred to in clause (i) of a handgun for law enforcement purposes (whether on or off duty); or

"(B) the transfer to, or possession by, a rail police officer employed by a rail carrier and certified or commissioned as a police officer under the laws of a State of a handgun for purposes of law enforcement (whether on or off duty);

"(C) the transfer to any person of a handgun listed as a curio or relic . . . ; or

"(D) the transfer to any person of a handgun for which a secure gun storage or safety device is temporarily unavailable. . . .

"(3) LIABILITY FOR USE.

"(A) IN GENERAL. Notwithstanding any other provision of law, a person who has lawful possession and control of a handgun, and who uses a secure gun storage or safety device with the handgun, shall be entitled to immunity from a qualified civil liability action.

"(B) PROSPECTIVE ACTIONS. A qualified civil liability action may not be brought in any Federal or State court.

"(C) DEFINED TERM. As used in this paragraph, the term 'qualified civil liability action'

"(i) means a civil action brought by any person against a person described in subparagraph (A) for damages resulting from the criminal or unlawful misuse of the handgun by a third party, if

"(I) the handgun was accessed by another person who did not have the permission or authorization of the person having lawful possession and control of the handgun to have access to it; and

"(II) at the time access was gained by the person not so authorized, the handgun had been made inoperable by use of a secure gun storage or safety device; and "(ii) shall not include an action brought against the person having lawful possession and control of the handgun for negligent entrustment or negligence per se.".

(2) CIVIL PENALTIES. — Section 924 of title 18, United States Code, is amended

. . . .

(B) by adding at the end the following:

"(p) PENALTIES RELATING TO SECURE GUN STORAGE OR SAFETY DEVICE.—

"(1) IN GENERAL.—

"(A) SUSPENSION OR REVOCATION OF LICENSE; CIVIL PENALTIES. With respect to each violation of section 922(z) (1) by a licensed manufacturer, licensed importer, or licensed dealer, the Secretary may, after notice and opportunity for hearing

"(i) suspend for not more than 6 months, or revoke, the license issued to the licensee under this chapter that was used to conduct the firearms transfer. . . .

. . . .

ARMOR PIERCING AMMUNITION.

(a) UNLAWFUL ACTS. Section 922(a) of title 18, United States Code, is amended by striking paragraphs (7) and (8) and inserting the following:

"(7) [It shall be unlawful] for any person to manufacture or import armor piercing ammunition, unless

"(A) the manufacture of such ammunition is for the use of the United States, any department or agency of the United States, any State, or any department, agency, or political subdivision of a State;

"(B) the manufacture of such ammunition is for the purpose of exportation; or

"(C) the manufacture or importation of such ammunition is for the purpose of testing or experimentation and has been authorized by the Attorney General;

"(8) [It shall be unlawful] for any manufacturer or importer to sell or deliver armor piercing ammunition, unless such sale or delivery

"(A) is for the use of the United States, any department or agency of the United States, any State, or any department, agency, or political subdivision of a State;

"(B) is for the purpose of exportation; or

"(C) is for the purpose of testing or experimentation and has been authorized by the Attorney General;"

(b) PENALTIES. Section 924(c) of title 18, United States Code, is amended by adding at the end the following:

"(5) Except to the extent that a greater minimum sentence is otherwise provided under this subsection, or by any other provision of law, any person who, during and in relation to any crime of violence or drug trafficking crime (including a crime of violence or drug trafficking crime that provides for an enhanced punishment if committed by the use of a deadly or dangerous weapon or device) for which the person may be prosecuted in a court of the United States, uses or carries armor piercing ammunition, or who, in furtherance of any such crime, possesses armor piercing ammunition, shall, in addition to the punishment provided for such crime of violence or drug trafficking crime or conviction under this section

"(A) be sentenced to a term of imprisonment of not less than 15 years; and

"(B) if death results from the use of such ammunition

"(i) if the killing is murder, be punished by death or sentenced to a term of imprisonment for any term of years or for life; and

"(ii) if the killing is manslaughter, be punished as provided in section 1112."

\* \* \*

## NOTES AND QUESTIONS

**1.** Apart from efforts by state and local governments to enact gun control legislation, some city and local governments have attempted to achieve some of the same objectives of gun control legislation through litigation claiming, among other things, that gun manufacturers and distributors are negligent in allowing the distribution of potentially dangerous products or liable for the inherent dangers of their products, or that gun manufacturers and distributors are creating a public nuisance. None of these government-sponsored lawsuits have been fully successful and most have been rejected or withdrawn. In that regard, the limited legal success (despite the ultimate political failure, as explained *infra*) of the city in *City of Cincinnati v. Beretta U.S.A. Corp.* is atypical, although the city's claims and arguments are fairly typical of the claims that have been pursued in various jurisdictions. The city focused most of its arguments on claims that this particular gun manufacturer had declined to incorporate safety devices into its guns, misled the public about the advantages of having a gun in the home, and engaged in distributional practices that fostered a large, illegitimate "secondary" market for guns. The majority and dissenting opinions reflect the opposing judicial responses to such arguments. Ultimately, a majority of the Ohio Supreme Court, unlike most other courts, allowed the city to proceed to trial. During the discovery process, however, political support for the lawsuit waned and the Cincinnati city council voted to drop the lawsuit.

For a similar lawsuit, see *City of Gary v. Smith & Wesson Corp.*, 801 N.E.2d 1222 (Ind. 2003). For lawsuits with different results, see *City of Chicago v. Beretta* U.S.A. Corp., 213 Ill. 2d 351, 821 N.E.2d 1099 (2004) (upholding trial court's granting of a motion to dismiss); *see also City of Philadelphia v. Beretta U.S.A. Corp.*, 277 F.3d 415 (3d Cir. 2002). For updates and references to additional lawsuits, see www.gunlawsuits.org/docket (last visited December 2006).

In an interesting and politically informative side-skirmish to the Chicago lawsuit, the city sought trace data (data identifying guns that had been identified as part of a criminal investigation) from the ATF. The ATF refused the city's request and the city sued the federal government agency under the Freedom of Information Act. In *City of Chicago v. Department of Treasury*, 384 F.3d 429 (7th Cir. 2004), the court ordered the ATF to release the data to the city. Congress, however, intervened, and amended the ATF appropriations bill to prohibit the expenditure of any funds to comply with the Seventh Circuit's order. What does this tell you about the politics of gun control?

From a public health policy point of view, does it make sense for cities and other local governments to pursue gun control through this type of litigation? Are these efforts to sidestep the political process? Would it make a difference if the plaintiff-governmental body were precluded from seeking regulatory gun control legislation by state preemption legislation? For that matter, what do you think the plaintiffs are trying to achieve: recovery of actual damages? limits on the distribution of guns? Would you feel differently if, in fact, these lawsuits were being orchestrated by a larger, nationwide "anti-gun conspiracy" and intended to force gun manufacturers or distributors out of business or into bankruptcy?

**2.** Lawsuits such as *Bryco,* brought by private individuals against gun manufacturers and gun sellers, have had somewhat more success — particularly where the factual claims focus on a particular incident or the dangers of a particular weapon, as in the *Bryco* case. In this regard, *Bryco* should be viewed as a rather narrow holding, tied to its specific facts, and not necessarily as a case that opens the door to many other lawsuits against many other defendants. (In fact, the defendant in *Bryco* has become notorious both for his often-malfunctioning products and his efforts to avoid liability; for a recounting of this story, see www.brandonsarms.org/ (last visited December 2006).

Nonetheless other plaintiffs have been successful. For example, the Ninth Circuit allowed that the surviving families of victims of a mass homicide could sue the distributors and manufacturers of the guns that were used in the incident for negligence and public nuisance, if the plaintiffs could show that the defendants knew they were over-saturating the market and creating an illegal secondary market for their products. *Ileto v. Glock, Inc.*, 349 F.3d 1191 (9th Cir. 2003). For decisions dismissing claims by victims of gun violence, see *Hamilton v. Beretta U.S.A. Corp.*, 264 F.3d 36 (2d Cir. 2000) (holding that New York state law does not allow survivors of a mass homicide to sue gun manufacturer or seller); *Merrill v. Navegar*, 26 Cal. 4th 465, 110 Cal. Rptr. 370, 28 P.3d 116 (2001) (under California state law, gun manufacturers and sellers are immune from liability).

In a case following the much-publicized "D.C. sniper" homicides in 2002, the families of the victims of John Mohammad and Lee Malvo sued the maker of the Bushmaster assault rifle used in the shootings and the gun shop which allowed Mohammad to obtain the rifle (in violation of various state and federal laws). The Washington state courts refused to dismiss the case and a trial was set for the Spring of 2005. In the Fall of 2004, a settlement was reached in which the gun manufacturer agreed to pay $2 million and to change some of their distributional practices; the gun shop agreed to pay $1 million to the

victims. A number of other lawsuits against gun manufacturers also have been
settled out-of-court.

**3.** Some of these government and privately initiated lawsuits have been
barred by state laws that provide gun manufacturers or sellers with immunity
from these types of lawsuits — immunity that was created by recent legislation clearly intended to short circuit precisely such lawuits.

At the federal level, in October of 2005 President Bush signed into law the
Protection of Lawful Commerce in Arms Act, Pub. L. No. 109-92. The new federal legislation preempts any cause of action in state or federal court against
manufacturers, distributors, dealers, or importers of firearms "resulting from
the criminal or unlawful use of a qualified product by a person or a third
party," subject to enumerated exceptions. A "qualified product" includes
firearms, their parts, or ammunition" — essentially eliminating many of the
pre-existing state common law and statutory remedies available to both governmental and private plaintiffs (with some notable exceptions). The federal
law also amended the pre-existing federal gun dealer licensing law to require
that new handguns be sold subject to certain "child safety" requirements; compliance with these requirements also triggers immunity from related state and
federal lawsuits.

What types of lawsuits against which defendants are still viable? Obviously
the new federal law limits many "upstream" lawsuits — *i.e.*, importers, manufacturers, dealers, and even sellers have been immunized from most lawsuits
resulting from harm caused by gun owners or possessors long after they have
passed through the stream of commerce, with rather limited and rather specific exceptions. Does this make sense (a) as a matter of law or (b) as a matter
of public policy? Are lawsuits attempting to impose a liability limitation on
commerce in guns? Or are they attempts to insure that guns only fall into the
hands of lawful consumers? Are we concerned that guns will be used, either
illegally or accidentally, in a way that we want to avoid, or that guns are
inherently dangerous even in the hands of lawful purchasers? Importers, manufacturers, dealers, and sellers are clearly links in the chain of events that
lead to various bad outcomes, ranging from homicides to accidental injuries.
Are they in the best position to break that chain of causation? Or are they
being blamed for something that is really caused — in the legal sense of the
term — by other actors?

Viewing the federal law somewhat more broadly, does the extension of
immunity incorporated into this law reflect policy judgments about the appropriate locus for liability, or was it a more crassly political decision? In this
regard, the extensive statements of purposes and findings at the beginning of
the statute are instructive. Congress has made some clear policy judgments
about the importance of commerce in guns, the legitimacy of judicial determinations of liability, and even the proper interpretation of the Second
Amendment.

# Chapter 8

## (BIO)TERRORISM

## A.  INTRODUCTION

For many Americans, time is divided by September 11, 2001; there is the world before and the world after. September 11 may not have "changed everything," but it has certainly changed a lot — including major changes in public health funding, laws, and structure. It has caused us to be concerned, even obsessed, with a disease the eradication of which has been seen as public health's greatest triumph: smallpox. It has refocused public health funding, led to new public health laws, and created an entirely new field, "public health preparedness." How should public health and public health lawyers react to the threat of terrorist attacks, including the possible use of a biological agent as a weapon, so-called "bioterrorism"?

This concluding chapter on a post-9/11 terrorism challenge to public health is designed as a case study to encourage students to apply the law highlighted in the preceding chapters in order to determine the most effective, efficient and civil-liberties-friendly responses. Because compulsory measures related to contagious disease epidemics, such as quarantine, are often discussed in the context of preparedness planning, the materials in Chapter Three will often be of particular relevance. Among the questions that are posed throughout are: Can public health funding really be "dual use" so that we need not sacrifice traditional public health activities for new ones, or will we have to develop new priorities? Does our current "all-hazards" approach to disaster planning make sense given our experience with it in failing to prepare for and respond effectively to Hurricane Katrina? What does "preparedness" mean, and how do we apply public health principles to preventing a bioterrorist attack? Should we expand public health surveillance over medical care in emergency departments and physician offices? Should we develop new rules restricting access to bacteria and viruses that can be used as weapons? Should we shift legal power from states and localities to the federal government, or even to multinational or global organizations? How can the trust of the public in public health be maintained and fostered? Is public health the ultimate global public good? Should public health encourage international cooperation and respect international law? And, ultimately, have we overreacted to 9/11, and if so, in what areas can or should we return to the pre-9/11 public health?

The materials in this Chapter begin with summaries and recommendations from the 9/11 Commission in Section B; Section C is devoted to the anthrax attacks that occurred just after 9/11; Section D details and explores the smallpox vaccination program initiated in the run-up to the Iraq war; Section E is devoted to the new and rapidly growing area of bioterror preparedness and research and its impact on public health and risk perception; Section F explores federal preparedness; and Section G addresses global health, including the emerging field of (public) "health and human rights."

## B.   9/11

### Craig R. Whitney, *Introduction*, THE 9/11
### INVESTIGATIONS
xx–xxi, xxxiii (Steven Strasser ed., 2004)

Until the cold war unraveled after the collapse of the Berlin Wall in 1989, the administrations of presidents Ronald Reagan and George H.W. Bush paid comparatively little attention to terrorism, despite the Hezbollah attack that killed 241 marines in Lebanon in October of 1983 and the Libyan sabotage of Pan American Flight 103 that killed 270 people over Lockerbie, Scotland in 1988. Before the first terrorist attack on the World Trade Center in New York City in 1993 — and the later discovery of a related plot to blow up the city's river tunnels and the United Nations building — terrorism had been considered only a marginal threat to the United States itself. It took time for the implications to sink in.

Not until 1995 did President Bill Clinton establish a working level "Counterterrorism Security Group" inside the White House, chaired by Richard A. Clarke. It was not until 1996, Clarke wrote in a controversial book published on the eve of his public testimony before the 9/11 commission, that the government figured out that it was up against an Islamic terrorist network of global dimensions led by a renegade from a wealthy Saudi Arabian family, Osama bin Laden. And only after terrorist suicide truck bombers destroyed the American embassies in Tanzania and Kenya in August 1998, killing 257 (including 12 Americans) and wounding 5,000 people in Nairobi, did President Clinton order the first direct response against al Qaeda, a cruise missile attack on its training grounds in Afghanistan.

Spending on U.S. defensive actions against terrorism increased in 1999 and 2000, but President Clinton was distracted by the Monica Lewinsky affair. Even after suicide bombers used a boat full of explosives to blow up the U.S.S. *Cole* in Aden on October 12, 2000, killing seventeen sailors and injuring thirty-nine, the Clinton administration did not retaliate against al Qaeda, unsure that it had carried out the attack. Clarke and other officials were left to try to persuade the incoming administration of President George W. Bush that the threat of terrorist strikes on American soil posed an urgent danger. President Bush's first national security briefings, Clarke said, were not about terrorism but about two issues that seemed more important to the president then — Iraq, where his father's administration had left Saddam Hussein in power after Operation Desert Storm, and missile defense.

Then came September 11 . . . September 11 was a warning, but also an opportunity to set in place defenses against new and even more terrible terrorist attacks. With the Arab world in turmoil over the war in Iraq and the Bush administration's unconditional backing of Israel in its showdown with the Palestinian Authority, al Qaeda metastasized rapidly despite losing its sanctuary in Afghanistan. After attacks in Indonesia, Thailand, the Philippines, and then Madrid in the spring of 2004, the threat of terrorism to the United States and its Middle Eastern and European allies seemed even greater than it had been in 2001. The worst scenario would be an attack using nuclear, biological, or chemical weapons, and al Qaeda and its spawn were known to have tried to acquire them.

\* \* \*

## NATIONAL COMMISSION ON TERRORIST ATTACKS UPON THE U.S., 9/11 COMMISSION REPORT
### 361–98 (2004)

Three years after 9/11, Americans are still thinking and talking about how to protect our nation in this new era. The national debate continues. Countering terrorism has become, beyond any doubt, the top national security priority for the United States. This shift has occurred with the full support of the Congress, both major political parties, the media, and the American people.

The nation has committed enormous resources to national security and to countering terrorism. Between fiscal year 2001, the last budget adopted before 9/11, and the present fiscal year 2004, total federal spending on defense (including expenditures on both Iraq and Afghanistan), homeland security, and international affairs rose more than 50 percent, from $354 billion to about $547 billion. The United States has not experienced such a rapid surge in national security spending since the Korean War.

This pattern has occurred before in American history. The United States faces a sudden crisis and summons a tremendous exertion of national energy. Then, as that surge transforms the landscape, comes a time for reflection and reevaluation. Some programs and even agencies are discarded; others are invented or redesigned. Private firms and engaged citizens redefine their relationships with government, working through the processes of the American republic. Now is the time for that reflection and reevaluation. The United States should consider *what to do* — the shape and objectives of a strategy. Americans should also consider *how to do it* — organizing their government in a different way.

### Defining the Threat

In the post-9/11 world, threats are defined more by the fault lines within societies than by the territorial boundaries between them. From terrorism to global disease or environmental degradation, the challenges have become transnational rather than international. That is the defining quality of world politics in the twenty-first century.

National security used to be considered by studying foreign frontiers, weighing opposing groups of states, and measuring industrial might. To be dangerous, an enemy had to muster large armies. Threats emerged slowly, often visibly, as weapons were forged, armies conscripted, and units trained and moved into place. Because large states were more powerful, they also had more to lose. They could be deterred.

Now threats can emerge quickly. An organization like al Qaeda, headquartered in a country on the other side of the earth, in a region so poor that electricity or telephones were scarce, could nonetheless scheme to wield weapons of unprecedented destructive power in the largest cities of the United States. In this sense, 9/11 has taught us that terrorism against American interests "over there" should be regarded just as we regard terrorism against America "over here." In this same sense, the American homeland is the planet.

But the enemy is not just "terrorism," some generic evil. This vagueness blurs the strategy. The catastrophic threat at this moment in history is more specific. It is the threat posed by *Islamist* terrorism — especially the al Qaeda network, its affiliates, and its ideology.

\* \* \*

Our enemy is twofold: al Qaeda, a stateless network of terrorists that struck us on 9/11; and a radical ideological movement in the Islamic world, inspired in part by al Qaeda, which has spawned terrorist groups and violence across the globe. The first enemy is weakened, but continues to pose a grave threat. The second enemy is gathering, and will menace Americans and American interests long after Usama Bin Ladin and his cohorts are killed or captured. Thus our strategy must match our means to two ends: dismantling the al Qaeda network and prevailing in the longer term over the ideology that gives rise to Islamist terrorism.

\* \* \*

Islam is not the enemy. It is not synonymous with terror. Nor does Islam teach terror. American and its friends oppose a perversion of Islam, not the great world faith itself. . . .

\* \* \*

The present transnational danger is Islamist terrorism. What is needed is a broad political-military strategy that rests on a firm tripod of policies to

- Attack terrorists and their organizations;

- Prevent the continued growth of Islamist terrorism; and

- Protect against and prepare for terrorist attacks.

## More than a War on Terrorism

Terrorism is a tactic used by individuals and organizations to kill and destroy. Our efforts should be directed at those individuals and organizations. Calling this struggle a war accurately describes the use of American and allied armed forces to find and destroy terrorist groups and their allies in the field, notably in Afghanistan. The language of war also evokes the mobilization for a national effort. Yet the strategy should be balanced.

The first phase of our post-9/11 efforts rightly included military action to topple the Taliban and pursue al Qaeda. This work continues. But long-term success demands the use of all elements of national power: diplomacy, intelligence, covert action, law enforcement, economic policy, foreign aid, public diplomacy, and homeland defense. If we favor one tool while neglecting others, we leave ourselves vulnerable and weaken our national effort.

Certainly the strategy should include offensive operations to counter terrorism. Terrorists should no longer find safe haven where their organizations can grow and flourish. America's strategy should be a coalition strategy that includes Muslim nations as partners in its development and implementation. Our effort should be accompanied by a preventive strategy that is as much, or more, political as it is military. The strategy must focus clearly on the Arab and Muslim world, in all its variety.

Our strategy should also include defenses. America can be attacked in many ways and has many vulnerabilities. No defenses are perfect. But risks must be calculated; hard choices must be made about allocating resources. Responsibilities for America's defense should be clearly defined. Planning does make a difference, identifying where a little money might have a large effect. Defenses also complicate the plans of attackers, increasing their risks of discovery and failure. Finally, the nation must prepare to deal with attacks that are not stopped.

### Measuring Success

What should Americans expect from their government in the struggle against Islamist terrorism? The goals seem unlimited: Defeat terrorism anywhere in the world. But Americans have also been told to expect the worst: An attack is probably coming; it may be terrible.

With such benchmarks, the justifications for action and spending seem limitless. Goals are good. Yet effective public policies also need concrete objectives. Agencies need to be able to measure success.

* * *

We do not believe it is possible to defeat all terrorist attacks against Americans, every time and everywhere. A president should tell the American people:

- No president can promise that a catastrophic attack like that of 9/11 will not happen again. History has shown that even the most vigilant and expert agencies cannot always prevent determined, suicidal attackers from reaching a target.

- But the American people are entitled to expect their government to do its very best. They should expect that officials will have realistic objectives, clear guidance, and effective organization. They are entitled to see some standards for performance so they can judge, with the help of their elected representatives, whether the objectives are being met.

* * *

**Recommendation: The U.S. government must define what the message is, what it stands for. We should offer an example of moral**

leadership in the world, committed to treat people humanely, abide by the rule of law, and be generous and caring to our neighbors. America and Muslim friends can agree on respect for human dignity and opportunity. To Muslim parents, terrorists like Bin Ladin have nothing to offer their children but visions of violence and death. America and its friends have a crucial advantage — we can offer these parents a vision that might give their children a better future. If we heed the views of thoughtful leaders in the Arab and Muslim world, a moderate consensus can be found.

That vision of the future should stress life over death: individual educational and economic opportunity. This vision includes widespread political participation and contempt for indiscriminate violence. It includes respect for the rule of law, openness in discussing differences, and tolerance for opposing points of view.

\* \* \*

Recommendation: The United States should engage its friends to develop a common coalition approach toward the detention and humane treatment of captured terrorists. New principles might draw upon Article 3 of the Geneva Conventions on the law of armed conflict. That article was specifically designed for those cases in which the usual laws of war did not apply. Its minimum standards are generally accepted throughout the world as customary international law.

\* \* \*

Recommendation: Our report shows that al Qaeda has tried to acquire or make weapons of mass destruction for at least ten years. There is no doubt the United States would be a prime target. Preventing the proliferation of these weapons warrants a maximum effort — by strengthening counterproliferation efforts, expanding the Proliferation Security Initiative, and supporting the Cooperative Threat Reduction program.

\* \* \*

Recommendation: At this time of increased and consolidated government authority, there should be a board within the executive branch to oversee adherence to the guidelines we recommend and the commitment the government makes to defend our civil liberties.

We must find ways of reconciling security with liberty, since the success of one helps protect the other. The choice between security and liberty is a false choice, as nothing is more likely to endanger America's liberties than the success of a terrorist attack at home. Our history has shown us that insecurity threatens liberty. Yet, if our liberties are curtailed, we lose the values that we are struggling to defend.

\* \* \*

Recommendation: Homeland security assistance should be based strictly on an assessment of risks and vulnerabilities. Now, in 2004, Washington, D.C., and New York City are certainly at the top of any such list. We **understand the contention that every state and city needs to have some minimum infrastructure for emergency response**. But **federal homeland security assistance should not remain a program for general revenue sharing**. It should **supplement state and local resources** based on the risks or vulnerabilities that merit additional support. Congress should not use this money as a pork barrel.

## NOTES AND QUESTIONS

**1.** The 9/11 Commission (officially known as "The National Commission on Terrorist Attacks Upon the U.S.") made 41 specific recommendations. Their final report was issued in July 2004 and is available in its entirety on a frozen website that is maintained by the National Archives at www.9-11 commission-gov/report/index.htm (last visited Aug. 2006). In December 2005 the Commission issued a report card on its recommendations, giving the government failing grades on many of its most important recommendations, including a "D" on developing critical infrastructure; an "F" on airline passenger pre-screening; a "D" on checked bag and cargo screening; a "D" on international collaboration on borders and document security, a "privacy and civil liberties oversight board, and on developing guidelines for sharing of personal information; and an "F" on "coalition detention standards." Dan Eggen, *U.S. Issued Failing Grades by 9/11 Panel,* WASHINGTON POST, Dec. 6, 2005, at A1.

Perhaps most strikingly, Congress continues to fund preparedness based on congressional districts rather than giving more funds to areas that are the most vulnerable. Editorial, *Hokum on Homeland Security,* N.Y. TIMES, Aug. 20, 2006, at WK9. For the inside story of the Commission by its co-chairs, see THOMAS H. KEAN & LEE H. HAMILTON, WITHOUT PRECEDENT: THE INSIDE STORY OF THE 9/11 COMMISSION (2006). Not everyone was enthusiastic about the Commission's recommendations. Richard Clarke, for example, thought that the quest for bipartisan unanimity led to the commission failing to "admit the obvious: we are less capable of defeating the jihadists because of the Iraq war. Unanimity has its value, but so do debate and dissent in a democracy facing a crisis. To fully realize the potential of the commission's report, we must see it not as the end of the discussion but as a partial blueprint for victory." Richard A. Clarke, *Honorable Commission, Toothless Report,* N.Y. TIMES, July 25, 2004, at A11. *See also,* RICHARD A. CLARKE, AGAINST ALL ENEMIES: INSIDE AMERICA'S WAR ON TERROR (2004).

**2.** One of the Commission's most striking findings was that the president had received a briefing on Bin Ladin's plans on August 6, 2001, raising the question of whether warnings and preparations can do much good. The Presidential Daily Brief Memo is reprinted on pages 261–262 of the final report, and contains the following observations about reports that Bin Ladin has wanted to hijack US aircraft since 1998:

FBI information since [1998] indicates patterns of suspicious activity in this country consistent with preparation for hijackings or other types of attacks, including recent surveillance of federal buildings in New York. The FBI is conducting approximately 70 full field investigations throughout the US that it considers Bin Ladin-related. CIA and the FBI are investigating a call to our embassy in the UAE in May saying that a group of Bin Ladin supporters was in the US planning attacks with explosives.

The Commission concluded that there were no further discussions "before September 11 among the President and his top advisors of the possibility of a threat of an al Qaeda attack on the United States." NAT'L COMM'N ON TERRORIST ATTACKS, *supra*, at 262.

Five years later the lesson seemed to have been learned, as the president said in a September 5, 2006 five-year anniversary speech on the global war on terror: "We know what the terrorists intend to do because they've told us — and we need to take their words seriously." (*available at* www.whitehouse.gov) On the role of al Qaeda see generally, LAWRENCE WRIGHT, THE LOOMING TOWER: AL-QAEDA AND THE ROAD TO 9/11 (2006).

**3.** *New York Times* columnist Tom Friedman has argued that dating America from September 11 is a major mistake, and that our country should remain the country of the 4th of July. In his view, globalization should continue to be seen as a positive force for the good of all, rather than as a threat to America. *See, e.g.*, THOMAS FRIEDMAN, THE WORLD IS FLAT: A BRIEF HISTORY OF THE TWENTY-FIRST CENTURY (Updated and expanded ed. 2006).

**4.** It is striking that the 9/11 Commission highlighted the importance of the Geneva Conventions in our response to 9/11. Only a few months after the attacks, the president signed an executive order declaring that the Geneva Conventions did not apply to the Taliban or to prisoners held at Guantanamo Bay, Cuba. This was the first time in U.S. history that a president has ever claimed an exception for the U.S. from this international treaty that covers the treatment of prisoners and civilians during wartime. In the summer of 2006 the U.S. Supreme Court had its first opportunity to decide if the president could unilaterally declare international law, specifically the Geneva Conventions, null. In what has been described as the most important case the Court has ever decided on the question of executive powers, the Court ruled that the Conventions must be followed as an integral part of international law. Justice Stevens wrote for the Court:

The [Court of Appeals] accepted the Executive's assertions that Hamdan was captured in connection with the United States war with al Qaeda and that war is distinct from the war with the Taliban in Afghanistan. It further reasoned that the war with al Qaeda evades the reach of the Geneva Conventions. *See* 415 F. 3d, at 41-42. We, like Judge Williams, disagree with the latter conclusion.

The conflict with al Qaeda is not, according to the Government, a conflict to which the full protections afforded detainees under the 1949 Geneva Conventions apply because Article 2 of those Conventions (which appears in all four Conventions) renders the full protections applicable only to "all cases of declared war or of any other armed conflict which may arise between two or more of the High Contracting Parties." 6 U.S.T., at 3318. Since Hamdan was captured and detained incident to the conflict with al Qaeda and not the conflict with the Taliban, and since al Qaeda, unlike Afghanistan, is not a "High Contracting Party" — *i.e.*, a signatory of the Conventions, the protections of those Conventions are not, it is argued, applicable to Hamdan.

We need not decide the merits of this argument because there is at least one provision of the Geneva Conventions that applies here even if the relevant conflict is not one between signatories. Article 3, often referred to as Common Article 3 because, like Article 2, it appears in all four Geneva Conventions, provides that in a "conflict not of an international character occurring in the territory of one of the High Contracting Parties, each Party to the conflict shall be bound to apply, as a minimum, certain provisions protecting "[p]ersons taking no active part in the hostilities, including members of armed forces who have laid down their arms and those placed *hors de combat* by . . . detention." One such provision prohibits "the passing of sentences and the carrying out of executions without previous judgment pronounced by a regularly constituted court affording all the judicial guarantees which are recognized as indispensable by civilized peoples."

The Court of Appeals thought, and the Government asserts, that Common Article 3 does not apply to Hamdan because the conflict with al Qaeda, being "'international in scope,'" does not qualify as a "'conflict not of an international character.'" 415 F. 3d, at 41. That reasoning is erroneous. The term "conflict not of an international character" is used here in contradistinction to a conflict between nations. So much is demonstrated by the "fundamental logic [of] the Convention's provisions on its application." (Williams, J., concurring). Common Article 2 provides that "the present Convention shall apply to all cases of declared war or of any other armed conflict which may arise between two or more of the High Contracting Parties." High Contracting Parties (signatories) also must abide by all terms of the Conventions vis-à-vis one another even if one party to the conflict is a nonsignatory "Power," and must so abide vis-à-vis the nonsignatory if "the latter accepts and applies" those terms. Common Article 3, by contrast, affords some minimal protection, falling short of full protection under the Conventions, to individuals associated with neither a signatory nor even a nonsignatory "Power" who are involved in a conflict "in the territory of" a signatory. The latter kind of conflict is distinguishable from the conflict described in Common Article 2 chiefly because it does not involve a clash between nations (whether signatories or not). In context, then, the phrase "not of an international character" bears its literal meaning.

*Hamdan v. Rumsfeld,* 126 S. Ct. 2749 (2006).

**5.** The complete text of Common Article 3 of the Geneva Conventions is:

In the case of armed conflict not of an international character occurring in the territory of one of the High Contracting Parties, each Party to the conflict shall be bound to apply, as a minimum, the following provisions:

(1) Persons taking no active part in the hostilities, including members of armed forces who have laid down their arms and those placed *hors de combat* by sickness, wounds, detention, or any other cause, shall in all circumstances be treated humanely, without any adverse distinction founded on race, color, religion or faith, sex, birth or wealth, or any other similar criteria.

To this end, the following acts are and shall remain prohibited at any time and in any place whatsoever with respect to the above-mentioned persons:

(a) violence to life and person, in particular murder of all kinds, mutilation, cruel treatment and torture;

(b) taking of hostages;

(c) outrages upon personal dignity, in particular, humiliating and degrading treatment;

(d) the passing of sentences and the carrying out of executions without previous judgment pronounced by a regularly constituted court affording all the judicial guarantees which are recognized as indispensable by civilized peoples.

(2) The wounded and sick shall be collected and cared for. An impartial humanitarian body, such as the International Committee of the Red Cross, may offer its services to the Parties to the conflict.

The Parties to the conflict should further endeavor to bring into force, by means of special agreements, all or part of the other provisions of the present Convention.

The application of the preceding provisions shall not affect the legal status of the Parties to conflict.

**6.** Taking human rights seriously in this context would have better sustained international support for the U.S. fight against terrorism. Moreover, following a convention-mandated screening process the United States could lawfully have questioned those prisoners (likely a majority) who did not qualify for POW status under the conventions. In short, little was gained, and much was lost, in the administration's attempt to trash the Geneva Conventions by putting pragmatism over principle.

The administration's decision to treat the Geneva Conventions as inapplicable helped create a sense that Guantanamo was a legal black hole to which neither U.S. nor international law applied. This attitude in turn helped produce the scandalous abuse and torture of Iraqi prisoners of war at Abu Ghraib prison. The photographs of their humiliating and degrading treatment made it appear that the United States was willing to fight terror with terror. Abu Ghraib negated any American claim of moral superiority in the world and destroyed all human rights rationales for the Iraq war. The "good guys" had become the "evildoers" on prime-time TV for the world to see.

Military physicians performed better when honoring both medical ethics and the human rights provisions of Geneva I, which covers wounded prisoners. After the fiercest battle in Afghanistan, (part of Operation Anaconda), for example, the surgeon in command of the U.S. Army field hospital at Bagram Air Base, Lt. Col. Ronald Smith, told reporters who asked him that the Taliban and al Qaeda wounded were being treated side by side with the American wounded at the hospital, noting that "the ethics of combat surgery" require it.

It is also worth noting that the Geneva Conventions themselves affirmatively protect medical ethics. For example, Article 16 of Protocol I (1977) states in relevant part:

(1) Under no circumstances shall any person be punished for carrying out medical *activities compatible with medical ethics,* regardless of the person benefiting therefrom.

(2) Persons engaged in medical activities shall not be compelled to perform acts or to carry out work contrary to the *rules of medical ethics* or to other medical rules designed for the benefit of the wounded and sick or to the provisions of the Conventions or this Protocol, or to refrain from performing acts or from carrying out work required by those rules and provisions. (emphasis added)

In short, under international humanitarian law, human rights and medical ethics requirements are symbiotic. *See, e.g.,* GEORGE J. ANNAS, AMERICAN BIOETHICS: CROSSING HUMAN RIGHTS AND HEALTH LAW BOUNDARIES 9-10 (2005); Edmund Pellegrino, *Medical Ethics Suborned by Tyranny and War,* 291 JAMA 1505 (2004).

**7.** Of course it is not just terrorism that has been globalized. As discussed in length in Chapter Three, diseases know no national boundaries, and pandemics like HIV/AIDS, SARS, and the avian flu are all inherently global diseases that, like the global environment, no country can deal with effectively on its own. *See, e.g.,* LAURIE GARRETT, THE COMING PLAGUE: NEWLY EMERGING DISEASE IN A WORLD OUT OF BALANCE (1994).

## C.  THE ANTHRAX ATTACKS

### Elin Gursky et al., *Anthrax 2001: Observations on the Medical and Public Health Response*
1 BIOSECURITY & BIOTERRORISM 97 (2003)

The immediate and continuing medical and public health response to the anthrax attacks of 2001 represents a singular episode in the history of public health . . .

The "response" to the anthrax attacks [which infected 22 people and killed 5] was extremely complex, and any analysis that purports to assess the response must account for this complexity. The unprecedented nature of the attacks and the context in which the response occurred are also crucial to understanding what happened and why. The long-standing neglect of federal, state, and local public health agencies, and the highly stressed condition of U.S. medical facilities, which routinely work at the limits of their capacity, are acknowledged by virtually all informed observers. That the medical and public health institutions involved in the response functioned as well as they did is a tribute to the extraordinary efforts of the individuals involved.

Despite the commitment and hard work of the individuals in these professional communities, what was revealed by the anthrax attacks was an unacceptable level of fragility in systems now properly recognized as vital to national defense. Too many citizens, elected leaders, and national security officials still have limited understanding of the degree to which 22 cases of anthrax rocked the public health agencies and hospitals involved in the response to this small bioterrorist attack. Most of the vulnerabilities in the medical and public health systems revealed by this response remain unaddressed. It is not the purpose of this article to praise or criticize individuals who responded to the 2001 anthrax attack. The emphasis here is on how to improve response *systems.* The article seeks to identify the strategic and organizational successes and shortcomings of the health response to the anthrax attacks so that medical and public health communities as well as elected officials can learn from this crisis. . . .

## CHRONOLOGY OF KEY EVENTS FOLLOWING THE ATTACKS

**October 2, 2001** — An infectious disease physician recognized a possible case of inhalational anthrax in a man hospitalized in Palm Beach County, Florida. This physician contacted the local health officer in Palm Beach County, who immediately began a public health investigation. By October 2, there were already 7 persons with cutaneous anthrax in the northeastern U.S., but none had yet been diagnosed.

**October 4** — The microbiologic diagnosis of *B. anthracis* was confirmed by the Florida Department of Health (FDH) and the Centers for Disease Control and Prevention (CDC), and the diagnosis was made public. Epidemiologic and environmental investigations were launched to determine the source of the patient's anthrax exposure. Evidence of contamination with *B. anthracis* was found at American Media Inc. (AMI) in Boca Raton, Florida where the first victim worked as a photo editor.

**October 5** — The first victim of the anthrax attacks died. A second AMI employee, who had been hospitalized for pneumonia on September 30, was diagnosed with inhalational anthrax. He was an employee in the AMI mailroom.

**October 6** — The Palm Beach County Health Department began to obtain nasal swabs from those who had been in the AMI building in an attempt to define exposure groups. Because nasal swab testing was known to be an insensitive diagnostic test, the health department also recommended prophylactic antibiotics for all those people who had been in the AMI building for at least one hour since August 1 regardless of the results of their nasal swab tests. Environmental samples taken from the mailroom showed evidence of *B. anthracis*.

**October 7** — A nasal swab was positive on another employee. A swab from the first victim's computer screen was positive. The AMI building was closed.

**October 9** — The New York City Department of Health notified CDC of a woman with a skin lesion consistent with cutaneous anthrax. The woman, an assistant to NBC anchor Tom Brokaw, had handled a powder-containing letter postmarked September 18 at her workplace.

**October 13** — Another cutaneous case of anthrax was recognized in a 7-month-old infant who had visited his mother's workplace, the ABC office building on West 66th Street in Manhattan, on September 28.

**October 13** — Symptoms of cutaneous and inhalational anthrax in New Jersey postal workers began to be observed and reported by physicians to the New York City Health Department. Diagnoses of anthrax are confirmed by the CDC on October 18 and 19.

**October 15** — A staff member in the office of Senator Daschle in the Hart Senate Office Building opened a letter (postmarked October 9) which contained a powder and a note identifying the powder as anthrax. The powder tested positive for *B. anthracis* on October 16. Nasal swab testing of anthrax spores was performed on 340 Senate staff members and visitors to the building who potentially were exposed and to approximately 5000 other people who self-referred for testing. This testing indicated exposure in 28 persons. Antimicrobial prophylaxis was administered on a broader scale and environmental testing was initiated.

**October 19** — CDC linked the four confirmed cases of anthrax to "intentional delivery of *B. anthracis* spores through mailed letters or packages."

**October 19–22** — Four postal workers at the Brentwood Mail Processing and Distribution Center in the District of Columbia were hospitalized with inhalational anthrax. The Brentwood facility was closed on October 21. On October 22 two of these four postal workers died.

**October 24** — CDC sent an advisory to state health officials via the Health Alert Network recommending antibiotic prophylaxis to prevent anthrax for all people who had been in the non-public mail operations area at the U.S. Postal Service's Brentwood Road Postal Distribution Center or who had worked in the non-public mail operations areas at postal facilities that had received mail directly from the Brentwood facility since October 11.

**October 27** — A CDC alert recommended antibiotic prophylaxis for workers in the mail facilities that supplied the CIA, the House office buildings, the Supreme Court, Walter Reed Army Institute of Research, the White House, and the Southwest Postal Station after preliminary environmental sampling revealed *B. anthracis* contamination in these mailrooms.

**October 31** — A 61-year-old female hospital stockroom worker in New York City died from inhalational anthrax after she had become ill with malaise and myalgias on October 25. The source of her exposure remains unknown despite extensive epidemiologic investigation.

November 16 — A 94-year-old woman residing in Oxford, Connecticut, was hospitalized with fever, cough, and weakness. She died on November 19. Her diagnosis was confirmed as *B. anthracis* on November 20 by the Connecticut Department of Public Health Laboratory. Subsequent environmental and epidemiological testing indicated exposure from cross-contaminated letters.

## Public health decision-making processes

The 2001 anthrax attacks challenged traditional decision-making processes of federal, state, and local public health authorities. Historically, most outbreaks of naturally occurring disease are first recognized in a limited geographic region; laboratory and clinical methods for accurately diagnosing and treating cases of an unfamiliar illness (*e.g.*, HIV/AIDS, Hanta virus, Legionnaire's Disease) often evolve over a period of months or even years. Data pertaining to the outbreak and the causes of the illness are collected and analyzed by scientists at CDC and other public health agencies and medical institutions, and these analyses are discussed in the academic public health and medical communities at conferences and in medical journals. With time, a consensus view usually emerges about the causes of a disease, who is at risk, and how the illness can best be diagnosed, treated, and prevented. These scientifically based guidelines often are published by CDC and/or professional medical societies and serve as the basis for state and local public health practice.

In October 2001, at the time of the initial discovery of a person with anthrax infection in Florida, public health officials worked closely with clinicians in Palm Beach County to rapidly confirm the medical diagnosis of anthrax and to initiate the epidemiologic investigation that followed. For many of the decisions and actions that would follow, traditional public health decision-making processes were not adequate to cope with the extent, pace, and complexities of events surrounding the attacks.

This was the first time that CDC had been called on to respond to outbreaks of illness occurring nearly simultaneously in five geographic epicenters. Because sending *B. anthracis* spores through the mail was clearly an act of terrorism, the FBI was involved, substantially increasing the number of people and organizations that needed to receive and interpret information pertinent to the disease investigation and remain "in the loop." In addition, because anthrax is virtually unknown in current medical practice, few local or federal public health officials had ever seen or been involved in evaluating a single case of *B. anthracis* infection, let alone a bioterrorist attack resulting in a series of cases.

Many public health policies — for example, whether to offer needle exchange programs to stem the spread of HIV/AIDS, or the nature and extent of prenatal care programs — routinely differ quite extensively from state to state and reflect variations in resources, expertise, and judgments about local priorities and needs. In the context of the anthrax attacks, however, policies and recommendations that differed between states, and between states and CDC, caused confusion. In some case, inconsistencies in the response were interpreted as evidence of incompetence or inequitable treatment, rather than as nuanced reactions to local situations or principled disagreement about what was the best course of action.

* * *

In some instances, state and local public health officials were reluctant to initiate public health actions, such as recommending prophylactic antibiotics, without benefit of specific CDC guidance. Other health departments made decisions prior to receiving CDC guidance, in some instances deciding to act in ways that conflicted with CDC recommendations. Such variations in states' decisions were especially notable in the context of determining who was at risk for exposure to *B. anthracis* spores and who should receive prophylactic antibiotics.

Confusion and contention surrounded both CDC's authority to mandate specific public health actions and state public health officials' responsibility to act on their own best judgments. Noted one state public health official, "We relied on CDC as a consultant. They gave us guidance and knowledge, but we used our own instincts. [We concluded that], if the environment had one spore, you are exposed." A local public health official expressed the view that although CDC's scientific expertise was valuable, CDC was "a research-based organization, far removed from how public health is delivered," and hence was not well placed to make operational decisions on the local level.

* * *

On some occasions during the response to the anthrax attacks of 2001, confusion about who was at risk of developing anthrax and ambiguities about the extent of public health officials' authority resulted in public health actions being influenced by political pressures. Several of those interviewed reported that in some locations elected officials had directed which groups of people should receive preventive antibiotics. In at least one case, differences among state health departments' recommendations about who should receive antibiotic prophylaxis caused great concern among elected federal representatives. One public health official noted, "The media would compare our decisions to those made [elsewhere]. It was extremely uncomfortable. Elected officials came down on us regarding fairness. One elected official said, "The only fair thing was to give every postal worker [in the state] Cipro even though state public health officials believed that the information available warranted a more limited distribution of antibiotics.". . .

In a number of areas targeted by the anthrax attacks, several different adjacent or overlapping public health agencies were simultaneously responding. City, county, and state health officials within states and across state borders, in many instances, had difficulty acquiring and sharing information and harmonizing their recommendations.

Medical and public health professionals from the greater Washington, DC, area reported many obstacles to reaching consensus decisions and to working collaboratively across the region. The Washington, DC, metropolitan area encompasses a complicated network of government jurisdictions. Many people who work in DC live in Maryland or Virginia. Three different health departments (Maryland, Virginia, and DC) were involved in the 2001 anthrax investigation and response. Although each was responsible for actions in their respective jurisdictions, the people at risk and the issues at stake often crossed geopolitical boundaries. In some instances, local public health officials working in these different jurisdictions were receiving contradictory recommendations from different sources. . . .

CDC's usual approach to investigating disease outbreaks — a careful, step-by-step gathering of evidence followed by deliberate scientific analysis — was not feasible in the context of a high-profile attack occurring in multiple epicenters that potentially placed thousands at risk and was causing massive disruption of government, business, and citizens' routines. The analytical challenges were compounded by the complexities of the investigation. For example, the FBI was in charge of studying the anthrax powder found in the identified envelopes — material that immediately became evidence in a criminal investigation. It is unclear how soon CDC became aware that the anthrax powder found in the letter to Senator Daschle had different physical properties from the anthrax powder in letters sent to ABC, which had been examined earlier. The Daschle material was more refined, "fluffier," and more likely to remain airborne, thus posing a greater threat of inhalation. . . .

In the days immediately following the discovery of the first case of inhalational anthrax in Florida, CDC scientists had judged that only opened envelopes posed a risk of spore exposure. The investigation to date had revealed that no postal workers were ill in the Florida facility "upstream" of the contaminated letter that was believed to have been the source of the first victim's exposure. Concerned about the potential side-effects of preventive antibiotics, and lacking information about what risks anthrax spores in sealed letters might pose to people working in the U.S. postal system, CDC initially recommended that only those in close proximity to *opened* anthrax-laden letters receive antibiotic prophylaxis. As the risks posed by sealed *B. anthracis*-laden envelopes became evident, prophylaxis recommendations were expanded to include mail handlers and others working in contaminated sites. . . . .

Postal workers also questioned the reliability of some of the CDC guidance. A representative of the postal workers noted, "The information [from CDC] changed every day. Nobody knew what was going on. I started a web page, but I would put something out and it would change. They said you need 10,000 spores to be ill, but we asked, 'Can't some people get sick with less?' They said, 'No. You have a better chance of getting hit by a bicycle.' We had a party [to celebrate] the end of 60 days [of Cipro] and then they came back [a few weeks later] and said there were spores still living in us. They held a lot of meetings. I sat in on each one. Every doctor and every story was different. They said the stuff [vaccine] was safe but we would have to sign all these papers and maybe we could lose our rights under workers comp. Then they said the military people used to get six shots but we were going to get less. Even that doctor said she had the six. If six was good for her, why not for us?"

The confusion caused by these scientific uncertainties was compounded by the poor communication among public health officials and the media and the public. As the investigation first evolved and CDC learned more about the nature of the anthrax powder, the risk posed by unopened envelopes working their way through post office sorting machines, and other technical issues that bore on who was at risk and the nature of the public health response, the public heard little from top federal health officials. The lack of a consistent, credible message emanating from CDC in the early days after the anthrax attacks has yet to be fully explained.

CDC thus faced daunting challenges. The world expected CDC to provide detailed, authoritative information about a disease with which it was not familiar, in the context of a deliberate attack during a criminal investigation, the scope of which was larger than anything CDC had ever handled. Key aspects of the investigation were not under CDC's control, and it is unclear to what extent CDC officials were free to speak to the public or the media.

\* \* \*

Faced with either poor access to public health officials or inadequate information, reporters scanned websites, downloaded articles, and attempted to identify experts. Without information from the public health authorities, one journalist noted that they had to assemble pieces of the anthrax puzzle from a variety of what they hoped would be credible sources. One reporter noted, "It was extremely difficult to get information [out of public health]. If I did not have a several-year relationship with officials, it would have been impossible. I have been in the business 25 years, but this was the fastest unfolding story. There was information, rumors, powders, and people on edge. It would have been useful to have a single person, point of contact, or continually updated website. Everyone was having meetings and things were hush-hush. They didn't know what was safe to say. The press relied on back channel contacts. We wanted to make sure we did not embellish. This took effort. The job of good reporting is a function of the reliability of data. There were many agencies involved that had conflicting information. You don't want reporters making scientific judgments."

The anthrax attacks of 2001 placed heavy and novel demands on a public health system that long has been recognized to lack resources commensurate with its responsibilities. Although some public health officials reported that experience with previous communicable disease outbreaks had helped to prepare them to respond to the anthrax attacks, most believed that the demands placed on public health authorities by the anthrax crisis made this different from past public health events. One state public health official noted, "Public health planning for West Nile Virus, Y2K and even 9/11 facilitated the development of systems and strategies, but we were under-prepared for the surge in demand [caused by the anthrax attacks]." A number of concerns were common across affected communities.

***Communications technology was inadequate.*** Equipment widely requested on an emergency basis by public health officials during the attacks included computers, software applications, conference call capability, wireless email, broadcast fax, and cell phones. . . .

***Systems for emergency procurement of critical resources were lacking.*** Few public health departments had emergency procurement systems. . . .

***Public health laboratories were stretched.*** State public health laboratories across the country were highly stressed by the quantity of potentially contaminated items brought in for testing. . . .

# NOTES AND QUESTIONS

**1.** The authors of this study/description of the public health reaction to the anthrax letter attacks drew five conclusions: (1) Expectations about federal, state, and local public health responsibilities require clarification; (2) Medical preparedness requires better communications among physicians and between medical and public health communities; (3) The public and medicine must recognize that response to bioterror attacks will evolve based on changing circumstances and new information; (4) Health officials must prepare to handle the media storm; and (5) Public health resources are barely adequate for a small-scale bioterror attack. Gursky et al., *supra*, at 107-09. The report stressed the need for more funding for public health and noted that "The smallpox immunization plan announced by the administration in December 2002 [*see infra*] has added great stress to public health agencies around the country." *Id.* at 109.

It is worth noting that this report identified no legal obstacles to public health response and recommended no changes in local, state, or federal law to enhance public health preparedness. Was this omission a mistake? Could specific legal changes have improved the quality of public health response to the anthrax mailings? If so, what changes would you recommend? Of course, the most critical pieces of information were scientific facts, such as how anthrax is spread. On the other hand, in an emergency there will never be time to obtain all the scientific facts before acting.

The authors conclude:

It will take considerable vision and leadership — and sustained funding — to build the medical and public health systems needed to appreciably improve the nation's capacity to mitigate the consequences of bioterrorist attacks. The anthrax attacks of 2001 demonstrated the feasibility of the use of biological weapons upon civilian populations. The SARS outbreak has again demonstrated the great responsibilities and challenges that the medical and public health systems bear in confronting disease epidemics, even when the overall number of cases remains relatively modest. Assessments of the response to the 2001 anthrax attacks and to other disease outbreaks such as SARS are critical to making wise decisions and strategic investments at the local, state, and federal levels concerning bioterrorism preparedness and response. Establishing the policy priorities, resources, and institutional capabilities to practice public health at a level of sophistication consistent with 21st century science and technology and commensurate with the threat posed by catastrophic bioterrorism is the task before us. *Id.* at 110.

2. Anthrax vaccine has been approved for use to prevent cutaneous anthrax and was mandatorily given to the troops in the Gulf War on the basis that it was an approved agent that could be given for an unapproved but closely-related use (inhalation anthrax). This vaccine was developed in 1970. After the Gulf War, DOD signed a sole source contract with a new company, Bioport, to produce anthrax vaccine. In 1998 Secretary of Defense William Cohen ordered that all active duty troops be given the anthrax vaccine, which was to be delivered in a series of six injections over an 18 month period. Some soldiers refused, and challenged the orders, arguing that the vaccine was experimental and thus could not be given without informed consent. Many of them were court-martialed. Anthrax vaccination was halted in 2001 when supplies ran out and the sole-source company was shut down by the FDA for failure to maintain proper manufacturing standards. Production and military vaccination resumed in 2002. There is no evidence of any military personnel or installation ever being attacked by anthrax anywhere in the world.

The bioterrorist anthrax attacks in the U.S. were on civilians, none of whom has been vaccinated. The recommended course of treatment for exposure to anthrax is 60 days of antibiotics, and antibiotics were made available to the 10,000 people potentially exposed. The anthrax vaccine was not available to civilians in October or November. In late December 2001, however, DOD agreed to supply sufficient vaccine to vaccinate the 10,000 exposed civilians. Of the 10,000 people eligible for the vaccine, only 152 eventually took it. Since the anthrax vaccine was an investigational drug when used for post-exposure inhalation anthrax, it could only be used in the context of a clinical trial, and then only with the informed consent of the subjects.

The FDA and CDC designed a consent form, together with a counseling process, for use in obtaining the consent of the exposed civilians to participate in the research project. Unlike the case of the military in the Gulf War, or even the peacetime military with the anthrax vaccine, in which the government required soldiers to be vaccinated, the choice was left entirely to individuals. Government officials did not even make a recommendation as to what they thought any individual should do. D.A. Henderson, the chief bioterrorist adviser to the Secretary of Health and Human Services (HHS), justified this failure to recommend for or against taking the anthrax vaccine by saying that there was insufficient information available to make a recommendation. But on what basis could individuals make a decision if those with the most experience with the anthrax vaccine refused even to advise them about what action was medically reasonable?

Although no survey of the exposed civilians has been conducted, it seems likely that the potential subjects mostly decided for themselves that their 60 days (or less) of antibiotics was sufficient protection. It is also unlikely that anyone who actually read and understood the information in the consent forms provided (for adults, adolescents, and children) would have chosen to take the vaccine. Specifically, the consent forms (which are essentially identical) are five-page, single-spaced documents. Designed for a clinical research trial, the forms are nonetheless captioned "Anthrax Vaccine and Drugs Availability Program for Persons Possibly Exposed to Inhaled Spores." Most of the form is in regular typeface, but the following information is in bold:

> **Before you decide to take part in this program, there are several important things that you should know. . .**
>
> - **Anthrax vaccine has not been shown to prevent infection** when given to people after exposure to anthrax spores. . .
>
> - The vaccine that you will receive in this program **has not been approved by the Food and Drug Administration (FDA) for this use and is considered investigational.** . .
>
> - FDA has not approved this lot of vaccine (Lot FAV-063) because the company's license to produce the vaccine is under review. . .
>
> - You should not consider the vaccine as a treatment for anthrax. The vaccine given in this program not been shown to give long term protection against anthrax.
>
> - You may have undesirable side effects from taking this vaccine.
>
> - . . . DHHS is not making any recommendation whether you should or should not take this vaccine. DHHS is making the vaccine available to you to allow you to decide whether or not you wish to use the vaccine.

* * *

The FDA does seem to have learned from its experience in the Gulf War, and did seem to understand that there could be no justification for waiving informed consent for competent adults, even in the face of a bioterrorist attack and uncertainty about the usefulness of the anthrax vaccine. Informed consent for research on competent adults is always feasible and is always ethically required. Informed consent is also required for treating competent adult civilians — only military personnel agree to accept reasonable and necessary approved medical procedures without specific consent. That is only one reason why it is dangerous to civilians to argue that after 9/11 "we are all soldiers now." George J. Annas, *Blinded by Bioterrorism: Public Health and Liberty in the 21st Century*, 13 HEALTH MATRIX 33, 38-41 (2003).

*See also* George J. Annas, *Protecting Soldiers from Friendly Fire: The Consent Requirement for Using Investigational Drugs and Vaccines in Combat*, 24 AM. J.L. & MED. 245 (1996); D.G. McNeil, *Drug Tested in Gulf War is Approved for Troops*, N.Y. TIMES, Feb. 6, 2003, at A19; Michael E. Frisina, *Medical Ethics in Military Biomedical Research, in* MILITARY MEDICAL ETHICS, VOL. 2, 533–63 (Thomas E. Beam & Linette R. Sparacino eds., 2003).

Lawsuits related to the military's anthrax vaccination program continue, as do production and safety questions.

**3.** It is worth noting that the first "bioterrorist" attack in the U.S. is generally credited to a small religious sect in Oregon, which followed Bhagwan Shree

Rajneesh, who lived on a ranch approximately a two-hour drive from The Dalles, Oregon. The "attack" took place on September 9, 1984, when members of the sect used agents ordered from the American Type Culture Collection, including *Salmonella typhimurium, Francisella tularensis, Enterobacter cloacae, Neisseria gonorrhoeae,* and *Shigella dysenteriae,* to poison salad bars at various restaurants in The Dallas. The idea was to make people sick in order to prevent them from voting in an election that could have been detrimental to their sect. The attack is described in JUDITH MILLER, STEPHEN ENGELBERG & WILLIAM BROAD, BIOLOGICAL WEAPONS AND AMERICA'S SECRET WAR: GERMS 15–33 (2001).

## D.  THE SMALLPOX VACCINATION PROGRAM

### INSTITUTE OF MEDICINE, COMMITTEE ON SMALLPOX VACCINATION PROGRAM IMPLEMENTATION, THE SMALLPOX VACCINATION PROGRAM: PUBLIC HEALTH IN AN AGE OF TERRORISM
### 123–61 (2005)

The last case of smallpox in the United States occurred in 1949. General vaccination against smallpox — accomplished with cutaneous administration of a closely related virus, vaccinia virus — ceased in the United States in 1972, when the threat of smallpox disease disappeared due to eradication efforts, which were declared complete by the World Health Organization on May 8, 1980. Only two official stocks of smallpox (variola) virus remained — under the auspices of the governments of the United States and the Soviet Union. It has often been rumored and suggested that some of the virus possessed by the Soviet Union could have been given illegally to people attempting to use the virus as a biological weapon, though factual evidence to support this concern has not been made public. The events of September and October 2001 increased U.S. concerns about all types of possible terrorism, including the potential for biological terrorism. Thus, attention turned to considerations of initiating vaccination against smallpox. CDC has been concurrently developing "post-event" vaccination plans (mass vaccinations after a smallpox release) and — the focus of this committee — "pre-event" plans (precautionary vaccination of smallpox response teams, first responders, and the general public).

On December 13, 2002, President Bush announced his policy on pre-event vaccination against smallpox. Vaccination of select military personnel, including the president in his role as Commander-in-Chief, began immediately thereafter. At the time of this writing, voluntary vaccination of state-based teams of public health disease investigators and of hospital-based teams of health care workers (who would respond to the first case of smallpox, should it ever appear) is scheduled to begin in late January 2003. The president has asked that this round of vaccinations be completed as quickly as possible and that a broader vaccination effort commence thereafter. As currently understood, the subsequent vaccinations will encompass the voluntary vaccination of all health care workers and those commonly defined as first responders, such as firefighters, police, and emergency medical personnel. Vaccination of the general public is specifically not recommended, but the president also announced the intent to provide vaccinations to those members of the public who request the intervention. The IOM's Committee on Smallpox Vaccination Program Implementation met for the first time December 18–20, 2002, to begin addressing their charge, stated most succinctly as providing advice on how best to implement the policy as announced by President Bush.

The committee has not been asked to, and will not, comment on the president's policy decision to recommend voluntary smallpox vaccination to health care, public health, and emergency personnel under a precautionary program, and to allow but not recommend access to the vaccine by people not included within those groups. The extensive expertise the committee brings to this issue will focus on program implementation.

The committee realizes that this is an atypical vaccination campaign, and that it is neither a research study nor an ideal public health program. Rather, it is a public health component of bioterrorism preparedness. . . .

\* \* \*

For practical reasons, the committee uses the term "phase I" to describe the planned vaccination of 500,000 public health and health care workers who volunteer to be part of smallpox response teams, and "phase II" to refer to the subsequent vaccination of 10 million health care and public health workers and other emergency responders. However, it is unclear what the rounds of vaccination are being called by CDC ("phases" seems most frequently used) and clarification also is needed about the target population for later vaccination efforts.

. . . Before addressing the specific items in its charge, the committee summarizes its key messages and then addresses some general considerations.

The committee urges CDC to:

1. Highlight the unique nature of the smallpox vaccination program as a public health component of a national bioterrorism preparedness policy, focusing on the delivery of clear, consistent, science-based information.

2. Proceed cautiously, allowing continuous opportunity for adequate and thoughtful deliberation, analysis, and evaluation. Embark on phase II only after adequate evaluation of phase I has occurred.

3. Use a wide range of methods for proactive communication, training, and education, and customize it to reach diverse audiences, including potential vaccines, all health care providers, and the general public.

4. Designate one credible, trusted scientist as key national spokesperson for the campaign, and sharpen and expand communication plans and strategies to ensure rapid, transparent, and sustained contact with the media throughout implementation.

\* \* \*

## Smallpox Vaccination Program Timeline

| Date | Event |
| --- | --- |
| **Date** | **Event** |
| June 2001 | "Dark Winter," a war game for senior-level officials, is conducted. . . .Exercise included a smallpox outbreak spreading to 25 states and 15 countries. . . . [*See* Chapter Three.] |
| September 2001 | Terrorist attacks in New York, Arlington (Virginia), and Pennsylvania |
| October 2001 | Letters containing anthrax spores delivered through U.S. mail |
| February 2002 | CDC asks ACIP to review its recommendations on smallpox vaccination |
| June 2002 | ACIP meets and drafts supplemental recommendations on smallpox vaccination (vaccinate up to 20,000 health care and public health workers) (ACIP, 2002). |
| | Public Health Security and Bioterrorism Preparedness and Response Act of 2002 signed into law. . . |
| October 2002 | ACIP meets again and updates recommendations on smallpox vaccination. ACIP also recommends offering vaccine to up to 500,000 health care and public health personnel. |
| November 2002 | President signs Homeland Security Act |
| | Designated CDC staff members receive smallpox vaccination (epidemiologic investigation teams). |
| | Mass media report that Bush administration intelligence review has concluded that four nations (Iraq, North Korea, Russia, and France) may possess covert and illegal stocks of smallpox virus. |
| December 2002 | States submit to CDC smallpox response plans and smallpox pre-event vaccination plans. |
| | President announces smallpox vaccination program |
| | HHS telebriefing on smallpox policy; initial goal: vaccinate 500,000 workers in 30 days. |
| January 2003 | Letter to White House issued by minority members of Senate calling for smallpox vaccine injury compensation. |
| | CDC begins shipping smallpox vaccine to states. |
| | Department of Homeland Security established. |
| | DHHS secretary authorizes civilian smallpox vaccinations. |
| | Civilian smallpox vaccination begins. |
| February 2003 | Media reports cite lack of a compensation plan as a barrier to smallpox vaccination. |
| | DHHS announces contracts to develop safer smallpox vaccines. |
| | DoD has vaccinated over 100,000 against smallpox |

| Date | Event |
|------|-------|
| | *Morbidity and Mortality Weekly Report (MMWR)* notifies of one case of angina 4 days after smallpox vaccination. |
| | DoD reports first cases of myocarditis among personnel recently immunized with smallpox vaccine. |
| March 2003 | First civilian instances of myo/pericarditis identified, later classified as suspected and probable |
| | DHHS proposes smallpox vaccination compensation plan |
| | Surgeon general, CDC director, and others are vaccinated against smallpox. |
| | War with Iraq begins on March 19, 2003. |
| | CDC accepts ACIP's exclusion criteria and revises fact sheets, screening materials, and informed consent form. |
| April 2003 | GAO report *Smallpox Vaccination: Implementation of National Program Faces Challenges* finds that 6% of target population has been vaccinated by week 10 of program; data are insufficient to assess safety. |
| | On April 30, 2003, president signs into law Smallpox Emergency Personnel Protection Act of 2003, which establishes no-fault Smallpox Vaccine Injury Compensation Program. |
| May 2003 | President declares end of major combat operations in Iraq. |
| | Media reports that in April and May, some states have begun offering smallpox vaccine to first responders. |
| June 2003 | ACIP recommends against expansion of smallpox vaccination program beyond "first phase" |
| December 2003 | Federal government issues interim final rule for Smallpox Emergency Personnel Protection Act of 2003 (SEPPA), plan for smallpox vaccine injury compensation. |
| January 2004 | HHS secretary's declaration regarding administration of smallpox countermeasures extended until and including January 23, 2005. |
| February 2004 | DoD reports that 581,183 service members received smallpox shots from December 13, 2002, to February 11, 2004. Seventy-two vaccinees, or about 1 in 8,072, suffered myopericarditis, and there were 30 cases of vaccinia infection in contacts of vaccinees. |
| June 2004 | DoD announces anthrax and smallpox vaccinations for all personnel deployed by Central Command and select units in Pacific Command. Since December 2002, 625,000 troops have been vaccinated against smallpox. |
| July 2004 | The Senate Select Committee on Intelligence issues report which describes evidence on Iraq's possession of smallpox as weak. |

October 2004       CIA . . . concludes that, although Iraq had capability to work
                   with smallpox virus, there is "no direct evidence that Iraq
                   either retained or acquired smallpox virus isolates or pro-
                   ceeded with any follow-up smallpox related research."

# NOTES AND QUESTIONS

1. In its final report, which also contains complete copies of the above "letter report" and its five subsequent reports, the Committee labels the smallpox
vaccination program "a case study at the intersection of public health and
national security, two fields brought together by the threat of bioterrorism." It
notes that the campaign involved federal agencies that usually do not work
together, and problems, such as classified information, that are not encountered in "typical public health programs." Most centrally, it emphasized that
"Bioterrorist attacks epitomize 'low-likelihood, high-consequence' events" for
which planning is especially problematic and difficult. INSTITUTE OF MEDICINE,
*supra*, at 5. Its two recommendations:

> Based on the lessons learned from the smallpox vaccination program,
> the committee concludes that a policy strategy and a mechanism are
> needed to balance the need for scientific evidence and public health
> analysis with the imperatives of national security, ensuring in the pro-
> cess that the authoritative voice of CDC, the nation's public health
> leader, will be preserved. The committee recommends that, in collabo-
> ration with its state and local partners and in the context of broad
> bioterrorism preparedness, CDC defines smallpox preparedness; set
> goals that reflect the best available scientific and public health reason-
> ing; conduct regular, comprehensive assessments of preparedness at
> the national level and by state; and communicate to the public about
> the status of preparedness efforts.

*Id.* at 6.

2. The military vaccination program was mandatory. The civilian one, however, was completely voluntary and relied on a combination of public trust and
informed consent. In its first report in January 2003, the committee noted specific problems that needed to be addressed, writing that the program was not
a "typical public health program" but rather "a matter of national public
health preparedness against a national security threat." There was no real
way of quantifying the actual threat and the benefit of the vaccine was
unknown — the question was how to communicate this. The committee specifically recommended: "all consent documents include a statement that the risks
of smallpox vaccine, which are very low, are predictably higher than the risks
associated with most other vaccines, but that the benefit is at present
unknown — possibly very low (absent exposure to smallpox) or very high (in
the event of exposure). The committee further recommends that informed consent forms included explicit notification of the availability, or lack thereof, of
compensation for adverse reactions." *Id.* at 136–38.

3. The major reason [for the failure of the smallpox vaccination program] is
that the administration failed to persuade physicians and nurses that the

known risks of serious side effects with the vaccine were justified given the fact that there is no evidence that Iraq (or anyone else) has both smallpox virus and the wish to use it in a terrorist attack. The Director of the Centers for Disease Control and Prevention (CDC), and the person in charge of the smallpox vaccination program, for example, told a U.S. Senate Appropriations Subcommittee on January 29, 2003, about a month after the smallpox vaccination campaign began,

> I can't discuss all of the details because some of the information is, of course, classified. However, I think our reading of the intelligence that we share with the intelligence community is that there is a real possibility of a smallpox attack either from nations that are likely to be harboring the virus or from individual entities, such as terrorist cells that could have access to the virus. Therefore, we know it is not zero. And, I think that's really what we can say with absolute certainty that there is not a zero risk of a smallpox attack.

This is wonderful doubletalk that proves nothing except that the CDC's director does not seem to know much about the risk of a smallpox attack. Most importantly, however, if the U.S. government knows that an individual, group, or nation has smallpox and is working to make it into a weapon, this information should be made public. It is the terrorists who want to keep their methods and intentions secret; the best defense for a potential target is to make this information public. George J. Annas, *The Statue of Security: Human Rights and Post-9/11 Epidemics*, 38 J. HEALTH L. 319, 330-31 (2005).

Gerberding's approach seems to have been guided by what has become known as the post-9/11 Cheney "One-Percent Doctrine." As described by author Ron Suskind, when asked how to respond to report that Pakistani scientists may be helping al Qaeda to build a nuclear weapon, Cheney responded, "If there's a one percent chance that Pakistani scientists are helping al Qaeda build or develop a nuclear weapon, we have to treat it as a certainty in terms of response. It's not about our analysis, or finding a preponderance of evidence. It's about our response." In Suskind's words,

> This doctrine — the one percent solution — divided what had largely been indivisible in the conduct of American foreign policy; analysisand action. Justified or not, fact-based or not, "our response" is what matters. As to "evidence," the bar was set so low that the word itself almost didn't apply.

RON SUSKIND, THE ONE PERCENT DOCTRINE: DEEP INSIDE AMERICA'S PURSUIT OF ITS ENEMIES SINCE 9/11 62 (2006). Marc Siegel applies the numbers to try to make sense of post-9/11 alarms regarding public health in his FALSE ALARM: THE TRUTH ABOUT THE EPIDEMIC OF FEAR (2005).

# E.   BIOTERROR PREPAREDNESS AND RESEARCH

## Hillel Cohen et al., *The Pitfalls of Bioterrorism Preparedness: The Anthrax and Smallpox Experiences*
### 94 AM. J. PUB. HEALTH 1667 (2004)

Recent Bioterrorism preparedness programs that illustrate irrational and dysfunctional responses to inadequately characterized risks should be of urgent concern to all members of the public health community. . . .

\* \* \*

Efforts by the United States to prepare for the use of biological agents in war based on flawed evaluations of risks have had serious health consequences for military personnel and have led to significant weakening of international agreements against the use of biological agents. Massive campaigns focusing on "bioterrorism preparedness" have had adverse health consequences and have resulted in the diversion of essential public health personnel, facilities, and other resources from urgent, real public health needs. Preparedness proponents argued that allocating major resources to what were admittedly low-probability events would not represent wastefulness and would instead heighten public awareness and promote "dual use" funding that would serve other public health needs. Public health resources are woefully inadequate, and the notion that bioterrorism funding would bolster public health capability seemed plausible to many, even though we and others have argued that the "dual use" rationale is illusory. An evaluation of recent experience concerning anthrax and smallpox can help illuminate these issues.

### Anthrax

Despite extensive work on the possible weaponization of anthrax, there has been no example of effective use of anthrax as a weapon of indiscriminant mass destruction. In 2001, shortly after the events of September 11, weapons-grade anthrax spores were mailed to several addressees, but none of the intended targets were injured. Of 11 people who developed inhalation anthrax, 5 died. Of the 12 who had cutaneous infections, all recovered after administration of antibiotics. Thousands of people in potentially exposed areas such as postal sorting centers were advised to use antibiotics prophylactically. Millions of people were terrified, and many thousands in areas where there was no possible risk of exposure also took antibiotics. Congress was closed for days, mail service was disrupted for months, and state and county public health laboratories were inundated with white powder samples that ranged from explicit anthrax hoaxes to spilled powdered sweeteners.

Despite early speculation linking the anthrax release to "foreign terrorists," evidence led investigators to suspect an individual who had been working in a US military facility that may have been in violation of the Biologic and Toxin Weapons Convention. Whether or not that specific individual was involved, it appears likely that the perpetrator or perpetrators were associated in some way with a US military program, that the motive for the extremely limited release was political, and that, without the existence of a US military laboratory, the material for the release would not have been available.

This experience supports the view that, as a consequence of the inherent difficulties in obtaining and handling such material, mass purposeful infection is highly improbable and the likely impact on morbidity and mortality limited. However, the nature of US "biodefense" programs may modify this prognosis; such programs may result in dangerous materials being more readily available, thus undermining the Biologic and Toxin Weapons Convention. Despite an absence of evidence of anthrax weapon stocks posing a threat to US military personnel, and despite problematic experiences of the military anthrax vaccination program, the US government announced plans to spend as much as $1.4 billion for millions of doses of an experimental anthrax vaccine that has not been proven safe or effective and the need for which has not been opened to public debate.

## Smallpox

The 2002-2003 campaign to promote smallpox as an imminent danger coincided with the Bush administration's preparations for war on Iraq and the now discredited claims that Iraq had amassed weapons of mass destruction and could launch a biological or chemical attack in "as little as 45 minutes." A media campaign describing the dangers of smallpox coincided with the buildup for war. An unprecedented campaign advocating "preevent" mass smallpox vaccinations, to be carried out in 2 phases — involving half a million members of the armed forces and half a million health workers in phase 1 and as many as 10 million emergency responders in phase 2 — was announced in December 2002.

Before then, the debate on smallpox had been whether the stocks of stored stand-by vaccine were adequate or whether they should be increased. The World Health Organization (WHO), the Centers for Disease Control and Prevention (CDC), and virtually every public health official took the position that the vaccine involved too many adverse events — was too dangerous — to warrant mass vaccination when no case of smallpox existed or had existed for more than 20 years. When the Bush administration announced support for mass vaccinations, WHO did not change its position, but the CDC and other US public health officials and organizations, including the American Public Health Association (APHA), decided to acquiesce.

The coincidence of the Bush war calendar and the smallpox vaccination calendar, while not conclusive, is nonetheless consistent with an inference that the war agenda was the driving force behind the smallpox vaccination campaign. Since the invasion, evidence has emerged that allegations regarding Iraqi weapons of mass destruction were deliberate exaggerations or lies. The evidence is highly suggestive that the smallpox vaccination program was launched primarily for public relations rather than public health reasons.

The vaccination campaign did not proceed as planned. Opposition arose on both safety and political grounds, and most front-line health professionals simply did not volunteer to participate. Of the 500,000 health professionals who were targeted for inoculations in phase 1, fewer than 8% participated. Despite efforts to avoid vaccination of those who might be at elevated risk, the CDC reported that there were 145 serious adverse events (resulting in hospitalization, permanent disability, life-threatening illness, or death) associated with smallpox vaccinations among civilians. Of these cases, at least 3 were deaths.

Three deaths resulting from thousands of inoculations would have been justifiable in preparation for a real threat of smallpox or in the midst of a smallpox outbreak, when vaccination could have saved many more lives. However, in the absence of any smallpox cases worldwide or any scientific basis for expecting an outbreak, these deaths and other serious adverse events are inexcusable. . . .

* * *

The smallpox vaccinations harmed others beyond those who suffered side effects. Considerable public health resources were used in the campaign. In a climate of state and local budget crises coinciding with the war and occupation, a downturn in employment, and a tax cut for the wealthy, public health services have been cut or are at serious risk. Funding for bioterrorism programs is not correcting the deficit, because such funds have been for the most part specifically earmarked for preparedness efforts and cannot be transferred to other public health programs. In general, federal increases in public health funding are much less extensive than state or local cuts. During the height of the smallpox vaccination effort, a number of state health officials complained that important work, including tuberculosis screening and standard children's inoculations, had to be scaled back. The siren song of dual use — that bioterrorism funding would strengthen public health infrastructure — has shown itself to be an empty promise, as preparedness priorities have weakened rather than strengthened public health.

## Broader Problems

Even worse, bioterrorism "preparedness" programs now under way include the development of a number of new secret research facilities that will store and handle dangerous materials, thus increasing the risk of accidental release or purposeful diversion. Reports of accidental leaks and improper disposal of hazardous wastes at the US Army facility at Fort Detrick serve as future warnings, as do revelations of mishandling of biological agents at the Plum Island, New York, facility that studies potential bioweapons that affect animals.

Most important, the proposed development of "biodefense" programs at sites, such as national nuclear weapons laboratories, that are traditionally secretive in their operations also provides an impetus for a potential global "biodefense race" that would likely spur proliferation of offensive biowarfare capabilities. Accidents or purposeful diversions from these facilities seem at least as likely as terrorist events, and perhaps more so, since the deadly materials are already present. The Patriot Act has greatly expanded the cloak of secrecy that shields these facilities from public awareness and oversight.

In short, bioterrorism preparedness programs have been a disaster for public health. Instead of leading to more resources for dealing with natural disease as had been promised, there are now fewer such resources. Worse, in response to bioterrorism preparedness, public health institutions and procedures are being reorganized along a military or police model that subverts the relationships between public health providers and the communities they serve.

\* \* \*

## UNITED STATES v. BUTLER
### 429 F.3d 140 (5th Cir. 2005), *cert. denied,* 126 S. Ct. 2049 (2006)

Before Wiener, DeMoss, and Prado, Circuit Judges.

## PER CURIAM

Appellant Dr. Thomas Butler was convicted on 47 of 69 counts of various criminal activity relating to work he performed as a medical researcher at the Texas Tech University Health Sciences Center ("HSC"). Of these 47 counts, Butler was convicted of 44 counts of contract-related crimes, including theft, fraud, embezzlement, mail fraud, and wire fraud, (collectively, the "Contract Counts"). Butler was also convicted of three counts relating to the transportation of human plague bacteria ("*Yersinia pestis*" or "YP"), including the illegal exportation of YP to Tanzania, the illegal transportation of hazardous materials, and making a false statement on the waybill accompanying the YP vials shipped to Tanzania, (collectively, the "Plague Counts"). The district court sentenced Butler to 24 months' imprisonment followed by 3 years' supervised release, a $15,000 fine, and ordered him to pay restitution to HSC in the amount of $38,675. Butler timely filed the instant appeal. For the reasons discussed below, we affirm.

Butler was a professor and Chief of Infectious Diseases in HSC's Internal Medicine Department since 1987. As part of Butler's pay structure, a percentage of his income was provided by the State of Texas while the remainder came from the Medical Practice Income Plan ("MPIP"). Under MPIP, a doctor earned money by seeing patients, receiving research grants, or conducting clinical studies under the auspices of HSC. The monies received from the patients a doctor treated and the funds paid out for the research/studies was remitted to HSC. Part of these monies paid for HSC's overhead costs and other expenses while another part was paid out as the non-state portion of the doctor's income. Any remaining funds from a clinical study was transferred to a developmental account for the researcher's department or division. The money in this account was earmarked for expenses such as professional dues and business travel, none of which was related to any particular project.

When a researcher at HSC was in a position to obtain a research grant or conduct a clinical study, it was required that the accompanying documentation be submitted to the institution for approval. Moreover, any monies paid out as a result of the research grant or clinical study were required to be paid directly to the institution. Consulting contracts, however, received different treatment from research grants or clinical studies. Specifically, a consulting contract was viewed by HSC as a means for a doctor to sell his or her expertise or advice directly to a third party, such as in designing a drug study. The consulting would not involve patient care or patient safety issues, and the consultant would not be using HSC's resources such as labs and personnel. Because of these considerations, consulting contracts were permissible without HSC's financial involvement or approval, unlike contracts covering clinical studies.

Between 1998 and 2001, Butler entered into several clinical study contracts with two different pharmaceutical companies, Pharmacia and Chiron. The first contract entered into with Pharmacia occurred in March 1998. Under this contract, Pharmacia agreed to pay HSC $2,400 for each patient enrolled in the clinical study. Apparently unbeknownst to HSC, however, Pharmacia and Butler entered into another "shadow" or "split" contract that provided Butler with an additional $2,400 per patient enrolled in the same study. A similar contract was entered into between Pharmacia and Butler in the spring of 2000 and again in the fall of 2000.

With respect to the contract in the fall of 2000, there was another HSC researcher, Dr. Casner, who was working on the same study as Butler. Dr. Casner's contract with Pharmacia was not split, and therefore it appeared that he had a budget twice the size of Butler's. A representative with HSC who was aware of Dr. Casner's contract, contacted Butler to inform him that she could get Butler a bigger budget. Butler allegedly refused the offer and informed the HSC representative that he would remain in charge of negotiating his own contracts. Butler had also negotiated two similar contracts with Chiron (another pharmaceutical company), using the contracts with Pharmacia as a template. The contracts with Chiron involved drug studies that were conducted in February 1999 and March 2000. Butler received payments under the contracts with Pharmacia and Chiron until August 2001.

The existence of the shadow contracts first came to the attention of HSC in July 2002, when an HSC representative learned from a Pharmacia representative that Butler was getting one-half of the money from the Pharmacia studies, while HSC received the other half. HSC initiated a preliminary investigation into the split contracts that continued until January 9, 2003, when HSC informed Butler by letter that an additional investigation by authorities charged with compliance issues was to begin. In the letter, HSC sought a response from Butler by no later than January 21, 2003. For the reasons discussed below, HSC never received the requested response.

In addition to his work at HSC in Texas, Butler conducted plague research in Tanzania in 2001.[1] Then, in April 2002, Butler returned to Tanzania where, for approximately 10 days, he worked on research of plague in human patients at clinics there. Part of his research involved personally culturing and subculturing specimens that he planned to bring back to the United States for additional studies.

Having returned to the United States with the *Yersinia pestis* cultures, Butler continued his research. Then, on January 13, 2003, four days after

---

[1] This work was reportedly encouraged by the Food and Drug Administration (the "FDA"), the Center for Disease Control and Prevention ("CDC"), and the United States Army.

receiving the letter from HSC auditors warning of the impending investigation into the alleged shadow contracts, Butler reported that 30 vials of the *Yersinia pestis* were missing from his HSC laboratory in Lubbock. The FBI was immediately notified and within hours descended upon Lubbock, where Butler was questioned. Eventually, Butler revealed that the *Yersinia pestis* was not actually missing, but that he had destroyed the vials accidentally.

In April 2003, a grand jury returned a 15-count indictment charging Butler with various crimes relating to his transporting of *Yersinia pestis*, the providing of false statements to FBI agents regarding *Yersinia pestis*, and a tax crime. A superceding indictment was returned by the grand jury in August 2003, in which Butler was charged with 54 additional criminal counts, including mail fraud, wire fraud, and embezzlement that arose out of Butler's agreements with the pharmaceutical companies and the Food and Drug Administration (the "FDA"). Butler filed a motion seeking to sever the Contract and Plague Counts, which the district court denied. After a three-week trial in November 2003, the jury returned a mixed-verdict against Butler, finding him guilty on most of the Contract Counts and not guilty on most of the Plague Counts and the tax count. On March 10, 2004, the district court sentenced Butler to 24 months' imprisonment, three years' supervised release, $15,000 in fines, and a $4,700 special assessment. Butler was also ordered to pay HSC restitution in the amount of $38,675. Butler timely filed the instant appeal.

## DISCUSSION

I.  Whether the district court erred by not severing the Contract Counts and the Plague Counts.

On appeal, Butler argues the Federal Rules of Criminal Procedure and this Circuit's case law prohibit the joinder of unrelated criminal categories charged; here, the Contract Counts and the Plague Counts. Butler contends that trying all the counts together caused him prejudice. Conversely, the Government maintains that joinder was proper because the charges in the superceding indictment were linked as transactions within a common scheme or plan.

The indictment specifically outlines Butler's research into non-plague-related diseases for Pharmacia and Chiron and his plague-related research for the FDA. The indictment's description of Butler's scheme to defraud explained how he failed to disclose material facts to HSC regarding not only the Pharmacia and Chiron contracts, but also the plague-related contracts with the FDA.

The introduction to the superseding indictment details how the FDA offered research opportunities to medical professionals regarding "the development and review of medications for the prevention and treatment of illness that could be caused by terrorists using biological agents." The FDA subsequently purchased Butler's professional service, and specifically, according to the indictment, "for the results of experimental research regarding the post-antibiotic effect of drugs on the microorganism *Yersinia pestis*," and later "to provide experimental results from [Butler]'s laboratory about the[] post-antibiotic effect of drugs on various strains of *Yersinia pestis* isolated from plague patients in Tanzania."

Meanwhile, the actual FDA fraud counts charged Butler with attempting to conceal the existence of his FDA contracts from HSC's administrative review and approval process. Butler was alleged to have subsequently obtained payments from the FDA without distributing any monies therefrom to HSC in accordance with HSC's relevant policies for doing so.

The superceding indictment clearly sets forth an alleged common scheme that connects both Butler's plague research and the Pharmacia/Chiron pharmaceutical contracts to the FDA fraud counts. In doing so, the superseding indictment, on its face, creates an overlap that logically intertwines the Contract Counts with the Plague Counts.

\* \* \*

## V.  Whether the Government presented sufficient evidence as to the Contract and Plague Counts.

. . . Butler maintains there was insufficient evidence to support the jury's finding that he willfully: (1) exported *Yersinia pestis* to Tanzania without a license; (2) described in a misleading manner the *Yersinia pestis* as "laboratory materials" on the FedEx waybill; and (3) violated federal hazardous material regulations when he shipped the *Yersinia pestis* to Tanzania.

As to the first sub-issue, the Government points this panel to evidence introduced at trial that Butler certified on the FedEx waybill that the samples were being "exported . . . in accordance with Export Administration Regulations," when in fact they were not. The Government notes that Butler had in his office a document downloaded from the Center for Disease Control website that clearly indicated a Department of Commerce permit was required to export *Yersinia pestis*. As further evidence of Butler's knowledge of export requirements, the Government observes that Butler previously signed four waybills shipping hazardous materials to Canada and checked the box indicating a Shipper's Export Declaration was not needed (which it is not in those circumstances). Moreover, the Government introduced evidence that during the 1990s, Butler properly shipped infectious substances and other dangerous goods more than 30 times. Based on this evidence, Butler's argument here must fail.

With regard to Butler's conviction for making a false statement by labeling the *Yersinia pestis* as "laboratory materials," he contends that because he did not intend to deceive anyone, he cannot be found to have acted willfully. The Government responds by noting that Butler also certified on that same label that he was not shipping dangerous goods. According to the Government, a reasonable person certainly could conclude that an accomplished researcher, who was the Chief of Infectious Diseases at HSC and had spent considerable time studying plague abroad, would have known that plague was a dangerous good requiring the proper identification thereof. Accordingly, Butler's sufficiency of the evidence argument on this sub-issue is also without merit.

Finally, Butler contends his conviction for violating hazardous material regulations required the Government to prove that his infraction could not have been due to a good faith mistake or misunderstanding of the law. The Government responds with an argument identical to its reason why there was sufficient evidence establishing Butler's unlawful export of *Yersinia pestis* to Tanzania without a license: Butler had successfully and legally shipped hazardous materials at least 30 times before making this particular shipment. Importantly, Butler comes forward with no specific evidence of his own on appeal refuting the Government's evidence, or establishing what about his actions warranted a finding that he made a good faith mistake or misunderstood the law. Without more, a reasonable trier of fact could have found that the evidence established guilt beyond a reasonable doubt.

Having carefully reviewed the entire record of this case, and having fully considered the parties' respective briefing and arguments, we conclude the district court did not commit reversible error by refusing to sever the Contract Counts from the Plague Counts. Moreover, the district court made appropriate discovery and evidentiary rulings. Also, there was sufficient evidence supporting Butler's convictions under the Contract Counts and the Plague Counts. . . . Accordingly, we AFFIRM Butler's conviction and sentence.

## NOTES AND QUESTIONS

**1.** On January 2, 2006, Butler completed his two-year sentence and was released. A scientific article detailing his plague research in Tanzania, completed while he was in prison, was published shortly thereafter. *See* William Mwengee, Thomas Butler et al., *Treatment of Plague with Gentamicin or Doxycycline in a Randomized Clinical Trial in Tanzania*, 40 CLINICAL INFECTIOUS DISEASE 614 (2006).

**2.** The case of physician-researcher Thomas Butler has been the subject of many commentaries — most arguing that his prosecution represents a gross overreaction on the part of federal authorities. Nonetheless, in an article in *Science*, Margaret A. Somerville and Ronald M. Atlas argued that Butler's prosecution "sent a clear signal to the research community, especially scientists and university researchers, that all ethical and legal requirements must be respected when undertaking research." They continued, "Biosafety regulations are not merely legal technicalities. They constitute some of the terms of the pact between science and the public that establishes public trust." *Ethics: A Weapon to Counter Bioterrorism,* 307 SCIENCE 1881 (2005).

Ethical guidelines for life sciences research that could be related to bioterrorism do seem critical, and the scientific community should be actively engaged in setting the standards for such research. As the National Research Council of the National Academy of Sciences has stated, "biological scientists have an affirmative moral duty to avoid contributing to the advancement of biowarfare or bioterrorism." It is reasonable for society to expect that scientists will adopt the equivalent of the physician's "do no harm" principle. Arguing for such an oath well before September 11, literary scholar Roger Shattuck noted that it could "help scientists scrutinize the proliferation of research in dubious areas" as well as "renew the confidence of ordinary citizens" in what is a potentially revolutionary endeavor. FORBIDDEN KNOWLEDGE 224 (1996).

But can an ethical code be effective? What should it say? Who should write it? Consider, for example, the National Research Council's seven classes of microbial experiments that should require special review:

*The experiments would:*

Demonstrate how to render a vaccine ineffective;

Confer resistance to therapeutically useful antibiotics or antiviral agents;

Enhance the virulence of a pathogen or render a nonpathogen virulent

Increase transmissibility of a pathogen;

Alter the host range of a pathogen;

Enable the evasion of diagnostic and detection methods;

Enable the weaponization of a biologic agent or toxin.

BIOTECHNOLOGY RESEARCH IN AN AGE OF TERRORISM 5 (2004).

**3.** The major approach the administration has taken toward potential bioterrorism since 9/11 has been to categorize biological agents according to their risks of being used as a terrorist weapon. The current scheme has three categories, and the fact that plague is in category A goes a long way to explaining why the FBI acted so strongly against Butler.

*Category A:*

Anthrax, botulism, plague, smallpox, tularemia, viral hemorrhagic fevers.

*Category B:*

Brucellosis, food safety threats, glanders, melioidosis, psittacosis, Q fever, ricin toxin, staphyloccococcal enterotoxin B, typhus fever, viral encephalitis, water safety threats.

*Category A*, or "high priority agents . . . pose a risk to national security because they can be easily disseminated or transmitted from person to person; result in high mortality rates and have the potential for major public health impact; might cause public panic and social disruption; and, require special action for public health preparedness.

*Category B* agents "include those that are moderately easy to disseminate; result in moderate morbidity rates and low mortality rates; and require specific enhancements of CDC's diagnostic capacity and enhanced disease surveillance.

There is also a *Category C* for those agents "that could be engineered for mass dissemination in the future because of availability; ease of production and dissemination; and potential for high morbidity and mortality rates and major health impact." CDC, BIOTERRORISM AGENTS/DISEASES, *available at* www.bt.ced.gov/agent/agentlist-category.asp (last visited Aug. 2006).

An Institute of Medicine committee has suggested that making such lists is not a useful way to counter bioterrorism because it takes no account of the future of science. In the Committee's words:

> First, the future is now. Even in the short time since the creation of the committee, we have seen the phenomenon of RNA Interference capture the collective consciousness of the life sciences community, providing entirely new insights into how human genes are normally regulated and how this regulation might be disrupted for malevolent purposes by those intent on doing harm.

> Similarly, "synthetic biology," an approach embraced and discussed by few at the time the Committee was formed, has now been redefined and promoted on the cover of one of the most widely read scientific journals. Neither of these developments could have been foretold ever a few years back, pointing to the futility of trying to predict with accuracy what will come in the next few years [the committee concluded, among other things, that we need a new threat reduction paradigm for the biological sciences].

INSTITUTE OF MEDICINE, COMMITTEE ON ADVANCES IN TECHNOLOGY AND THE PREVENTION OF THEIR APPLICATION TO NEXT GENERATION BIOWARFARE THREATS: GLOBALIZATION, BIOSECURITY, AND THE FUTURE OF THE LIFE SCIENCES viii (2006). On the risks to public health from concentrating too much on preparedness, see TERRORISM AND PUBLIC HEALTH: A BALANCED APPROACH TO STRENGTHENING SYSTEMS AND PROTECTING PEOPLE (BARRY S. LEVY & VICTOR W. SIDEL, eds., 2003)

**4.** There are other examples of an arguably overly-aggressive FBI that seems to see bioterrorism in activities, including art, that it would not have seen them pre-9/11, and wastes time, effort, and resources that could almost certainly be better spent in trying to identify real bioterrorist threats:

> Shortly after Butler's trial, in another part of the country — Buffalo, New York — FBI agents were called in to investigate a suspected act of bioterrorism in the home of Steve Kurtz, a professor and artist at the State University of New York at Buffalo. Kurtz awoke on May 11, 2004, to find his wife dead beside him. Kurtz and his wife previously had cofounded the Critical Art Ensemble, an artists' collective "dedicated to exploring the intersections between art, technology, radical politics and critical theory." Kurtz liked to distinguish what he did from the emerging field of "bioart," which is perhaps best known to the public because of the notoriety of Alba, a rabbit that glowed green because of the insertion of a jellyfish gene. Kurtz thinks of bioart as

consisting of stunts and his own art as an exploration of "the political economy of biotechnology." He had previously argued against the introduction of genetically modified food, and he had encouraged activists to oppose it by means of "fuzzy biological sabotage" — for instance, by releasing genetically mutated and deformed flies at restaurants to stir up paranoia.

The day after his wife's death, the FBI raided his home in full biohazard gear. Kurtz had been studying the history of germ warfare for a new project. In connection with this project, he was growing bacterial cultures that he was planning to use to simulate attacks with anthrax and plague. He had obtained the bacteria samples (*Serratia marcescens* and *Bacillus atrophaeus*) from a colleague, Professor Robert Ferrell, a geneticist at the University of Pittsburgh Medical Center, who had ordered them for him from the American Type Culture Collection. Kurtz and Ferrell were suspected almost immediately of being involved in a bioterror ring and were thoroughly investigated. Once the New York Department of Health determined that the bacteria were harmless and that Kurtz's wife had died of natural causes, the bioterrorism investigation was dropped. The Justice Department nonetheless charged both Ferrell and Kurtz with four counts of wire fraud and mail fraud. The allegation was that Ferrell, at Kurtz's request, defrauded the University of Pittsburgh and the American Type Culture Collection by representing that the bacteria samples he ordered would be used in his University of Pittsburgh laboratory. [As of January 2007] neither case has yet gone to trial.

Exactly what Kurtz was planning to do with the bacteria is unclear, but serratia, which is known for its ability to form bright red colonies, has been used in biowarfare simulations in the past. Perhaps its most well-known use was a 1950 simulation in which an offshore naval vessel blanketed a 50-square-mile section of San Francisco with an aerosol spray containing serratia to determine what dose could be delivered effectively to the population. Whether using a similar technique as an art exhibit would constitute bioart, biotechnology, or biohazard (or even bioterrorism) may be in the eye of the beholder even more than in the eye of the artist or scientist.

Bioart is not bioterrorism, but the two are related politically. As bioart curator and commentator Jens Hauser has said, bioart aims "at the heart of our fears" and is meant to "disturb." He notes, "these artists expose the gulf between the apologetic official discourse about technoscience on the one hand, and paranoia on the other." Like defensive and offensive bioweapons research, bioart and biotechnology may be impossible to distinguish by anything other than the researcher's or creator's intent. Thus, Alba, the bunny with the inserted jellyfish gene, is considered to be and is accepted as a creation of bioart, at least in the contemporary art community; whereas ANDi, the monkey with the inserted jellyfish gene, is considered to be a creation of science, at least in the biotechnology community. Hauser was referring to paranoia in the face of the "rapid acceleration of technical prowess." On the basis of the reaction of federal law enforcement to the actions of Thomas Butler and Steve Kurtz, however, although the advances of biotechnology that have potential applications to bioterrorism and biowarfare are scary, even scarier are the responses — in the name of preventing bioterrorism — of law-enforcement agencies to legitimate scientists and artists whose actions pose no threat to the public.

Butler's arrest came about one year after a simulated bioterrorism event in Lubbock, Texas; this simulation involved the use of aerosolized plague at a civic center. Simulations have been a centerpiece of efforts to prepare for acts of bioterrorism. As we should have learned from our obsession with building bomb shelters during the cold war, however, simulations promote fear of worst-case scenarios and make them look much more likely. Bioterrorism simulations such as Dark Winter (smallpox) and Top Officials (TOPOFF) involve more art than science and are likely to provoke a response based more on fear than logic. They should probably be classified as bioart in the sense of performance art, and they should have their most socially useful outlet not in federal law-enforcement agencies or biosafety laboratories but in television dramas like *24*.

George J. Annas, *Bioterror and "Bioart" – A Plague o' Both Your Houses,* 354 NEW ENG. J. MED. 2715 (2006).

Do you agree? Are law enforcement agencies overreacting or underreacting to the threat of bioterrorism?

Annas concludes:

One reasonable response to the dispute between Butler and the Justice Department and the dispute between Kurtz and the Justice Department could be Mercutio's retort in *Romeo and Juliet*: "A plague o' both your houses." This is because the public is currently more victim and bystander than participant and seems much more likely to be harmed than helped by much of the research. Members of the public recognize this probability, and their skepticism of federal authorities, of the effectiveness of countermeasures, of the existence of weapons of mass destruction in Iraq, and of the entire bioterrorism scare is well illustrated by the few people who took drugs to treat anthrax that were offered after the anthrax attacks. This same skepticism, combined with the lack of evidence of stockpiles of smallpox in Iraq and the certainty of side effects from the drugs, also explains the small number of health professionals who volunteered to take the smallpox vaccine immediately before and shortly after the commencement of the war in Iraq.

*Id.* at 2719.

**5.** At least some over-reactions can be traced to books highlighting the dangers of a bioterrorist attack. President Bill Clinton, for example, said he first became focused on this risk when he read Richard Preston's novel, THE COBRA EVENT (1997), in 1997. Preston later wrote a nonfiction book on the dangers of a smallpox attack, THE DEMON IN THE FREEZER: A TRUE STORY (2002). Perhaps more frightening to public health officials were the books by the former Soviet

head of bioweapons development, KEN ALIBEK, BIOHAZARD: THE CHILLING TRUE
STORY OF THE LARGEST COVERT BIOLOGICAL WEAPONS PROGRAM IN THE World —
TOLD FROM INSIDE BY THE MAN WHO RAN IT (1999), and by Minnesota epidemiologist MICHAEL OSTERHOLM (WITH JOHN SCHWARTZ), LIVING TERRORS: WHAT
AMERICANS NEEDS TO KNOW TO SURVIVE THE COMING BIOTERRORIST
CATASTROPHE (2000). All of these books portray what might be described as
worst case scenarios, and the value of concentrating on worse cases (instead of
likely cases) is debatable. Of course the nuclear arms race provided the background for over-reaction, complete with its "mutually assured destruction" scenarios, home fallout shelters, and "duck and cover" grade school exercises. *See,
e.g.,* HERMAN KAHN, ON THERMONUCLEAR WAR (2d ed. 1961), and SHARON
GHAMARI-TABIZI, THE WORLDS OF HERMAN KAHN: THE INTUITIVE SCIENCE OF
THERMONUCLEAR WAR (2005).

"Worst case scenarios" are not only popular in emergency preparedness
training exercises, but also in more mundane public health problems such as
deciding if a particular site for a new post-9/11 research laboratory is safe for
the public. Controversy continues, for example, over Boston University's plan
to build a post-9/11 BSL-4 laboratory on the Boston Medical Center campus in
the city of Boston. The following is from a Superior Court decision examining
the adequacy of an environmental impact report prepared for the laboratory.
The report was required by the Massachusetts Environmental Policy Act (G.L.
c. 30, secs.61-62H).

## TEN RESIDENTS OF BOSTON v. BOSTON
## REDEVELOPMENT AUTHORITY
### Suffolk Sup. Ct., 05-0109-BLS2 (July 31, 2006)

Gants, J.

. . . The Secretary specifically directed that the Final EIR [Environmental
Impact Report] address only four issues: (1) "discuss the design features that
the biocontainment building will employ to enhance safety," (2) "document
how the facility would meet any applicable state and federal regulations
regarding safety of the facility," (3) "evaluate a 'worst case' safety event involving the loss of the physical integrity of the containment systems," and
(4) "address safety considerations related to any transport of potentially hazardous biological agents to and from the Biocontainment facility." In providing
this guidance, the Secretary failed to focus on the difference in risk posed by
pathogens which can be spread through the air and may be fatal if inhaled but
are not contagious (such as anthrax or, more precisely, its infectious agent —
bacillus anthracis), versus those pathogens which are infectious and can be
spread through person-to-person contact, such as:

- Smallpox, which can be spread by "direct and fairly prolonged face-to-
  face contact" or "direct contact with infected bodily fluids or contaminated objects, such as bedding or clothing,"

- Severe Acute Respiratory Syndrome, known as SARS, which can be
  spread "through respiratory droplets,"

- Ebola hemorrhagic fever, which can be spread "through direct contact
  with infected blood secretions, organs or semen."

Since the "worst case safety event" was limited to "the loss of the physical integrity of the containment systems," University Associates reasonably understood that the focus should be on pathogens that can be spread by airborne inhalation if the ventilation containment system at the BSL-4 laboratory were to fail, and therefore provided the scenario involving the dropped vial of purified anthrax inside the laboratory.

There were two substantial failures in the risk assessment that arose from limiting the "worst case safety event" to a failure of the ventilation containment system. First, no "worst case safety event" was analyzed regarding any release of a contagious disease from the laboratory, even though such a release potentially may occur, not from a complete failure of the ventilation containment system, but simply from a laboratory staff member becoming infected with the infectious pathogen. The risk of such an infection, while small, cannot be characterized as nonexistent.

Appendix 4 of the Final EIR contains two reports prepared by Karl M. Johnson, M.D. on October 15, 2003. The first, entitled "Biosafety at National Institute of Allergy and Infectious Disease: 1982-2003," examines the number of accidental exposures to infectious agents during this period at BSL-2 and BSL-3 laboratories operated by the National Institute in three locations — Bethesda and Rockville, Maryland, and Hamilton, Montana. Dr. Johnson found one clinical infection, four silent infections, and 24 other accidents which did not lead to infections in more than three million hours of working with these organisms. While Dr. Johnson justly concludes that the safety record for these laboratories is "outstanding" and specifically notes that "[n]o agent has escaped from any laboratory to cause infection in adjacent civilian communities," his report demonstrates that there is a small, but significant, risk of infections and accidental exposures over the life of these facilities. Dr. Johnson's second report, entitled "Biosafety at BSL-4: More than 20 Years Experience at Three Major Facilities," examined the number of laboratory accidents at three BSL-4 laboratories — Fort Detrick, Maryland, the CDC laboratory in Atlanta, and a laboratory in Johannesburg, South Africa operated by the South African National Institute for Communicable Diseases. Dr. Johnson found that, at Fort Detrick, in the early years of the laboratory, an unspecified number of "invasive accidents resulted in treatment with human plasma containing specific antibodies to virus in question, as well as confinement in an isolation suite in one building. . . ." Two invasive accidents were of the greatest concern, one in which a staff member's finger was accidentally punctured with a needle on a syringe loaded with the Lassa virus and another in which a bone fragment of a monkey infected with the Junin virus punctured a staff member's finger. Fortunately, no infection occurred in either incident. At the CDC facility, various laboratory accidents were identified, none of which resulted in an infection. Among these accidents were: a rodent infected with Hantavirus bit a staff member; a needle pricked a worker who was setting up an inoculation with a mouse-adapted Ebola virus; and "multiple events over the years of outer gloves or suits developing tears or holes detected during work." At the Johannesburg laboratory, Dr. Johnson learned of a bat bite through double gloves, which did not produce an infection, and "multiple other accidents," during which "[t]hose exposed are monitored closely for 21 days, during which time they are not permitted to leave town — as are all employees after their last day of work inside BSL-4 space." No infections were reported from these accidents. Here, too, Dr. Johnson could justly conclude that no clinical infections had occurred at these facilities despite nearly half a million hours of working with these organisms, and that no infectious agent had escaped into a neighboring community. However, Dr. Johnson does not negate the possibility of infection to either laboratory workers or the outside community. Rather, he states, "The zero numerator of infections in these three laboratories and the huge denominator of exposure hours make it impossible to provide a number for 'risk of infection' to either laboratory workers or outside communities. Nevertheless, that number must be small."

Dr. Johnson did not identify any instance of intentional infection by a laboratory employee, such as a laboratory worker who intended to infect himself or a co-worker, or of the intentional removal of a pathogen from the laboratory to commit extortion or provide to a terrorist organization. This risk, too, is surely small but, equally surely, the risk must be recognized to exist. To be sure, the Final EIR observes that background and security checks will be conducted on all employees before being assigned to the Biolab. However, all CIA and FBI agents are subject to background and security checks as well, perhaps more intensive than any contemplated by NIH, but there are at least two documented instances in the past two decades of a CIA agent (Aldrich Ames) and FBI agent (Robert Hanssen) each with compartmentalized top secret clearances, providing classified secrets to the then-Soviet Union that risked (and probably cost) the lives of various confidential informants. If the CIA and FBI, with their expertise in background checks, cannot ensure that none of their carefully selected agents will betray their trust, there is no good reason to assume that University Associates need not fear this risk.

* * *

In short, the Final EIR demonstrated that there was a small, but significant, risk of a laboratory accident that could result in the infection of a laboratory worker with a contagious disease, but the Final EIR did not contain any "worst case" scenario that explored the potential consequences of such an accident. Nor did it contain any "worst case" scenario that explored the potential consequences of the release of a contagious pathogen arising from a suicidal, criminal, or terrorist act.

* * *

. . . Any reasonable evaluation of a risk requires an understanding of the probability of the risk occurring over the life of the Project and the magnitude of harm that could arise if it were to occur. From the Final EIR, the agencies could evaluate the probability of an accidental or malevolent release of a contagious pathogen and recognize it to be small, but the Final EIR did not provide any guidance as to the magnitude of harm that could result if that small risk were sadly to occur. Since, as noted earlier, "[a]ny finding required by [Section 61] shall be limited to those matters which are within the scope of the environmental impact report," G.L. c. 30 § 62A, the absence of this information regarding the potential environmental impact meant that it could not be addressed in the Section 61 finding. Even worse, the Final EIR permitted the agencies to act upon the belief that even the "worst case safety event" posed only a negligible risk of public harm. Therefore, the absence of any "worst case" scenario involving the accidental or malevolent release of a contagious disease-causing organism meant that the Final EIR failed to inform the relevant public agencies making financial and permitting decisions regarding the Project of the potential for catastrophic harm posed by the Project. To be sure, the small risk of even catastrophic harm does not suggest that any public agency should kill the Project, especially when, as here, the Project itself will conduct research designed to combat bioterrorism. But it is necessary that a public agency considering such a Project come to grips with the true risks posed by the Project and not be lulled by the Final EIR into ignoring the small possibility of enormous public harm.

\* \* \*

## F. FEDERAL PREPAREDNESS

### PUBLIC HEALTH SECURITY AND BIOTERRORISM PREPAREDNESS AND RESPONSE ACT OF 2002
Pub. L. No. 107-188

Title I — NATIONAL PREPAREDNESS FOR BIOTERRORISM AND OTHER PUBLIC HEALTH EMERGENCIES

Subtitle A — National Preparedness and Response Planning, Coordinating, and Reporting

Sec. 2801. NATIONAL PREPAREDNESS PLAN.

(a) In General. —

(1) Preparedness and response regarding public health emergencies. — The Secretary [of HHS] shall further develop and implement a coordinated strategy, building upon the core public health capabilities established pursuant to section 319A, for carrying out health-related activities to prepare for and respond effectively to bioterrorism and other public health emergencies, including the preparation of a plan under this section. The Secretary shall periodically thereafter review and, as appropriate, revise the plan.

(2) National approach. — In carrying out paragraph (1), the Secretary shall collaborate with the States toward the goal of ensuring that the activities of the Secretary regarding bioterrorism and other public health emergencies are coordinated with activities of the States, including local governments.

(3) Evaluation of progress. — The plan under paragraph (1) shall provide for specific benchmarks and outcome measures for evaluating the progress of the Secretary and the States, including local governments, with respect to the plan under paragraph (1), including progress toward achieving the goals specified in subsection (b).

(b) Preparedness Goals. — The plan under subsection (a) should include provisions in furtherance of the following:

(1) Providing effective assistance to State and local governments in the event of bioterrorism or other public health emergency.

(2) Ensuring that State and local governments have appropriate capacity to detect and respond effectively to such emergencies, including capacities for the following:

(A) Effective public health surveillance and reporting mechanisms at the State and local levels.

(B) Appropriate laboratory readiness.

(C) Properly trained and equipped emergency response, public health, and medical personnel.

(D) Health and safety protection of workers responding to such an emergency.

(E) Public health agencies that are prepared to coordinate health services (including mental health services) during and after such emergencies.

(F) Participation in communications networks that can effectively disseminate relevant information in a timely and secure manner to appropriate public and private entities and to the public.

(3) Developing and maintaining medical countermeasures (such as drugs, vaccines and other biological products, medical devices, and other supplies) against biological agents and toxins that may be involved in such emergencies.

(4) Ensuring coordination and minimizing duplication of Federal, State, and local planning, preparedness, and response activities, including during the investigation of a suspicious disease outbreak or other potential public health emergency.

(5) Enhancing the readiness of hospitals and other health care facilities to respond effectively to such emergencies.

* * *

# DEPARTMENT OF HOMELAND SECURITY, NATIONAL RESPONSE PLAN
(December 2004)

## Introduction

The Nation's domestic incident management landscape changed dramatically following the terrorist attacks of September 11, 2001. Today's threat environment includes not only the traditional spectrum of manmade and natural hazards — wildland and urban fires, floods, oil spills, hazardous materials releases, transportation accidents, earthquakes, hurricanes, tornadoes, pandemics, and disruptions to the Nation's energy and information technology infrastructure — but also the deadly and devastating terrorist arsenal of chemical, biological, radiological, nuclear, and high-yield explosive weapons.

These complex and emerging 21st century threats and hazards demand a unified and coordinated national approach to domestic incident management. The National Strategy for Homeland Security; Homeland Security Act of 2002; and Homeland Security Presidential Directive-5 (HSPD-5), Management of Domestic Incidents, establish clear objectives for a concerted national effort to prevent terrorist attacks within the United States; reduce America's vulnerability to terrorism, major disasters, and other emergencies; and minimize the damage and recover from attacks, major disasters, and other emergencies that occur.

## Development and Implementation of a National Response Plan

Achieving these homeland security objectives is a challenge requiring bold steps and adjustments to established structures, processes, and protocols. An important initiative called for in the above documents is the development and implementation of a National Response Plan (NRP), predicated on a new National Incident Management System (NIMS), that aligns the patchwork of Federal special-purpose incident management and emergency response plans into an effective and efficient structure. Together, the NRP and the NIMS integrate the capabilities and resources of various governmental jurisdictions, incident management and emergency response disciplines, nongovernmental organizations (NGOs), and the private sector into a cohesive, coordinated, and seamless national framework for domestic incident management.

The NRP, using the NIMS, is an all-hazards plan that provides the structure and mechanisms for national-level policy and operational coordination for domestic incident management. . . .

\* \* \*

## Purpose

The purpose of the NRP is to establish a comprehensive, national, all-hazards approach to domestic incident management across a spectrum of activities including prevention, preparedness, response, and recovery.

The NRP incorporates best practices and procedures from various incident management disciplines — homeland security, emergency management, law enforcement, firefighting, hazardous materials response, public works, public health, emergency medical services, and responder and recovery worker health and safety — and integrates them into a unified coordinating structure.

The NRP provides the framework for Federal interaction with State, local, and tribal governments; the private sector; and NGOs in the context of domestic incident prevention, preparedness, response, and recovery activities. It describes capabilities and resources and establishes responsibilities, operational processes, and protocols to help protect the Nation from terrorist attacks and other natural and manmade hazards; save lives; protect public health, safety, property, and the environment; and reduce adverse psychological consequences and disruptions. . . .

\* \* \*

## Incidents of National Significance

As the principal Federal official for domestic incident management, the Secretary of Homeland Security declares Incidents of National Significance . . . and provides coordination for Federal operations and/or resources, establishes reporting requirements, and conducts ongoing communications with Federal, State, local, tribal, private-sector, and nongovernmental organizations to maintain situational awareness, analyze threats, assess national implications of threat and operational response activities, and coordinate threat or incident response activities.

---

The NRP bases the definition of Incidents of National Significance on situations related to the following four criteria . . . :

1. A Federal department or agency acting under its own authority has requested the assistance of the Secretary of Homeland Security.

2. The resources of State and local authorities are overwhelmed and Federal assistance has been requested by the appropriate State and local authorities. Examples include:

   ● Major disasters or emergencies as defined under the Stafford Act; and

   ● Catastrophic incidents

3. More than one Federal department or agency has become substantially involved in responding to an incident. Examples include:

   ● Credible threats, indications or warnings of imminent terrorist attack, or acts of terrorism directed domestically against the people, property, environment, or political or legal institutions of the United States or its territories or possessions; and

   ● Threats or incidents related to high-profile, large-scale events that present high-probability targets such as National Special Security Events (NSSEs) and other special events as determined by the Secretary of Homeland Security, in coordination with other Federal departments and agencies.

4. The Secretary of Homeland Security has been directed to assume responsibility for managing a domestic incident by the President.

---

## Incident Management Activities

. . . Examples of incident management actions from a national perspective include:

● Increasing nationwide public awareness;

● Assessing trends that point to potential terrorist activity;

- Elevating the national Homeland Security Advisory System (HSAS) alert condition and coordinating protective measures across jurisdictions;

- Increasing countermeasures such as inspections, surveillance, security, counterintelligence, and infrastructure protection;

- Conducting public health surveillance and assessment processes and, where appropriate, conducting a wide range of prevention measures to include, but not be limited to, immunizations;

- Providing immediate and long-term public health and medical response assets;

- Coordinating Federal support to State, local, and tribal authorities in the aftermath of an incident;

- Providing strategies for coordination of Federal resources required to handle subsequent events;

- Restoring public confidence after a terrorist attack; and

- Enabling immediate recovery activities, as well as addressing long-term consequences in the impacted area.

### George J. Annas, *The Statue of Security: Human Rights and Post-9/11 Epidemics*
### 38 J. HEALTH L. 319 (2005)

*Our enemies are innovative and resourceful, and so are we. They never stop thinking about new ways to harm our country and our people, and neither do we.*

President George W. Bush on signing the Defense Appropriations Act, August 5, 2004

Immediately after 9/11 the U.S. government closed the Statue of Liberty to the public. It took almost three years to reopen Liberty Island, just in time for the Republican National Convention. The public can again visit, but little is the same. Those wishing to take the ferry to the island, for example, must submit to airport-like screening, as well as bag checks, including bomb-sniffing dogs, upon arrival. And on the boat trip, the National Park Service has a new recorded "welcome" which asserts that although historically the Statue of Liberty symbolized freedom, it is now "a symbol of America's freedom, safety, and security." Similar screening is also required to view the Liberty Bell in Philadelphia. We have not yet renamed the Statue of Liberty, the "Statue of Security"; or the Liberty Bell, the "Safety Bell," but safety and security have been consistently promoted as at least as important as liberty, and often more important, since 9/11.

The next stop after Liberty Island is Ellis Island, the site of screening for more than 2 million immigrants to America in the early 20th century. The most rigorous part of screening immigrants involved federal uniformed public health service physicians whose main duty was to prevent immigrants with contagious diseases from entering the country. Few federal public health officials other than the Surgeon General any longer wear military uniforms, and most public health activities now are done under state or local jurisdiction. But 9/11 has affected public health as well, as public health has been called upon to prepare the nation for a "bioterrorist attack" utilizing lethal disease agents, like smallpox or anthrax. Many public health officials hope that public health can take advantage of the new funding available for terrorism preparedness, and not only do its part in national security, but also make "dual use" of the funding to help it fulfill its core missions of protecting the publics' health and preparing for "natural" epidemics.

September 11 was an event, not an epidemic, but the U.S. reacted to it as if it portends an actual epidemic of terrorist attacks against us. In this way, September 11 has been viewed by many in the public health community as a signal of a coming pandemic: akin to the rise of SARS in China, or a novel form of bird flu in Asia. And public health has been asked to prepare for both natural and terrorist-induced epidemics simultaneously. Does 9/11 mean we must make fundamental changes in public health practice regarding epidemic control and revert to 19th century Ellis Island-type quarantine and forced treatment? Must we trade off human rights and civil liberties for increased safety and security? These are important and complex questions. In this article I argue that the answer to both of these questions is no, and that the movement in public health toward the adoption of a modern health and human rights ethical framework begun before 9/11 should continue.

Osama bin Laden and his homicidal Qaeda followers present a real danger to Americans, and the US should bring them to justice for their crimes. The U.S. is more vulnerable to terrorist attacks than we had believed; and we should strengthen our defenses. But we should not undermine our lives and our values by overreacting to the threat of terrorism. Preserving a human rights framework in the war on terrorists both preserves core American values, and makes it more likely that we will prevail in the long run. Ignoring or marginalizing human and constitutional rights, and treating Americans themselves as suspects or actual enemies is counterproductive and dangerous in itself — a conclusion I will support in this article with specific post-9/11 examples, such as public health preparedness plans for mass smallpox vaccination, the experiences of public health in the SARS epidemic, the enactment of new state public health vaccination and quarantine laws, and the use of torture on terrorist suspects and prisoners of war. Public health professionals are the "good guys" and rightly want to protect the publics' health. But the world has changed since the early 19th century, and reliance on coercion rather than education is no longer either legally justifiable or likely to be effective. In this regard, what might be labeled "public health fundamentalism," is as dangerous to the health and safety of Americans as Islamic religious fundamentalism.

The language of human rights also has the great advantage of being universal and thus global. Neither the fight against terrorists, nor the fight against epidemics, can be successfully waged on a local, state, or even national level alone: both can easily cross national boundaries and both can only be effectively confronted by a global, cooperative, strategy. "Safety first" is a good thought, as is the Hippocratic injunction, "first, do no harm"; but neither safety nor inaction are ends in themselves, but only means to promote health and human rights. Sacrificing human rights for safety is almost never necessary and almost always counterproductive in a free society. Benjamin Franklin went further in expressing an American thought from "the land of the free and the home of the brave," saying, "Those who would give up an essential liberty to purchase temporary security deserve neither liberty nor security."

* * *

### Bioterrorism

In the immediate aftermath of 9/11 it was easy for human rights advocates and civil libertarians to despair. Congress almost immediately passed the Orwellian-named USA Patriot Act, and authorized an international (and *1984*-like perpetual) global war on terror, and the Bush Administration also announced that it would disregard not only the United Nations but also fundamental international human rights and humanitarian law as expressed in the Geneva Conventions.

More recently, however, the tide seems to be changing, and many governmental actions are now met with considerable skepticism and even active resistance. The color-coded terrorist warning system has been all but abandoned as too vague to do any more than scare the public. A proposal to enlist mail carriers and TV repair persons as "tipsters" (the so-called "tips" program) has been abandoned. Duct tape and plastic sheeting remain punch lines in jokes about personal protection from chemical and biological agents.

We continue to be bombarded with bioterrorism doomsday scenarios, although the major terrorist threats are not from biological agents. Rather they are from conventional weapons (*e.g.*, firearms and bombs — including "dirty bombs," conventional explosives containing radioactive material), delivered either in trucks or by individual suicide bombers, as evidenced by terrorist activities in Israel for decades, by insurgent attacks in Iraq, and by terrorists worldwide. These create panic, but the most dangerous weapons are not chemical or biological, but nuclear. Our government knows this. Although there were many inconsistent rationales given for going to war with Iraq, no one suggested it was because they possessed chemical or biological weapons: we have known about these weapons for more than two decades, and Iraq has actually used their chemical weapons on both civilian and military targets. It was the future prospect of possessing nuclear weapons that ultimately moved us to war.

Bioterrorism, nonetheless, continues to be hyped beyond all scientific or historic reality, even in the public health community which should know better. A leading public health lawyer, for example, has asserted that "a single gram of crystalline botulinum toxin, evenly disperse and inhaled, could kill more than 1 million people." But, when looking at actual data, that same lawyer admits that in fact, when Aum Shinrikyo, the Japanese terrorist cult, actually "attempted to disperse aerosolized botulinum toxin both in Tokyo and at several military installations in Japan" the result was not millions dead, or even thousands or hundreds: rather all of these attacks "failed to kill anyone."

Likewise, it has been asserted that the release of 100 kilograms of aerosolized anthrax over Washington, D.C. could kill up to three million people. The real anthrax attacks through the U.S. mails were highly effective in sowing terror in the populations, but resulted in only 5 deaths (the number killed in American hospitals by negligence every 30 minutes, or on our nation's highways every hour).

The scariest scenario involves smallpox because, unlike botulinum or anthrax, smallpox can be transmitted from one person to another. This is why the Bush administration used the threat of a smallpox attack from Iraq as one reason for us to fear Iraq, and as the almost sole justification for its massive three-phase smallpox vaccination program. That now-abandoned program was a public policy and public relations disaster, vaccinating only about 40,000 of the initially-proposed 500,000 health care workers the government planned to have vaccinated with the smallpox vaccine during phase one (phase two would have encompassed up to 10 million first responders and public safety personnel, and phase three would have included all willing civilians).

I think the major reason is that the administration failed to persuade physicians and nurses that the known risks of serious side effects with the vaccine were justified given the fact that there is no evidence that Iraq (or anyone else) has both smallpox virus and the wish to use it in a terrorist attack. The information provided on this issue to the physicians and nurses was in the same spirit as the Iraq nuclear threat information, except that it contained no facts at all, not even misleading or phony ones.

* * *

## Bioterrorism and Epidemics

But what about a "real" epidemic, such as a new, worldwide pandemic? A repeat of the 1918 flu epidemic is likely at some point, and could prove devastating. We can and should produce vaccines against the annual flu epidemics. Our new emphasis on bioterrorism, however, has actually drained public health resources away from this effective vaccine. As the World Health Organization warned in late-2004, we need much better planning, and international cooperation, to prepare for an influenza pandemic. Instead we are diverting funds away from this traditional public health concern which involves tens of thousands of deaths a year in the U.S. alone, and a predictable worldwide pandemic at some point, to trying to protect against an extremely unlikely bioterrorist attack. And it is here that we can determine whether or not "dual use" is a reality or just a marketing slogan. I agree with those who say that public health infrastructure generally must be improved for the sake of the nation's health. But where I disagree is on what effect bioterrorism preparation will actually have on public health infrastructure.

I wrongly and naively (it turns out) expected the federal government to provide increased funding for public health in the wake of 9/11. There has been some funding for bioterrorism, but mostly public health departments have been struggling with more unfunded federal mandates and suggestions, and have had to actually divert funds from public health programs we know work to save lives and improve health, to bioterrorism preparation which has little or no public health payoff.

My own state of Massachusetts, for example, always a national leader in public health, has made major cuts in tobacco control, domestic violence prevention, and immunizations against pneumonia and hepatitis A and B. Public health dollars have shrunken $30 million in two years, during which time Massachusetts has received $21 million for bioterrorism-related activities, some of which could be categorized as "dual-use." Public health expert David Ozonoff of the Boston University School of Public Health accurately describes what is happening: "The whole bioterrorism initiative and what it's doing to public health is a cancer, it's hollowing out public health from within. . . . This is a catastrophe for American public health." This was dramatically demonstrated nationally in the fall of 2004 when the U.S. experienced a shortage of flu vaccine and was forced to ration it to Americans most at risk of death and hospitalization from the flu. Cartoonist Matt Davies caught the irony in his cartoon picturing a citizen coming to the door of the "Homeland Security Bio-Terror Readiness Unit" only to be greeted by a note pinned to the door reading, "Out with the Flu."

Other public health experts have put the weakening of public health in even most disturbing terms, noting "Worse, in response to bioterrorism preparedness, public health institutions are being reorganized along a military or police model that subverts the relationships between public health providers and the communities they serve." To the extent that these experts are correct, and I think they are, exaggerated fear of bioterrorism is resulting in overreaction that is already counterproductive in that it is harming both public health's effectiveness and its relationship with the communities public health serves.

Exaggerated risks produce extreme responses that are based more on fear than facts, so it is not surprising that they have unintended consequences. Public health planning should be based on science not free-floating anxiety and fear. Instead of using the tools of public health, especially epidemiology to gather data and risk-assessment, to identify most likely risks and work on them, our government seems to have adopted the bizarre notion that all threats are equal and that all states and localities should equally prepare for all of them. This philosophy has produced two interrelated epidemics in the U.S. today: an epidemic of fear, and an epidemic of security screening.

In the midst of concern over bioterrorism, but after the SARS epidemic, the New York Academy of Medicine did a survey of the American public asking how they would respond to two types of terrorist attacks: smallpox and a dirty bomb. Published in September 2004, the surveys' results support two lessons that were apparent on 9/11: (1) the primary concern Americans have in a crisis is the safety of their family members; and (2) the most important predictor of whether they will follow the advice of public officials is if they trust them to be telling the truth and to be guided by their welfare. Specifically, the survey found that only 40% of Americans would go to a vaccination site in a smallpox outbreak if told to do so, and only 60% would shelter in place for as long as they were told to in the event of a dirty bomb explosion.

The reasons given for not following advice are instructive. In the smallpox scenario, 60% had worries about the safety of the vaccine itself — twice as many who worried about getting smallpox themselves. The respondents also suggested ways to make them more likely to cooperate. For smallpox, overwhelming majorities (94% and 88%) wanted to speak with someone who knew a lot about smallpox and who they trusted to want what was best for them. A physician not working for the government would fit the bill. In the dirty bomb case, the primary concern respondents had was the safety of their family members. 75% of those who would not shelter in place said they would do so if they could communicate with people they care about or if they knew they were safe. Overall the study concluded that "people are more likely to follow official instructions when they have a lot of trust in what officials tell them to do and are confident that their community is prepared to meet their needs if a terrorist attack occurs."

These survey results are consistent with past bioterrorist exercises as well. As Senator Sam Nunn, who played the part of the president in the smallpox exercise, Dark Winter, in which mass quarantine failed, observed: "There is no force on earth that can make Americans do something that they do not believe is in their own best interests and that of their families."

Given the data from real world events, public opinion surveys, and mock exercises, it is quite remarkable that some public health officials are still at home with draconian 19th century quarantine and compulsory treatment methods. This is likely because public health officials, who believe all their actions are designed to protect the public, are much more concerned with false negatives (failing to treat or detain someone who actually has a communicable disease) than with false positives (detaining someone who actually does not have a communicable disease), and believe that brute force can effectively control the behavior of Americans in an epidemic or bioterrorist attack. To the extent this faith in coercion remains alive in the public health community, it is predictable that public health officials with the power to arbitrarily quarantine large numbers of people in an emergency will use it immediately, whether it is warranted or not. From their perspective, protecting public health is more important than protecting liberty, and as public health officials they may really believe they have nothing to lose. But abuse of power will predictably destroy public trust and instill panic. Even totalitarian dictatorships like China cannot control their populations in epidemics by fear alone in the 21st century.

It cannot be emphasized enough that the primary goal and purpose of public health is prevention of disease in the first place. In the case of bioterrorism, this means prevention of the attack is much more important (to public health) than responding to it after the fact. And contemporary public health prevention of epidemics and bioterrorism is not primarily a local or state issue at all, but is fundamentally a global security issue that must be dealt with by the community of nations working together. National laws and treaties, with realistic inspection and sanctions, devoted to preventing the development and production of biological weapons are the most important tool in the prevention of bioterrorism. We are also right to want to modernize the World Health Organization's International Health Regulations: but, as WHO recognizes, to be effective revised regulations must be founded on respecting and protecting human rights, not trampling them.

State laws, no matter what they say, and no matter what the CDC says, simply cannot prevent or control bioterrorism. Moreover, by seeming to grant unconstitutional power over citizens lives and liberty, bad state public health emergency laws undermine public trust and are thus a danger to public health itself. Florida's crude summary of CDC's-sponsored "model act" which seeks to trade off human rights for safety and security, provides the country's starkest example, and thus helps illustrate why honoring rather than destroying human rights is essential to effective public health action in the 21st century. . . . [for material from this article on the U.S. reaction to SARS, and the Florida statute based on the model act, see Chapter Three.]

**Conclusion**

At the outset of the 21st century bioterrorism, although only one threat to public health, can be the catalyst to effectively federalize and integrate much of what is now uncoordinated and piecemeal state and local public health programs. This should include a renewed effort for national health insurance, national licensure for physicians, nurses, and allied health professionals, and national patient safety standards. Federal public health leadership will also encourage us to look outward, and to recognize that prevention of future bioterrorist attacks and even ordinary epidemics will require international cooperation. As the SARS epidemic illustrates, it is time to not only federalize public health, but to globalize it as well. And universal human rights is the proper foundation for a global public health ethic.

Our new kind of war against bioterrorism should be built on a goal of protecting liberty, not depriving Americans of it. There is a knee jerk tendency in times of war and national emergencies to restrict civil liberties as the most effective way to counteract the threat. But history has taught us that such restrictions are almost always useless and often counterproductive, and we usually wind up with deep regrets for our action. The tendency to return to the days before liberty and informed consent were taken seriously has been evident in the immediate aftermath of 9/11. Arbitrary and unlawful responses have not, however, helped make Americans safer or more secure, instead they threaten the very liberties that make our country worth protecting. It is wrong and dangerous for our government to treat its citizens either as enemies to be controlled by force or children to be pacified with platitudes.

America is strong because its people are free, and to be both moral and effective public planning for war and public health emergencies must be based on respecting freedom and trusting our fellow citizens. The United States should lead the world in proclaiming a new, global public health, based on transparency, trust, and science, and most importantly, based on respect for human rights. We don't need a new Statue of Security; the Statue of Liberty is just fine.

## NOTES AND QUESTIONS

**1.** The National Plan has defined roles for state and local officials as well:

Police, fire, public health and medical, emergency management, public works, environmental response, and other personnel are often the first to arrive and the last to leave an incident site. In some instances, a Federal agency in the local area may act as a first responder, and the local assets of Federal agencies may be used to advise or assist local officials in accordance with agency authorities and procedures. Mutual aid agreements provide mechanisms to mobilize and employ resources from neighboring jurisdictions to support the incident command.

When State resources and capabilities are overwhelmed, Governors may request Federal assistance under a Presidential disaster or emergency declaration. Summarized below are the responsibilities of the Governor, Local Chief Executive Officer, and Tribal Chief Executive Officer.

## Governor

As a State's chief executive, the Governor is responsible for the public safety and welfare of the people of that State or territory. The Governor:

- Is responsible for coordinating State resources to address the full spectrum of actions to prevent, prepare for, respond to, and recover from incidents in an all-hazards context to include terrorism, natural disasters, accidents, and other contingencies;

- Under certain emergency conditions, typically has police powers to make, amend, and rescind orders and regulations;

- Provides leadership and plays a key role in communicating to the public and in helping people, businesses, and organizations cope with the consequences of any type of declared emergency within State jurisdiction;

- Encourages participation in mutual aid and implements authorities for the State to enter into mutual agreements with other States, tribes, and territories to facilitate resource-sharing;

- Is the Commander-in-Chief of State military forces . . .; and

- Requests Federal assistance when it becomes clear that State or tribal capabilities will be insufficient or have been exceeded or exhausted.

## Local Chief Executive Officer

A mayor or city or county manager, as a jurisdiction's chief executive, is responsible for the public safety and welfare of the people of that jurisdiction. The Local Chief Executive Officer:

- Is responsible for coordinating local resources to address the full spectrum of actions to prevent, prepare for, respond to, and recover from incidents involving all hazards including terrorism, natural disasters, accidents, and other contingencies;

- Dependent upon State and local law, has extraordinary powers to suspend local laws and ordinances, such as to establish a curfew, direct evacuations, and, in coordination with the local health authority, to order a quarantine;

- Provides leadership and plays a key role in communicating to the public, and in helping people, businesses, and organizations cope with the consequences of any type of domestic incident within the jurisdiction;

- Negotiates and enters into mutual aid agreements with other jurisdictions to facilitate resource-sharing; and

- Requests State and, if necessary, Federal assistance through the Governor of the State when the jurisdiction's capabilities have been exceeded or exhausted.

**2.** The post-9/11 approach has been an "all-hazards" one. What are the pros and cons to this type of "one-size fits all" planning? Is it really true, as President Bush has said, that planning for a pandemic flu will build our capacity to respond to a chemical attack?

**3.** President Eisenhower, when he was commanding general in Europe, is credited with observing before the D-Day invasion: "It's not the plan, it's the planning." Explain. In March, 1942, Winston Churchill observed, "One cannot always provide against the worse assumptions, and to try to do so prevents the best disposition of limited resources." What did these leaders mean and are these observations from World War II relevant today?

**4.** The most notorious example of a complete failure of the national preparedness plan was the response to Hurricane Katrina, despite the fact that only a year earlier the agencies responsible for responding to a hurricane/flood in New Orleans had participated in a simulation of just such a catastrophe, called "Hurricane Pam." Under new rules that existed at the time, the Department of Homeland Security was to be the lead agency, but it did not get involved until days after the flooding. On the day the levees broke, Secretary Chertoff traveled to Atlanta to take part in exercises designed to get the country ready for an avian flu pandemic. Almost a year later Chertoff announced the Department's new plan, which was that:

> People should be prepared to sustain themselves for up to 72 hours after a disaster — because first responders might not be able to reach every single person within the first day. That means individuals — especially those in the Gulf states — need to have an emergency plan and an emergency kit with adequate supplied of food, water, and other essentials like a flashlight, first-aid, and medicine.

In the words of Christopher Cooper and Robert Block, who quote this speech from Chertoff to conclude their study of Katrina in DISASTER: HURRICANE KATRINA AND THE FAILURE OF HOMELAND SECURITY (2006): "In the end Chertoff unwittingly defined the most important lesson of all to emerge from Hurricane Katrina: When disaster strikes, we are all on our own." *Id.* at 306. On the actual response of local, state and federal officials during the week after Katrina struck, see DOUGLAS BRINKLEY, THE GREAT DELUGE: HURRICANE KATRINA, NEW ORLEANS, AND THE MISSISSIPPI GULF COAST (2006).

# Richard Horton, *Public Health: A Neglected Counterterrorist Measure*
## 358 LANCET 1112 (2001)

The war against terrorism, announced by President Bush and endorsed by western political leaders in the immediate aftermath of the Sept. 11 assault on America, will fail. No matter how much international collaboration is achieved between governments, intelligence services, and police networks, terrorists will never be wholly eradicated from society. Such is the nature of terrorism. A declaration of war, deemed necessary to reassure an anxious public, has raised false expectations of victory. The western response will not only come to be discredited but also may foster the very terrorist activity it is designed to prevent.

Paul Pillar, a former counterterrorism policymaker at the US Central Intelligence Agency, has studied American covert and foreign-policy approaches to terrorist threats. . . . He argues that war metaphors. . . drive "a tendency toward absolute solutions and a rejection of accommodation and finesse." He views traditional counterterrorist policies — diplomatic, legal, military, and economic — as ineffective and counterproductive. The best hope we have, he concludes, is not triumph, but containment. Terrorism is a problem managed, never solved.

In response to the present crisis there has been a curious failure to discuss the root causes of terrorism, except for some rather blunt criticism of America itself. Action so far has been confined to three fronts. First, the capabilities of terrorist groups have been targeted. Their organization is being disrupted, their members sought. Second, the intentions of terrorists have been scrutinized. A capability to attack might well be available, but what makes the terrorist decide to act? Encouraging terrorists not to attack involves deterrence and diplomacy. The third front is occupying most political airtime right now — namely, defence. Airport and aircraft security, homeland protection, and military force are all important defensive instruments. None of these efforts gets close to the cause of the problem.

\* \* \*

No single counterterrorist measure will succeed alone. But the existing narrow range of options could be broadened to find ways of engaging and helping rather than punishing populations at risk.

\* \* \*

Afghanistan has been the victim of two decades of savage exploitation by several of those countries now urging a war against terrorism. The hypocrisy of these governments is breathtaking, the consequences predictable and tragic.

In addition to the welcome promises of aid by western powers, there must be three longer-term revisions of policy. First, foreign-policy goals should incorporate health, development, and human rights as key strategic objectives. Too often, foreign policy is reduced to little more than short-term alliances for political or military advantage. These limited goals sow the seeds for later terrorist — and humanitarian — crises.

Second, the application of sanctions must be judged more wisely. In Afghanistan, UN sanctions were aimed at forcing the Taliban government to hand over Osama bin Laden. The health effects have been crushing, while the political objective has failed entirely. Third, western powers must recommit themselves to international agencies, such as the UN, and to international treaties, such as those on criminal justice and the environment. . . .

The discipline of public health therefore adds fresh perspectives on foreign policy and counterterrorism measures. Principles of harm reduction are more realistic and practicable than false notions of a war on terrorism. Attacking hunger, disease, poverty, and social exclusion might do more good than air marshals, asylum restrictions, and identity cards. Global security will be achieved only by building stable and strong societies. Health is an undervalued measure of our global security.

# NOTES AND QUESTIONS

**1.** Horton makes a strong case in his editorial. Is he correct about the importance of public health to combat terrorism? Former UN Commissioner for Human Rights, Mary Robinson, has argued that our world is continually becoming less secure because of the increase in global public health problems. She quotes from the 2004 HUMAN DEVELOPMENT REPORT from the United Nations:

> More than 800 million people suffer from undernourishment. Some 100 million children who should be in school are not, 60 million of them girls. More than a billion people survive on less than one dollar a day. . . . And about 900 million people belong to ethnic, religious, racial or linguistic groups that face discrimination. . . . An unprecedented number of countries saw development slide backwards in the 1990s. In 46 countries people are poorer today than in 1990. In 25 countries more people go hungry today than a decade ago. *Id.* at 129.

Robinson goes on to note that in the last six years approximately 25,000 people have died from terrorist attacks. During that same time period, approximately 25,000 people die each day from hunger, malaria, and other preventable diseases. Mary Robinson, *Connecting Human Rights, Human Development, and Human Security, in* HUMAN RIGHTS AND THE "WAR ON TERROR" 311 (Richard Ashly Wilson ed., 2005).

**2.** Economist Amartya Sen, cited by Robinson, has also directly linked health, especially public health, to freedom and economic development. For example, in his DEVELOPMENT AS FREEDOM 4 (1999) he writes:

> Sometimes the lack of substantive freedoms relates directly to economic poverty, which robs people of the freedom to satisfy hunger, or to achieve sufficient nutrition, or to obtain remedies for treatable illnesses, or the opportunity to be adequately clothed and sheltered, or to enjoy clean water or sanitary facilities. In other cases, the unfreedom links closely to the lack of public facilities and social care, such as the absence of epidemiological programs, or of organized arrangements for health care or educational facilities. . . .

See also on the relationship between health and development, THE WORLD BANK, WORLD DEVELOPMENT REPORT 1993: INVESTING IN HEALTH (1993).

# G.  GLOBAL HEALTH

## Sofia Gruskin & Daniel Tarantola, *Health and Human Rights, in* PERSPECTIVES ON HEALTH AND HUMAN RIGHTS 3–57 (Gruskin et al., eds., 2005)

Since the creation of the United Nations over 50 years ago, international responsibility for health and for human rights has been increasingly acknowledged. Yet the actual links between health and human rights had not been recognized even a decade ago. Generally thought to be fundamentally antagonistic, these two worlds had evolved along parallel but distinctly separate tracks until a number of recent events helped to bring them together.

Conceptually one can point to the HIV/AIDS pandemic, to women's health issues, including violence, and to the blatant violations of human rights which occurred in such places as the Balkans and the Great Lakes region in Africa as having brought attention to the intrinsic connections that exist between health and human rights. Each of these issues helped to illustrate distinct, but linked, pieces of the health and human rights paradigm. While the relationship between health and human rights with respect to these and similar issues may always have made sense intuitively, the development of a 'health and human rights' language in the last few years has allowed for the connections between health and human rights to be explicitly named, and therefore for conceptual, analytical, policy, and programmatic work to begin to bridge these disparate disciplines and to move forward. In the last few years human rights have increasingly been at the centre of analysis and action in regard to health and development issues. The level of institutional and state political commitment to health and human rights has, in fact, never been higher. This is true within the work of the United Nations system but, even more importantly, can also be seen in the work of governments and non-governmental organizations at both the national and international level.

The importance of the HIV/AIDS pandemic as a catalyst for beginning to define some of the structural connections between health and human rights cannot be overemphasized. The first time that human rights were explicitly named in a public health strategy was only in the late 1980s, when the call for human rights and for compassion and solidarity with people living with HIV/AIDS was embodied in the first World Health Organization (WHO) global response to AIDS. This approach was motivated by moral outrage but also, even more importantly, by the recognition that protecting the human rights of people living with HIV/AIDS was a necessary element of the worldwide public health response to the emerging epidemics. The implications of this call were far reaching. Framing this public health strategy in human rights terms — although initially focused on the rights of people living with HIV/AIDS rather than on the broad array of human rights influencing people's vulnerability to the epidemic — allowed it to become anchored in international law, thereby making governments and intergovernmental organizations publicly accountable for their actions towards people living with HIV/AIDS. The groundbreaking contribution of this era lies in the recognition of the applicability of international law to HIV/AIDS issues and in the attention this approach then generated to the links between other health issues and human rights — and therefore to the ultimate responsibility and accountability of the state under international law for issues relating to health and well being.

\* \* \*

While human rights thinking and practice has a long history, the importance of human rights for governmental action and accountability was first widely recognized only after the Second World War. Agreement between nation-states that all people are "born free and equal in dignity and rights" was reached in 1945 when the promotion of human rights was identified as a principal purpose of the newly created United Nations. The United Nations Charter established general obligations that apply to all its member states, including respect for human rights and dignity. Then, in 1948, the Universal Declaration of Human Rights was adopted as a common standard of achievement for all peoples and nations. The basic characteristics of human rights are that they are the rights of individuals, which inhere in individuals because they are human, that they apply to people everywhere in the world, and that they are principally concerned with the relationship between the individual and the state. In practical terms, international human rights law is about defining what governments can do to us, cannot do to us, and should do for us. For example, governments obviously should not do things like torture people, imprison them arbitrarily, or invade their privacy. Governments should ensure that all people in a society have shelter, food, medical care, and basic education.

The Universal Declaration of Human Rights can well be understood to be the cornerstone of the modern human rights movement. The preamble to the Universal Declaration of Human Rights proposes that human rights and dignity are self-evident, the "highest aspiration of the common people," and the "foundation of freedom, justice and peace." "Social progress and better standards of life" including the "prevention of barbarous acts which have outraged the conscience of mankind," and, broadly speaking, individual and collective well being, are understood to depend on the "promotion of universal respect for and observance of human rights." Although the Universal Declaration of Human Rights is not a legally binding document, nations have endowed it with a tremendous legitimacy through their actions, including invoking it legally and politically at the national and international levels. Portions of the Universal Declaration of the Human Rights are cited in the majority of national constitutions drafted since it came into being, and governments often cite the Universal Declaration of Human Rights in their negotiations with other governments, as well as in their accusations against each other of violating human rights. Under the auspices of the United Nations, more than 20 multilateral human rights treaties have been formulated since the adoption of the Universal Declaration of Human Rights. These treaties create legally binding obligations on the nations that have ratified them, thereby giving them the status and power of international law. . . .

The rights that form the corpus of human rights law are found in the international human rights documents. While it is possible to identify different categories of rights, it is also critical to rights discourse and action to recognize that all rights are interdependent and interrelated, and that individuals rarely suffer neglect or violation of a particular right in isolation. . . .

\* \* \*

Health and government responsibility for health is codified in these documents in several ways. The right to the highest attainable standard of health appears in one form or another in most of them. More importantly, nearly every article of every document can be understood to have clear implications for health. While the rights to information, education, housing, and safe working conditions, and social security, for example, are particularly relevant to the health and human rights relationship, specific reference must be made to three rights: the right to non-discrimination, the right to the benefits of scientific progress, and the right to health.

\* \* \*

Governments are responsible not only for not directly violating rights, but also for ensuring the conditions which enable individuals to realize their rights as fully as possible. This is understood as an obligation to respect, protect, and fulfill rights, and governments are legally responsible for complying with this range of obligations for every right in every human rights document they have ratified.

Governmental obligations towards ensuring the right to health are summarized below as an illustration of the range of issues relevant to respecting, protecting, and fulfilling human rights.

1.  *Respecting* the right means that a state cannot violate the right directly. A government violates its responsibility to respect the right to health when it is immediately responsible for providing medical care to certain populations, such as prisoners or the military, and it arbitrarily decides to withhold that care.

2.  *Protecting* the right means that a state has to prevent violations of rights by non-state actors and offer some sort of redress that people know about and can access if a violation occurs. This means that the state would be responsible for making it illegal to deny insurance or health care to people on the basis of a health condition, and that they would be responsible for ensuring safety nets and some system of redress that people know about and can access if a violation does occur.

3.  *Fulfilling* the right means that a state has to take all appropriate measures — including but not limited to legislative, administrative, budgetary, and judicial — toward fulfillment of the right, including to promote the right in question. A state could be found to be in violation of the right to health if it failed to allocate sufficient resources incrementally to meet the public health needs of all the communities within its borders.

In all countries, resource and other constraints can make it impossible for a government to fulfill all rights immediately and completely. The human rights machinery recognizes this and acknowledges that, in practical terms, a commitment to the right to health requires more than just passing a law. It will require financial resources, trained personnel, facilities, and, more than anything else, a sustainable infrastructure. Therefore, realization of rights is generally understood to be a matter of progressive realization of making steady progress toward a goal. The principle of "progressive realization" is fundamental to the achievement of human rights. This is critical for resource-poor countries that are responsible for striving towards human rights goals to the maximum extent possible. It is also of relevance to wealthier countries in that they are responsible for respecting, protecting, and fulfilling human rights not only within their own borders, but through their engagement in international assistance and cooperation.

* * *

In spite of the importance attached to human rights, there are situations where it is considered legitimate to restrict rights in order to achieve a broader public good. As described in the International Covenant on Civil and Political Rights, the public good can take precedence to "secure due recognition and respect for the rights and freedoms of others; meet the just requirements of morality, public order, and the general welfare; and in times of emergency, when there are threats to the life of the nation" (ICCPR Article 4). Public health is one such recognized public good. (The specific power of the state to restrict rights in the name of public health can be understood to be derived from Article 12(c) of the ICESCR, which gives governments the right to take the steps they deem necessary for the "prevention, treatment, and control of epidemic, endemic, occupational, and other diseases.") Traditional public health measures have generally focused on curbing the spread of disease by imposing restrictions on the rights of those already infected or thought to be most vulnerable to becoming infected. In fact, coercion, compulsion, and restriction have historically been significant components of public health measures. Although the restrictions on rights that have occurred in the context of public health have generally had as their first concern protection of the public's health, it is also true that the measures taken have often been excessive. Interference with freedom of movement when instituting quarantine or isolation for a serious communicable disease — for example, Ebola fever, syphilis, typhoid, or untreated tuberculosis — is an example of a restriction on rights that may in certain circumstances be necessary for the public good and therefore could be considered legitimate under international human rights law. Conversely, arbitrary measures taken by public health authorities that fail to consider other valid alternatives may be found to be abusive of both human rights principles and public health "best practice." In recent times, measures taken around the world in response to HIV/AIDS provides some examples of this type of abuse.

Certain rights are absolute, which means that restrictions may never be placed on them, even if justified as necessary for the public good. These include such rights as the right to be free from torture, slavery, or servitude, the right to a fair trial, and the right to freedom of thought. (See, for example,

Article 4 of the ICCPR, which states that "[n]o derogation from articles 6, 7, 8 (paragraphs 1 and 2), 11, 15, 16, 18 may be made under this provision.") Paradoxically, the right to life, which might at first glance appear to be inalienable, is not absolute; what is forbidden is the arbitrary deprivation of life. Interference with most rights can be legitimately justified as necessary under narrowly defined circumstances in many situations relevant to public health. (See, for example, Article 4 of the ICCPR, which states that "[I]n time of public emergency which threatens the life of the nation and the existence of which is officially proclaimed, the States Parties to the present Covenant may take measures derogating from their obligations under the present Covenant to the extent strictly required by the exigencies of the situation, provided that such measures are not inconsistent with their other obligations under international law and do not involve discrimination solely on the ground of race, color, sex, language, religion, or social origin.")

Limitations on rights, however, are considered a serious issue under international human rights law, regardless of the apparent importance of the public good involved. When a government limits the exercise or enjoyment of a right, this action must be taken as a last resort and will only be considered legitimate if the following criteria are met.

1. The restriction is provided for and carried out in accordance with the law;

2. The restriction is in the interest of a legitimate objective of general interest;

3. The restriction is strictly necessary in a democratic society to achieve the objective;

4. There are no less intrusive and restrictive means available to reach the same goal; and

5. The restriction is not imposed arbitrarily, i.e., in an unreasonable or otherwise discriminatory manner.

This approach, often called the Siracusa Principles because they were conceptualized at a meeting in Siracusa, Italy, has long been recognized by those concerned with human rights monitoring and implementation as relevant to analyzing a government's actions, and it has also recently begun to be considered a useful tool by those responsible within government for health-related policies and programs. This framework, although still rudimentary, may be helpful in identifying public health actions that are abusive, whether intentionally or unintentionally.

At the outset of the twenty-first century, the translation of the right to health into guidelines and other tools useful to national and international monitoring of governmental and intergovernmental obligations is still in its infancy. The ICESCR General Comment on the Right to the Highest Attainable Standard of Health, which was adopted in 2000, may help to provide some useful guidelines. In parallel, as described below, the WHO is developing a new set of tools and recommendations aimed at redirecting the attention given to monitoring global health indicators from disease-specific morbidity and mortality trends towards others that are more reflective of the degree to which health and human rights principles are respected, protected, and fulfilled. How and to what extent these instruments will be put to use and how effective they will be in advancing the health and human rights agenda has yet to be seen, but there are several factors that, even at this early stage, allow for guarded optimism. First, the treaty bodies and international organizations concerned with health are doing this work based on open dialogue and a degree of collaboration that greatly exceeds the level and quality if interagency collaboration traditionally observed within the United Nations machinery. This is exemplified by the sharing of goals and the collective technical co-operation that has prevailed in the current processes of defining obligations and monitoring methods and standards relevant to health and human rights in the process of operationalizing both the international treaties and the recommendations promulgated at the international conferences. Potentially, this work will help not only to monitor what governments are doing, but also to build their capacity to incorporate health and human rights principles into their policies and programs.

In several countries, including Brazil, Thailand, and South Africa, human rights principles relevant to health have recently found their way into national legislation and new constitutions, thereby ensuring citizens the right to seek fulfillment of their right to care, for example, through national juridical means.

\* \* \*

Over 50 years ago, the Constitution of the WHO projected a vision of health as a state of complete physical, mental, and social well being — a definition of health that is more relevant today than ever. It recognized that the enjoyment of the highest attainable standard of health was one of the fundamental rights of every human being and that governments have a responsibility for the health of their peoples, which can be fulfilled only through the provision of adequate health and social measures. The 1978 Alma-Ata Declaration called on nations to ensure the availability of the essentials of primary health care, including:

- Education concerning health problems and the methods for preventing and controlling them

- Promotion of food supply and proper nutrition

- An adequate supply of safe water and basic sanitation

- Maternal and child health care, including family planning

- Immunization against major infectious diseases

- Prevention and control of locally endemic diseases

- Appropriate treatment of common disease and injuries

- Provision of essential drugs.

In 1998, the World Health Assembly reaffirmed the commitment of nations to strive towards these goals in a World Health Declaration that stressed the

'will to promote health by addressing the basic determinants and prerequisites for health' and the urgent priority 'to pay the greatest attention to those most in need, burdened by ill health, receiving inadequate services for health or affected by poverty.'. . .

WHO [has attempted] to measure health on the national or international level selectively [using] morbidity, mortality, and disability indicators. This exercise was severely constrained by incomplete national data, differences in measurement methods across countries, and, even more importantly, an inability to relate health outcomes to the performance of health systems. Furthermore, most of these indicators were applied at a national aggregate level with insufficient attempts to disaggregate the data collected to reveal the disparities that exist within nations. It has been understood that measurement indicators and benchmarks that focus on the aggregate (national) level may not reveal important differentials that may be associated with a variety of human rights violations — in particular, discrimination.

In order to improve the knowledge and understanding of health status and trends, and to relate these trends to health system performance, the WHO . . . developed the following five global indicators [in 2000].

1.  Healthy life expectancy: a composite indicator incorporating mortality, morbidity, and disability in a disability-adjusted life years measure. This indicator will reflect time spent in a state of less than full health.

2.  Health inequalities: the degree of disparity in healthy life expectancy within the population.

3.  Responsiveness of health systems: a composite indicator reflecting the protection of dignity and confidentiality in and by health systems, and people's autonomy (that is, their individual capacity to effect informed choice in health matters).

4.  Responsiveness inequality: the disparity in responsiveness within health systems, bringing out issues of low efficiency, neglect, and discrimination.

5.  Fairness in financing: measured by the level of health financing contribution of households.

The WHO has stated that it will collect this data through built-in health information systems, demographic and health surveys conducted periodically within countries, and other survey instruments. Data will thus be analyzable by sex, age, race/birth (if warranted under national law), population groups (for example, indigenous populations), educational achievement, and other variables.

The WHO has also expressed its commitment to working with countries toward increasing their capacity to collect this information and also to determine additional data and targets that may be specifically suited to country-specific situations and needs. The WHO and other institutions concerned with health have stated their desire to use these data to assess trends in the performance of national health systems, inform national and international policies and programs, make comparisons across countries, and monitor global health.

# Who Is WHO?

The World Health Organization (WHO) was established in 1948 under the auspices of the United Nations. The United Nations Charter and the WHO Constitution grant WHO the authority to monitor world health. The WHO Constitution allows WHO to address various public health issues by adopting conventions, agreements, and regulations through its supreme decision-making body, the World Health Assembly (Health Assembly). Any member of the United Nations may become a member of WHO by accepting its Constitution. Membership is available to other countries by application, if approval is given by a majority vote of the Health Assembly. There are currently 192 WHO member countries. Each WHO member sends a delegation to meetings of the Health Assembly, typically held in Geneva in May of each year. A 32-member Executive Board meets in January to set the agenda for the upcoming meeting. The Secretariat of WHO is responsible for implementation. The Secretariat has a staff of approximately 3500 at its Geneva headquarters, in six regional offices, and in specific countries. Its head is the Director-General, who is appointed by the Health Assembly on the nomination of the Executive Board.

Articles 19-22 of the WHO Constitution delineate the specific areas of authority of the Health Assembly. Article 21 empowers the Health Assembly to adopt regulations in areas including sanitary and quarantine requirements and other procedures designed to prevent the international spread of disease; nomenclature with respect to diseases; causes of death and public health practices; and standards for diagnostic procedures. After notice of adoption is given, regulations come into force for all member countries, with the caveat that the notice of adoption will specify a period for members to reject or register reservations with the Director-General. The member countries are bound by a set of regulations, and any reservations are typically listed in annexes to the official text.

The control of infectious diseases is one of the areas in which international law has been developed and implemented by WHO. These efforts have culminated in the body of regulations referred to as the International Health Regulations (IHRs). The precursors of today's IHRs were adopted in 1951 as the International Sanitary Regulations . . . and were given their current name in 1969. The IHRs have been modified twice since their enactment, in 1973 and in 1981. The IHRs are intended to maximize security against the global spread of disease while minimizing interference with global movement.

The IHRs require member countries to notify WHO of all cases of certain infectious diseases in humans. Currently [as of 2003], the list of notifiable diseases is limited to cholera, plague, and yellow fever. The IHRs also provide health-related rules for travel and commerce; require health documentation of those traveling from infected to non-infected places; require other travel documentation, such as maritime declaration of health; and establish guidelines for de-ratting, disinfecting, and adopting other hygiene measures related to travel and commerce. The IHRs not only mandate certain public health activities, they also set limits on the measures member countries may take to protect public health, especially if these impede international traffic For example, with respect to quarantine, the IHRs allow for surveillance or isolation of infected persons only for the duration of the incubation period based on the date of last exposure or arrival.

For many years, there has been debate on the need to revise and strengthen the IHRs to reflect the current concerns about the rapidity with which infectious disease can spread under contemporary social conditions as well as the emergence of new and dormant infections. The SARS outbreak has given a new impetus to the effort needed to update provisions and standards related to reporting and controlling infectious disease on a global level . . . [See *infra*, Section G, Note 7.]

The Department of Communicable Disease Surveillance and Response (CSR) at WHO houses its global alert and response activities. The mission of CSR is to provide support for global health security and epidemic alert and response. . . . The IHRs provide the basic framework for CSR and are the only set of binding. international legal rules on infectious disease control. . . .

The Global Outbreak Alert and Response Network (GOARN) was established by WHO in 2000 with the assistance of the Canadian government. GOARN is a collaboration of institutions and networks around the world that provides coordination and logistical support in the form of standardized protocols, agreed standards, procedures for alert and verifications process, communications, coordination of response, specialist equipment, medical supplies, emergency evacuation, research, evaluation, and relations with media. It is supported administratively by the office of Alert and Response Operations within CSR. Through GOARN, WHO and partners aim to enhance the coordinated delivery of international assistance in support of local efforts; strengthen local infrastructure and capacity to reduce illness, death, and prevent disease spread. . . .

. . . GOARN functions under guiding principles developed through international consensus with the IHRs as the overarching framework. . . . Although GOARN has played a central role in keeping the global community informed and updated as to changes and progress regarding SARS, its effectiveness has been limited by the voluntary nature of countries reporting beyond the three notifiable diseases under the IHRs. . . .

WHO maintains a number of specific mechanisms that assist member countries in detecting, responding to, and sharing information about disease outbreaks. The Global Public Health Intelligence Network is an electronic system that continuously searches websites, newswires and media sites, public health e-mail services, national government websites, public health institutions, non-governmental organizations, and specialized discussion groups to identify information regarding epidemic threats and rumors. . . . Support for effective response to threats comes from Global Alert and Response Teams, which draw on the expertise of personnel from WHO country offices, WHO regional response teams, alert and response operation center teams, and disease specialists. . . . The Outbreak Verification List is a weekly electronic report of confirmed and unconfirmed reports of outbreaks of international public health importance. . . . The Disease Outbreak News is a web-based system providing public information about officially confirmed outbreaks of international importance.

From MARK A. ROTHSTEIN et al., QUARANTINE AND ISOLATION: LESSONS LEARNED FROM SARS 27–32 (2003). *See also* www.who.int.

## UNIVERSAL DECLARATION OF HUMAN RIGHTS
### (1948)

Whereas recognition of the inherent dignity and of the equal and inalienable rights of all members of the human family is the foundation of freedom, justice and peace in the world,

Whereas disregard and contempt for human rights have resulted in barbarous acts which have outraged the conscience of mankind, and the advent of a world in which human beings shall enjoy freedom of speech and belief and freedom from fear and want has been proclaimed as the highest aspiration of the common people,

Whereas it is essential, if man is not to be compelled to have recourse, as a last resort, to rebellion against tyranny and oppression, that human rights should be protected by the rule of law,

Whereas it is essential to promote the development of friendly relations between nations,

Whereas the peoples of the United Nations have in the Charter reaffirmed their faith in fundamental human rights, in the dignity and worth of the human person and in the equal rights of men and women and have determined to promote social progress and better standards of life in larger freedom,

Whereas Member States have pledged themselves to achieve, in co-operation with the United Nations, the promotion of universal respect for and observance of human rights and fundamental freedoms,

Whereas a common understanding of these rights and freedoms is of the greatest importance for the full realization of this pledge,

Now, Therefore THE GENERAL ASSEMBLY proclaims THIS UNIVERSAL DECLARATION OF HUMAN RIGHTS as a common standard of achievement for all peoples and all nations, to the end that every individual and every organ of society, keeping this Declaration constantly in mind, shall strive by teaching and education to promote respect for these rights and freedoms and by progressive measures, national and international, to secure their universal and effective recognition and observance, both among the peoples of Member States themselves and among the peoples of territories under their jurisdiction.

### Article 1.

All human beings are born free and equal in dignity and rights. They are endowed with reason and conscience and should act towards one another in a spirit of brotherhood.

**Article 2.**

Everyone is entitled to all the rights and freedoms set forth in this Declaration, without distinction of any kind, such as race, colour, sex, language, religion, political or other opinion, national or social origin, property, birth or other status. Furthermore, no distinction shall be made on the basis of the political, jurisdictional or international status of the country or territory to which a person belongs, whether it be independent, trust, non-self-governing or under any other limitation of sovereignty.

**Article 3.**

Everyone has the right to life, liberty and security of person.

**Article 4.**

No one shall be held in slavery or servitude; slavery and the slave trade shall be prohibited in all their forms.

**Article 5.**

No one shall be subjected to torture or to cruel, inhuman or degrading treatment or punishment.

**Article 6.**

Everyone has the right to recognition everywhere as a person before the law.

**Article 7.**

All are equal before the law and are entitled without any discrimination to equal protection of the law. All are entitled to equal protection against any discrimination in violation of this Declaration and against any incitement to such discrimination.

**Article 8.**

Everyone has the right to an effective remedy by the competent national tribunals for acts violating the fundamental rights granted him by the constitution or by law.

**Article 9.**

No one shall be subjected to arbitrary arrest, detention or exile.

**Article 10.**

Everyone is entitled in full equality to a fair and public hearing by an independent and impartial tribunal, in the determination of his rights and obligations and of any criminal charge against him.

**Article 11.**

(1) Everyone charged with a penal offence has the right to be presumed innocent until proved guilty according to law in a public trial at which he has had all the guarantees necessary for his defense.

(2) No one shall be held guilty of any penal offence on account of any act or omission which did not constitute a penal offence, under national or international law, at the time when it was committed. Nor shall a heavier penalty be

imposed than the one that was applicable at the time the penal offence was committed.

### Article 12.

No one shall be subjected to arbitrary interference with his privacy, family, home or correspondence, nor to attacks upon his honour and reputation. Everyone has the right to the protection of the law against such interference or attacks.

### Article 13.

(1) Everyone has the right to freedom of movement and residence within the borders of each state.

(2) Everyone has the right to leave any country, including his own, and to return to his country.

### Article 14.

(1) Everyone has the right to seek and to enjoy in other countries asylum from persecution.

(2) This right may not be invoked in the case of prosecutions genuinely arising from non-political crimes or from acts contrary to the purposes and principles of the United Nations.

### Article 15.

(1) Everyone has the right to a nationality.

(2) No one shall be arbitrarily deprived of his nationality nor denied the right to change his nationality.

### Article 16.

(1) Men and women of full age, without any limitation due to race, nationality or religion, have the right to marry and to found a family. They are entitled to equal rights as to marriage, during marriage and at its dissolution.

(2) Marriage shall be entered into only with the free and full consent of the intending spouses.

(3) The family is the natural and fundamental group unit of society and is entitled to protection by society and the State.

### Article 17.

(1) Everyone has the right to own property alone as well as in association with others.

(2) No one shall be arbitrarily deprived of his property.

### Article 18.

Everyone has the right to freedom of thought, conscience and religion; this right includes freedom to change his religion or belief, and freedom, either alone or in community with others and in public or private, to manifest his religion or belief in teaching, practice, worship and observance.

**Article 19.**

Everyone has the right to freedom of opinion and expression; this right includes freedom to hold opinions without interference and to seek, receive and impart information and ideas through any media and regardless of frontiers.

**Article 20.**

(1) Everyone has the right to freedom of peaceful assembly and association.

(2) No one may be compelled to belong to an association.

**Article 21.**

(1) Everyone has the right to take part in the government of his country, directly or through freely chosen representatives.

(2) Everyone has the right of equal access to public service in his country.

(3) The will of the people shall be the basis of the authority of government; this will shall be expressed in periodic and genuine elections which shall be by universal and equal suffrage and shall be held by secret vote or by equivalent free voting procedures.

**Article 22.**

Everyone, as a member of society, has the right to social security and is entitled to realization, through national effort and international co-operation and in accordance with the organization and resources of each State, of the economic, social and cultural rights indispensable for his dignity and the free development of his personality.

**Article 23.**

(1) Everyone has the right to work, to free choice of employment, to just and favorable conditions of work and to protection against unemployment.

(2) Everyone, without any discrimination, has the right to equal pay for equal work.

(3) Everyone who works has the right to just and favorable remuneration ensuring for himself and his family an existence worthy of human dignity, and supplemented, if necessary, by other means of social protection.

(4) Everyone has the right to form and to join trade unions for the protection of his interests.

**Article 24.**

Everyone has the right to rest and leisure, including reasonable limitation of working hours and periodic holidays with pay.

**Article 25.**

(1) Everyone has the right to a standard of living adequate for the health and well-being of himself and of his family, including food, clothing, housing and medical care and necessary social services, and the right to security in the

event of unemployment, sickness, disability, widowhood, old age or other lack of livelihood in circumstances beyond his control.

(2) Motherhood and childhood are entitled to special care and assistance. All children, whether born in or out of wedlock, shall enjoy the same social protection.

### Article 26.

(1) Everyone has the right to education. Education shall be free, at least in the elementary and fundamental stages. Elementary education shall be compulsory. Technical and professional education shall be made generally available and higher education shall be equally accessible to all on the basis of merit.

(2) Education shall be directed to the full development of the human personality and to the strengthening of respect for human rights and fundamental freedoms. It shall promote understanding, tolerance and friendship among all nations, racial or religious groups, and shall further the activities of the United Nations for the maintenance of peace.

(3) Parents have a prior right to choose the kind of education that shall be given to their children.

### Article 27.

(1) Everyone has the right freely to participate in the cultural life of the community, to enjoy the arts and to share in scientific advancement and its benefits.

(2) Everyone has the right to the protection of the moral and material interests resulting from any scientific, literary or artistic production of which he is the author.

### Article 28.

Everyone is entitled to a social and international order in which the rights and freedoms set forth in this Declaration can be fully realized.

### Article 29.

(1) Everyone has duties to the community in which alone the free and full development of his personality is possible.

(2) In the exercise of his rights and freedoms, everyone shall be subject only to such limitations as are determined by law solely for the purpose of securing due recognition and respect for the rights and freedoms of others and of meeting the just requirements of morality, public order and the general welfare in a democratic society.

(3) These rights and freedoms may in no case be exercised contrary to the purposes and principles of the United Nations.

### Article 30.

Nothing in this Declaration may be interpreted as implying for any State, group or person any right to engage in any activity or to perform any act aimed at the destruction of any of the rights and freedoms set forth herein.

# INTERNATIONAL COVENANT ON CIVIL AND POLITICAL RIGHTS
## (1966)

**Article 1.**

    1.  All peoples have the right of self-determination . . .

**Article 4.**

    1.  In time of public emergency which threatens the life of the nation and the existence of which is officially proclaimed, the States Parties to the present Covenant may take measures derogating from their obligations under the present Covenant to the extent strictly required by the exigencies of the situation, provided that such measures are not inconsistent with their other obligations under international law and do not involve discrimination solely on the ground of race, colour, sex, language, religion or social origin.

    2.  No derogation from articles 6, 7, 8 (paragraphs 1 and 2), 11, 15, 16 and 18 may be made under this provision.

    3.  Any State Party to the present Covenant availing itself of the right of derogation shall immediately inform the other States Parties to the present Covenant, through the intermediary of the Secretary-General of the United Nations, of the provisions from which it has derogated and of the reasons by which it was actuated . . .

**Article 6.**

    1.  Every human being has the inherent right to life. This right shall be protected by law. No one shall be arbitrarily deprived of his life. . .

**Article 7.**

No one shall be subjected to torture or to cruel, inhuman or degrading treatment or punishment. In particular, no one shall be subjected without his free consent to medical or scientific experimentation.

**Article 8.**

    1.  No one shall be held in slavery; slavery and the slave-trade in all their forms shall be prohibited.

    2.  No one shall be held in servitude . . .

**Article 11.**

No one shall be imprisoned merely on the ground of inability to fulfill a contractual obligation.

**Article 15.**

No one shall be held guilty of any criminal offence on account of any act or omission which did not constitute a criminal offence, under national or international law, at the time when it was committed . . .

## Article 16.

Everyone shall have the right to recognition everywhere as a person before the law.

## Article 18.

Everyone shall have the right to freedom of thought, conscience, and religion. . . .

# INTERNATIONAL COVENANT ON ECONOMIC, SOCIAL, AND CULTURAL RIGHTS
### (1966)

## Article 2.

1. Each State Party to the present Covenant undertakes to take steps, individually and through international assistance and co-operation, especially economic and technical, to the maximum of its available resources, with a view to achieving progressively the full realization of the rights recognized in the present Covenant by all appropriate means, including particularly the adoption of legislative measures . . .

## Article 11.

1. The States Parties to the present Covenant recognize the right of everyone to an adequate standard of living for himself and his family, including adequate food, clothing and housing, and to the continuous improvement of living conditions . . .

## Article 12.

1. The States Parties to the present Covenant recognize the right of everyone to the enjoyment of the highest attainable standard of physical and mental health.

2. The steps to be taken by the States Parties to the present Covenant to achieve the full realization of this right shall include those necessary for:

   (a) The provision for the reduction of the stillbirth-rate and of infant mortality and for the healthy development of the child;

   (b) The improvement of all aspects of environmental and industrial hygiene;

   (c) The prevention, treatment and control of epidemic, endemic, occupational and other diseases;

   (d) The creation of conditions which would assure to all medical service and medical attention in the event of sickness.

## Article 13.

1. The States Parties to the present Covenant recognize the right of everyone to education. . . .

# NOTES AND QUESTIONS

**1.** The United Nations was formed at the end of World War II as a permanent peace-keeping organization. The charter of the United Nations, signed by the 50 original member nations in San Francisco on June 26, 1945, spells out the organization's goals. The first two goals are "to save succeeding generations from the scourge of war . . . and to reaffirm faith in fundamental human rights, in the dignity and worth of the human person, in the equal rights of men and women and of nations large and small." After the charter was signed, the adoption of an international bill of rights with legal authority proceeded in three steps: a declaration, treaty-based covenants, and implementation measures.

**2.** The Universal Declaration of Human Rights was adopted by the United Nations General Assembly in 1948, with 48 member states voting in favor of adoption and 8 (Saudi Arabia, South Africa, and the Soviet Union together with 5 other countries whose votes it controlled) abstaining. The declaration was adopted as a "common standard for all people and nations." As Henry Steiner notes, "No other document has so caught the historical moment, achieved the same moral and rhetorical force, or exerted so much influence on the human rights movement as a whole." The rights enumerated in the declaration "stem from the cardinal axiom that all human beings are born free and equal, in dignity and rights, and are endowed with reason and conscience. All the rights and freedoms belong to everybody." These points are spelled out in Articles 1 and 2. Nondiscrimination is the overarching principle. Article 7, for example, is explicit: "All are equal before the law and are entitled without any discrimination to equal protection of the law." Other articles prohibit slavery, torture, and arbitrary detention and protect freedom of expression, assembly, and religion, the right to own property, and the right to work and receive an education. Of special importance to health care professionals is Article 25, which states, in part, "Everyone has the right to a standard of living adequate for the health and well-being of himself and his family, including food, clothing, housing, and medical care and necessary social services."

Human rights are primarily rights individuals have in relation to governments. Human rights require governments to refrain from doing certain things, such as torturing persons or limiting freedom of religion, and also require that they take actions to make people's lives better, such as providing education and nutrition programs. The United Nations adopted the Universal Declaration of Human Rights as a statement of aspirations. The legal obligations of governments were to derive from formal treaties that member nations would individually sign and incorporate into domestic law. On the development of the UDHR, see MARY ANN GLENDON, A WORLD MADE NEW: ELEANOR ROOSEVELT AND THE UNIVERSAL DECLARATION OF HUMAN RIGHTS (2002).

**3.** Because of the cold war, with its conflicting ideologies, it took almost 20 years to reach an agreement on the texts of the two human-rights treaties. On December 16, 1966, both the International Covenant on Civil and Political Rights and the International Covenant on Economic, Social, and Cultural Rights were adopted by the General Assembly and offered for signature and ratification by the member nations. The United States ratified the

International Covenant on Civil and Political Rights in 1992, but not surprisingly, given our capitalist economic system with its emphasis on private property, we have yet to act on the International Covenant on Economic, Social, and Cultural Rights. The division of human rights into two separate treaties illustrates the tension between liberal states founded on civil and political rights and socialist and communist welfare states founded on solidarity and the government's obligation to meet basic economic and social needs.

The rights spelled out in the International Covenant on Civil and Political Rights include equality, the right to liberty and security of person, and freedom of movement, religion, expression, and association. The International Covenant on Economic, Social, and Cultural Rights focuses on well-being, including the right to work, the right to receive fair wages, the right to make a decent living, the right to work under safe and healthy conditions, the right to be free from hunger, the right to education, and "the right of everyone to the enjoyment of the highest attainable standard of physical and mental health."

Given the horrors of poverty, disease, and civil wars over the past 50 years, it is easy to dismiss the rights enunciated in these documents as empty gestures. Indeed, Amnesty International, in marking the 50th anniversary of the Universal Declaration of Human Rights, labeled the rights it articulates "little more than a paper promise" for most people in the world. It is certainly true that unadulterated celebration is not in order, but as Kunz noted almost 60 years ago in writing about the birth of the declaration, "In the field of human rights as in other actual problems of international law it is necessary to avoid the Scylla of a pessimistic cynicism and the Charybdis of mere wishful thinking and superficial optimism." Joseph L. Kunz, *The United Nations Declaration of Human Rights*, 43 AM. J. INT'L L. 316, 321 (1949).

**4.** The right to health has been given more precise definition in a report of the Committee on Economic, Social, and Cultural Rights, the treaty entity formed to help implement the International Covenant on Economic, Social, and Cultural Rights. The document is known as General Comment No. 14 and was issued in 2000. Among its most important provisions are the following:

Health is a fundamental human right indispensable for the exercise of other human rights . . .

4. . . . the right to health embraces a wide range of socio-economic factors that promote conditions in which people can lead a healthy life, and extends to the underlying determinants of health, such as food and nutrition, housing, access to safe and potable water and adequate sanitation, safe and healthy working conditions, and a healthy environment.

8. The right to health is not to be understood as a right to be healthy. The right to health contains both freedoms and entitlements. The freedoms include the right to control one's health and body, including sexual and reproductive freedom, and the right to be free from interference, such as the right to be free from torture, non-consensual medical treatment and experimentation. By contrast, the entitlements include the right to a system of health protection which provides

equality of opportunity for people to enjoy the highest attainable level of health.

11. . . . the right to health . . . [is] an inclusive right extending not only to timely and appropriate health care but also to the underlying determinants of health, such as access to safe and potable water and adequate sanitation, an adequate supply of safe food, nutrition and housing, healthy occupational and environmental conditions, and access to health-related education and information, including on sexual and reproductive health . . .

12. The right to health in all its forms and at all levels contains the following interrelated and essential elements, the precise application of which will depend on the conditions prevailing in a particular State party:

(a) *Availability.* Functioning public health and health-care facilities, goods and services, as well as programs, have to be available. . . .

(b) *Accessibility.* Health facilities, goods and services have to be accessible to everyone without discrimination . . . physical accessibility . . . economic accessibility (affordability). . . information accessibility. . . .

(c) *Acceptability* . . . All health facilities, goods and services must be respectful of medical ethics and culturally appropriate . . .

(d) *Quality* . . . must also be scientifically and medically appropriate and of good quality. This requires, *inter alia*, skilled medical personnel, scientifically approved and unexpired drugs and hospital equipment, safe and potable water, and adequate sanitation.

17. The right to health facilities . . . [includes] the provision of . . . equal and timely access to basic preventive, curative, rehabilitative health services and health education; regular screening programs; appropriate treatment of prevalent diseases, illnesses, injuries and disabilities, preferably at community level; the provision of essential drugs; and appropriate mental health treatment and care . . .

33. The right to health, like all human rights, imposes three types or levels of obligations on States parties: the obligations to *respect, protect* and *fulfill*.

34. States are under the obligation to *respect* the right to health by, *inter alia*, refraining from denying or limiting equal access for all persons, including prisoners or detainees, minorities, asylum seekers and illegal immigrants, to preventive, curative and palliative health services; abstaining from enforcing discriminatory practices as a State policy; and abstaining from imposing discriminatory practices relating to women's health status and needs. . . .

35. Obligations to *protect* include, *inter alia*, the duties of States to adopt legislation or to take other measures ensuring equal access to health care and health-related services provided by third parties; to ensure that privatization of the health sector does not constitute a

threat to the availability, accessibility, acceptability and quality of health facilities, goods and services; to control the marketing of medical equipment and medicines by third parties; and to ensure that medical practitioners and other health professionals meet appropriate standards of education, skill and ethical codes of conduct. . .

36. The obligation to *fulfill* requires States parties, *inter alia*, to give sufficient recognition to the right to health in the national political and legal systems, preferably by way of legislative implementation, and to adopt a national health policy with a detailed plan for realizing the right to health. States must ensure provision of health care, including immunization programs against the major infectious diseases, and ensure equal access for all to the underlying determinants of health, such as nutritiously safe food and potable drinking water, basic sanitation and adequate housing and living conditions. Public health infrastructures should provide for sexual and reproductive health services, including safe motherhood, particularly in rural areas. . . .

43. . . . core obligations [minimum essential level of the right] include at least the following obligations:

(a) To ensure the right of access to health facilities, goods and services on a nondiscriminatory basis, especially for vulnerable or marginalized groups;

(b) To ensure access to the minimum essential food which is nutritionally adequate and safe, to ensure freedom from hunger to everyone;

(c) To ensure access to basic shelter, housing, and sanitation, and an adequate supply of safe and potable water;

(d) To provide essential drugs, as from time to time defined under the WHO Action Program on Essential Drugs;

(e) To ensure equitable distribution of all health facilities, goods and services;

(f) To adopt and implement a national public health strategy and plan of action, on the basis of epidemiological evidence, addressing the health concerns of the whole population; the strategy and plan of action shall be devised, and periodically reviewed, on the basis of a participatory and transparent process; they shall include methods, such as right to health indicators and benchmarks, by which progress can be closely monitored; the process by which the strategy and plan of action are devised, as well as their content, shall give particular attention to all vulnerable or marginalized groups.

47. . . . a State party cannot, under any circumstances whatsoever, justify its noncompliance with the core obligations set out in paragraph 43, which are non-derogable.

**5.** World War II, arguably the first truly global war, led many nations to acknowledge the universality of human rights and the responsibility of governments to promote them. Jonathan Mann perceptively noted that the AIDS epidemic can be viewed as the first global epidemic, because it is taking place at a time when all countries are linked both electronically and by easy transportation. Like World War II, this tragedy requires us to think in new ways and to develop effective methods to prevent and treat disease on a global level. Globalization is a mercantile and ecologic fact; it is also a reality in health care. The challenge facing medicine and health care is to develop a global language and strategy to improve the health of all the world's citizens.

Clinical medicine is practiced one patient at a time. The language of medical ethics is the language of self-determination and beneficence: doing what is in the best interests of the patient with the patient's informed consent. This language is powerful, but often has little application in countries where physicians are scarce and medical resources very limited.

Public health deals with populations and prevention of disease — the necessary frame of reference in the global context. In the context of clinical practice, the treatment of human immunodeficiency virus infection with a combination of antiviral medicines makes sense. In the context of worldwide public health, however, such treatment may be available to less than 5 percent of people with AIDS. To control AIDS, it has become necessary to deal directly with discrimination, immigration status, and access to health care. It is clear that population-based prevention is required to address the AIDS epidemic effectively on a global level (as well as, for example, tuberculosis, malaria, and tobacco-related illness). Nonetheless, it has been much harder to articulate a global public health ethic. The field of public health itself has had an extraordinarily difficult time developing its own ethical language. This problem of language has two basic causes: the incredibly large array of factors that influence health at the population level, and the emphasis by contemporary public health professionals on individualism and market forces rather than on the collective responsibility for social welfare. Because of its universality and its emphasis on equality and dignity, the language of human rights is well suited to public health.

On the 50th anniversary of the Universal Declaration of Human Rights, George Annas, following the lead of Jonathan Mann, the father of the "health and human rights" field, suggested that the declaration itself sets forth the ethics of public health, since its goal is to provide the conditions under which people can flourish. This is also the goal of public health. The unification of public health and human-rights efforts throughout the world could be a powerful force to improve the lives of every person. George J. Annas, *The Universal Declaration of Human Rights at 50*, 339 NEW ENG. J. MED 1778 (1998).

**6.** The "Siracusa Principles" describe the conditions under which emergency powers can be used by the state to limit human rights. U.N., ECONOMIC AND SOCIAL COUNCIL, SUB-COMMISSION ON PREVENTION OF DISCRIMINATION AND PROTECTION OF MINORITIES, SIRACUSA PRINCIPLES ON THE LIMITATION AND DEROGATION OF PROVISIONS IN THE INTERNATIONAL COVENANT ON CIVIL AND POLITICAL RIGHTS, U.N. Doc. E/CN4/1984/4, Annex (1984):

## LIMITATION CLAUSES

### A.  General Interpretative Principles Relating to the Justification of Limitations

1.  No limitations or grounds for applying them to rights guaranteed by the Covenant are permitted other than those contained in the terms of the Covenant itself.

2.  The scope of a limitation referred to in the Covenant shall not be interpreted so as to jeopardize the essence of the right concerned.

3.  All limitation clauses shall be interpreted strictly and in favor of the rights at issue.

All limitations shall be interpreted in the light and context of the particular right concerned.

\* \* \*

9. No limitation on a right recognized by the Covenant shall discriminate contrary to Article 2, paragraph 1.

10.  Whenever a limitation is required in the terms of the Covenant to be "necessary," this term implies that the limitation:

(a) is based on one of the grounds justifying limitations recognized by the relevant article of the Covenant,

(b) responds to a pressing public or social need,

(c) pursues a legitimate aim, and

(d) is proportionate to that aim.

Any assessment as to the necessity of a limitation shall be made on objective considerations.

11.  In applying a limitation, a state shall use no more restrictive means than are required for the achievement of the purpose of the limitation.

12. The burden of justifying a limitation upon a right guaranteed under the Covenant lies with the state.

*B.  Interpretative Principles Relating to Specific Limitation Clauses. . .*

*iv. "public health"*

25.  Public health may be invoked as a ground for limiting certain rights in order to allow a state to take measures dealing with a serious threat to the health of the population or individual members of the population. These measures must be specifically aimed at preventing disease or injury or providing care for the sick and injured.

26.  Due regard shall be had to the international health regulations of the World Health Organization.

**7.** International Health Regulations, promulgated by the WHO, have always been problematic because the WHO itself is founded on the theory that each state party retains its complete sovereignty. As noted in Chapter Three in the discussion on SARS, this can be a major problem if a country wants to prevent an investigation of an outbreak by WHO because it is worried about things like trade and tourism. After the SARS epidemic, the International Health Regulations were amended in 2005, and take effect June 15, 2007. WORLD HEALTH ORG., APPLICATION OF THE INTERNATIONAL HEALTH REGULATIONS (2005), www.who.int/gb/ebwha/pdf_files/WHA59_2-en.pdf (last visited Jan. 2007). *See, e.g.*, Lawrence Gostin, *International Infectious Disease Law: Revision of the World Health Organization's International Health Regulations*, 291 JAMA 2623 (2004). The new regulations are designed, among other things, to encourage the development of more effective public health surveillance methods and to encourage information sharing, especially for "potential public health emergencies of international concern" defined as "an extraordinary event which is determined, as provided in these regulations, (i) to constitute a public health threat to other States through the international spread of disease, and (ii) to potentially require a coordinated response." Other provisions include:

### Article 5, Surveillance

Each State Party shall develop, strengthen and maintain, as soon as possible but not later than five years from the entry into force of these Regulations for that State Party, the capacity to detect, assess, notify and report events in accordance with these Regulations, as specified in Annex 1 [of the regulations].

### Article 6, Notification

1. Each State Party shall assess events occurring within its territory by using the decision instrument in Annex 2. Each State Party shall notify WHO, by the most efficient means of communication available, by way of the National IHR Focal Point, and within 24 hours of assessment of public health information, of all events which may constitute a public health emergency of international concern, within its territory in accordance with the decision instrument, as well as any health measure implemented in response to those events . . .

2. Following a notification, a State Party shall continue to communicate to WHO timely, accurate and sufficiently detailed public health information available to it on the notified event, where possible including case definitions, laboratory results, source and type of the risk, number of cases and deaths, conditions affecting the spread of the disease and the health measures employed; and report, when necessary, the difficulties faced and support needed in responding to the potential public health emergency of international concern.

**8.** There are also treaties that apply directly to bioterrorism and biowarfare, the most important of which is the 1972 Biological and Toxin Weapons Convention. Article I sets forth its basic operative language:

Each State Party to this Convention undertakes never in any circumstance to develop, produce, stockpile or otherwise acquire or retain:

(1) Microbial or other biological agents, or toxins whatever their origin or method of production, of types and in quantities that have no justification for prophylactic, protective or other peaceful purposes;

(2) Weapons, equipment or means of delivery designed to use such agents or toxins for hostile purposes or in armed conflict.

# MINISTER OF HEALTH v. TREATMENT ACTION CAMPAIGN
## South Africa Constitutional Court, 2002(10) BCLR 1033(CC)

The HIV/AIDS pandemic in South Africa has been described as "an incomprehensible calamity" and "the most important challenge facing South Africa since the birth of our new democracy" and government's fight against "this scourge" as "a top priority". It "has claimed millions of lives, inflicting pain and grief, causing fear and uncertainty, and threatening the economy." These are not the words of alarmists but are taken from a Department of Health publication in 2000 and a ministerial foreword to an earlier departmental publication.

This appeal is directed at reversing orders made in a High Court against government because of perceived shortcomings in its response to an aspect of the HIV/AIDS challenge. The court found that government had not reasonably addressed the need to reduce the risk of HIV-positive mothers transmitting the disease to their babies at birth. More specifically the finding was that government had acted unreasonably in (a) refusing to make an antiretroviral drug called Nevirapine available in the public health sector where the attending doctor considered it medically indicated, and (b) not setting out a timeframe for a national program to prevent mother-to-child transmission of HIV.

The case started as an application in the High Court in Pretoria on 21 August 2001. The applicants were a number of associations and members of civil society concerned with the treatment of people with HIV/AIDS and with the prevention of new infections. In this judgment they are referred to collectively as "the applicants." The principal actor among them was the Treatment Action Campaign (TAC). The respondents were the national Minister of Health and the respective members of the executive councils (MECs) responsible for health in all provinces save the Western Cape. They are referred to collectively as "the government" or "government."

Government, as part of a formidable array of responses to the pandemic, devised a program to deal with mother-to-child transmission of HIV at birth and identified Nevirapine as its drug of choice for this purpose. The program imposes restrictions on the availability of Nevirapine in the public health sector. This is where the first of two main issues in the case arose. The applicants contended that these restrictions are unreasonable when measured against the Constitution, which commands the State and all its organs to give effect to the rights guaranteed by the Bill of Rights. This duty is put thus by sections 7(2) and 8(1) of the Constitution respectively:

7(2) The State must respect, protect, promote and fulfill the rights in the Bill of Rights.

. . .

8(1) The Bill of Rights applies to all law, and binds the legislature, the executive, the judiciary and all organs of State.

At issue here is the right given to everyone to have access to public health care services and the right of children to be afforded special protection. These rights are expressed in the following terms in the Bill of Rights:

27(1) Everyone has the right to have access to —

(a) health care services, including reproductive health care;. . .

(2) The State must take reasonable legislative and other measures, within its available resources, to achieve the progressive realization of each of these rights. . .

28(1) Every child has the right -. . .

(c) to basic nutrition, shelter, basic health care services and social services.

The second main issue also arises out of the provisions of sections 27 and 28 of the Constitution. It is whether government is constitutionally obliged and had to be ordered forthwith to plan and implement an effective, comprehensive and progressive program for the prevention of mother-to-child transmission of HIV throughout the country. * * *

The State is obliged to take reasonable measures progressively to eliminate or reduce the large areas of severe deprivation that afflict our society. The courts will guarantee that the democratic processes are protected so as to ensure accountability, responsiveness and openness, as the Constitution requires in section 1. As the Bill of Rights indicates, their function in respect of socio-economic rights is directed towards ensuring that legislative and other measures taken by the State are reasonable. As this Court said in *Grootboom,* "[i]t is necessary to recognize that a wide range of possible measures could be adopted by the State to meet its obligations. . . ." As was said in *Soobramoney*: "The State has to manage its limited resources in order to address all these claims. There will be times when this requires it to adopt a holistic approach to the larger needs of society rather than to focus on the specific needs of particular individuals within society."

Courts are ill-suited to adjudicate upon issues where court orders could have multiple social and economic consequences for the community. The Constitution contemplates rather a restrained and focused role for the courts, namely, to require the State to take measures to meet its constitutional obligations and to subject the reasonableness of these measures to evaluation. Such determinations of reasonableness may in fact have budgetary implications, but are not in themselves directed at rearranging budgets. In this way the judicial, legislative and executive functions achieve appropriate constitutional balance.

We therefore conclude that section 27(1) of the Constitution does not give rise to a self-standing and independent positive right enforceable irrespective of the considerations mentioned in section 27(2). Sections 27(1) and 27(2) must be read together as defining the scope of the positive rights that everyone has and the corresponding obligations on the State to "respect, protect, promote and fulfill" such rights. The rights conferred by sections 26(1) and 27(1) are to have "access" to the services that the State is obliged to provide in terms of sections 26(2) and 27(2). . . .

It is the applicants' case that the measures adopted by government to provide access to health care services to HIV-positive pregnant women were deficient in two material respects: first, because they prohibited the administration of Nevirapine at public hospitals and clinics outside the research and training sites; and second, because they failed to implement a comprehensive program for the prevention of mother-to-child transmission of HIV . . . The applicants' contentions raise two questions, namely, is the policy of confining the supply of Nevirapine reasonable in the circumstances; and does government have a comprehensive policy for the prevention of mother-to-child transmission of HIV.

In deciding on the policy to confine Nevirapine to the research and training sites, the cost of the drug itself was not a factor. . . . In substance four reasons were advanced in the affidavits for confining the administration of Nevirapine to the research and training sites. First, concern was expressed about the efficacy of Nevirapine where the "comprehensive package" is not available. . . . Secondly, there was a concern that the administration of Nevirapine to the mother and her child might lead to the development of resistance to the efficacy of Nevirapine and related antiretrovirals in later years. Thirdly, there was a perceived safety issue. Nevirapine is a potent drug and it is not known what hazards may attach to its use. Finally, there was the question whether the public health system has the capacity to provide the package. It was contended on behalf of government that Nevirapine should be administered only with the "full package" and that it was not reasonably possible to do this on a comprehensive basis because of the lack of trained counselors and counseling facilities and also budgetary constraints which precluded such a comprehensive scheme being implemented.

We deal with each of these issues in turn. First, the concern about efficacy. It is clear from the evidence that the provision of Nevirapine will save the lives of a significant number of infants even if it is administered without the full package and support services that are available at the research and training sites. Mother-to-child transmission of HIV can take place during pregnancy, at birth and as a result of breastfeeding. . . . The wealth of scientific material produced by both sides makes plain that sero-conversion of HIV takes place in some, but not all, cases and that Nevirapine thus remains to some extent efficacious in combating mother-to-child transmission even if the mother breastfeeds her baby. As far as resistance is concerned, the only relevance is the possible need to treat the mother and/or the child at some time in the future. Although resistant strains of HIV might exist after a single dose of Nevirapine, this mutation is likely to be transient. At most there is a possibility of such resistance persisting, and although this possibility cannot be excluded, its weight is small in comparison with the potential benefit of providing a single tablet of Nevirapine to the mother and a few drops to her baby at the time of birth. The prospects of the child surviving if infected are so slim and the nature of the suffering so grave that the risk of some resistance manifesting at some time in the future is well worth running.

The evidence shows that safety is no more than a hypothetical issue. The only evidence of potential harm concerns risks attaching to the administration of Nevirapine as a chronic medication on an ongoing basis for the treatment of HIV-positive persons. There is, however, no evidence to suggest that a dose of Nevirapine to both mother and child at the time of birth will result in any harm to either of them. . . . The policy of confining Nevirapine to research and training sites fails to address the needs of mothers and their newborn children who do not have access to these sites. It fails to distinguish between the evaluation of programs for reducing mother-to-child transmission and the need to provide access to health care services required by those who do not have access to the sites.

In *Grootboom* (*supra*) this Court held that: "[t]o be reasonable, measures cannot leave out of account the degree and extent of the denial of the right they endeavor to realize. Those whose needs are the most urgent and whose ability to enjoy all rights therefore is most in peril, must not be ignored by the measures aimed at achieving realization of the right. . . .

In evaluating government's policy, regard must be had to the fact that this case is concerned with newborn babies whose lives might be saved by the administration of Nevirapine to mother and child at the time of birth. . . . the provision of a single dose of Nevirapine to mother and child where medically indicated is a simple, cheap and potentially lifesaving medical intervention.

## Children's rights

There is another consideration that is material. This case is concerned with newborn children. Sections 28(1) (b) and (c) of the Constitution provide that

[e]very child has the right —

(b) to family care or parental care, or to appropriate alternative care when removed from the family environment;

(c) to basic nutrition, shelter, basic health care services and social services.

The provision of a single dose of Nevirapine to mother and child for the purpose of protecting the child against the transmission of HIV is, as far as the children are concerned, essential. Their needs are "most urgent" and their inability to have access to Nevirapine profoundly affects their ability to enjoy all rights to which they are entitled. Their rights are "most in peril" as a result of the policy that has been adopted and are most affected by a rigid and inflexible policy that excludes them from having access to Nevirapine.

The State is obliged to ensure that children are accorded the protection contemplated by section 28 that arises when the implementation of the right to parental or family care is lacking. Here we are concerned with children born in public hospitals and clinics to mothers who are for the most part indigent and unable to gain access to private medical treatment which is beyond their means. They and their children are in the main dependent upon the State to make health care services available to them. . . .

We are also conscious of the daunting problems confronting government as a result of the pandemic. And besides the pandemic, the State faces huge demands in relation to access to education, land, housing, health care, food, water and social security. These are the socio-economic rights entrenched in the Constitution, and the State is obliged to take reasonable legislative and other measures within its available resources to achieve the progressive realization of each of them. In the light of our history this is an extraordinarily difficult task. Nonetheless it is an obligation imposed on the State by the Constitution. . . .

South African courts have a wide range of powers at their disposal to ensure that the Constitution is upheld. These include mandatory and structural interdicts. How they should exercise those powers depends on the circumstances of each particular case. Here due regard must be paid to the roles of the legislature and the executive in a democracy. What must be made clear, however, is that when it is appropriate to do so, courts may — and if need be must — use their wide powers to make orders that affect policy as well as legislation.* * * In the present case we have identified aspects of government policy that are inconsistent with the Constitution. The decision not to make Nevirapine available at hospitals and clinics other than the research and training sites is central to the entire policy. Once that restriction is removed, government will be able to devise and implement a more comprehensive policy that will give access to health care services to HIV-positive mothers and their newborn children, and will include the administration of Nevirapine where that is appropriate. The policy as reformulated must meet the constitutional requirement of providing reasonable measures within available resources for the progressive realization of the rights of such women and newborn children. This may also require, where that is necessary, that counselors at places other than at the research and training sites be trained in counseling for the use of Nevirapine. We will formulate a declaration to address these issues. . . .

It is essential that there be a concerted national effort to combat the HIV/AIDS pandemic. The government has committed itself to such an effort. We have held that its policy fails to meet constitutional standards because it excludes those who could reasonably be included where such treatment is medically indicated to combat mother-to-child transmission of HIV.*** We consider it important that all sectors of the community, in particular civil society, should co-operate in the steps taken to achieve this goal. In our view that will be facilitated by spelling out the steps necessary to comply with the Constitution. We will do this on the basis of the policy that government has adopted as the best means of combating mother-to-child transmission of HIV, which is to make use of Nevirapine for this purpose. Government must retain the right to adapt the policy, consistent with its constitutional obligations, should it consider it appropriate to do so. The order that we make has regard to this. . . . We accordingly make the following orders:

1. The orders made by the High Court are set aside and the following orders are substituted.

2. It is declared that:

(a) Sections 27(1) and (2) of the Constitution require the government to devise and implement within its available resources a comprehensive and co-ordinated program to realize progressively the rights of pregnant women and their newborn children to have access to health services to combat mother-to-child transmission of HIV.

(b) The program to be realized progressively within available resources must include reasonable measures for counseling and testing pregnant women for HIV, counseling HIV-positive pregnant women on the options open to them to reduce the risk of mother-to-child transmission of HIV, and making appropriate treatment available to them for such purposes.

(c) The policy for reducing the risk of mother-to-child transmission of HIV as formulated and implemented by government fell short of compliance with the requirements in subparagraphs (a) and (b) in that:

(i) Doctors at public hospitals and clinics other than the research and training sites were not enabled to prescribe Nevirapine to reduce the risk of mother-to-child transmission of HIV even where it was medically indicated and adequate facilities existed for the testing and counseling of the pregnant women concerned.

(ii) The policy failed to make provision for counselors at hospitals and clinics other than at research and training sites to be trained in counseling for the use of Nevirapine as a means of reducing the risk of mother-to-child transmission of HIV.

3. Government is ordered without delay to:

(a) Remove the restrictions that prevent Nevirapine from being made available for the purpose of reducing the risk of mother-to-child transmission of HIV at public hospitals and clinics that are not research and training sites.

(b) Permit and facilitate the use of Nevirapine for the purpose of reducing the risk of mother-to-child transmission of HIV and to make it available for this purpose at hospitals and clinics when in the judgment of the attending medical practitioner acting in consultation with the medical superintendent of the facility concerned this is medically indicated, which shall if necessary include that the mother concerned has been appropriately tested and counseled.

(c) Make provision if necessary for counselors based at public hospitals and clinics other than the research and training sites to be trained for the counseling necessary for the use of Nevirapine to reduce the risk of mother-to-child transmission of HIV.

(d) Take reasonable measures to extend the testing and counseling facilities at hospitals and clinics throughout the public health sector to facilitate and expedite the use of Nevirapine for the purpose of reducing the risk of mother-to-child transmission of HIV.

4. The orders made in paragraph 3 do not preclude government from adapting its policy in a manner consistent with the Constitution if equally appropriate or better methods become available to it for the prevention of mother-to-child transmission of HIV. . . .

# NOTES AND QUESTIONS

**1.** The provisions in the South African constitution discussed in this case are modeled on those in the International Covenant on Economic, Social and Cultural Rights — and placing the provisions of this international treaty in legislation and constitutional provisions of individual states is an especially effective way of making international law integral to national law. Note that Article 12 of the Covenant includes not only appropriate health care, but also the underlying determinants of health, including clean water, sanitation, safe food, housing, and health-related education. In addition, South Africa's constitution adopts specific provisions in the Convention on the Rights of the Child, which, of course, have special application in this case.

**2.** The decision in the Nevirapine case illustrates both the strength and the weakness of relying on courts to determine specific applications of the right to health. The strength is that the right to health is a legal right, and since there can be no legal right without a remedy, courts will provide a remedy for violations of the right to health. In this regard, it is worth noting not only that the right to health and access to health care articulated in the Universal Declaration of Human Rights has been given more specific meaning in the International Covenant on Economic, Social, and Cultural Rights and other internationally binding documents on human rights, but also that these rights have been written into the constitutions of many countries, including South Africa. The widespread failure of governments to take the right to health seriously, however, means that we are still a long way from the realization of this right. Nonetheless, the activism of many nongovernmental organizations, such as the Treatment Action Campaign, in the area of health rights, provides some ground for optimism that government inaction will not go unchallenged.

The weakness of relying on courts is that the subject matter of the right to health in a courtroom struggle is likely to be narrow, involving interventions such as kidney dialysis or Nevirapine therapy. The HIV epidemic demands a comprehensive strategy of treatment, care, and prevention, including education, adequate nutrition, clean water, and nondiscrimination. The government of South Africa has so far been unwilling to designate the HIV epidemic as a national emergency or to take steps to make the prevention and treatment of HIV infection its highest health priority.

**3.** This was the third case in which the Constitutional Court had been asked to enforce a socioeconomic right under the South African constitution. The first, *Soobramoney v. Minister of Health*, was also a right-to-health case, 1997 (12) BCLR 1696 (CC). It involved a 41-year-old man with chronic renal failure and a history of stroke, heart disease, and diabetes, who was not eligible for a kidney transplant and therefore required lifelong dialysis to survive. The renal-dialysis unit in the region where he lived, which had 20 dialysis machines — not nearly enough to provide dialysis for everyone who required it — had a policy of accepting only patients with acute renal failure. The health department argued that this policy met the government's duty to provide emergency care under the constitution. Patients with chronic renal failure, like the petitioner, did not automatically qualify.

In considering whether the constitution required the health department to provide a sufficient number of machines to offer dialysis to everyone whose life could be saved by it, the court observed that under the constitution, the state's obligation to provide health care services was qualified by its "available resources." The court noted that offering extremely expensive medical treatments to everyone would make "substantial inroads into the health budget . . . to the prejudice of the other needs which the state has to meet." The Constitutional Court ultimately decided that the administrators of provincial health services, not the courts, should set budgetary priorities and that the courts should not interfere with decisions that are rational and made "in good faith by those political organs and medical authorities whose responsibility it is to deal with such matters."

Likewise, in *South Africa v. Grootboom*, 2000 (11) BCLR 1169 (CC), a case involving the right to housing, the Constitutional Court determined that although the state is obligated to act positively to ameliorate the conditions of the homeless, it "is not obligated to go beyond available resources or to realize these rights immediately." The constitutional requirement is that the right to housing be "progressively realized." Nonetheless, the court noted, there is "at the very least, a negative obligation placed upon the state and all other entities and persons to desist from preventing or impairing the right of access to adequate housing."

Applying the rulings in these two cases to the Nevirapine case, the Constitutional Court reasonably concluded that the right to health care services "does not give rise to a self-standing and independent fulfillment right" that is enforceable irrespective of available resources. Nonetheless, the government's obligation to respect rights, as articulated in the housing case, applies equally to the right to health care services. *See* George J. Annas, *The Right to Health and the Nevirapine Case in South Africa*, 348 NEW ENG. J. MED. 750 (2003). For a discussion of a similar case from Venezuela, see Mary Ann Torres, *The Human Right to Health, National Courts, and Access to HIV/AIDS Treatment: A Case Study from Venezuela*, 3 CHICAGO J. INT'L L. 1 (2002).

**4.** Jonathan Mann was the first to observe that "health and human rights are inextricably linked," Jonathan M. Mann, *Human Rights and AIDS: The Future of the Pandemic*, in HEALTH AND HUMAN RIGHTS: A READER 216-26 (Jonathan M. Mann et al. eds., 1999), and Paul Farmer has argued that "the most important question facing modern medicine involves human rights." Farmer noted that many poor people have no access to modern medicine and concluded, "The more effective the treatment, the greater the injustice meted out to those who do not have access to care." Paul Farmer, *The Major*

*Infectious Diseases in the World — To Treat or Not to Treat?* 345 N. ENG. J
MED. 208 (2001). *See also* PAUL FARMER, INFECTIONS AND INEQUALITIES: THE
MODERN PLAGUES (Updated ed. 1999); AMARTYA SEN, DEVELOPMENT AS
FREEDOM (1999); and LAURIE WERMUTH, GLOBAL INEQUALITY AND HUMAN
NEEDS: HEALTH AND ILLNESS IN AN INCREASINGLY UNEQUAL WORLD (2003).

**5.** Access to treatment for infection with the human immunodeficiency virus
(HIV) and AIDS has been problematic in most countries, but especially in
South Africa, where almost 5 million people are infected with HIV and the government's attitude toward the epidemic has been described as pseudoscientific
and dangerous. M.W. Makgoba, *HIV/AIDS: The Peril of Pseudoscience*, 288
SCIENCE 1171 (2000). Political resistance by the South African government to
outside funders who want to set the country's health care agenda is, of course,
understandable in the context of racism and colonialism. But even understandable politics cannot excuse the government's failure to act more decisively in the face of an unprecedented epidemic.

**6.** A major concern, of course, is that the entire human rights movement
could fall victim to the "war on terror." As Richard Falk has expressed it:

> By highlighting "terrorism" there is an almost unavoidable tendency
> to perceive issues through the lens of the September 11 attacks, and to
> downplay such other issues as are associated with the inequities aris-
> ing from the operation of the world economy or with the practices that
> produce environmental decay. In these respects from the perspective
> of human rights' priorities, the highlighting of the security agenda
> inevitably leads to a downplaying of economic and social rights, the
> right of self-determination, health issues, and rights associated with
> environmental protection. It is to be expected that academic discus-
> sions of security would take different forms in other parts of the world,
> that the American context of discussion is in this respect rather the
> exception than the rule.

Richard Falk, *Human Rights: A Descending Spiral*, *in* HUMAN RIGHTS IN THE
"WAR ON TERROR" 229 (Richard Ashby Wilson ed., 2005).

## Jim Kim & Paul Farmer, *AIDS in 2006 — Moving Toward One World, One Hope?*
### 355 NEW ENG. J. MED. 645 (2006)

For the past two decades, AIDS experts — clinicians, epidemiologists, policymakers, activists, and scientists — have gathered every two years to confer
about what is now the world's leading infectious cause of death among young
adults. This year, the International AIDS Society is hosting the meeting in
Toronto from August 13 through 18. The last time the conference was held in
Canada, in 1996, its theme was "One World, One Hope." But it was evident to
conferees from the poorer reaches of the world that the price tag of the era's
great hope — combination antiretroviral therapy — rendered it out of their
reach. Indeed, some African participants that year made a banner reading,
"One World, No Hope."

Today, the global picture is quite different. The claims that have been made for the efficacy of antiretroviral therapy have proved to be well founded: in the United States, such therapy has prolonged life by an estimated 13 years — a success rate that would compare favorably with that of almost any treatment for cancer or complications of coronary artery disease. In addition, a number of lessons, with implications for policy and action, have emerged from efforts that are well under way in the developing world. During the past decade, we have gleaned these lessons from our work in setting global AIDS policies at the World Health Organization in Geneva and in implementing integrated programs for AIDS prevention and care in places such as rural Haiti and Rwanda. As vastly different as these places may be, they are part of one world, and we believe that ambitious policy goals, adequate funding, and knowledge about implementation can move us toward the elusive goal of shared hope.

The first lesson is that charging for AIDS prevention and care will pose insurmountable problems for people living in poverty, since there will always be those unable to pay even modest amounts for services or medications, whether generic or branded. Like efforts to battle airborne tuberculosis, such services should be seen as a public good for public health. Policymakers and public health officials, especially in heavily burdened regions, should adopt universal access plans and waive fees for HIV care. Initially, this approach will require sustained donor contributions, but many African countries have recently set targets for increased national investments in health, a pledge that could render ambitious programs sustainable in the long run.

As local investments increase, the price of AIDS care is decreasing. The development of generic medications means that antiretroviral therapy can now cost less than 50 cents per day, and costs continue to decrease to affordable levels for public health officials in developing countries. All antiretroviral medications — first-line, second-line, and third-line — must be made available at such prices. Manufacturers of generic drugs in China, India, and other developing countries stand ready to provide the full range of drugs. Whether through negotiated agreements or use of the Agreement on Trade-Related Aspects of Intellectual Property Rights, full access to all available antiretroviral drugs must quickly become the standard in all countries.

Second, the effective scale-up of pilot projects will require the strengthening and even rebuilding of health care systems, including those charged with delivering primary care. In the past, the lack of a health care infrastructure has been a barrier to antiretroviral therapy; we must now marshal AIDS resources, which are at last considerable, to rebuild public health systems in sub-Saharan Africa and other HIV-burdened regions. . . . Only the public sector, not nongovernmental organizations, can offer health care as a right.

Third, a lack of trained health care personnel, most notably doctors, is invoked as a reason for the failure to treat AIDS in poor countries. The lack is real, and the brain drain continues. But one reason doctors flee Africa is that they lack the tools of their trade. AIDS funding offers us a chance not only to recruit physicians and nurses to underserved regions, but also to train community health care workers to supervise care, for AIDS and many other diseases within their home villages and neighborhoods. . . .

Fourth, extreme poverty makes it difficult for many patients to comply with antiretroviral therapy. Indeed, poverty is far and away the greatest barrier to the scale-up of treatment and prevention programs. Our experience in Haiti and Rwanda has shown us that it is possible to remove many of the social and economic barriers to adherence but only with what are sometimes termed "wrap-around services": food supplements for the hungry, help with transportation to clinics, child care and housing. In many rural regions of Africa, hunger is the major coexisting condition with AIDS or tuberculosis, and these consumptive diseases cannot be treated effectively without food supplementation. . . .

* * *

Fifth, investments in efforts to combat the global epidemics of AIDS and tuberculosis are much more generous than they were five years ago, but funding must be increased and sustained if we are to slow these increasingly complex epidemics. . . .

The unglamorous and difficult process of increasing access to prevention and care needs to be our primary focus if we are to move toward the lofty goal of equitably distributed medical services in a world riven by inequality. Without such goals, the slogan "One World, One Hope" will remain nothing more than a dream.

## NOTES AND QUESTIONS

**1.** Kim and Farmer approach the HIV/AIDS pandemic from the perspective they would describe as "social justice." How does this perspective differ from a "health and human rights" perspective? Jonathan Mann, the founder of the health and human rights field, has observed that most of the problems of health are problems of poverty — nonetheless he also noted that framing them as poverty problems makes them seem insurmountable and intractable. Better, he thought, to focus on the basic human rights which most people support and whose recognition can dramatically improve health status. See MADISON POWERS & RUTH FADEN, SOCIAL JUSTICE (2006). In 2006 the American Public Health Association made human rights the theme of their Annual Meeting, and Paul Farmer gave the keynote address in which he linked human rights and social justice.

**2.** Kim and Farmer (and the World Health Organization generally) have argued that we must make treatment available to all who are infected with HIV as soon as possible. This is a reasonable goal, but how can it be achieved? Most recently, for example, WHO failed in its attempt, labeled "3x5" to enroll 3 million new HIV patients in treatment programs by the end of 2005. It seems reasonable to note that in this same period of time more than five million new HIV infections occurred. The point needs to be emphasized: treatment is critical, but from a public health perspective, prevention is overwhelmingly vital. Consider how treatment and prevention go hand in hand. Assuming that not everyone can get access to treatment immediately, how should public health officials prioritize who should get access first? Do we need an explicit rationing scheme that puts parents, workers, children, or some other group at the top of

the priority list? How should such a list be constructed and who should construct it? Would it be an inherent violation of the nondiscrimination basis of
the human rights movement?

Of course, these same issues will be faced in the event of an epidemic or
bioterrorist attack — who should be treated first with available drugs and vaccines? In this regard, the CDC has suggested priorities for flu vaccinations,
both in the yearly flu (when supplies are short) and in the event of an avian
pandemic, when vaccine will not be immediately available to anyone. Who
should be at the top of the distribution list and why? *See, e.g.,* Alfred I. Tauber,
*Medicine, Public Health, and the Ethics of Rationing*, 45 PERSPECTIVES IN
BIOLOGY & MED. 16 (2002); Ezekiel Emanuel & Alan Wertheimer, *Who Should
Get Influenza Vaccine When Not All Can?*, 312 SCIENCE 854 (2006); and George
J. Annas, *The Prostitute, the Playboy, and the Poet: Rationing Schemes for
Organ Transplantation*, 75 AM. J. PUB. HEALTH 187 (1985).

**3.** The editor of the *Lancet*, Richard Horton, was far less impressed by the
August 2006 International AIDS meeting in Toronto than others. The meeting, for example, committed to a goal of "universal access to comprehensive
prevention programs, treatment, care and support by 2010."

Unfortunately, as Horton notes,

> . . . the opportunity to produce a roadmap to reach the 2010 target
> of universal access was squandered. Rarely has there been a meeting
> that felt so disengaged from a global predicament of such historic pro-
> portions. The agenda in Toronto was unfocused, giving prime air time
> to celebrities, such as Bill Gates and Bill Clinton, while largely ignor-
> ing Africa [even though] Africa bears the greatest burden of AIDS
> today — 24.5 million of 38.6 million people with HIV.

Horton went on to raise ten specific questions that he believes need answers
now, including: 1. Why do we refuse to admit that there is still no genuine
global commitment to scale up our response to AIDS?; 2. Why are the wider
health, economic, social and cultural contexts of AIDS still being ignored?;
6. Why do health agencies and programs still base their prevention messages
on the outdated and scientifically corrupt idea of abstinence?; and 7. Why are
civil society and NGOs still not being given the credit they deserve as vital
levers in the global AIDS response?

The next International AIDS meeting will be in Mexico in 2008. In Horton's
view, "The litmus test for Mexico's success will be the degree to which the conference can be transformed from a scientific meeting and global beacon for
AIDS, to a coordinating mechanism to drive advances in prevention, treatment, and care at the country level. Talking is easy. Doing will demand a revolution." Richard Horton, *A Prescription for AIDS 2006-10*, 368 LANCET 726-28
(2006). Horton's essay echoes the more generalized arguments of LAURIE
GARRETT, BETRAYAL OF TRUST: THE COLLAPSE OF GLOBAL PUBLIC HEALTH (2000),
a critical pre-9/11 look at global public health dedicated to Jonathan Mann.

**4.** As Horton notes, the stars of the 2006 AIDS meeting were Bill Gates and
Bill Clinton, based largely on their recent work in donating and raising private
funds for AIDS research and treatment. Their activities and status raise some

fundamental questions for public health advocates. Why do governments fail to adequately fund public health programs? And what is the role of the private sector in public health? Are public-private partnerships the future of public health? See Public Health, Ethics, and Equity (Sudhir Anand et al. eds, 2004).

Of course, global public health problems demand global approaches. And even the *Wall Street Journal* has taken note that these issues have yet to be resolved, and that what decisions are made in late 2006 to fill the positions of Director-General of WHO, Executive Director of the Global Fund to Combat AIDS, Tuberculosis, and Malaria, and the Senior VP for Health Development of the World Bank "will help determine the world's strategy for confronting health threats ranging from AIDS to pandemic flu for years to come." Betsy McKay, *Three Top Jobs in Global Health Face Vacancies*, WALL ST. J., September 5, 2006, at A16.

Bill Gates has recently concluded that his foundation will put most of its resources into global health initiatives, especially HIV/AIDS, because he believes that this is the area in which you can get the most return on your investment in terms of lives saved. Warren Buffet, the second richest man in the US after Gates, has announced that he will leave most of his fortune to the Gates Foundation because he believes they have the right approach and his own foundation could not do it better. Private charity is to be admired and foundations funding is almost always welcome. But what does this say about public health to note that the Gates Foundation annually provides more funding for public health initiatives than the entire budget of the World Health Organization? Gates has said that he got most of his philanthropic investment ideas from reading a report by the World Bank, which is still well worth reading. WORLD BANK, WORLD DEVELOPMENT REPORT 1993: INVESTING IN HEALTH (1993).

The Bill and Melinda Gates Foundation has so far been primarily interested in developing an AIDS vaccine, although the foundation has branched out more recently. Vaccines are, of course, the most basic of successful public health interventions, in that they can prevent disease in populations. Nonetheless, even the limited quest to provide already existing and effective vaccines to the world's children has been consistently overwhelmed by politics. *See, e.g.*, WILLIAM MURASKIN, THE POLITICS OF INTERNATIONAL HEALTH: THE CHILDREN'S VACCINE INITIATIVE AND THE STRUGGLE TO DEVELOP VACCINES FOR THE THIRD WORLD (1998).

**5.** One of the major legal issues involving world health of the past decade has been the debate around pharmaceutical patenting and profits. Although almost everyone now realizes that just providing drugs, without a public health infrastructure to deliver them and care for patients is not feasible, nonetheless the cost of drugs remains a critical issue to providing decent care, especially for HIV/AIDS, in many countries. An excellent introduction to this subject is contained in Symposium, *Globalization of Pharmaceuticals: International Regulatory Issues*, 32 AM. J.L. & MED. 153 (2006) *See also* Ellen 't Hoen, *TRIPS, Pharmaceuticals Patents, and Access to Essential Medicines: A Long Way from Seattle to Doha*, 3 CHI. J. INT'L L. 27 (2002); Kevin Outterson, *Pharmaceutical Arbitrage: Balancing Access and Innovation in International Prescription Drug Markets*, 5 YALE J. HEALTH POL'Y L. & ETHICS 193 (2005).

**6.** Norman Daniels has argued persuasively that bioethics should move to broaden its agenda from the doctor-patient relationship to include public health and population problems, and should do so based on a social justice rather than a human rights perspective. The last three items he urges bioethicists to add to their agenda are to:

> 10) assess the implications of the obligation not to harm for reducing health inequalities internationally;

> 11) develop an account of justice for the evolving international institutions and rule-making bodies that have an impact on international health inequalities; and

> 12) examine Promethean challenges from the perspective of their impact on international health inequalities and obligations of justice regarding them.

Norman Daniels, *Equity and Population Health: Toward a Broader Bioethics Agenda*, 36(4) HASTINGS CENTER REP. 22, 33 (2006).

**7.** Other commentators prefer to keep bioethics at some distance from public health. Jonathan Mann, for example, has written that he believes bioethics is the correct language for medicine, but that human rights is the proper language for public health. *See, e.g.,* Jonathan Mann, *Medicine and Public Health, Ethics and Human Rights*, 27(3) HASTINGS CENTER REP. 6 (1997). Ron Bayer and Amy Fairchild would go much further, arguing that modern bioethics has no place in public health ethics. In their words, "Bioethics cannot serve as a basis for thinking about the balances required in the defense of the public's health. As we commence the process of shaping an ethics of public health, it is clear that bioethics is the wrong place to start." Ronald Bayer & Amy L. Fairchild, *The Genesis of Public Health Ethics*, 18 BIOETHICS 473, 492 (2004).

Of course, the real answer may be that when medicine and public health work together (usually the case) public health must take account of bioethics (sometimes called simply "medical ethics"), and that in real life there are no sharp borders between health law, bioethics, and human rights in public health practice. *See, e.g.,* GEORGE J. ANNAS, AMERICAN BIOETHICS: CROSSING HUMAN RIGHTS AND HEALTH LAW BOUNDARIES (2005); BRITISH MEDICAL ASSOCIATION, THE MEDICAL PROFESSION AND HUMAN RIGHTS: HANDBOOK FOR A CHANGING AGENDA (2001); and DAVID J. ROTHMAN & SHEILA M. ROTHMAN, TRUST IS NOT ENOUGH: BRINGING HUMAN RIGHTS TO MEDICINE (2006).

# TABLE OF CASES

[Principle cases appear in italics.]

# INDEX

[References are to pages.]

[References are to pages.]